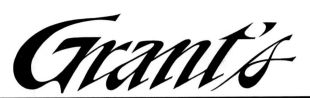

Atlas of Anatomy
Tenth Edition

1

2

3

4

5

6

7

8

9

CCHB

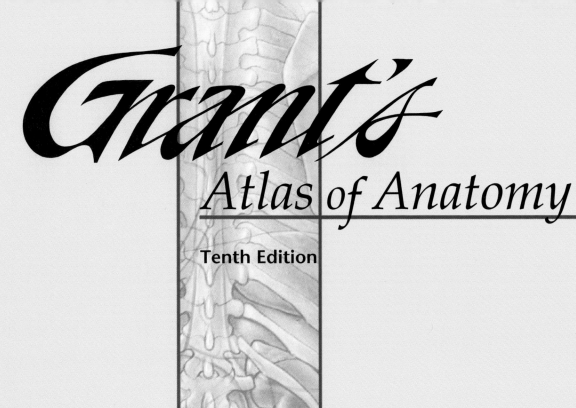

Grant's
Atlas of Anatomy

Tenth Edition

Anne M.R. Agur, B.Sc. (OT), M.Sc.

Associate Professor in Division of Anatomy, Department of Surgery
Department of Physical Therapy and Department of Occupational Therapy
Division of Biomedical Communications, Department of Surgery
Faculty of Medicine
University of Toronto
Toronto, Ontario
Canada

Ming J. Lee, M.D.

Senior Tutor in Division of Anatomy, and Division of Biomedical
Communications, Department of Surgery
Faculty of Medicine
University of Toronto
Toronto, Ontario
Canada

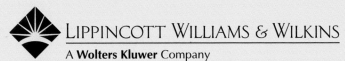

LIPPINCOTT WILLIAMS & WILKINS
A **Wolters Kluwer** Company

Philadelphia • Baltimore • New York • London
Buenos Aires • Hong Kong • Sydney • Tokyo

Editor: Paul J. Kelly
Managing Editor: Crystal Taylor
Development Editor: Nancy J. Peterson
Marketing Manager: Christine Kushner
Production Manager: Susan Rockwell
Design Coordinator: Mario Fernandez

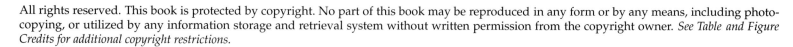

Copyright © 1999 Lippincott Williams & Wilkins

351 West Camden Street
Baltimore, Maryland 21201-2436 USA

227 East Washington Square
Philadelphia, PA 19106

Printed in Canada

By J.C.B. Grant:
First Edition, 1943
Second Edition, 1947
Third Edition, 1951
Fourth Edition, 1956
Fifth Edition, 1962
Sixth Edition, 1972
By J.E. Anderson:
Seventh Edition, 1978
Eighth Edition, 1983
By A.M.R. Agur:
Ninth Edition, 1991

Library of Congress Cataloging-in-Publication Data

Agur, A. M. R.
    Grant's atlas of anatomy. — 10th ed. / Anne M.R. Agur, Ming J.
Lee.
        p. cm.
    Includes bibliographical references and index.
    Includes bibliographical references and index.
    ISBN 0-683-30264-7 (pbk.)
    I. Lee, Ming J. II. Grant, J. C. Boileau (John Charles Boileau),
1886–1973. III. Title. IV. Title: Atlas of anatomy.
    [DNLM: 1. Human anatomy Atlases. 2. Anatomy, Regional—atlases.
QS 17 A284g 1999]
611'.0022'2—dc21
DNLM/DLC
for Library of Congress   99–25481
                                                                CIP

The publishers have made every effort to trace the copyright holders for borrowed material. If they have inadvertently overlooked any, they will be pleased to make the necessary arrangements at the first opportunity.

To purchase additional copies of this book, call our customer service department at **(800) 638-3030** or fax orders to **(301) 824-7390**. For other book services, including chapter reprints and large quantity sales, ask for the Special Sales department.

For all other calls originating outside of the United States, please call **(301) 714-2324**.

Visit Lippincott Williams & Wilkins on the Internet: **http://www.lww.com** . Lippincott Williams & Wilkins customer service representatives are available from 8:30 am to 6:00 pm, EST, Monday through Friday, for telephone access.

99 00 01 02 03
2 3 4 5 6 7 8 9 10

To Dr. Carlton G. Smith and Professor Marguerite Harland Smith
and
To my husband Enno, and for my children, Erik and Kristina

DR. JOHN CHARLES BOILEAU GRANT
1886—1973

by Dr. Carlton G. Smith M.D., PH.D
Professor Emeritus, Division of Anatomy
Department of Surgery
Faculty of Medicine
University of Toronto, Canada

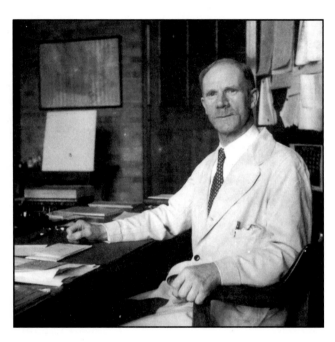

Dr. J.C.B. Grant in his office, McMurrich building, University of Toronto, 1946.

Editor's Note: With the 10th edition of this classic anatomy atlas, we felt it appropriate to pay tribute to Dr. J.C. Boileau Grant. Through his textbooks, Dr. Grant made an indelible impression on the teaching of anatomy throughout the world.

The life of J.C. Boileau Grant has been likened to the course of the seventh cranial nerve as it passes out of the skull: complicated, but purposeful. [1] He was born in the parish of Lasswade in Edinburgh, Scotland, on February 6, 1886. Dr. Grant studied medicine at the University of Edinburgh from 1903 to 1908. Here, his skill as a dissector in the laboratory of the renowned anatomist, Dr. Daniel John Cunningham (1850–1909), earned him a number of awards.

Following graduation, Dr. Grant was appointed the resident house officer at the Infirmary in Whitehaven, Cumberland. From 1909 to 1911, Dr. Grant demonstrated anatomy in the University of Edinburgh, followed by two years at the University of Durham, at Newcastle-on-Tyne in England, in the laboratory of Professor Robert Howden, editor of *Gray's Anatomy.*

With the outbreak of World War I in 1914, Dr. Grant joined the Royal Army Medical Corps and served with distinction. He was mentioned in dispatches in September 1916, received the Military Cross in September 1917 for "conspicuous gallantry and devotion to duty during attack," and received a bar to the Military Cross in August 1918. [1]

In October 1919, released from the Royal Army, he accepted the position of Professor of Anatomy at the University of Manitoba in Winnipeg, Canada. With the front-line medical practitioner in mind, he endeavored to "bring up a generation of surgeons who knew exactly what they were doing once an operation had begun." [1] Devoted to research and learning, Dr. Grant took interest in other projects, such as performing anthropometric studies of Indian tribes in northern Manitoba during the 1920s. In Winnipeg Dr. Grant met Catriona Christie, whom he married in 1922.

Dr. Grant was known for his reliance on logic, analysis, and deduction as opposed to rote memory. While at the University of Manitoba, Dr. Grant began writing *A Method of Anatomy, Descriptive and Deductive*, which was published in 1937. [2]

In 1930, Dr. Grant accepted the position of Chair of Anatomy at the University of Toronto. He stressed the value of a "clean" dissection, with the structures well defined. This required the delicate touch of a sharp scalpel, and students soon learned that a dull tool was an anathema. Instructive dissections were made available in the Anatomy Museum, a means of student review on which Dr. Grant placed a high priority. Many of these illustrations have been included in *Grant's Atlas of Anatomy.*

The first edition of the *Atlas*, published in 1943, was the first anatomical atlas to be published in North America. [3] *Grant's Dissector* preceded the Atlas in 1940. [4]

Dr. Grant remained at the University of Toronto until his retirement in 1956. At that time, he became Curator of the Anatomy Museum in the University. He also served as Visiting Professor of Anatomy at the University of California at Los Angeles, where he taught for 10 years.

Dr. Grant died in 1973 of cancer. Through his teaching method, still presented in the *Grant's* textbooks, Dr. Grant's life interest—human anatomy—lives on. In their eulogy, colleagues and friends Ross MacKenzie and J. S. Thompson said:

"Dr. Grant's knowledge of anatomical fact was encyclopedic, and he enjoyed nothing better than sharing his knowledge with others, whether they were junior students or senior staff. While somewhat strict as a teacher, his quiet wit and boundless humanity never failed to impress. He was, in the very finest sense, a scholar and a gentleman."[1]

PREFACE

Planning for the new edition of an atlas—even a classic with as long and rich a history as *Grant's Atlas of Anatomy*—requires intensive research and creativity. It is not enough to rely on a solid reputation. Medical education and the role of anatomy instruction within it are continually changing as educational models and the health-care environment evolve. In addition, publishing technology rapidly advances, offering better possibilities for presenting content.

Vision

The revision process began by evaluating the existing content of the *Atlas* and, with the publisher, soliciting and analyzing feedback from medical students and faculty members from around the world. Then we developed those ideas to provide you with this 10th edition of *Grant's Atlas of Anatomy*. You will find the *Atlas* to be:

- A companion in the dissecting room, guiding you through each step of exploring and exposing structures;
- A portable "anatomical museum," useful in determining relationships when superficial structures have been removed; reviewing regions when away from the dissection lab; and preparing for examinations; and
- A lifetime companion as a reference book for all fields of medicine.

Key Features

Classic Dissection Illustrations. A unique feature of *Grant's Atlas of Anatomy* is that, rather than providing an idealized view of human anatomy, the classic illustrations represent actual dissections that the student can readily relate to the specimen in the lab. In this edition, we have reintroduced several key dissection illustrations from the Grant's collection that have been found to be particularly instructive over the years. The accuracy, simplicity, and beauty of these illustrations have always been an acclaimed feature of the *Atlas*.

Schematic Illustrations. Full-color schematic illustrations supplement the dissection figures to clarify anatomical concepts, show the relationships of structures, and give an overview of the body region being studied. Many new schematic illustrations have been added to this edition. All labeled illustrations were reviewed to ensure that they conform with Grant's desire to "keep it simple"; extraneous labels were deleted, and some labels were added to identify key structures and make the illustrations as useful as possible to students. In addition, many new, simple orientation drawings were added for ease of identifying dissected regions.

Neuroanatomy. The coverage of neuroanatomy was significantly expanded in this edition by adding serial dissections and other illustrations of the human brain.

Diagnostic Images. Because medical imaging has taken on increased importance in the diagnosis and treatment of injuries and illnesses, diagnostic imaging sections have been added to the end of each chapter, featuring approximately 100 clinically relevant magnetic resonance images (MRIs), computed tomography (CT) scans, ultrasound scans, and corresponding orientation drawings.

Muscle Tables. With this edition, we have introduced muscle tables to provide students with a concise overview of muscles and attachments while studying.

Legends and Clinical Comments. Admittedly, artwork is the focus of any atlas; however, the Grant's legends have long been considered a unique and valuable feature of the *Atlas*. The observations and comments that accompany the illustrations draw attention to salient points and significant structures that might otherwise escape notice. Their purpose is to interpret the illustrations without providing exhaustive description. Readability, clarity, and practicality were emphasized in the editing of this edition. Clinical comments, which deliver practical "pearls" that link anatomic features with their significance in health care practice, are italicized within the figure legends.

Organization and Layout. The organization and layout of the *Atlas* has always been determined with ease-of-use as the goal. Although the basic organization by body region was maintained in this edition, every figure within every chapter was scrutinized to ensure that its placement is logical and effective. To further clarify the organization of figures, chapter subtitles were added to each page.

We believe that the 10th edition of *Grant's Atlas of Anatomy* has met our goal of safeguarding its historical strengths while bringing the content up to date and enhancing its usefulness to the student.

Anne M.R. Agur
University of Toronto
May 1999

ACKNOWLEDGMENTS

During the over 50-year history of this work, many people have given generously of their talents and expertise and I acknowledge their participation with heartfelt gratitude. Most of the original carbon dust halftones on which this book is based were created by Dorothy Foster Chubb, a pupil of Max Brödel, and one of Canada's first professionally trained medical artists. She was later joined by Nancy Joy, who is Professor Emeritus in the Department of Art as Applied to Medicine, University of Toronto. Mrs. Chubb was mainly responsible for the artwork of the first two editions and the sixth edition; Miss Joy for those in between. In subsequent editions, additional line and half-tone illustrations by Elizabeth Blackstock, Elia Hopper Ross, and Marguerite Drummond were added. Much credit is also due to Charles E. Storton for his role in the preparation of the majority of the original dissections and preliminary photographic work. I also wish to acknowledge the work of Dr. James Anderson, a pupil of Dr. Grant, under whose stewardship the seventh and eighth editions were published. The individuals listed below also provided invaluable contributions to the previous editions of the *Atlas*, and are gratefully acknowledged:

C.A. Armstrong	P. George	A.J.A. Noronha
P.G. Ashmore	R.K. George	S. O'Sullivan
D. Baker	M.G. Gray	W. Pallie
D.A. Barr	B.L. Guyatt	W.M. Paul
J.V. Basmajian	C.W. Hill	C.H. Sawyer
S. Bensley	W.J. Horsey	A.I. Scott
D. Bilbey	B.S. Jaden	J.S. Simpkins
J. Bottos	G.F. Lewis	J.S. Simpson
W. Boyd	I.B. MacDonald	C.G. Smith
J. Callagan	D.L. MacIntosh	I.M. Thompson
H.A. Cates	R.G. MacKenzie	J.S. Thompson
S.A. Crooks	S. Mader	N.A. Watters
M. Dickie	K.O. McCuaig	R.W. Wilson
J.W.A. Duckworth	D. Mazierski	B. Vallecoccia
F.B. Fallis	W.R. Mitchell	K. Yu
J.B. Francis	K. Nancekivell	
J.S. Fraser		

Tenth Edition

I am indebted to my colleagues and my former professors for their encouragement—especially Dr. K.L. Moore for his expert advice; Dr. C.G. Smith for his generosity and support; Dr. N. Hunt McKee for her friendly help and patience; and Drs. E.K. Sauerland, C. Pincus, and A. Colthurst and for their invaluable input. My sincere appreciation to Drs. M.A. Haider, D. Salonen, E. Becker, and D. Armstrong for their enthusiastic support in providing most of the radiological material. Thanks also to Drs. W. Kucharczyk, A.M. Arenson, A. Toi, M. Asch, and P. Bobechko.

I extend my gratitude to the medical artists who contributed to the tenth edition: Corinne Sandone, Duckwall Productions, David Rini, and Valerie Oxorn. Special thanks go to everyone at Lippincott Williams & Wilkins—especially Crystal Taylor, Managing Editor; Nancy Peterson, Development Editor; Paul Kelly, Acquisitions Editor; Tim Satterfield, Executive Vice President, Education and Reference; Susan Rockwell, Production Manager, Copyediting; Wayne Hubbel, Pre-press Coordinator; Michael Standen, Editorial Assistant; and Danielle Jablonski, Development Assistant. To Crystal Taylor and Nancy Peterson my sincere thanks for nurturing this project; your efforts and expertise are much appreciated.

I would like to acknowledge the reviewers who provided expert advice on the development of this edition:

Edward T. Bersu, Ph.D., Associate Professor, Department of Anatomy, University of Wisconsin-Madison

Michael Binder, M.D., Assistant Professor of Anatomy, Dartmouth Medical School, Hanover

Martin D. Cassell, Ph.D., Associate Professor, Department of Anatomy and Cell Biology, University of Iowa, College of Medicine, Iowa City

Richard L. Drake, Ph.D., Professor and Vice-Chairman, Department of Cell Biology, Neurobiology, and Anatomy, University of Cincinnati

Andrew P. Evan, Ph.D., Professor of Anatomy, Department of Anatomy, Indiana University School of Medicine, Indianapolis

Daniel O. Graney, Ph.D., Associate Professor, Department of Biological Structure, University of Washington School of Medicine, Seattle

John A. Negulesco, MA, Ph.D., Professor of Anatomy, Department of Anatomy and Medical Education, The Ohio State University, College of Medicine and Public Health, Columbus

Bruce A. Richardson, Ph.D., Dean and Professor, Division of Basic Medical Sciences, California College of Podiatric Medicine, San Francisco

William J. Swartz, Ph.D., Marilyn L. Zimny Professor of Anatomy, Department of Cell Biology and Anatomy, LSU Medical Center, New Orleans

Anna Bloxham, Medical Student, University of California at San Francisco

William Strohman, Student, MCP Hahnemann School of Medicine, Philadelphia

Lori M. Sweitzer, Student, Philadelphia College of Osteopathic Medicine

Finally, I would like to thank the hundreds of instructors and students who have, over the years, communicated via the publisher their suggestions and advice as to how this *Atlas* might be improved. These suggestions have been passed on to me and I have tried to consider all of them. I hope readers will find many of these suggestions incorporated and will continue to provide their input.

Anne M.R. Agur

CONTENTS

TABLE AND FIGURE CREDITS

TABLE AND FIGURE CREDITS

Tables

All tables that appear in this atlas are reproduced from: Moore KL, Dalley AF. Clinically Oriented Anatomy. 4th ed. Philadelphia: Lippincott Williams & Wilkins, 1999 and/or Moore KL, Agur AMR. Essential Clinical Anatomy. Baltimore: Williams & Wilkins, 1995.

Figures

page vi Photograph of Dr. J. C. B. Grant courtesy of Dr. C. G. Smith.

Chapter 1

1.7A,B	Courtesy of Dr. K. Bukhanov, University of Toronto, Canada.
1.24	Courtesy of Dr. M.A. Haider, University of Toronto, Canada.
1.25D	Courtesy of Dr. W. Kucharczyk, University of Toronto, Canada.
1.31A	Courtesy of Dr. D.E. Sanders, University of Toronto, Canada.
1.31B	Courtesy of Dr. S. Herman University of Toronto, Canada.
1.31C	Courtesy of Dr. E.L. Lansdown, University of Toronto, Canada.
1.36	Courtesy of Dr. J. Heslin, Toronto, Canada.
1.40B	Moore KL, Dalley AF. Clinically Oriented Anatomy. 4th ed., 1999:293 (Fig. 270B).
1.47B,D	Courtesy of Dr. I. Morrow, University of Manitoba, Canada.
1.48B	Courtesy of Dr. J. Heslin, Toronto, Canada.
1.50B	Courtesy of Dr. E.L. Lansdown, University of Toronto, Canada.
1.75A–F	MRIs courtesy of Dr. M.A. Haider, University of Toronto, Canada; orientation drawing from Moore KL, Agur AMR. Essential Clinical Anatomy, 1995:56 (Fig. 2.12A).
1.76A–C	MRIs courtesy of Dr. M.A. Haider, University of Toronto, Canada; orientation drawing from Moore KL, Agur AMR. Essential Clinical Anatomy, 1995:71 (Fig. 2.16).
1.77A,B	MRIs courtesy of Dr. M.A. Haider, University of Toronto, Canada.

Chapter 2

2.25	Courtesy of Dr. E.L. Lansdown, University of Toronto, Canada.
2.26A	Courtesy of Dr. J. Heslin, Toronto, Canada.
2.26B,C	Courtesy of Dr. E.L. Lansdown, University of Toronto, Canada.
2.27	Courtesy of Dr. J. Heslin, Toronto, Canada.
2.38A,B	Courtesy of Dr. J. Heslin, Toronto, Canada.
2.40A,B	Courtesy of Dr. G.B. Haber, University of Toronto, Canada.
2.48	Courtesy of Dr. A.M. Arenson, University of Toronto, Canada.
2.50B	Courtesy of Dr. E.L. Lansdown, University of Toronto, Canada.
2.59	Courtesy of Dr. G.B. Haber, University of Toronto, Canada.
2.64A	Courtesy of Dr. C.S. Ho, University of Toronto, Canada.
2.64B	Courtesy of Dr. E.L. Lansdown, University of Toronto, Canada.
2.64C	Courtesy of Dr. W. Kucharczyk, University of Toronto, Canada.
2.69	Courtesy of Dr. E.L. Lansdown, University of Toronto, Canada.
2.71	Courtesy of Dr. J. Heslin, Toronto, Canada.
2.73	Courtesy of Dr. K. Sniderman, University of Toronto, Canada.
2.84B	Courtesy of Dr. E.L. Lansdown, University of Toronto, Canada.
2.85A	Courtesy of Dr. M. Asch, University of Toronto, Canada.
2.86B	Pyelogram courtesy of Dr. M. Asch, University of Toronto, Canada.
2.94A,B	From Moore KL, Dalley AF. Clinically Oriented Anatomy. 4th ed., 1999. Photographs © J/B Woolsey Associates, Pennsylvania.
2.99D–E	Ultrasounds courtesy of J. Lai, University of Toronto, Canada.; bottom orientation drawing on page 163 from Moore KL, Agur AMR. Essential Clinical Anatomy, 1995:125.
2.102A–D	MRIs courtesy of Dr. M.A. Haider, University of Toronto, Canada.
2.103A–F	CTs courtesy of Dr. M.A. Haider, University of Toronto, Canada.

2.104A–D   MRIs courtesy of Dr. M.A. Haider, University of Toronto, Canada.

Table 2.2   Illustration from Moore KL, Agur AMR. Essential Clinical Anatomy, 1995:133 (Fig. 3.22).

Chapter 3

3.2D   Orientation drawing from Moore KL, Agur AMR. Essential Clinical Anatomy, 1995:146 (Fig. 4.1).

3.12A–C   From Moore KL, Dalley AF. Clinically Oriented Anatomy. 4th ed., 1999:386,387 (Fig. 3.30A,B;3.31B).

3.16B   From Moore KL, Dalley AF. Clinically Oriented Anatomy. 4th ed., 1999:361 (Fig. 3.16C).

3.18   Ultrasound courtesy of Dr. A. Toi, University of Toronto, Canada.

3.19   Courtesy of Dr. K. Sniderman, University of Toronto, Canada.

3.22C   From Moore KL, Dalley AF. Clinically Oriented Anatomy. 4th ed., 1999.

3.24B   From Moore KL, Agur AMR. Essential Clinical Anatomy, 1995:166 (Fig. 4.12B).

3.31B   Orientation drawing from Moore KL, Agur AMR. Essential Clinical Anatomy, 1995:168 (Fig. 4.13B).

3.33A   Courtesy of Dr. A.M. Arenson, University of Toronto, Canada.

3.33B   From Moore KL, Dalley AF. Clinically Oriented Anatomy. 4th ed., 1999:419 (Fig. 3.52A).

3.35C,D   From Moore KL, Agur AMR. Essential Clinical Anatomy, 1995:160,170 (Figs. 4.9B, 4.15B).

3.37A–E   From Moore KL, Dalley AF. Clinically Oriented Anatomy. 4th ed., 1999.

3.38A,B   From Moore KL, Dalley AF. Clinically Oriented Anatomy. 4th ed., 1999.

3.52A–F   Courtesy of Dr. M.A. Haider, University of Toronto, Canada.

3.53A–C   Courtesy of Dr. M.A. Haider, University of Toronto, Canada.

3.54   Ultrasounds courtesy of Dr. M.A. Haider, University of Toronto, Canada.

3.55A,B   Ultrasounds courtesy of Dr. A. Toi, University of Toronto, Canada.

3.56I,M,L   Courtesy of Dr. M.A. Haider, University of Toronto, Canada.

3.57A,B   Ultrasounds courtesy of Dr. A.M. Arenson, University of Toronto, Canada.

3.58A–E   MRIs courtesy of Dr. M.A. Haider, University of Toronto, Canada.

3.59A,B   Courtesy of Dr. M.A. Haider, University of Toronto, Canada.

Table 3.1   Bottom illustration from Moore KL, Dalley AF. Clinically Oriented Anatomy. 4th ed., 1999:343 (Table 3.2D).

Chapter 4

4.1B   Courtesy of Dr. D. Salonen, University of Toronto, Canada.

4.3B,E   Courtesy of Dr. D. Armstrong, University of Toronto, Canada.

4.7A–C   Courtesy of Drs. E. Becker and P. Bobechko, University of Toronto, Canada.

4.8B,D   Courtesy of Dr. J. Heslin, Toronto, Canada.

4.13D   Courtesy of Dr. E. Becker, University of Toronto, Canada.

4.14   Courtesy of Dr. E. Becker, University of Toronto, Canada.

4.15A   Courtesy of Dr. E. Becker, University of Toronto, Canada.

4.18A,B   Courtesy of Dr. E. Becker, University of Toronto, Canada.

4.21B,C   Courtesy of Dr. E. Becker, University of Toronto, Canada.

4.24B   From Moore KL, Agur AMR. Essential Clinical Anatomy, 1995:200 (bottom).

4.43C   From Moore KL, Agur AMR. Essential Clinical Anatomy, 1995:27 (Fig. 1.15A).

4.56A,B   Courtesy of Dr. D. Armstrong, University of Toronto, Canada.

4.56C,D   Courtesy of Dr. D. Salonen, University of Toronto, Canada.

4.56E   Courtesy of Dr. D. Armstrong, University of Toronto, Canada.

4.56F–M   Courtesy of Dr. D. Salonen, University of Toronto, Canada.

Table 4.1   Left illustration from Moore KL, Agur AMR. Essential Clinical Anatomy, 1995:205 (Fig. 5.3).

Table 4.2   Bottom illustration (anterior view) from Moore KL, Agur AMR. Essential Clinical Anatomy, 1995:425.

Chapter 5

5.2C,D   Courtesy of Dr. P. Babyn, University of Toronto, Canada.

5.4C   From Moore KL, Agur AMR. Essential Clinical Anatomy, 1995:227 (Fig. 6.5A).

5.5A,B   From Moore KL, Agur AMR. Essential Clinical Anatomy, 1995:227 (Figs. 6.5A,C).

5.9A   Courtesy of Dr. E.L. Lansdown, University of Toronto, Canada.

5.30,5.33   Orientation illustrations from Moore KL, Agur AMR. Essential Clinical Anatomy, 1995:10 (Fig. 1.3).

5.35B   From Moore KL, Agur AMR. Essential Clinical Anatomy, 1995:268 (top).

5.39   Courtesy of Dr. E. Becker, University of Toronto, Canada.

5.40B   Courtesy of Dr. D. Salonen, University of Toronto, Canada.

5.48A,B	Courtesy of Dr. P. Bobechko, University of Toronto, Canada.
5.51A	Courtesy of Dr. D. Salonen, University of Toronto, Canada.
5.51B	Courtesy of Dr. P. Bobechko, University of Toronto, Canada.
5.58,5.59	Orientation drawings from Basmajian JV, Slonecker CE. Grant's Method of Anatomy: A Clinical Problem-Solving Approach. 11th ed. Baltimore: Williams & Wilkins, 1989:xix,xviii.
5.58B,C	Courtesy of Dr. D. Salonen, University of Toronto, Canada.
5.59B,C	Courtesy of Dr. D. Salonen, University of Toronto, Canada.
5.72	Courtesy of Dr. K. Sniderman, University of Toronto, Canada.
5.85A	Courtesy of Dr. P. Bobechko University of Toronto, Canada.
5.85B,D	Courtesy of Dr. E. Becker, University of Toronto, Canada.
5.91B	Courtesy of Dr. W. Kucharczyk, University of Toronto, Canada.
5.92B	Courtesy of Dr. W. Kucharczyk, University of Toronto, Canada.
5.101A,B	Courtesy of Dr. D. Salonen, University of Toronto, Canada; orientation drawing from Moore KL, Agur AMR. Essential Clinical Anatomy, 1995:246 (Fig. 6.11C).
5.103A–C	Courtesy of Dr. D. Salonen, University of Toronto, Canada; orientation drawing from Moore KL, Agur AMR. Essential Clinical Anatomy, 1995:253 (Fig. 6.14D).
5.104A,B	Courtesy of Dr. D. Salonen, University of Toronto, Canada.
Table 5.2	From Moore KL, Agur AMR. Essential Clinical Anatomy, 1995 (Fig. 6.6D).
Table 5.8	Illustrations from Moore KL, Agur AMR. Essential Clinical Anatomy, 1995:257 (Figs. 6.16C,D).

Chapter 6

6.3B	Courtesy of Dr. D. Armstrong, University of Toronto, Canada.
6.4A,D	From Moore KL, Agur AMR. Essential Clinical Anatomy, 1995:291 (Figs. 7.5A,B).
6.11B	From Moore KL, Agur AMR. Essential Clinical Anatomy, 1995:288 (Fig. 7.3A).
6.16B	Courtesy of Dr. D. Salonen, University of Toronto, Canada.
6.18	Courtesy of Dr. D. Armstrong, University of Toronto, Canada.
6.22B	From Moore KL, Agur AMR. Essential Clinical Anatomy, 1995:291 (Fig. 7.6B inset).
6.40A	Courtesy of Dr. E. Becker, University of Toronto, Canada.

6.40B	Courtesy of Dr. D. Salonen, University of Toronto, Canada.
6.44	From Moore KL, Agur AMR. Essential Clinical Anatomy, 1995.
6.48C–F	Courtesy of Dr. E. Becker, University of Toronto, Canada.
6.48G	Courtesy of Dr. D. Salonen, University of Toronto, Canada.
6.52A,B	Radiographs courtesy of Dr. J. Heslin, Toronto, Canada; orientation drawings from Moore KL, Agur AMR. Essential Clinical Anatomy, 1995:338,339.
6.53A	Courtesy of Dr. K. Sniderman, University of Toronto, Canada.
6.61A–C	From Moore KL, Agur AMR. Essential Clinical Anatomy, 1995:325.
6.64A	Courtesy of Dr. D. Armstrong, University of Toronto, Canada.
6.65B	From Moore KL, Agur AMR. Essential Clinical Anatomy, 1995:330 (left).
6.79F	Courtesy of Dr. E. Becker, University of Toronto, Canada.
6.82A,B	Courtesy of Dr. E. Becker, University of Toronto, Canada.
6.82C	Courtesy of Dr. D. Armstrong, University of Toronto, Canada.
6.93A–C	Courtesy of Dr. D. Salonen, University of Toronto, Canada.
6.94A–C	Courtesy of Dr. D. Salonen, University of Toronto, Canada; orientation drawing from Moore KL, Dalley AF. Clinically Oriented Anatomy. 4th ed., 1999:800 (Fig. 6.72 left).
6.95B,C	Courtesy of Dr. D. Salonen, University of Toronto, Canada.
6.96C,D	Courtesy of Dr. D. Salonen, University of Toronto, Canada.
Table 6.1	Illustration from Moore KL, Agur AMR. Essential Clinical Anatomy, 1995:298 (top).
Table 6.2	Illustration from Moore KL, Agur AMR. Essential Clinical Anatomy, 1995:302 (Fig. 7.8).
Table 6.5	Illustration from Moore KL, Agur AMR. Essential Clinical Anatomy, 1995:324.
Table 6.7	Illustration from Moore KL, Agur AMR. Essential Clinical Anatomy, 1995:326 (right).

Chapter 7

7.5A,B	Courtesy of Dr. E. Becker, University of Toronto, Canada.
7.6A,C	Courtesy of Dr. D. Armstrong, University of Toronto, Canada.
7.7A–D	Courtesy of Dr. D. Armstrong, University of Toronto, Canada.
7.12A,B	From Moore KL, Agur AMR. Essential Clinical Anatomy, 1995:351,356(top).

7.18B | From Moore KL, Agur AMR. Essential Clinical Anatomy, 1995:362,356.

7.21B,C | Courtesy of Dr. D. Armstrong, University of Toronto, Canada.

7.22 | Orientation drawing from Moore KL, Dalley AF. Clinically Oriented Anatomy. 4th ed., 1999 (Table 9.1).

7.26–7.31 | (*Except* 7.27C, 7.28B, 7.30B) Colorized from photographs provided courtesy of Dr. C. G. Smith, which appeared in Smith CG. Serial Dissections of the Human Brain. Baltimore: Urban & Schwarzenberg, Inc and Toronto: Gage Publishing Ltd., 1981. (©Carlton G. Smith)

7.27C | Colorized from an illustration provided courtesy of Dr. C. G. Smith, which appeared in Smith CG. Basic Neuroanatomy. 2nd ed. Toronto: University of Toronto Press, 1971. (©Carlton G. Smith)

7.33A–D | Colorized from photographs provided courtesy of Dr. C. G. Smith, which appeared in Smith CG. Serial Dissections of the Human Brain. Baltimore: Urban & Schwarzenberg, Inc and Toronto: Gage Publishing Ltd., 1981. (©Carlton G. Smith)

7.35A–C | Courtesy of Dr. D. Armstrong, University of Toronto, Canada.

7.36A | From Moore KL, Dalley AF. Clinically Oriented Anatomy. 4th ed., 1999:895 (Table 7.7C).

7.37 | Orientation drawing colorized from an illustration provided courtesy of Dr. C. G. Smith, which appeared in Smith CG. Serial Dissections of the Human Brain. Baltimore: Urban & Schwarzenberg, Inc and Toronto: Gage Publishing Ltd., 1981. (©Carlton G. Smith)

7.40B | From Moore KL, Agur AMR. Essential Clinical Anatomy, 1995:360 (Figs. 8.10B).

7.45C | Courtesy of Dr. W. Kucharczyk, University of Toronto, Canada.

7.48B | Courtesy of Dr. W. Kucharczyk, University of Toronto, Canada.

7.52 | Courtesy of Dr. J.R. Buncic, University of Toronto, Canada.

7.55,7.56 | Orientation drawings from Moore KL, Agur AMR. Essential Clinical Anatomy, 1995:382 (Table 8.8).

7.67C | From Moore KL, Agur AMR. Essential Clinical Anatomy, 1995:396 (Figs. 8.22B).

7.69 | Orientation drawing from Moore KL, Agur AMR. Essential Clinical Anatomy, 1995:389 (Figs. 8.21A).

7.78C | Courtesy of M.J. Pharoah, University of Toronto, Canada

7.88A,B | Courtesy of Dr. E. Becker, University of Toronto, Canada.

7.88D | Courtesy of Dr. D. Armstrong, University of Toronto, Canada.

7.106B | From Moore KL, Agur AMR. Essential Clinical Anatomy, 1995:352 (Figs. 8.6B).

7.107A–C | Courtesy of Dr. W. Kucharczyk, University of Toronto, Canada.

7.108A,B | Courtesy of Dr. W. Kucharczyk, University of Toronto, Canada.

7.109A–E | MRIs courtesy of Dr. D. Armstrong, University of Toronto, Canada; orientation drawing from Moore KL, Dalley AF. Clinically Oriented Anatomy. 4th ed., 1999:888 (Fig. 7.25B).

7.110A–F | MRIs courtesy of Dr. D. Armstrong, University of Toronto, Canada; orientation drawing from Moore KL, Dalley AF. Clinically Oriented Anatomy. 4th ed., 1999:888 (Fig. 7.25B).

7.111A–F | MRIs courtesy of Dr. D. Armstrong, University of Toronto, Canada; orientation drawing from Moore KL, Dalley AF. Clinically Oriented Anatomy. 4th ed., 1999:888 (Fig. 7.25A).

7.112A–C | MRIs courtesy of Dr. D. Armstrong, University of Toronto, Canada; orientation drawing from Moore KL, Dalley AF. Clinically Oriented Anatomy. 4th ed., 1999:888 (Fig. 7.25, superior view).

Table 7.4 | MRIs courtesy of Dr. W. Kucharczyk, University of Toronto, Canada.

Table 7.5 | Illustrations from Moore KL, Agur AMR. Essential Clinical Anatomy, 1995:382 (Table 8.8).

Table 7.7 | Illustration from Moore KL, Agur AMR. Essential Clinical Anatomy, 1995:388 (Figs. 8.20B).

Chapter 8

8.2A | From Moore KL, Dalley AF. Clinically Oriented Anatomy. 4th ed., 1999 (Fig. 8.4B).

8.2B | From Moore KL, Agur AMR. Essential Clinical Anatomy, 1995:410 (Figs. 9.1A,B).

8.3 | From Moore KL, Dalley AF. Clinically Oriented Anatomy. 4th ed., 1999:1004 (Table 8.2B).

8.21B | From Moore KL, Dalley AF. Clinically Oriented Anatomy. 4th ed., 1999:945 (Fig. 7.58).

8.28B | Courtesy of Dr. W. Kucharczyk, University of Toronto, Canada.

8.39,8.40 | Orientation drawings from Moore KL, Agur AMR. Essential Clinical Anatomy, 1995:440 (Figs. 9.10).

8.43B | From Liebgott B. The Anatomical Basis of Dentistry. Philadelphia: WB Saunders Co. 1982.

8.60A,B | Courtesy of Dr. W. Kucharczyk, University of Toronto, Canada.

8.60C (left) | Courtesy of Dr. D. Salonen, University of Toronto, Canada.

8.61 | Orientation drawing from Moore KL, Agur AMR. Essential Clinical Anatomy, 1995.

8.61A–C   Courtesy of Dr. D. Salonen, University of Toronto, Canada.

8.63A   Courtesy of Dr. D. Salonen, University of Toronto, Canada.

8.63B   Courtesy of Dr. W. Kucharczyk, University of Toronto, Canada.

Table 8.1   Illustration from Moore KL, Agur AMR. Essential Clinical Anatomy, 1995:413.

Table 8.2   Illustration from Moore KL, Agur AMR. Essential Clinical Anatomy, 1995:418 (top).

Chapter 9

9.2A   From Moore KL, Dalley AF. Clinically Oriented Anatomy. 4th ed., 1999.

9.2B   From Parent A. Carpenter's Human Neuroanatomy. 9th ed. Baltimore: Williams & Wilkins, 1996 (fig. 12.15).

9.3B   From Moore KL, Agur AMR. Essential Clinical Anatomy, 1995:449 (Figs. 10.2B).

9.11C   From Moore KL, Agur AMR. Essential Clinical Anatomy, 1995:456 (Figs. 10.6B).

9.12C   From Moore KL, Dalley AF. Clinically Oriented Anatomy. 4th ed., 1999.

9.14C   From Moore KL, Agur AMR. Essential Clinical Anatomy, 1995:459 (Table 10.2).

9.15   From Moore KL, Dalley AF. Clinically Oriented Anatomy. 4th ed., 1999:1101 (Table 9.4).

9.17A–F   Courtesy of Dr. W. Kucharczyk, University of Toronto, Canada.

9.18A–C   Courtesy of Dr. W. Kucharczyk, University of Toronto, Canada.

Table 7.4   Illustration From Moore KL, Dalley AF. Clinically Oriented Anatomy. 4th ed., 1999:926 (Table 7.11).

REFERENCES

Tribute to Dr Grant

1. Robinson C. Canadian Medical Lives: J.C. Boileau Grant: Anatomist Extraordinary. Markham, Ontario, Canada: Associated Medical Services Inc./Fithzenry & Whiteside, 1993.
2. Grant JCB. A Method of Anatomy, Descriptive and Deductive. Baltimore: Williams & Wilkins Co., 1937. (11th edition, J. Basmajian and C. Slonecker, 1989)
3. Grant JCB. Grant's Atlas of Anatomy. Baltimore: Williams & Wilkins Co., 1943 (10th Edition, A. Agur and L. Ming, 1999)
4. Grant JCB, Cates HA. Grant's Dissector (A Handbook for Dissectors). Baltimore: Williams & Wilkins Co., 1940 (12th edition, E.K. Sauerland, 1999)

Chapter 1

[1] (Fig. 1.51) Anson, B.H. The aortic arch and its branches, *Cardiology*. New York: McGraw-Hill, vol 1: 1963.

Chapter 2

[1] (Fig. 2.45) Couinaud C. Lobes et segments hepatiques: Note sur l'architecture anatomique et chirurgicale du foie. Presse Med 1954;62:709.

[2] (Fig. 2.45) Healy JE, Schroy PC. Anatomy of the biliary ducts within the human liver: Analysis of the prevailing pattern of branchings and the major variations of the biliary ducts. Arch Surg 1953;66:599.

[3] (Fig. 2.86B) Campbell M. Ureteral reduplication (double ureter). Urology, Vol. Philadelphia: WB Saunders, 1954:309.

Chapter 3

[1] (Fig. 3.38A) Oelrich TM. The urethral sphincter muscle in the male. Am J Anat 1980;158:229.

[2] (Fig. 3.38B) Oelrich TM. The striated urogenital sphincter muscle in the female. Anat Rec 1983;205:223.

Chapter 4

[1] (Fig. 4.47) Jit I, Charnakia VM. The vertebral level of the termination of the spinal cord. J Anat Soc India 1959;8:93.

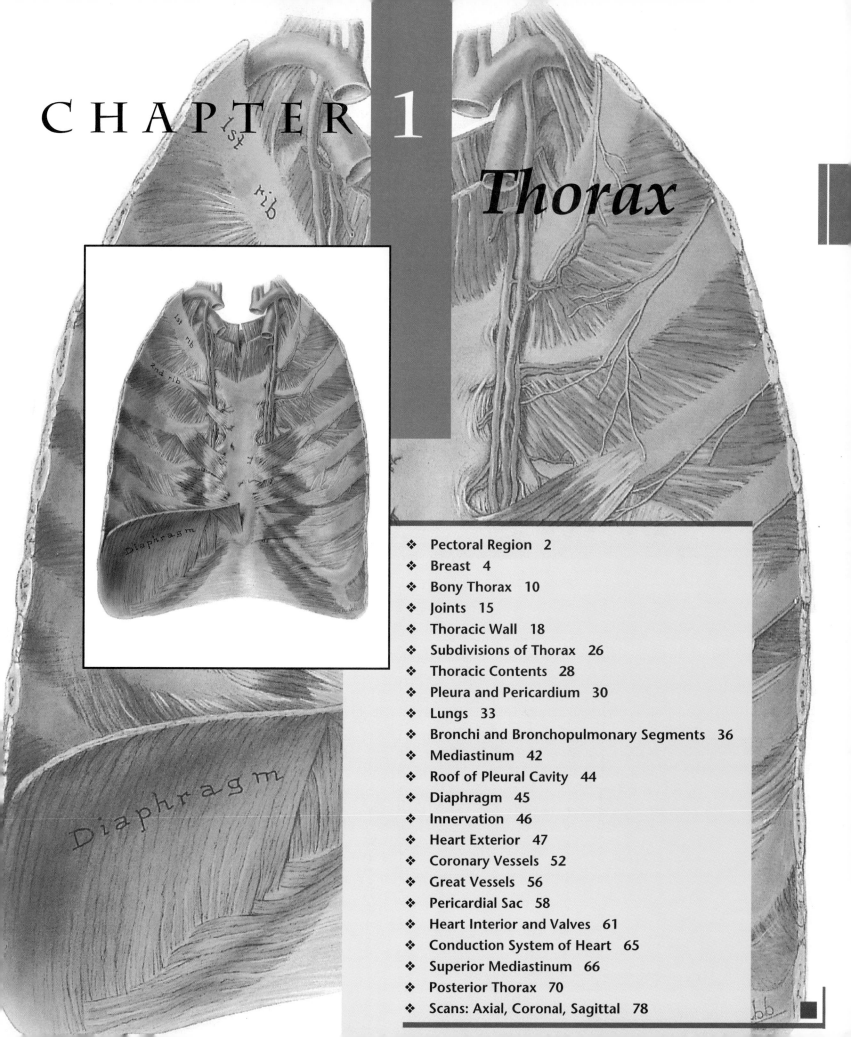

C H A P T E R 1

Thorax

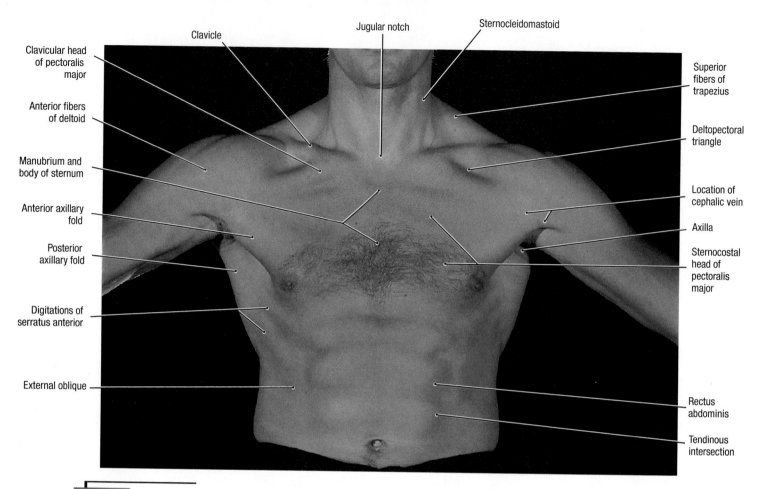

Clavicular head
of pectoralis
major

Anterior fibers
of deltoid

Manubrium and
body of sternum

Anterior axillary
fold

Posterior
axillary fold

Digitations of
serratus anterior

External oblique

Clavicle

Jugular notch

Sternocleidomastoid

Superior
fibers of
trapezius

Deltopectoral
triangle

Location of
cephalic vein

Axilla

Sternocostal
head of
pectoralis
major

Rectus
abdominis

Tendinous
intersection

1.1 ## Surface anatomy of male pectoral region, anterior view

The subject is adducting the shoulders against resistance to demonstrate the pectoralis major muscle and anterior fibers of the deltoid muscle.

OBSERVE:
1. The pectoralis major muscle: the sternal part of the sternocostal head originates from the manubrium and body of the sternum, and the clavicular head originates from the medial half of the anterior surface of the clavicle;
2. The anterior axillary fold is formed by the inferior border of the pectoralis major muscle;
3. The deltopectoral triangle (infraclavicular fossa) is bounded by the clavicle superiorly, the deltoid muscle laterally, and the pectoralis major muscle medially.

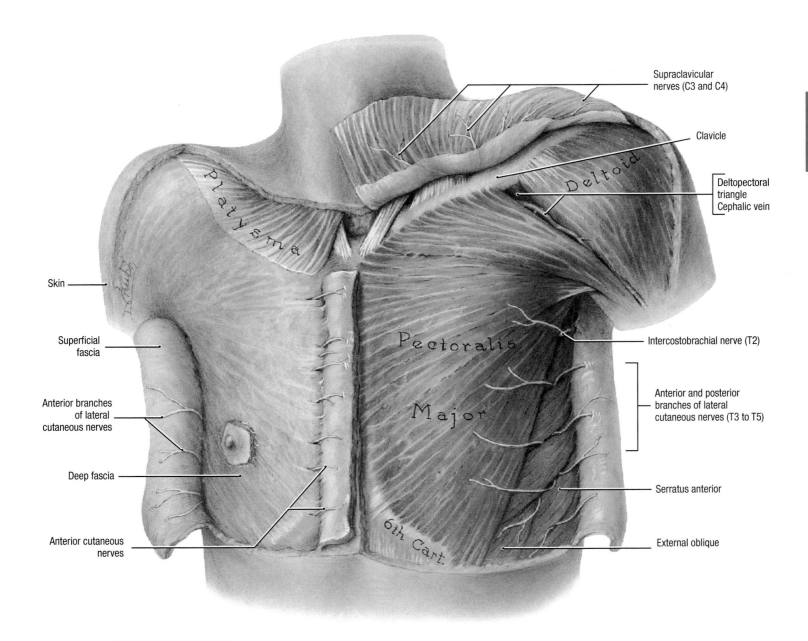

Supraclavicular nerves (C3 and C4)

Clavicle

Deltoid

Deltopectoral triangle
Cephalic vein

Platysma

Skin

Superficial fascia

Pectoralis

Intercostobrachial nerve (T2)

Anterior branches of lateral cutaneous nerves

Major

Anterior and posterior branches of lateral cutaneous nerves (T3 to T5)

Deep fascia

6th Cart.

Serratus anterior

Anterior cutaneous nerves

External oblique

1.2 Superficial dissection, male pectoral region, anterolateral view

The platysma muscle, which descends to the 2nd or 3rd rib, is cut short on the right side; together with the supraclavicular nerves, it is reflected on the left side.

OBSERVE:
1. The deep fascia covering the pectoralis major muscle is filmy;
2. The intermuscular bony strip of the clavicle is subcutaneous and subplatysmal;
3. The cephalic vein passes deeply to join the axillary vein in the deltopectoral triangle;
4. The cutaneous innervation of the pectoral region by the supraclavicular nerves (C3 and C4) and upper thoracic nerves (T2 to T6); the brachial plexus (C5, C6, C7, C8, and T1) does not supply cutaneous branches to the pectoral region.

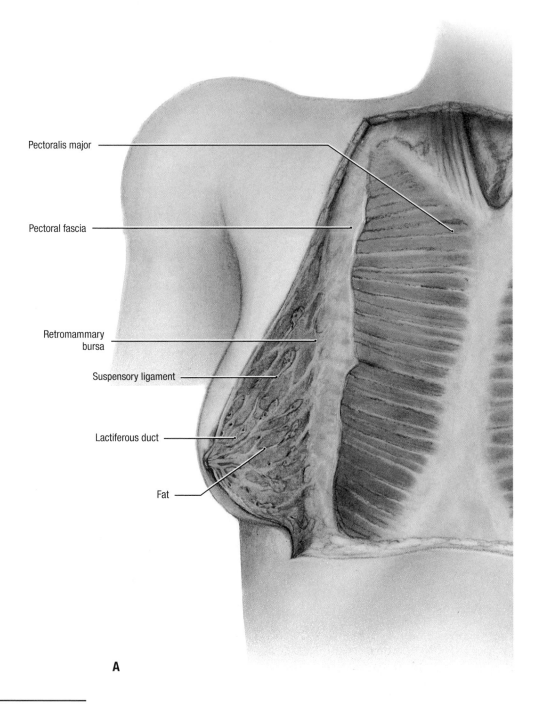

Pectoralis major

Pectoral fascia

Retromammary bursa

Suspensory ligament

Lactiferous duct

Fat

A

1.3   Superficial dissection, female pectoral region

A. Sagittal section. **B.** Anterior view.

OBSERVE IN **A:**
1. The lactiferous ducts (usually 15 to 20 in number) run dorsally in the long axis of the nipple, enveloped in an areolar cuff, and then spread radially and drain the glandular tissue.
2. The suspensory ligaments of the breast extend from the deep (pectoral) fascia to the skin;
3. Pectoral fascia covers the pectoralis major muscle;
4. A region of loose connective tissue between the deep (pectoral) fascia and the deep surface of the breast (the retromammary bursa) permits the breast to move on the deep fascia.

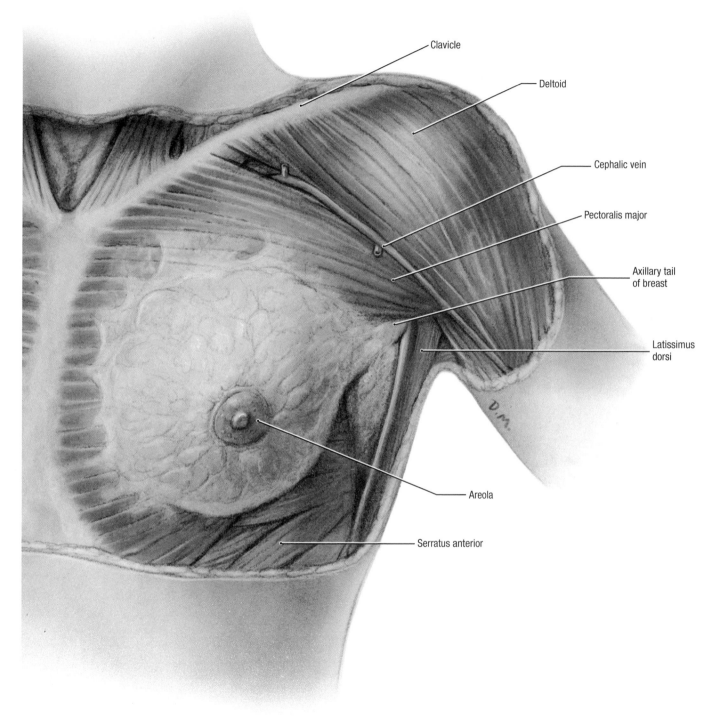

Clavicle

Deltoid

Cephalic vein

Pectoralis major

Axillary tail
of breast

Latissimus
dorsi

Areola

Serratus anterior

B

OBSERVE IN **B:**
5. The breast extends from the 2nd to the 6th rib, and the axillary tail projects into the axilla;
6. The pectoralis major and latissimus dorsi muscles form the boundaries of the axilla;
7. The cephalic vein drains deeply into the axillary vein at the deltopectoral triangle.

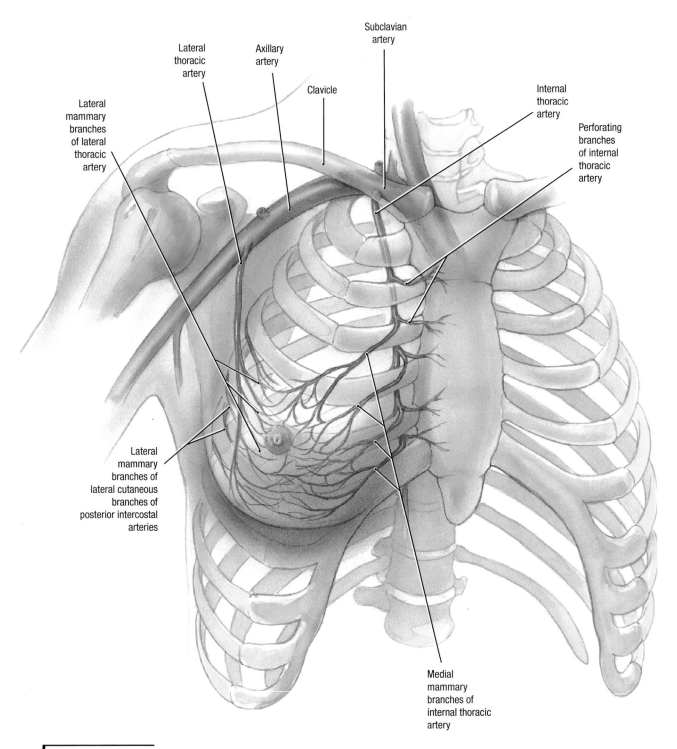

1.4   Arterial supply of the breast, anterior view

OBSERVE:

1. The arteries enter the breast from its superomedial and superolateral aspects; vessels also penetrate the deep surface of the breast;
2. The arteries branch profusely and anastomose with each other;
3. The blood supply is from the medial mammary branches of the internal thoracic artery, lateral mammary branches from the lateral thoracic artery and lateral mammary branches of lateral cutaneous branches of the posterior intercostal arteries (Fig. 1.20).

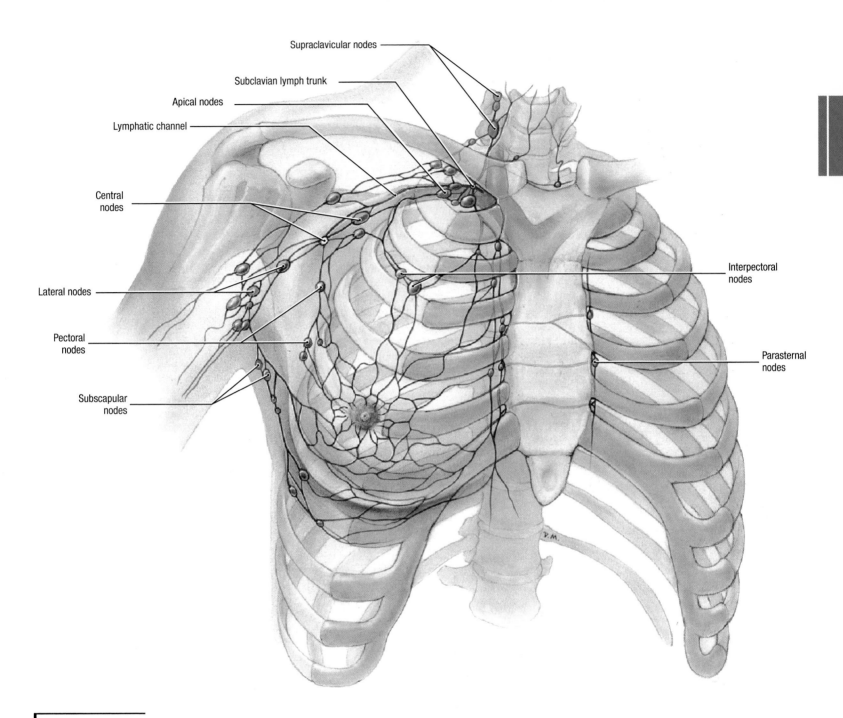

Supraclavicular nodes

Subclavian lymph trunk

Apical nodes

Lymphatic channel

Central nodes

Lateral nodes

Pectoral nodes

Subscapular nodes

Interpectoral nodes

Parasternal nodes

1.5   Lymphatic drainage of breast, anterior view

Drainage of lymph from the upper limb and breast passes through nodes arranged irregularly in groups: a) pectoral, along the inferior border of the pectoralis minor muscle; b) subscapular, along the subscapular artery and veins; c) lateral, along the distal part of the axillary vein; d) central, at the base of the axilla embedded in axillary fat; and e) apical, along the axillary vein between the clavicle and the pectoralis minor muscle. Most of the breast is drained through this system to the subclavian lymph trunk, which joins the venous system at the junction of the subclavian and internal jugular veins. The medial part of the breast drains to the parasternal nodes, which follow the internal thoracic vessels. *Parasternal nodes are less accessible surgically. When blockage of the lymphatic system occurs, as in cancer, drainage may go to the opposite breast and its nodes or inferiorly along the anterior abdominal wall to the inguinal nodes.*

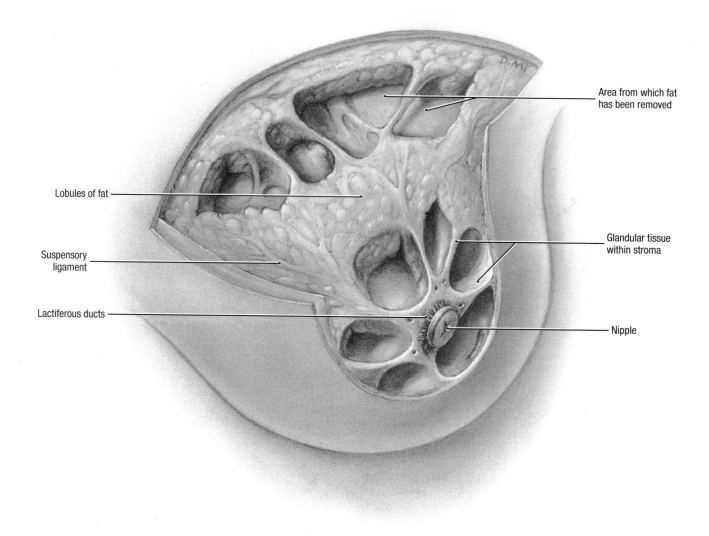

Area from which fat has been removed

Lobules of fat

Suspensory ligament

Lactiferous ducts

Glandular tissue within stroma

Nipple

1.6 Female mammary gland, anterior view

The breast, or mammary gland, lies in the superficial fascia and varies in size and shape. The nonlactating breast consists primarily of fat compartmentalized in connective and glandular tissue septa. (With the rounded handle of the scalpel, collections of superficial fat were scooped out of their compartments between septa.)

OBSERVE:
1. The lactiferous ducts open on the nipple;
2. The glandular tissue lies within a dense (fibro-) areolar stroma, from which suspensory ligaments extend to the deeper layers of the skin. *Breast cancer can result in fibrosis of the suspensory ligaments and subsequent retraction and pitting of the skin; the cancerous breast may lose its mobility and adhere to the underlying pectoralis major muscle if the tumor invades the deep fascia.*

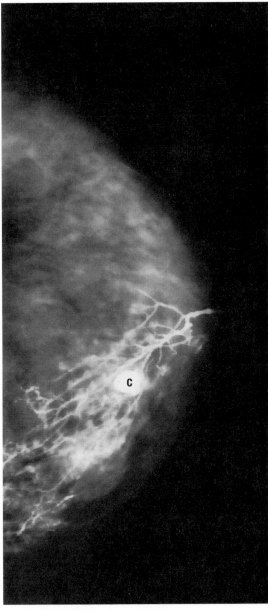

A

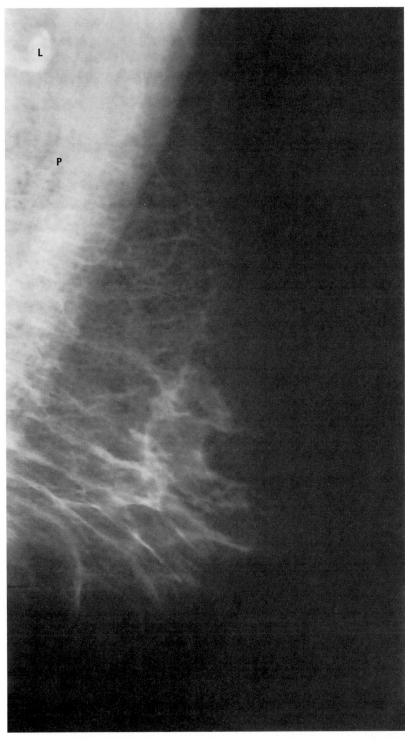

B

1.7   Imaging of breast

A. Galactogram. Contrast has been injected into a lactiferous duct, outlining the branching pattern of its tributaries. Note the presence of a ductal cyst (*C*).

B. Normal mammogram. Observe the connective tissue network of the breast. The fatty tissue provides a natural contrast medium for the connective tissue and glandular stroma. The stroma is radiopaque and changes with age and during lactation. Pectoralis major muscle (*P*) and an axillary lymph node (*L*) can also be seen.

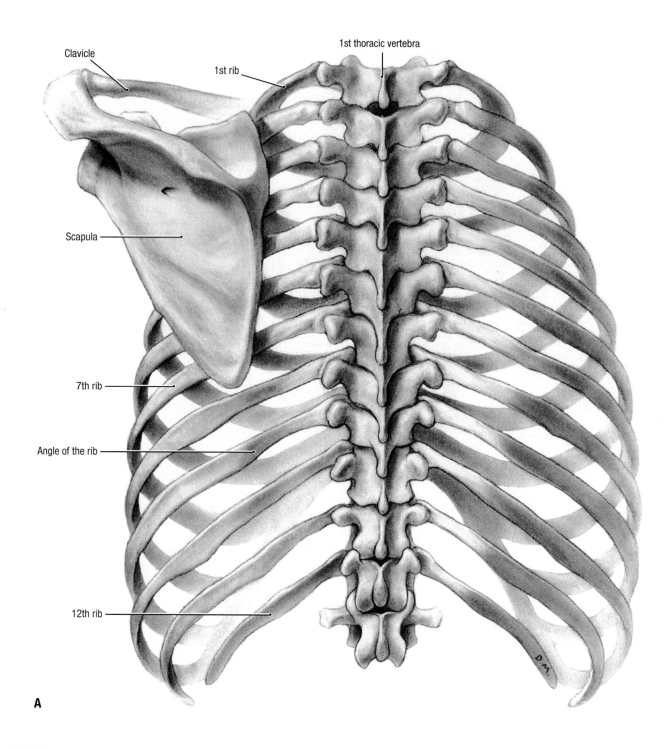

Clavicle

1st rib

1st thoracic vertebra

Scapula

7th rib

Angle of the rib

12th rib

A

1.8   Bony thorax

A. Posterior view. **B.** Anterior view.

OBSERVE:
1. The skeleton of the thorax consists of 12 thoracic vertebrae, 12 pairs of ribs and costal cartilages, and the sternum;
2. Each rib articulates posteriorly with the vertebral column;

3. Anteriorly, the superior seven costal cartilages articulate with the sternum; the 8th, 9th, and 10th cartilages articulate with the cartilage above; the 11th and 12th are "floating" ribs, i.e., their cartilages do not articulate anteriorly;
4. Posteriorly, all ribs angle inferiorly; anteriorly, the 3rd to 10th costal cartilages angle superiorly;

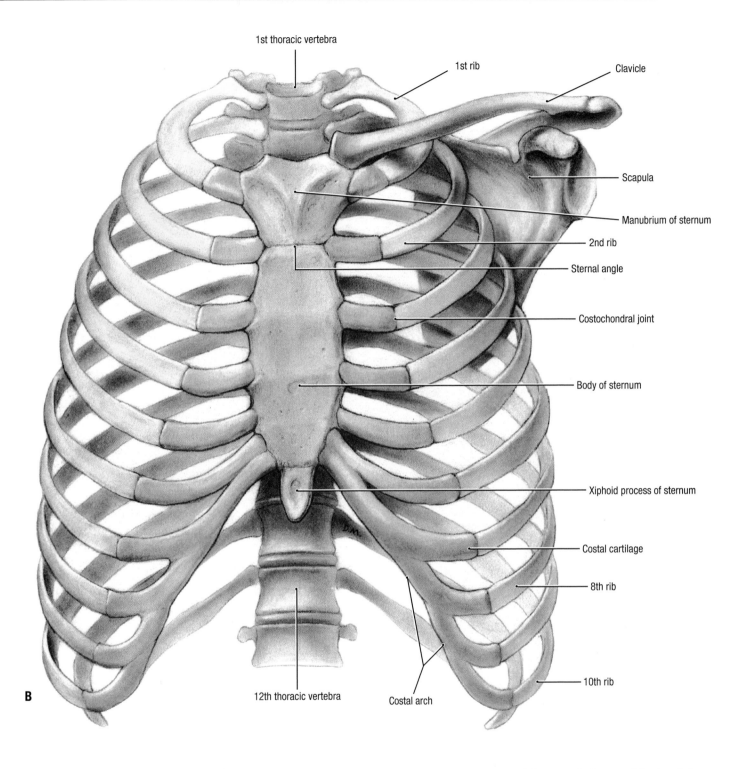

1st thoracic vertebra

1st rib

Clavicle

Scapula

Manubrium of sternum

2nd rib

Sternal angle

Costochondral joint

Body of sternum

Xiphoid process of sternum

Costal cartilage

8th rib

10th rib

B

12th thoracic vertebra

Costal arch

5. The superior thoracic aperture (thoracic inlet) is the doorway between the thoracic cavity and the neck region; it is bounded by the 1st thoracic vertebra, the 1st ribs and their cartilages, and the manubrium of the sternum.
6. The clavicle lies over the anterosuperior aspect of the 1st rib, making it difficult to palpate;
7. The 2nd rib is easy to locate because its costal cartilage articulates with the sternum at the sternal angle; find this important bony element

vation at the junction of the manubrium and body of the sternum (Fig. 1.11B);
8. The 3rd to 10th ribs can be palpated in sequence inferolaterally from the 2nd rib; the fused costal cartilages of the 7th to 10th ribs form the costal arch (margin), and the tips of the 11th and 12th ribs can be palpated posterolaterally;
9. The scapula is suspended from the clavicle and crosses the 2nd to 7th ribs.

1.9   Ribs

A. "Typical" and "atypical" ribs, posterior view.

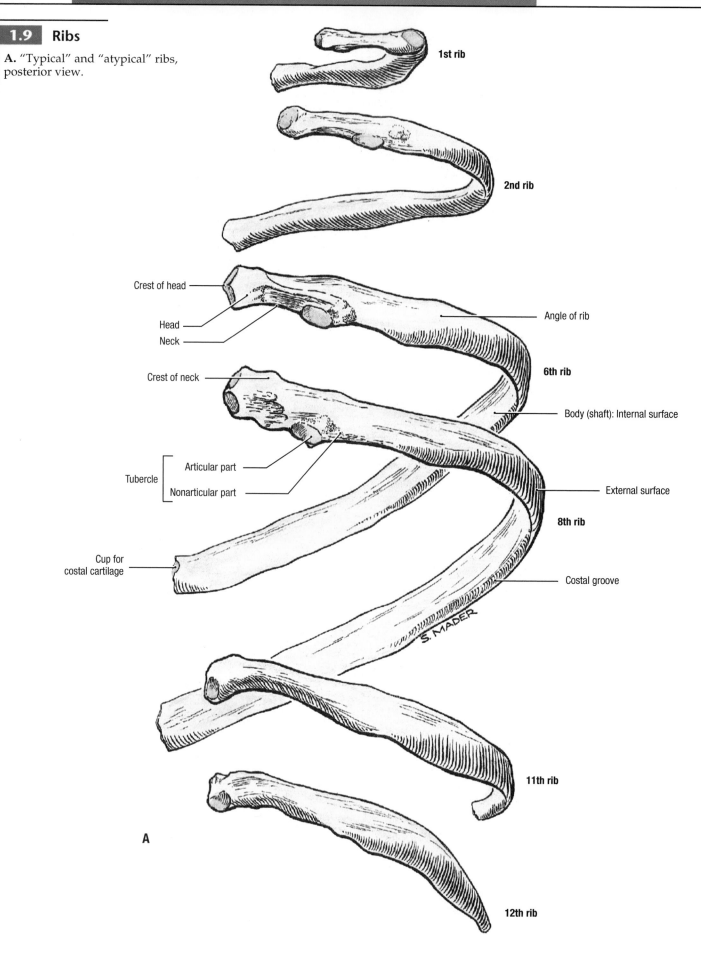

1st rib

2nd rib

Crest of head

Head

Neck

Angle of rib

Crest of neck

6th rib

Body (shaft): Internal surface

Tubercle — Articular part

Nonarticular part

External surface

8th rib

Cup for costal cartilage

Costal groove

S. MADER

11th rib

A

12th rib

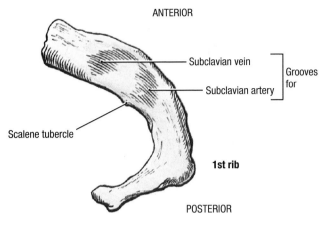

B. First rib, superior view.

OBSERVE IN **A**, RIBS 3 THROUGH 10, WHICH ARE CONSIDERED "TYPICAL," AS REPRESENTED BY RIBS 6 AND 8:
1. The head of the rib is wedge-shaped and has two articular facets separated by the crest of the head;
2. The tubercle of the rib consists of articular and nonarticular parts;
3. The costal groove shelters the intercostal vein, artery, and nerve;
4. The posterior part of the shaft (body) is rounded, the anterior part is flattened, and the sternal end has a cup-shaped area for articulation with costal cartilage.

OBSERVE IN **A**, RIBS 1, 2, 11, AND 12, WHICH ARE CONSIDERED "ATYPICAL":
5. The 1st rib is the shortest, broadest, and most curved; the head has a single facet;
6. The 2nd rib has a poorly marked costal groove and a rough tuberosity;
7. The 11th and 12th ribs, or "floating" ribs, have a single facet on the head, no tubercle, and a tapering anterior end.

OBSERVE IN **B**:
8. The grooves for the subclavian vein and artery;
9. The scalene tubercle for the scalenus anterior muscle.

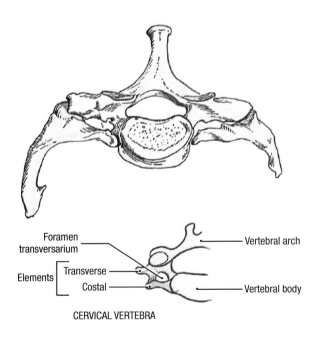

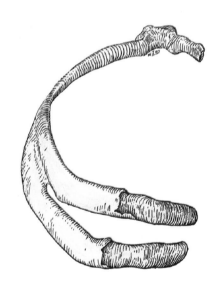

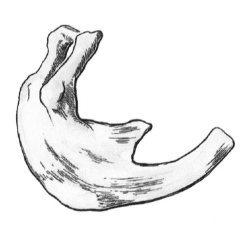

1.10   Rib anomalies

A. Cervical ribs. This is an enlarged costal element of the 7th cervical vertebra. It can be unilateral or bilateral, and large and palpable, or detectable only radiologically. It can be asymptomatic or, through pressure on the most inferior root of the brachial plexus, can produce sensory and motor changes over the distribution of the ulnar nerve.
B. Bicipital rib. In this specimen, there has been partial fusion of the first two thoracic ribs. A similar condition can result from the partial fusion of a cervical rib with the 1st thoracic rib.
C. Bifid rib. The superior component of this 3rd rib is supernumerary and articulated with the lateral aspect of the 1st sternebra (Fig. 1.11A) of the body of the sternum. The inferior component articulated at the junction of the 1st and 2nd sternebrae.

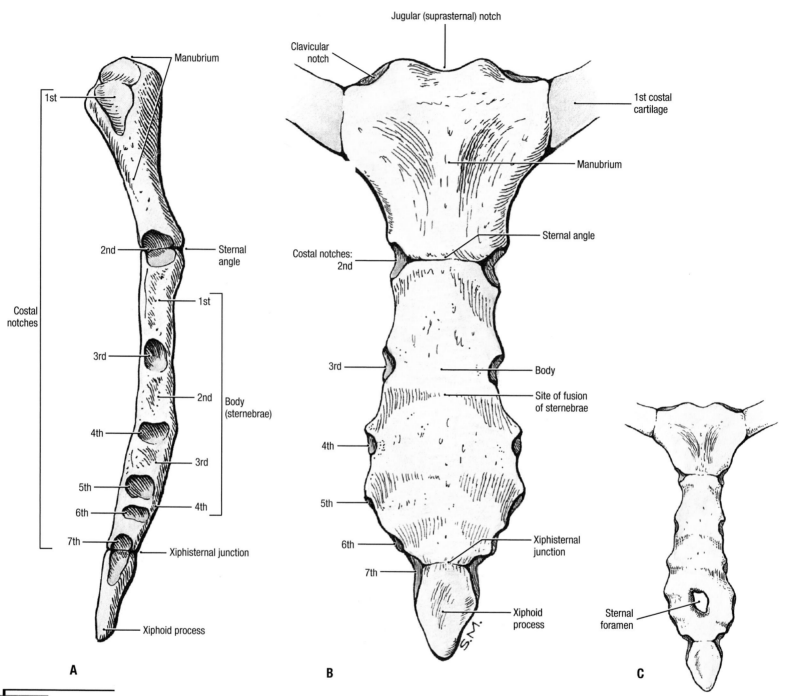

A. Lateral view. **B.** Anterior view. **C.** Sternal foramen, anterior view.

1.11 Sternum

OBSERVE:

1. The jugular (suprasternal) notch is between the clavicular notches. *A finger placed in this notch palpates the trachea*;
2. The sternal angle is at the junction of the manubrium and body. This is a palpable landmark that guides location of the 2nd costal cartilage;
3. The body is composed of four fused sternebrae; lines marking the sites of fusion can be seen crossing the anterior surface of the body;

4. The sharp inferior edge of the body at the xiphisternal junction is palpable. *Forceful displacement of the xiphoid process endangers the underlying liver*;
5. Seven costal cartilages articulate with the sternum at the costal notches; the 1st with the manubrium, and the 6th with the lateral aspect of the 4th sternebra; all others articulate at junctions of the manubrium, the four sternebrae, and the xiphoid process.
6. In **C**: *This malformation results from a defect of ossification and can be misdiagnosed as a bullet wound.*

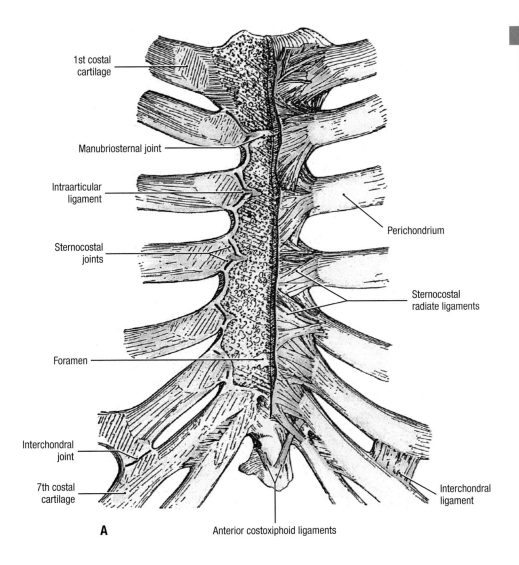

1st costal cartilage

Manubriosternal joint

Intraarticular ligament

Sternocostal joints

Foramen

Interchondral joint

7th costal cartilage

Perichondrium

Sternocostal radiate ligaments

Interchondral ligament

Anterior costoxiphoid ligaments

A

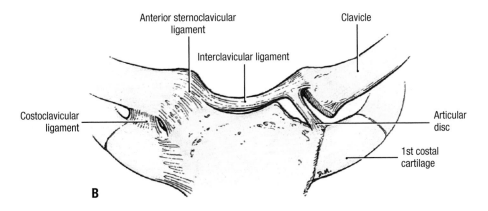

Anterior sternoclavicular ligament

Interclavicular ligament

Clavicle

Costoclavicular ligament

Articular disc

1st costal cartilage

B

1.12 Sternocostal, interchondral, and sternoclavicular joints

A. Sternocostal and interchondral joints, anterior view. On the right side, the cortex of the sternum and the external surface of the costal cartilages have been shaved away; to obtain a specimen of bone marrow, a sternal puncture is done through the thin cortical bone into the area of cancellous (spongy) bone.

OBSERVE:
1. On the left side, dissection shows that the fibers of the perichondrium of the costal cartilages terminate as sternocostal radiate ligaments;
2. Three types of joints are demonstrated: synchondroses between the 1st costal cartilage and manubrium, and between the 7th costal cartilage and the sternum (in this case); symphysis at the manubriosternal joint; and synovial joints at the other sternocostal joints and the interchondral joints.

B. Sternoclavicular joint, anterior view. The sternoclavicular joint is the only articulation between the appendicular skeleton of the upper limb and the axial skeleton of the trunk. *Fractures of the clavicle are more common than dislocation of the medial end of the clavicle because of the strength of the articular disc within the joint and the surrounding ligaments.*

OBSERVE ON THE RIGHT SIDE:
3. The anterior sternoclavicular ligament reinforces the joint capsule anteriorly;
4. The interclavicular ligament connects the medial ends of the clavicles and reinforces the superior aspect of the joint;
5. The short, fibrous costoclavicular ligament joins the 1st rib and costal cartilage to the inferior surface of the clavicle.

OBSERVE ON THE LEFT SIDE:
6. The joint capsule is removed, revealing the articular disc, which attaches superiorly to the clavicle and inferiorly to the 1st costal cartilage;
7. The articular surface of the clavicle is larger than that of the manubrium.

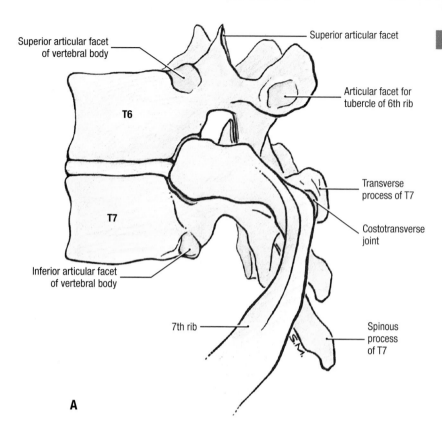

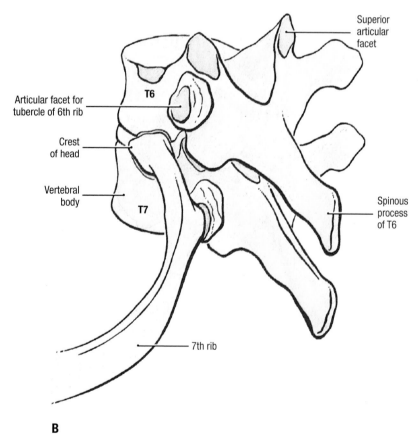

A

B

1.13 Costovertebral articulations

A. Lateral view. **B.** Posterolateral view. **C.** Costotransverse joints.

OBSERVE:

1. The costovertebral articulations include the articulation of the head of the rib with two adjacent vertebral bodies and the tubercle of the rib with the transverse process of a vertebra;
2. There are two articular facets on the head of the rib: a larger, inferior one for articulation with the vertebral body of its own number, and a smaller, superior facet for the vertebral body above;
3. The crest of the head of the rib separates the two articular facets;
4. The smooth articular part of the tubercle of the rib articulates with the transverse process of the same numbered vertebra at the costotransverse joint.
5. In **C:** At the 1st to 7th costotransverse joints, the ribs rotate; at the 8th, 9th, and 10th, they glide, increasing the transverse diameter of the upper abdomen.

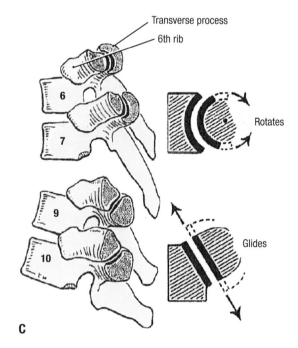

C

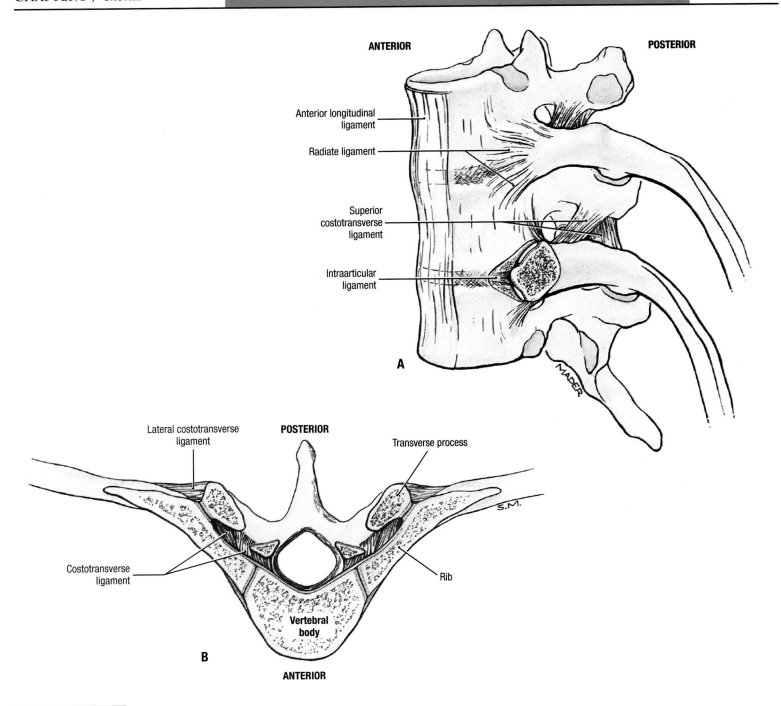

1.14 Ligaments of costovertebral articulations

A. Lateral view. **B.** Superior view.

OBSERVE IN **A:**
1. The radiate ligament joins the head of the rib to two vertebral bodies and the interposed intervertebral disc;
2. The superior costotransverse ligament joins the crest of the neck of the rib to the transverse process above;
3. The intraarticular ligament joins the crest of the head of the rib to the intervertebral disc.

OBSERVE IN **B:**
4. The vertebral body, transverse processes, superior articulating processes, and posterior elements of the articulating ribs have been transversely sectioned to visualize the joint surfaces and ligaments;
5. The costotransverse ligament joins the posterior aspect of the neck of the rib to the adjacent transverse process;
6. The lateral costotransverse ligament joins the nonarticulating part of the tubercle of the rib to the tip (apex) of the transverse process;
7. The articular surfaces (blue) of the synovial plane costovertebral joints.

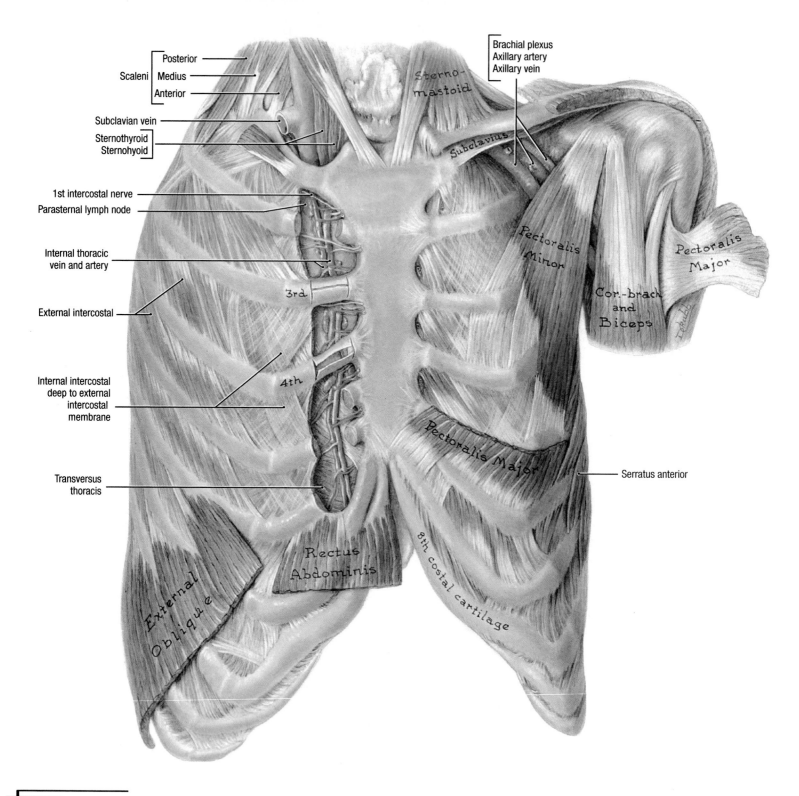

Brachial plexus
Axillary artery
Axillary vein

Posterior
Scaleni Medius
Anterior

Sterno-
mastoid

Subclavian vein

Sternothyroid
Sternohyoid

Subclavius

1st intercostal nerve

Parasternal lymph node

Pectoralis
Minor

Pectoralis
Major

Internal thoracic
vein and artery

3rd

External intercostal

4th

Cor-brach
and
Biceps

Internal intercostal
deep to external
intercostal
membrane

Pectoralis Major

Serratus anterior

Transversus
thoracis

Rectus
Abdominis

8th costal cartilage

External
Oblique

1.15   Thoracic wall, anterior view

OBSERVE:

1. The internal thoracic (internal mammary) vessels run inferiorly just lateral to the edge of the sternum and providing intercostal branches;

2. The parasternal lymph nodes (green) receive lymphatic vessels from the intercostal spaces, the costal pleura and diaphragm, and the medial part of the breast. *By this route, cancer of the breast can spread to the lungs and mediastinum;*

3. The subclavian vessels are "sandwiched" between the 1st rib and clavicle (padded by the subclavius muscle);

4. The H-shaped cut through the perichondrium of the 3rd and 4th cartilages was made to shell out segments of cartilage. *Similarly, in a thoracotomy, the surgeon may shell a segment of rib out of its periosteum; later, bone regenerates from this periosteum.*

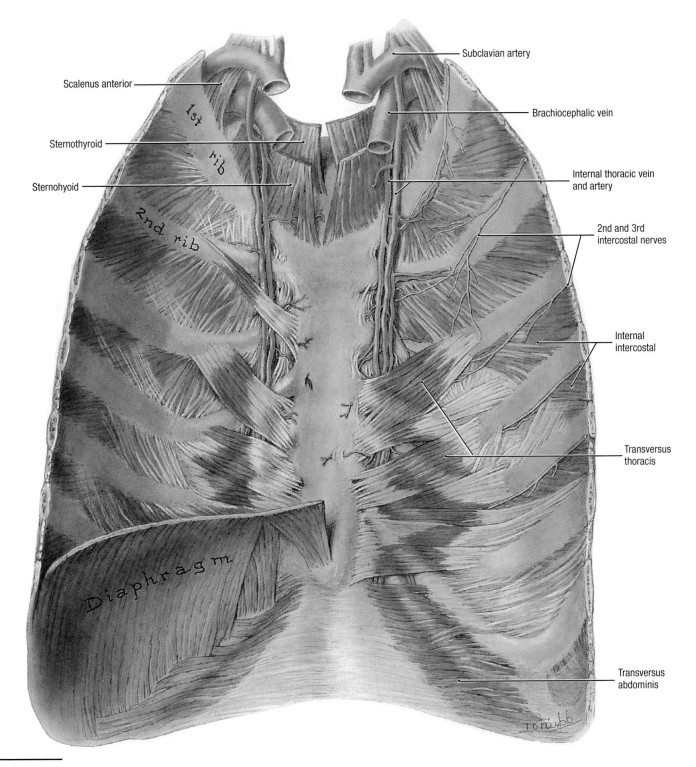

Labels on image: Subclavian artery; Scalenus anterior; 1st rib; Sternothyroid; Brachiocephalic vein; Sternohyoid; 2nd rib; Internal thoracic vein and artery; 2nd and 3rd intercostal nerves; Internal intercostal; Transversus thoracis; Diaphragm; Transversus abdominis

1.16   Anterior thoracic wall, posterior view

OBSERVE:
1. The transversus thoracis muscle is continuous with the transversus abdominis muscle; these form the innermost layer of the three flat muscles of the thoracoabdominal wall;
2. The internal thoracic (internal mammary) artery arises from the subclavian artery, accompanied by two veins (venae comitantes) up to the 2nd costal cartilage and, superior to this, by the single internal thoracic vein, which drains into the brachiocephalic vein;
3. The inferior portions of the internal thoracic vessels are covered posteriorly by the transversus thoracis muscle; the superior portions are in contact with parietal pleura (removed).

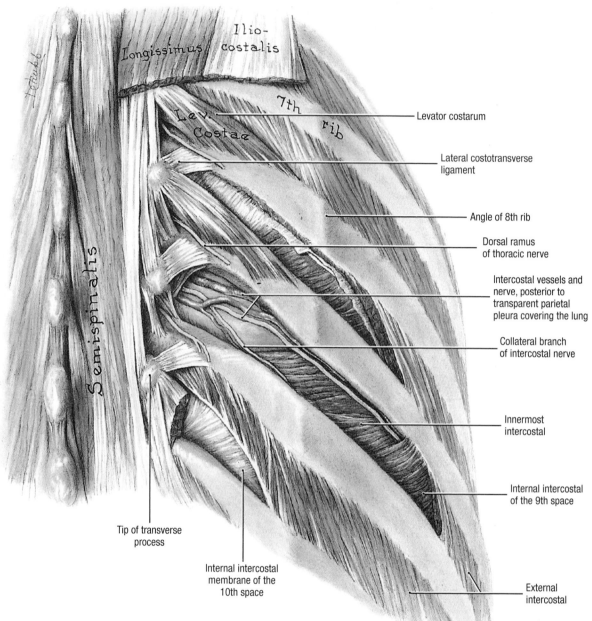

Levator costarum

Lateral costotransverse ligament

Angle of 8th rib

Dorsal ramus of thoracic nerve

Intercostal vessels and nerve, posterior to transparent parietal pleura covering the lung

Collateral branch of intercostal nerve

Innermost intercostal

Internal intercostal of the 9th space

External intercostal

Tip of transverse process

Internal intercostal membrane of the 10th space

1.17   Posterior ends of inferior intercostal spaces, posterior view

The iliocostalis and longissimus muscles have been removed, exposing the levator costarum muscle. Of the five intercostal spaces shown, the superior two (6th and 7th) are intact. In the 8th and 10th spaces, varying portions of the external intercostal muscle have been removed to reveal the underlying internal intercostal membrane, which is continuous with the internal intercostal muscle. In the 9th space, the levator costarum muscle has been removed to show the intercostal vessels and nerve.

OBSERVE:

1. The intercostal vessels and nerve appear medially between the superior costotransverse ligament and the transparent parietal pleura covering the lung; they disappear laterally between the internal and innermost intercostal muscles;
2. The intercostal nerve is the most inferior of the trio and the least sheltered in the intercostal groove; a collateral branch arises near the angle of the rib. *To avoid damage to the intercostal nerve and vessels, the needle is inserted superior to the rib, high enough to avoid the collateral branches.*

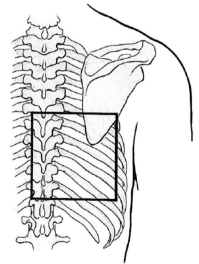

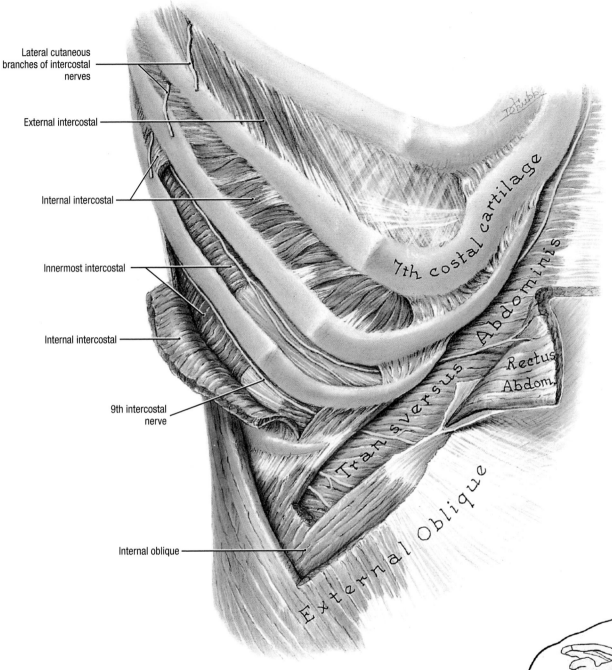

Lateral cutaneous branches of intercostal nerves

External intercostal

Internal intercostal

Innermost intercostal

Internal intercostal

9th intercostal nerve

Internal oblique

7th costal cartilage

Transversus Abdominis

Rectus Abdom.

External Oblique

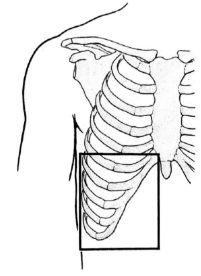

1.18 **Anterior ends of inferior intercostal spaces, anterior view**

OBSERVE:
1. The fibers of the external intercostal and external oblique muscles run inferomedially;
2. The internal intercostal and internal oblique muscles are in continuity at the ends of the 9th, 10th, and 11th intercostal spaces;
3. The intercostal nerves lie deep to the internal intercostal muscle but superficial to the innermost intercostal muscle; anteriorly, these nerves lie superficial to the transversus abdominis or transversus thoracis muscles;
4. Intercostal nerves run parallel to their ribs and costal cartilages; on reaching the abdominal wall, nerves T7 and T8 continue superiorly, T9 continues nearly horizontally, and T10 continues inferomedially toward the umbilicus. These nerves provide cutaneous innervation in overlapping segmental bands.

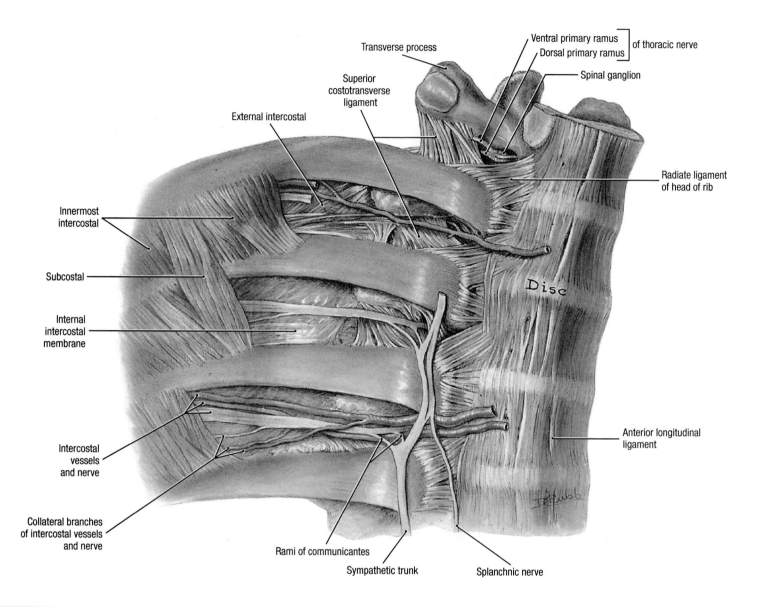

Transverse process

Superior costotransverse ligament

External intercostal

Ventral primary ramus ⎤ of thoracic nerve
Dorsal primary ramus ⎦

Spinal ganglion

Innermost intercostal

Radiate ligament of head of rib

Subcostal

Disc

Internal intercostal membrane

Intercostal vessels and nerve

Anterior longitudinal ligament

Collateral branches of intercostal vessels and nerve

Rami of communicantes

Sympathetic trunk

Splanchnic nerve

1.19   Vertebral ends of intercostal spaces, anterior view

OBSERVE:

1. Portions of the innermost intercostal muscle that bridge two intercostal spaces are called subcostal muscles;
2. External intercostal muscle in the most superior space;
3. Internal intercostal membrane in the middle space, continuous medially with the superior costotransverse ligament;
4. Order of the structures in the most inferior space: intercostal vein, artery, and nerve; note their collateral branches;

5. Thoracic nerve near the top of the illustration; the ventral primary ramus crosses anterior to the superior costotransverse ligament; the dorsal primary ramus is posterior to it;
6. The attachment of intercostal nerves to the sympathetic trunk by the rami communicantes; the splanchnic nerve is a visceral branch of the trunk.

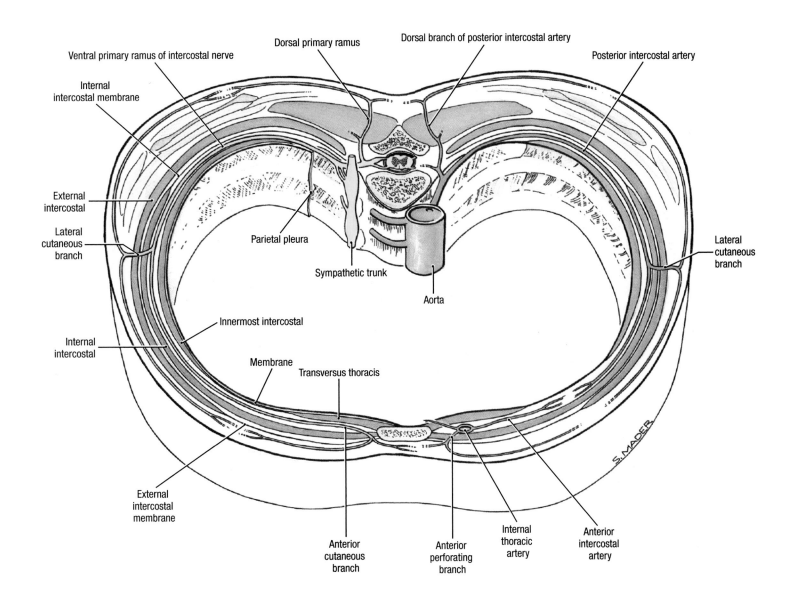

Ventral primary ramus of intercostal nerve

Dorsal primary ramus

Dorsal branch of posterior intercostal artery

Posterior intercostal artery

Internal intercostal membrane

External intercostal

Lateral cutaneous branch

Parietal pleura

Sympathetic trunk

Aorta

Lateral cutaneous branch

Innermost intercostal

Internal intercostal

Membrane

Transversus thoracis

External intercostal membrane

Anterior cutaneous branch

Anterior perforating branch

Internal thoracic artery

Anterior intercostal artery

S. MADER

1.20   Contents of intercostal space, transverse section

This diagram is simplified by showing nerves on the right and arteries on the left.

OBSERVE:
1. Three muscular layers: (a) external intercostal muscle and membrane, (b) internal intercostal muscle and membrane, (c) innermost intercostal and transversus thoracis muscles and the membrane connecting them;
2. The dorsal primary ramus innervates the deep back muscles and skin adjacent to the vertebral column;
3. The intercostal nerves are the ventral primary rami of spinal nerves T1 to T11; the ventral primary ramus of spinal nerve T12 is the sub-costal nerve;

4. The upper intercostal vessels and nerves run in the plane between the middle and innermost layers of muscles; the lower intercostal vessels and nerves occupy a corresponding plane in the abdominal wall as shown in Figure 1.18.
5. Posterior intercostal arteries are branches of the aorta (the superior two spaces are supplied from the superior intercostal branch of the costocervical trunk); anterior intercostal arteries are branches of the internal thoracic artery.

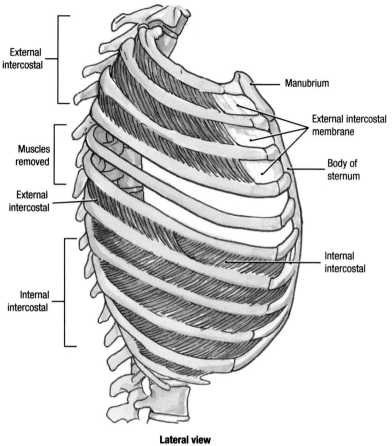

External intercostal

Muscles removed

External intercostal

Internal intercostal

Manubrium

External intercostal membrane

Body of sternum

Internal intercostal

Lateral view

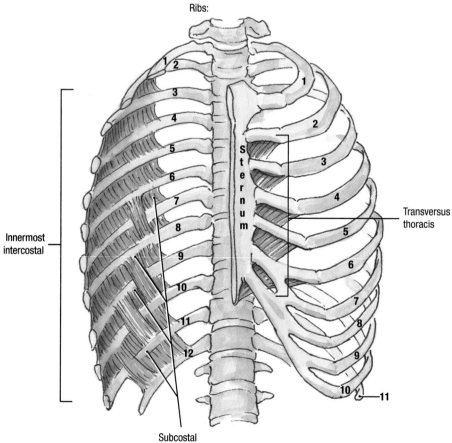

Ribs:

Innermost intercostal

Sternum

Transversus thoracis

Subcostal

Anterior view

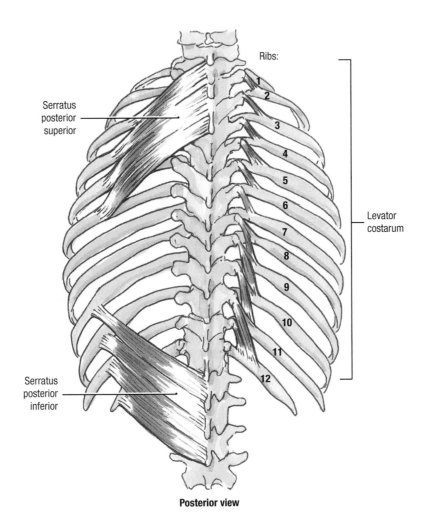

Ribs:
1
2
3
4
5
6
7
8
9
10
11
12

Serratus posterior superior

Levator costarum

Serratus posterior inferior

Posterior view

Table 1.1. Muscles of thoracic wall

Muscles	Superior Attachment	Inferior Attachment	Innervation	Action[a]
External intercostal	Inferior border of ribs	Superior border of ribs below Superior border of ribs below	Intercostal nerve	Elevate ribs
Internal intercostal	Inferior border of ribs	Superior border of ribs below	Intercostal nerve	Depress ribs
Innermost intercostal	Inferior border of ribs	Internal surface of costal carilages 2–6	Intercostal nerve	Probably elevate ribs
Transversus thoracis	Posterior surface of lower sternum	Superior borders of 2nd or 3rd ribs below	Intercostal nerve	Depress ribs
Subcostal	Internal surface of lower ribs near their angles	Subjacent ribs between tubercle and angle	Intercostal nerve	Elevate ribs
Levator costarum	Transverse processes of T7–T11	Superior borders of 2nd to 4th ribs	Dorsal primary rami of C8–T11 nerves	Elevate ribs
Serratus posterior superior	Ligamentum nuchae, spinous processes of C7 to T3 vertebrae	Inferior borders of 8th to 12th ribs near their angles	Second to fifth intercostal nerves	Elevate ribs
Serratus posterior inferior	Spinous processes of T11 to L2 vertebrae		Ventral rami of ninth to twelfth thoracic spinal nerves	Depress ribs

[a] All intercostal muscles keep intercostal spaces rigid, thereby preventing them from bulging out during expiration and from being drawn in during inspiration. Role of individual intercostal muscles and accessory muscles of respiration in moving the ribs is difficult to interpret despite many electromyographic studies.

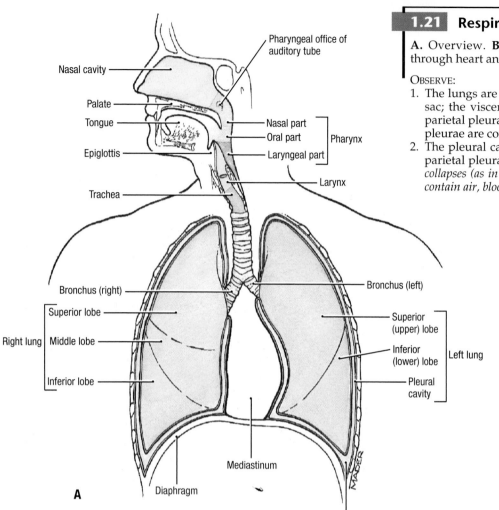

1.21 Respiratory system

A. Overview. **B.** Pleural cavity and pleura **C.** Coronal section through heart and lungs.

OBSERVE:
1. The lungs are invaginated by a continuous membranous pleural sac; the visceral (pulmonary) pleura covers the lungs, and the parietal pleura lines the thoracic cavity. The visceral and parietal pleurae are continuous at the root of the lung;
2. The pleural cavity is a potential space between the visceral and parietal pleurae that contains a thin layer of fluid. *When the lung collapses (as in B), the pleural cavity becomes a "real" space and may contain air, blood, etc.*
3. The left pleural cavity is smaller than the right because of the projection of the heart into the left side;
4. The parietal pleura can be divided regionally into the costal, diaphragmatic, mediastinal, and cervical pleura; note the costomediastinal recess between the costal and diaphragmatic parietal pleura.

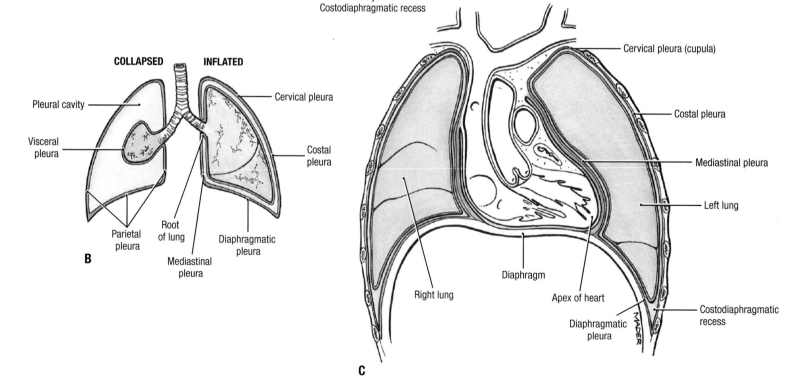

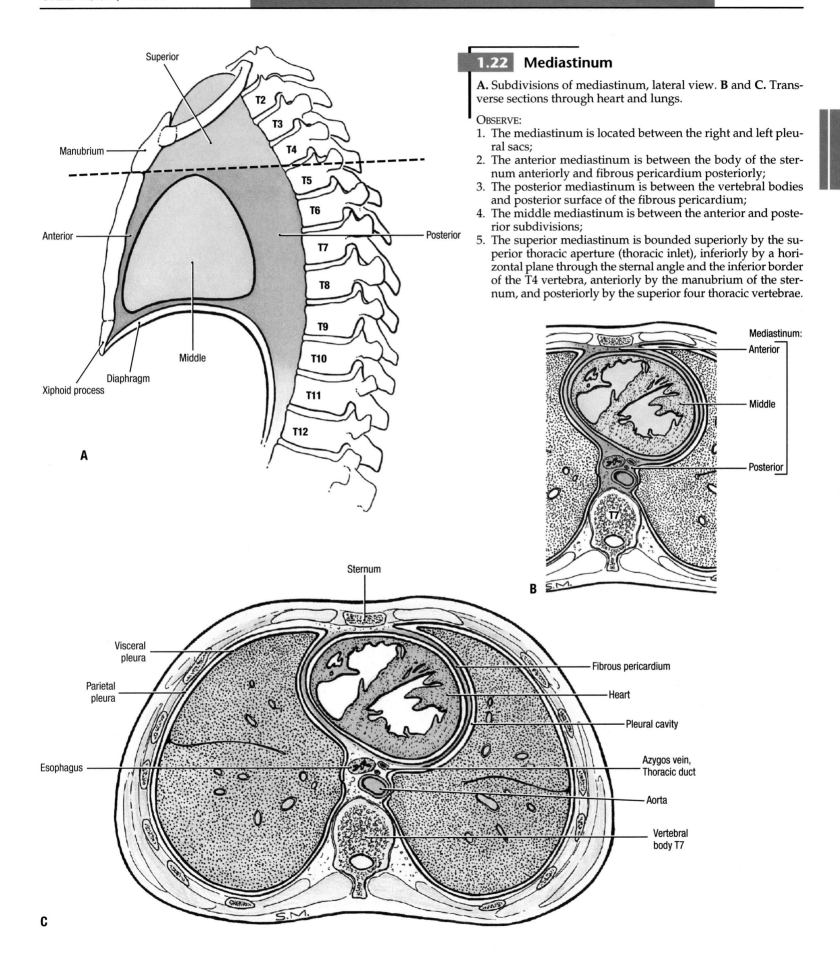

1.22 Mediastinum

A. Subdivisions of mediastinum, lateral view. **B** and **C.** Transverse sections through heart and lungs.

OBSERVE:

1. The mediastinum is located between the right and left pleural sacs;
2. The anterior mediastinum is between the body of the sternum anteriorly and fibrous pericardium posteriorly;
3. The posterior mediastinum is between the vertebral bodies and posterior surface of the fibrous pericardium;
4. The middle mediastinum is between the anterior and posterior subdivisions;
5. The superior mediastinum is bounded superiorly by the superior thoracic aperture (thoracic inlet), inferiorly by a horizontal plane through the sternal angle and the inferior border of the T4 vertebra, anteriorly by the manubrium of the sternum, and posteriorly by the superior four thoracic vertebrae.

Labels for figure A: Superior, Manubrium, Anterior, Xiphoid process, Diaphragm, Middle, Posterior, T2, T3, T4, T5, T6, T7, T8, T9, T10, T11, T12

Labels for figure B: Mediastinum: Anterior, Middle, Posterior, T7

Labels for figure C: Sternum, Visceral pleura, Parietal pleura, Esophagus, Fibrous pericardium, Heart, Pleural cavity, Azygos vein, Thoracic duct, Aorta, Vertebral body T7

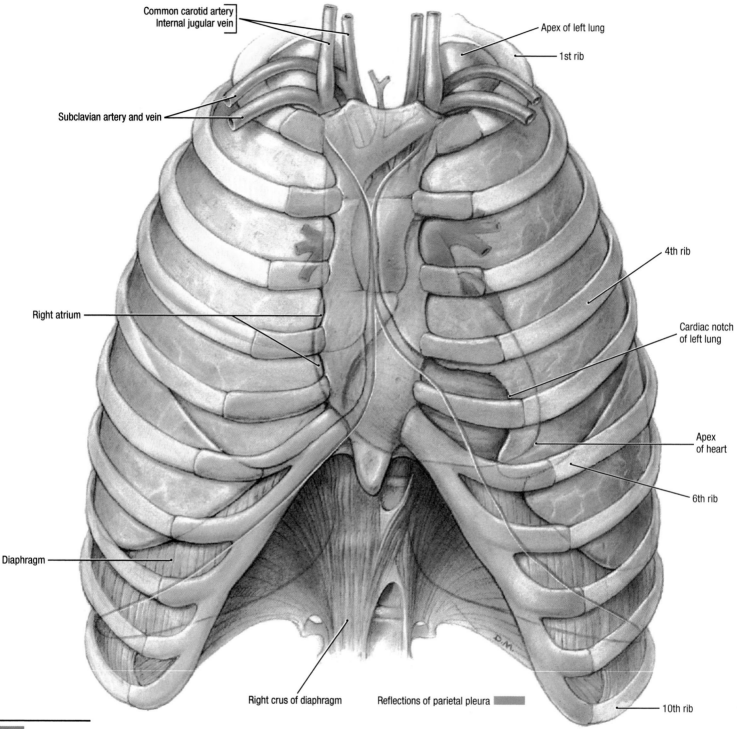

1.23   **Thoracic contents, anterior view**

OBSERVE:

1. The apex of the lungs is at the level of the neck of the 1st rib, and the inferior border of the lungs is the 6th rib in the left midclavicular line and the 8th rib at the lateral aspect of the bony thorax at the midaxillary line;

2. The cardiac notch of the left lung and the deviation of the parietal pleura away from the median plane toward the left side in the region of the notch;

3. The reflection of parietal pleura inferiorly at the 8th costochondral junction at the midclavicular line, at the 10th rib in the midaxillary

line, and at the level of the neck of the 12th rib on each side of the vertebral column;

4. The apex of the heart is in the 5th interspace at the left midclavicular line;

5. The right atrium forms the right border of the heart and extends just beyond the lateral margin of the sternum;

6. The great vessels of the heart and their branches, which pass through the superior thoracic aperture.

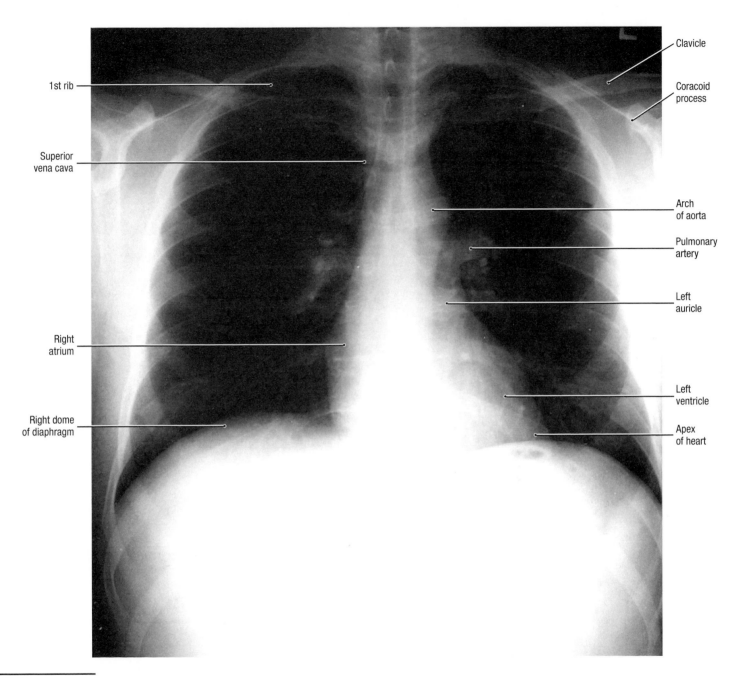

Clavicle

Coracoid process

1st rib

Superior vena cava

Arch of aorta

Pulmonary artery

Left auricle

Right atrium

Left ventricle

Right dome of diaphragm

Apex of heart

1.24 Radiograph of chest

Using Figure 1.23 for reference, observe in this posteroanterior projection:
1. Body of the 1st thoracic vertebra (T1) and articulation of the 1st rib with the vertebral body; follow the 1st rib, which curves laterally and then medially to cross the clavicle;
2. The dome of the diaphragm is higher on the right;

3. The convexity of the right mediastinal border is formed by the right atrium; above this, the superior vena cava produces a less convex shape.
4. The left mediastinal border is formed by the arch of the aorta, pulmonary trunk, left auricle (not prominent on a normal chest radiograph), and left ventricle.

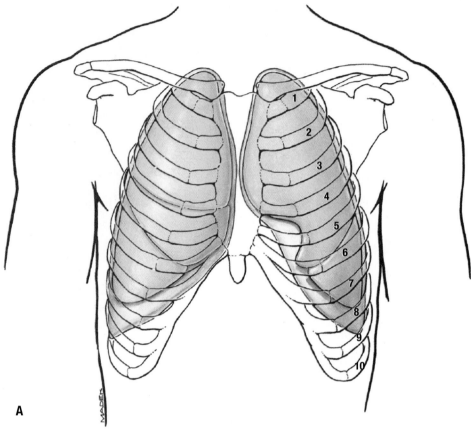

A

1.25   Outline of pleura and lungs

A. Anterior view. **B.** Posterior view.

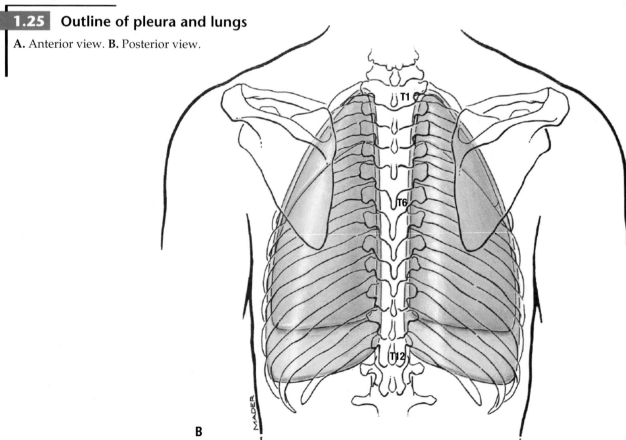

B

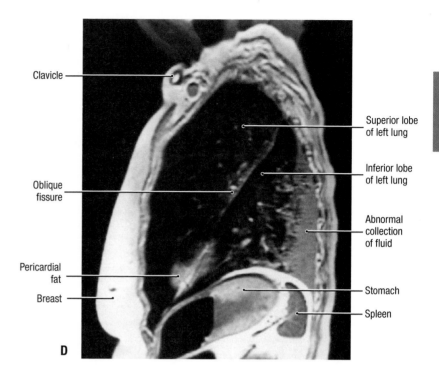

Clavicle

Superior lobe
of left lung

Oblique
fissure

Inferior lobe
of left lung

Abnormal
collection
of fluid

Pericardial
fat

Stomach

Breast

Spleen

D

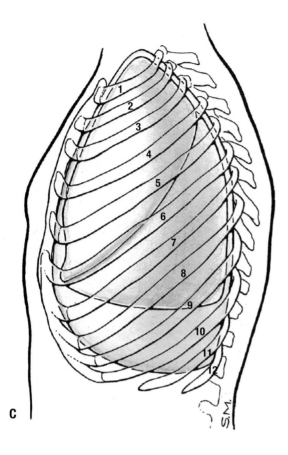

C

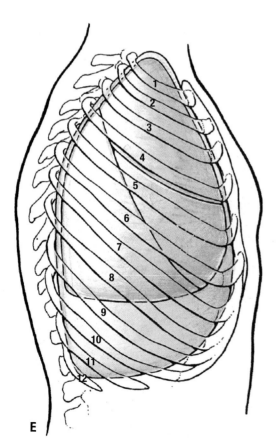

E

C. Left lateral view. **D.** MRI. **E.** Right lateral view.

Trace the outline of the lung covered with visceral pleura (pink) and the outline of the parietal pleura (blue) as observed in quiet respiration.

OBSERVE:

1. The apices of the lungs and cervical pleura extend to the neck of the 1st rib;
2. The apices and anterior borders of the lungs lie directly adjacent to the parietal pleura as far as the 4th costal cartilage. At this level, the left lung has a well-defined cardiac notch spanning horizontally along the 4th costal cartilage and rib to the midclavicular line and then curving inferiorly to the 6th rib or costal cartilage;
3. At the 6th costal cartilage, the parietal pleura passes laterally to reach the midclavicular line at the level of the 8th costal cartilage, the 10th rib at the midaxillary line, the 12th rib at the midscapular line, and the spinous process of T12;
4. The parietal pleura extends approximately two ribs inferior to the lung;
5. The oblique fissure of the right and left lungs extends from the level of the spinous process of T2 posteriorly to the 6th costal cartilage anteriorly; the horizontal fissure of the right lung extends from the oblique fissure along the 4th rib and costal cartilage anteriorly. Compare the left lateral view **(C)** to the MRI **(D)**.

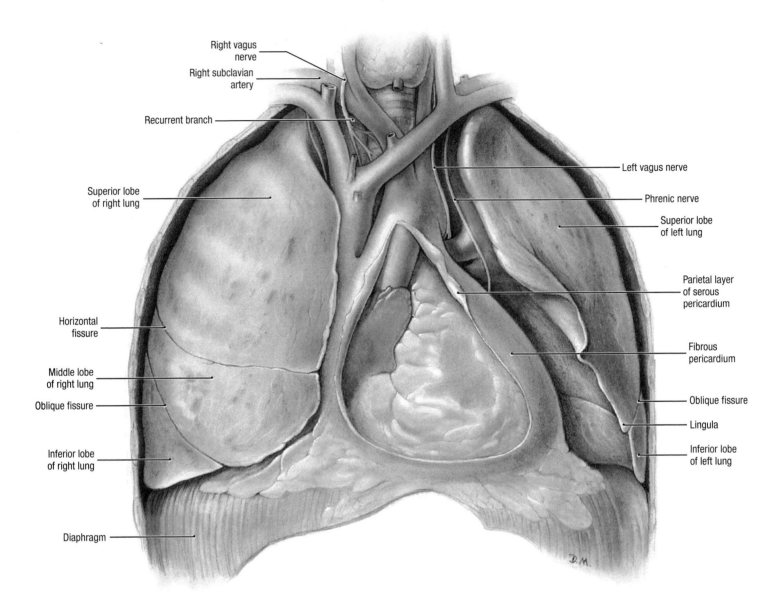

Right vagus
nerve

Right subclavian
artery

Recurrent branch

Left vagus nerve

Phrenic nerve

Superior lobe
of right lung

Superior lobe
of left lung

Parietal layer
of serous
pericardium

Horizontal
fissure

Fibrous
pericardium

Middle lobe
of right lung

Oblique fissure

Oblique fissure

Lingula

Inferior lobe
of right lung

Inferior lobe
of left lung

Diaphragm

D.M.

1.26   Thoracic contents in situ, anterior view.

The fibrous pericardium, lined by the parietal layer of serous pericardium, is removed anteriorly to expose the heart and great vessels.

OBSERVE:
1. The right lung has three lobes; the superior lobe is separated from
   the middle lobe by the horizontal fissure, and the middle lobe is
   separated from the inferior lobe by the oblique fissure;
2. The left lung has two lobes, superior and inferior, separated by the
   oblique fissure. The anterior border of the left lung is reflected laterally to visualize the phrenic nerve passing anterior to the root of

the lung and the vagus nerve lying anterior to the arch of the aorta
and then passing posterior to the root of the lung;
3. The right vagus nerve passes anterior to the right subclavian artery,
   where it gives off the recurrent branch and then divides to contribute fibers to the esophageal, cardiac, and pulmonary plexuses.

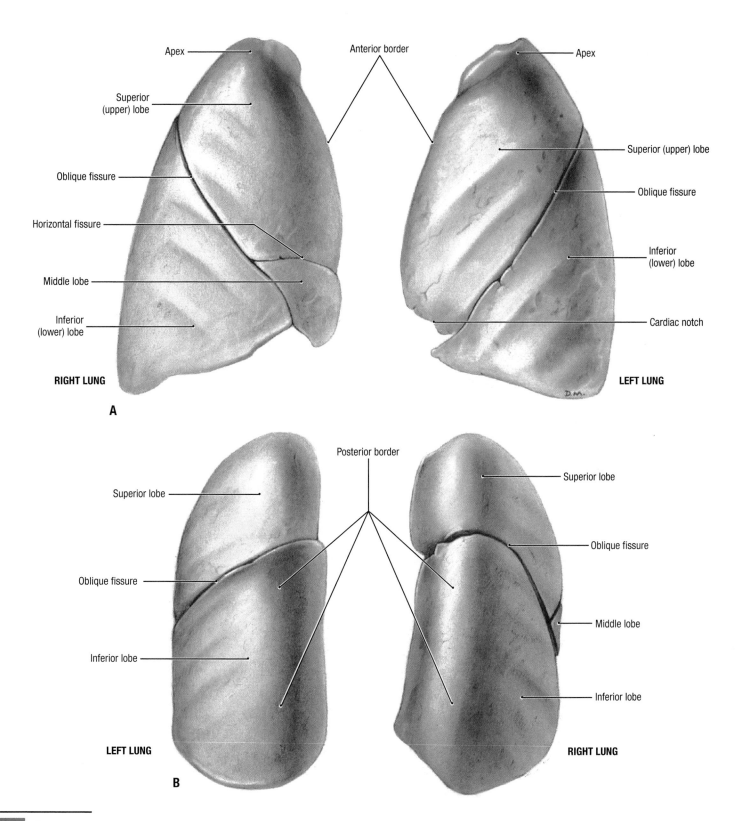

1.27 Lungs

A. Lateral view. **B.** Posterior view.

OBSERVE:

1. The three lobes of the right lung and two lobes of the left;
2. The deficiency of the superior (upper) lobe of the left lung, called the cardiac notch;
3. The oblique and horizontal fissures of the right lung, and the oblique fissure of the left lung; the fissures may be incomplete or absent on some specimens;
4. The sharp anterior border and rounded posterior border of the lungs;
5. The impressions of the ribs on the anterior and lateral aspects of the lung.

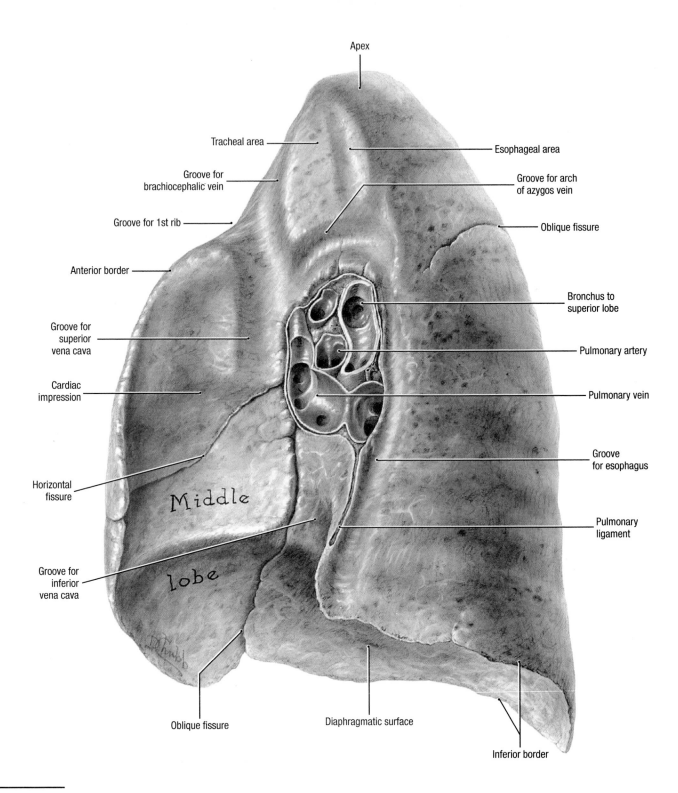

Apex

Tracheal area

Esophageal area

Groove for brachiocephalic vein

Groove for arch of azygos vein

Groove for 1st rib

Oblique fissure

Anterior border

Bronchus to superior lobe

Groove for superior vena cava

Pulmonary artery

Cardiac impression

Pulmonary vein

Groove for esophagus

Horizontal fissure

Middle

lobe

Pulmonary ligament

Groove for inferior vena cava

Oblique fissure

Diaphragmatic surface

Inferior border

1.28   Mediastinal (medial) surface of right lung

OBSERVE:

1. The embalmed lung shows impressions of the structures with which it comes into contact clearly demarcated as surface features; the base is contoured by the domes of the diaphragm; the costal surface bears the impressions of the ribs; distended vessels leave their mark, but nerves do not;

2. The somewhat pear-shaped root of the lung near the center of the

mediastinal surface, and the pulmonary ligament descending like a stalk from the root;

3. The groove for (or line of contact with) the esophagus throughout the length of the lung, except where the arch of the azygos vein intervenes; this groove passes posterior to the root and the pulmonary ligament, which separates it from the groove for the inferior vena cava;

4. The oblique fissure is incomplete here, but complete in Figure 1.29.

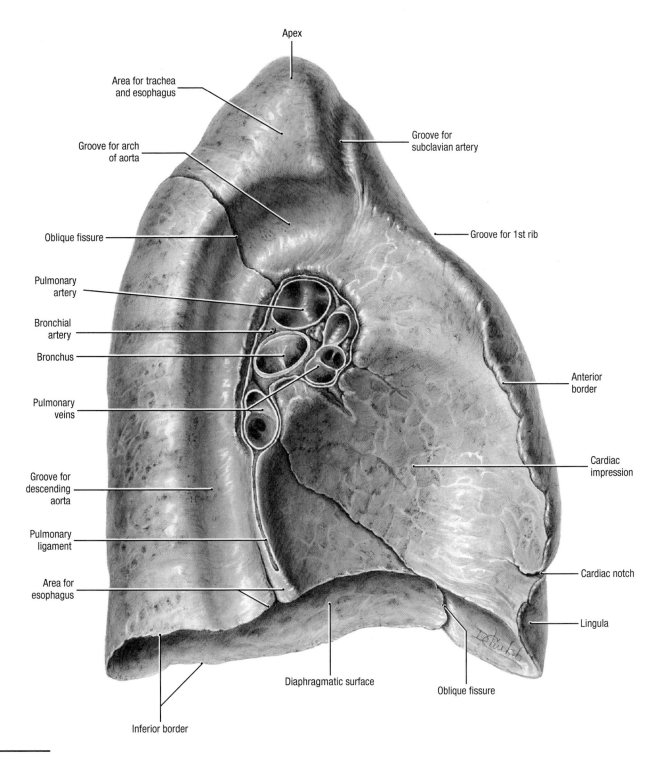

Apex

Area for trachea
and esophagus

Groove for arch
of aorta

Oblique fissure

Pulmonary
artery

Bronchial
artery

Bronchus

Pulmonary
veins

Groove for
descending
aorta

Pulmonary
ligament

Area for
esophagus

Inferior border

Groove for
subclavian artery

Groove for 1st rib

Anterior
border

Cardiac
impression

Cardiac notch

Lingula

Diaphragmatic surface

Oblique fissure

1.29   Mediastinal (medial) surface of left lung

OBSERVE:
1. Near the center, the root of the lung and the pulmonary ligament descending from it;
2. The site of contact with the esophagus, between the descending aorta and the inferior end of the pulmonary ligament;
3. The oblique fissure, cutting completely through the lung substance;

4. In the right and left roots, the artery is superior, the bronchus is posterior, one vein is anterior, and the other is inferior; in the right root, the bronchus to the superior lobe, also called the eparterial bronchus, is the most superior structure.

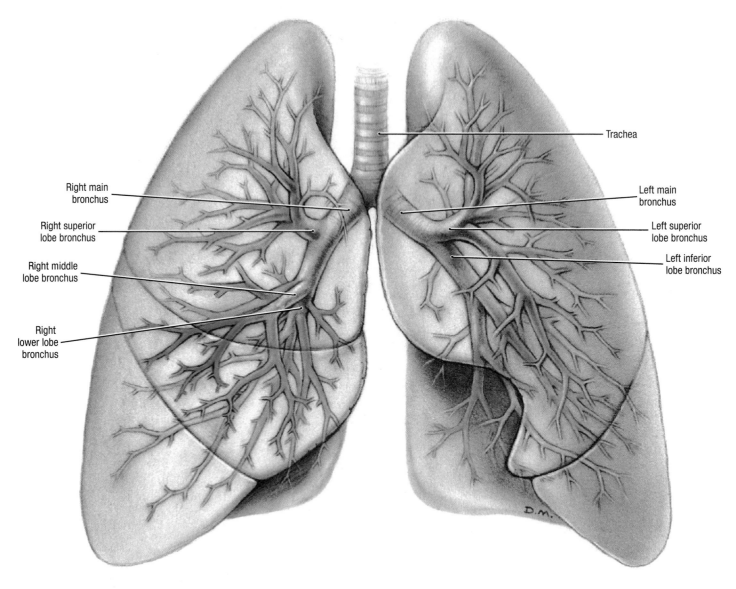

Trachea

Right main bronchus

Right superior lobe bronchus

Right middle lobe bronchus

Right lower lobe bronchus

Left main bronchus

Left superior lobe bronchus

Left inferior lobe bronchus

1.30 **Trachea and bronchi in situ, anterior view**

OBSERVE:

1. The trachea bifurcates into right and left main (primary) bronchi;
2. The right main bronchus is shorter, wider, and more vertical than the left. *Therefore, it is more likely that foreign objects will become lodged in the right main bronchus;*
3. The right main bronchus gives off the right superior lobe bronchus (eparterial bronchus) before entering the hilum (hilus) of the lung; after entering the hilum, the right middle and inferior lobe bronchi branch off;
4. The left main bronchus divides into the left superior and left inferior lobe bronchi; the left superior lobe bronchus also supplies the lingula (Fig. 1.29).
5. The lobar bronchi further divide into segmental (tertiary) bronchi. The segmental bronchi are color coded.

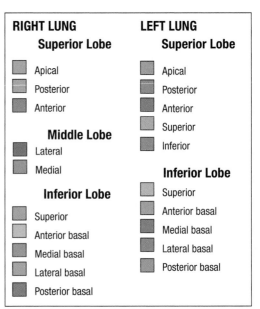

RIGHT LUNG	**LEFT LUNG**
Superior Lobe	**Superior Lobe**
☐ Apical	☐ Apical
☐ Posterior	☐ Posterior
☐ Anterior	☐ Anterior
	☐ Superior
Middle Lobe	☐ Inferior
☐ Lateral	
☐ Medial	**Inferior Lobe**
	☐ Superior
Inferior Lobe	☐ Anterior basal
☐ Superior	☐ Medial basal
☐ Anterior basal	☐ Lateral basal
☐ Medial basal	☐ Posterior basal
☐ Lateral basal	
☐ Posterior basal	

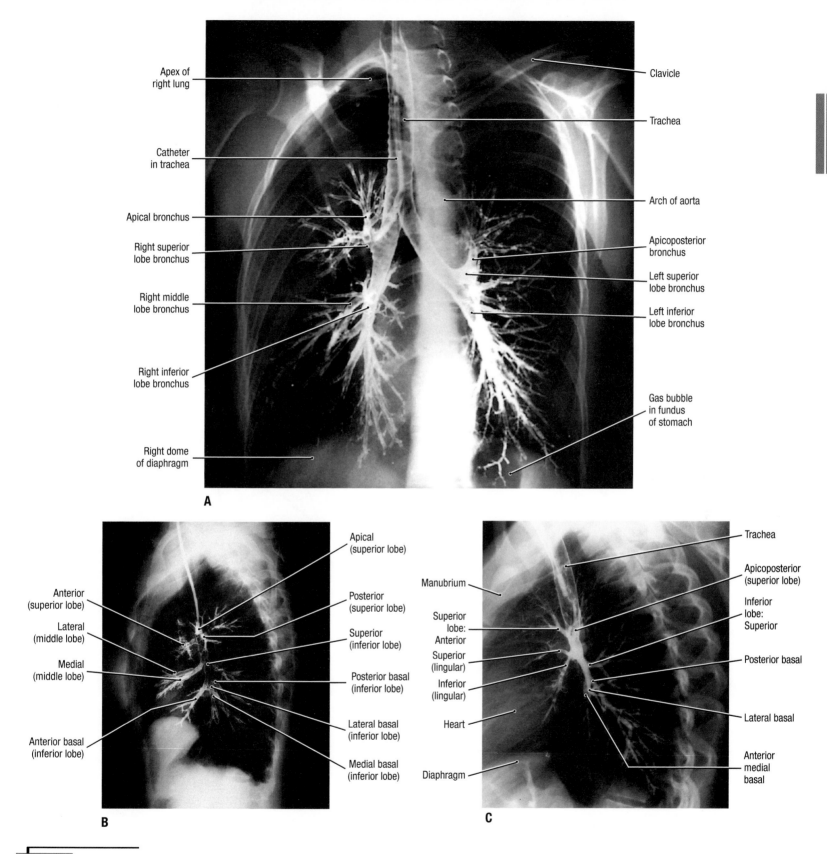

1.31 Bronchograms

A. Bronchogram of right and left bronchial trees. This is a slightly oblique, posteroanterior view.

B. Right lateral bronchogram, showing segmental bronchi. **C.** Left lateral bronchogram, showing segmental bronchi.

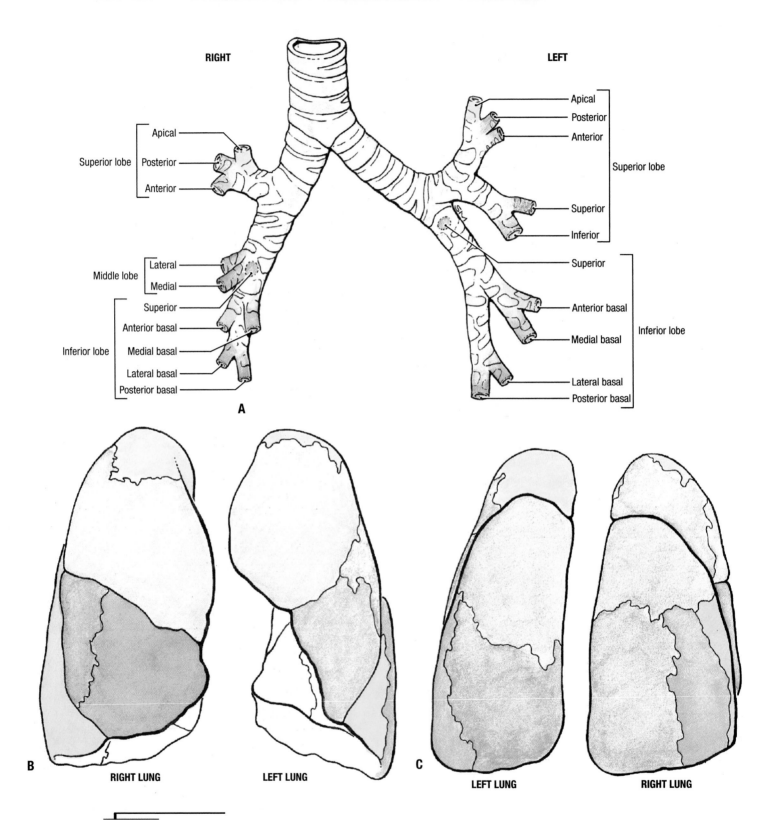

RIGHT

LEFT

Apical
Posterior
Anterior
} Superior lobe

Apical
Posterior
Anterior
Superior lobe

Superior
Inferior

Lateral
Medial
} Middle lobe

Superior

Superior
Anterior basal
Medial basal
Lateral basal
Posterior basal
} Inferior lobe

Anterior basal
Medial basal
Lateral basal
Posterior basal
Inferior lobe

A

B   RIGHT LUNG   LEFT LUNG   **C**   LEFT LUNG   RIGHT LUNG

1.32   Segmental bronchi and bronchopulmonary segments

A. Segmental bronchi, anterior view. There are 10 tertiary or segmental bronchi on the right, and 8 on the left. Note that on the left, the apical and posterior bronchi arise from a single stem, as do the anterior basal and medial basal. **B.** Anterior view. **C.** Posterior view.

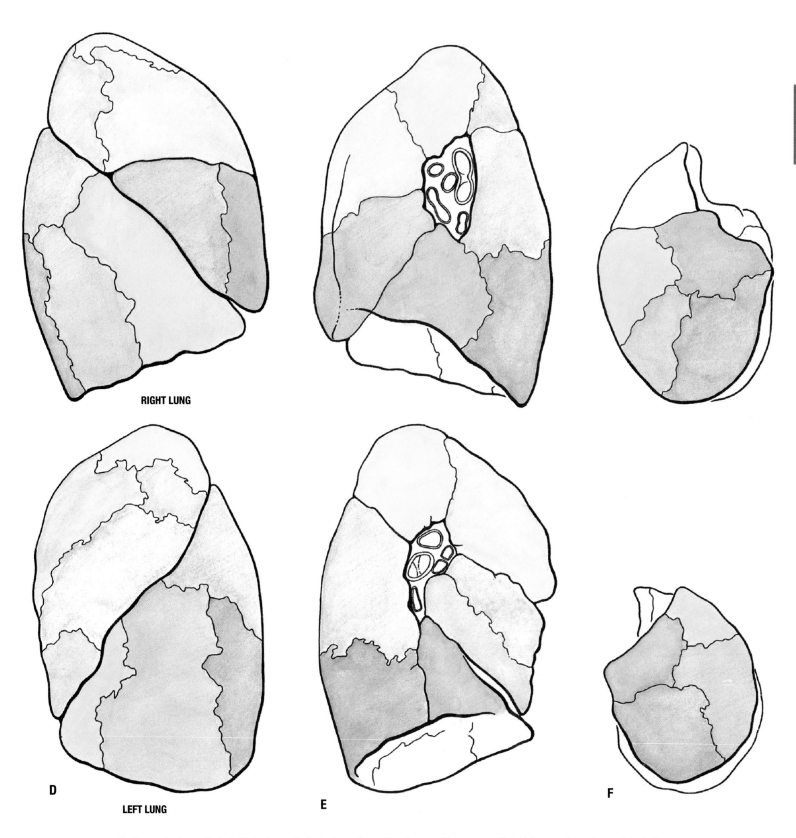

RIGHT LUNG

LEFT LUNG

D

E

F

D. Lateral view. **E.** Medial view. **F.** Inferior view. Portions of lung ventilated by tertiary bronchi. A bronchopulmonary segment consists of a tertiary bronchus, the portion of lung it ventilates, an artery, and a vein. *These structures are surgically separable to allow segmental resection of the lung.* To prepare these specimens, the tertiary bronchi of fresh lungs were isolated within the hilus and injected with latex of various colors. Minor variations in the branching of the bronchi result in variations in the surface patterns.

1.33 Bronchi and pulmonary veins, medial view

A. Right lung. **B.** Left lung.

The pulmonary veins (purple) of fresh lungs were filled with latex, and the bronchi (gray) were inflated with air under low pressure until thoroughly dry, thereby assuring their natural form. The tissues surrounding the bronchi and veins were then moistened and cut away. The tertiary (segmental) bronchi are labeled.

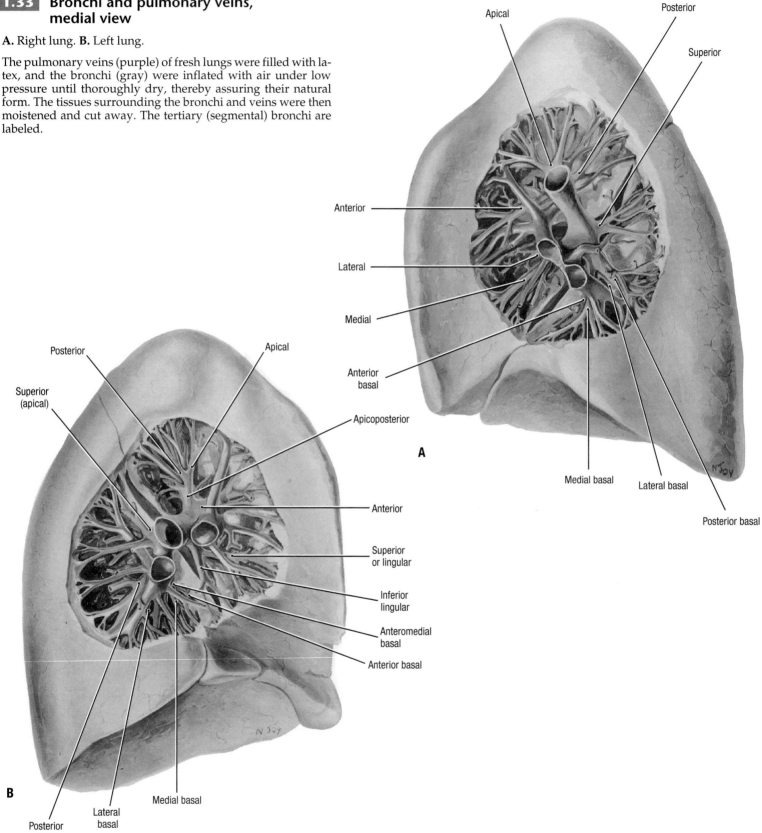

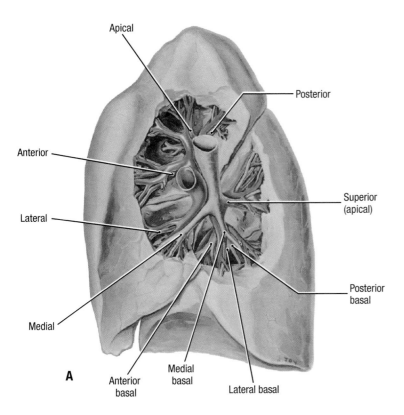

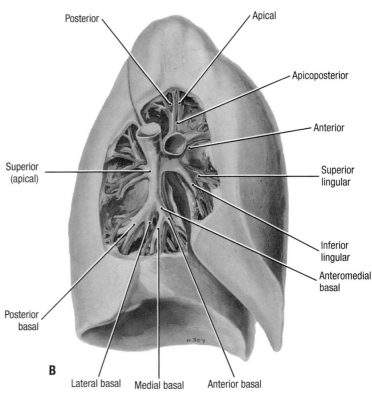

1.34   Bronchi and pulmonary arteries, medial view

A. Right lung. **B.** Left lung.

The pulmonary arteries (blue) of the lungs were filled with latex, and the bronchi (gray) were kept inflated and treated, as for Figure 1.33.

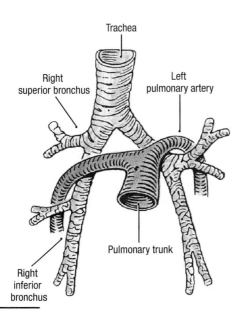

1.35   Relationship of bronchi and pulmonary arteries, anterior view

The right pulmonary artery at the root of the lung lies between the secondary bronchi to the upper and middle lobes; the left pulmonary artery arches anterior to the left primary bronchus.

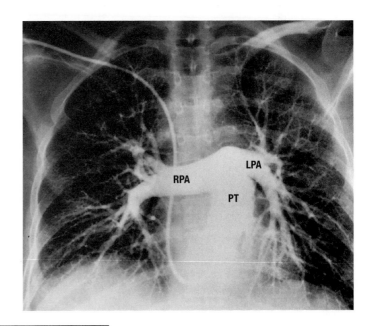

1.36   Pulmonary angiogram

Observe the catheter located in the right ventricle and pulmonary trunk *(PT)*; the pulmonary trunk dividing into a longer right pulmonary artery *(RPA)* and shorter left pulmonary artery *(LPA)*; and the branches of the right and left pulmonary arteries following the corresponding segmental bronchi.

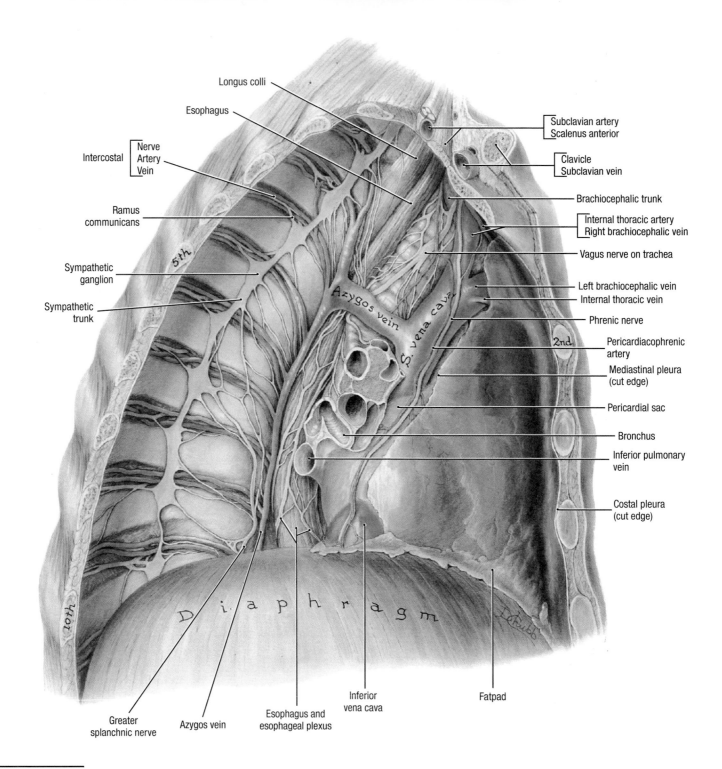

Longus colli

Esophagus

Intercostal
- Nerve
- Artery
- Vein

Ramus communicans

Sympathetic ganglion

Sympathetic trunk

5th

10th

Subclavian artery
Scalenus anterior

Clavicle
Subclavian vein

Brachiocephalic trunk

Internal thoracic artery
Right brachiocephalic vein

Vagus nerve on trachea

Left brachiocephalic vein
Internal thoracic vein

Phrenic nerve

Pericardiacophrenic artery

Mediastinal pleura (cut edge)

Pericardial sac

Bronchus

Inferior pulmonary vein

Costal pleura (cut edge)

Azygos vein

S. vena cava

2nd

Diaphragm

Greater splanchnic nerve

Azygos vein

Esophagus and esophageal plexus

Inferior vena cava

Fatpad

1.37   Mediastinum, right side

The costal and mediastinal pleurae have mostly been removed, exposing the underlying structures. Compare with the mediastinal surface of the right lung in Figure 1.28.

OBSERVE:

1. The right side of the mediastinum is the "blue side," dominated by the arch of the azygos vein and the superior vena cava;
2. When the mediastinal pleura is removed, the phrenic nerve is free; follow its medial relationships to the diaphragm;
3. The trachea and esophagus are visible;
4. On entering the mediastinum, the right vagus nerve travels on the medial surface of the trachea, passes medial to the arch of the azygos vein, and then slightly posteriorly to travel along the medial aspect of the esophagus;
5. The sympathetic trunk and its ganglia, the greater splanchnic nerve, and the esophageal plexus.

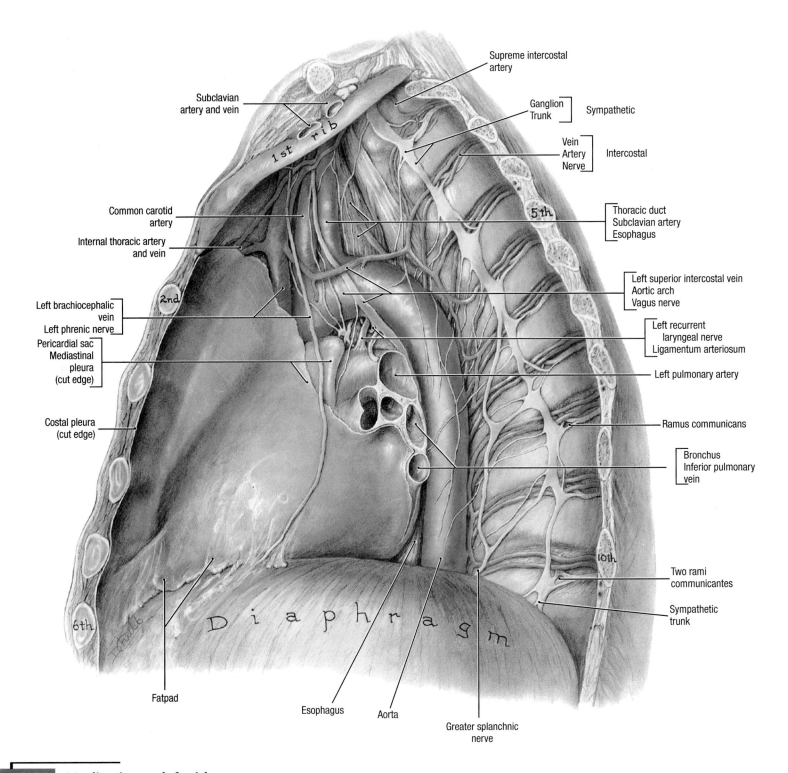

Supreme intercostal artery

Subclavian artery and vein

1st rib

Ganglion Trunk | Sympathetic

Vein / Artery / Nerve | Intercostal

Common carotid artery

Internal thoracic artery and vein

5th

Thoracic duct / Subclavian artery / Esophagus

2nd

Left superior intercostal vein / Aortic arch / Vagus nerve

Left brachiocephalic vein

Left phrenic nerve

Pericardial sac / Mediastinal pleura (cut edge)

Left recurrent laryngeal nerve / Ligamentum arteriosum

Left pulmonary artery

Costal pleura (cut edge)

Ramus communicans

Bronchus / Inferior pulmonary vein

10th

6th

Two rami communicantes

Sympathetic trunk

Diaphragm

Fatpad

Esophagus　　Aorta

Greater splanchnic nerve

1.38 　Mediastinum, left side

Compare with the mediastinal surface of the left lung in Figure 1.29.

OBSERVE:

1. The left side of the mediastinum is the "red side," dominated by the arch and descending portion of the aorta, the left common carotid, and subclavian arteries;
2. The phrenic nerve, freed by removal of pleura, passes anterior to the root of the lung;
3. The thoracic duct on the esophagus;
4. The left vagus nerve passes posterior to the root of the lung, sending its recurrent laryngeal branch around the ligamentum arteriosum posterior to the aortic arch;
5. The sympathetic trunk is attached to intercostal nerves by rami communicantes.

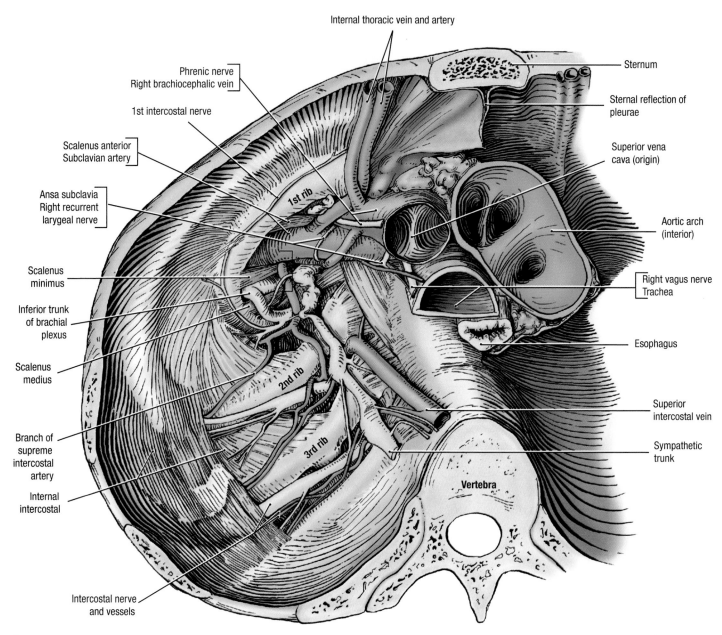

Internal thoracic vein and artery

Phrenic nerve
Right brachiocephalic vein

1st intercostal nerve

Scalenus anterior
Subclavian artery

Ansa subclavia
Right recurrent
larygeal nerve

Scalenus
minimus

Inferior trunk
of brachial
plexus

Scalenus
medius

Branch of
supreme
intercostal
artery

Internal
intercostal

Intercostal nerve
and vessels

1st rib

2nd rib

3rd rib

Vertebra

Sternum

Sternal reflection of
pleurae

Superior vena
cava (origin)

Aortic arch
(interior)

Right vagus nerve
Trachea

Esophagus

Superior
intercostal vein

Sympathetic
trunk

A

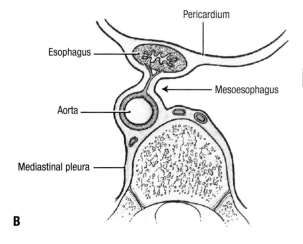

Pericardium

Esophagus

Mesoesophagus

Aorta

Mediastinal pleura

B

1.39   Roof of pleural cavity

A. Roof of pleural cavity with pleura removed, inferior view.

OBSERVE IN **A**:
1. The first part of the subclavian artery disappears at the first rib;
2. The internal thoracic artery and vein;
3. The ansa subclavia from the sympathetic trunk and recurrent laryngeal nerve from the vagus nerve loop around the subclavian artery;
4. The inferior trunk of the brachial plexus.

B. The mesoesophagus. Between the inferior part of the esophagus and the aorta, the right and left layers of mediastinal pleura form a dorsal mesoesophagus.

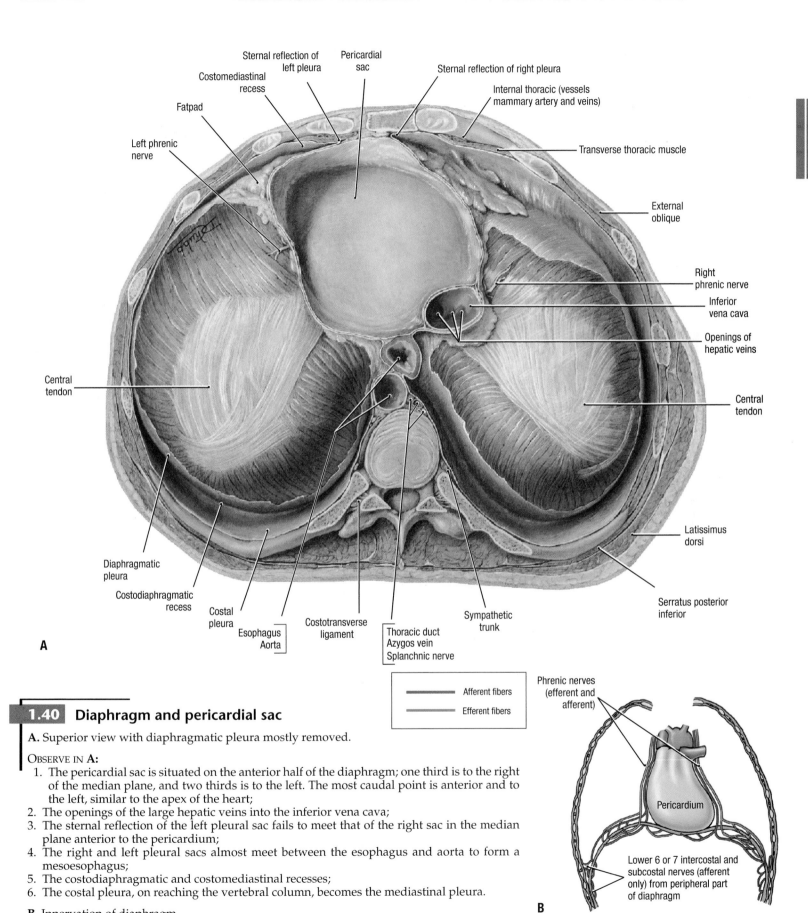

A. Superior view with diaphragmatic pleura mostly removed.

OBSERVE IN **A:**
1. The pericardial sac is situated on the anterior half of the diaphragm; one third is to the right of the median plane, and two thirds is to the left. The most caudal point is anterior and to the left, similar to the apex of the heart;
2. The openings of the large hepatic veins into the inferior vena cava;
3. The sternal reflection of the left pleural sac fails to meet that of the right sac in the median plane anterior to the pericardium;
4. The right and left pleural sacs almost meet between the esophagus and aorta to form a mesoesophagus;
5. The costodiaphragmatic and costomediastinal recesses;
6. The costal pleura, on reaching the vertebral column, becomes the mediastinal pleura.

B. Innervation of diaphragm.

1.40   Diaphragm and pericardial sac

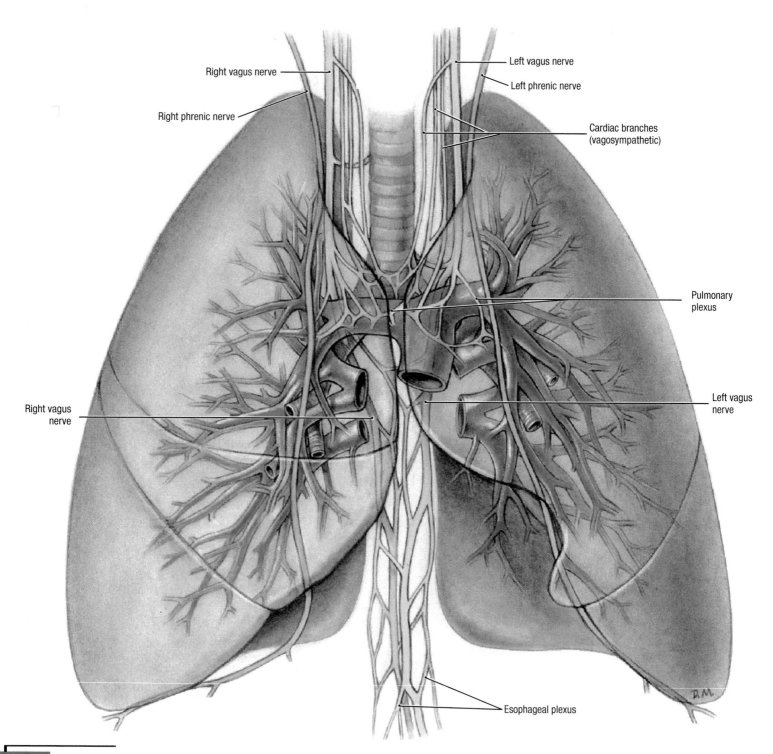

Right vagus nerve

Right phrenic nerve

Left vagus nerve

Left phrenic nerve

Cardiac branches
(vagosympathetic)

Pulmonary
plexus

Right vagus
nerve

Left vagus
nerve

Esophageal plexus

1.41   Innervation of lungs, anterior view

OBSERVE:

1. The pulmonary plexuses, located anterior and posterior to the roots of the lungs, receive sympathetic contributions from the right and left sympathetic trunks (2nd to 5th thoracic ganglia), not shown, and parasympathetic contributions from the right and left vagus nerves;

2. The right and left vagus nerves pass inferiorly from the posterior pulmonary plexus to contribute fibers to the esophageal plexus;

3. Branches from the pulmonary plexuses continue along the bronchi and pulmonary vasculature to the lungs;

4. The phrenic nerves pass anterior to the root of the lung to the diaphragm.

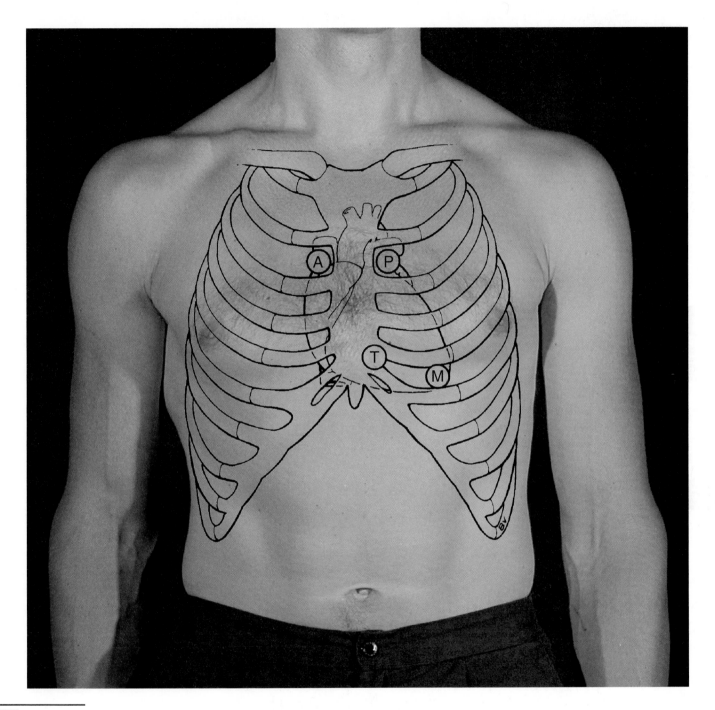

1.42 **Surface markings of heart and auscultation areas, anterior view**

OBSERVE:
1. The superior border of the heart is represented by a slightly oblique line joining the 3rd costal cartilages; the convex right side of the heart projecting lateral to the sternum and inferiorly lying at the 6th or 7th costochondral junction; and the inferior border of the heart lying superior to the central tendon of the diaphragm and sloping slightly inferiorly to the apex at the 5th interspace at the midclavicular line;

2. *Auscultation areas are where sounds from each of the heart's valves can be heard most distinctly through a stethoscope.*
3. *The aortic (A) and pulmonary (P) auscultation areas are in the 2nd interspace to the right and left of the sternal border; the tricuspid area (T) is near the left sternal border in the 5th or 6th interspace; the mitral valve (M) is heard best near the apex in the 5th intercostal space in the midclavicular line.*

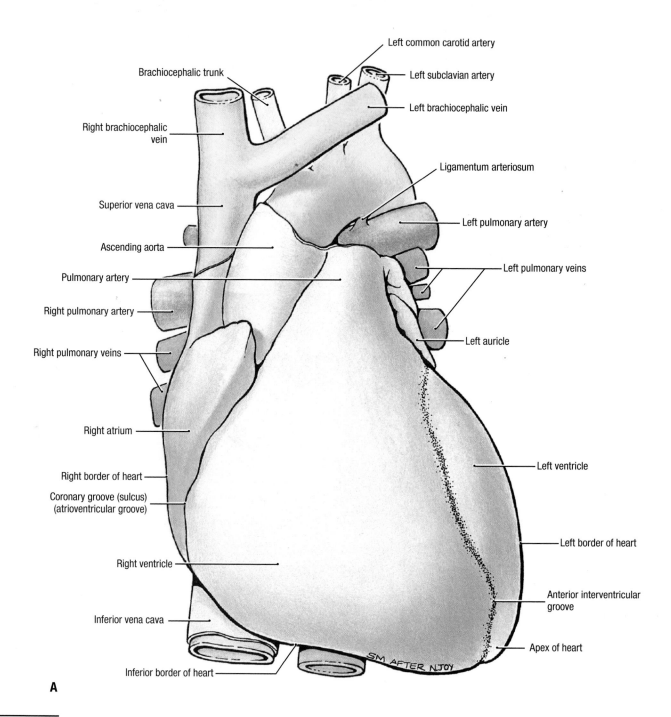

Brachiocephalic trunk

Left common carotid artery

Left subclavian artery

Left brachiocephalic vein

Right brachiocephalic vein

Ligamentum arteriosum

Superior vena cava

Left pulmonary artery

Ascending aorta

Pulmonary artery

Left pulmonary veins

Right pulmonary artery

Right pulmonary veins

Left auricle

Right atrium

Right border of heart

Left ventricle

Coronary groove (sulcus) (atrioventricular groove)

Left border of heart

Right ventricle

Anterior interventricular groove

Inferior vena cava

Apex of heart

Inferior border of heart

SM AFTER N.JOY

A

1.43 Heart and great vessels

A. Anterior view. **B.** Posterior view.

OBSERVE IN **A:**

1. The right border, formed by the right atrium, is slightly convex and almost in line with the superior vena cava and inferior vena cava. *Enlargement of the right atrium shows as a bulging of the right border of the heart;*

2. The inferior border is formed primarily by the right ventricle and a small part of the left ventricle;

3. The left border is formed primarily by the left ventricle and a small portion by the left auricle. *When the left ventricle is dilated, the apex of the heart extends further to the left;*

4. The pulmonary artery bifurcates inferior to the arch of the aorta into the right and left pulmonary arteries;

5. The ligamentum arteriosum passes from the origin of the left pulmonary artery to the arch of the aorta.

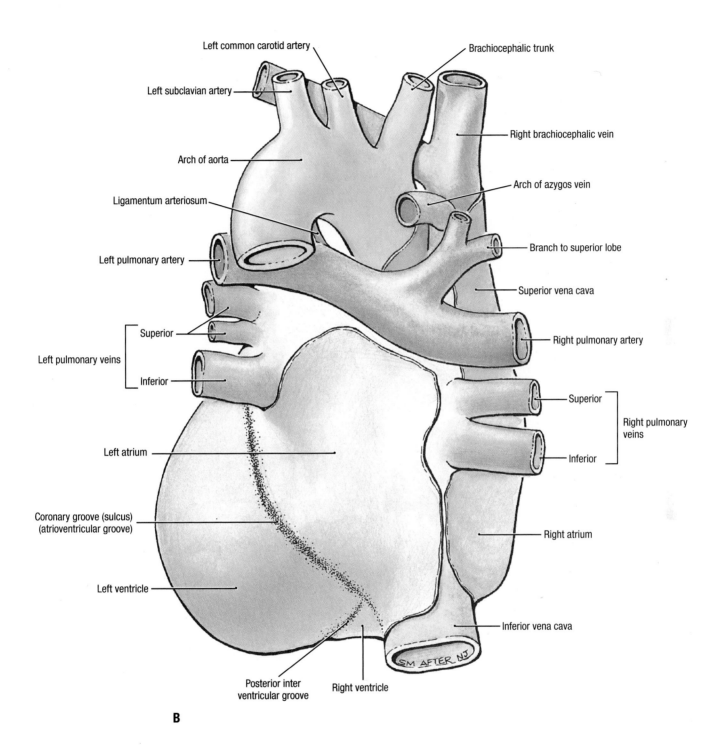

Left common carotid artery

Left subclavian artery

Arch of aorta

Ligamentum arteriosum

Left pulmonary artery

Left pulmonary veins

Superior

Inferior

Left atrium

Coronary groove (sulcus)
(atrioventricular groove)

Left ventricle

Posterior inter
ventricular groove

Right ventricle

Brachiocephalic trunk

Right brachiocephalic vein

Arch of azygos vein

Branch to superior lobe

Superior vena cava

Right pulmonary artery

Superior

Inferior

Right pulmonary
veins

Right atrium

Inferior vena cava

SM AFTER NJ

B

OBSERVE IN **B:**

6. Most of the left atrium, much of the left ventricle, a little of the right atrium, and almost none of the right ventricle are visible from posterior;

7. The right and left pulmonary veins converge to open into the left atrium;

8. The right and left pulmonary arteries are just superior and parallel to the pulmonary veins, and incline from the left side inferiorly to the right; hence, the root of the right lung is more inferior than the left;

9. The aorta arches over the left pulmonary vessels (and bronchus); the azygos vein arches over the right pulmonary vessels (and bronchus);

10. The arch of the aorta is arched in two planes: superiorly and to the left. The convexity to the left is molded on the esophagus and trachea;

11. The atrioventricular groove or coronary groove (sulcus) is between the left atrium and left ventricle.

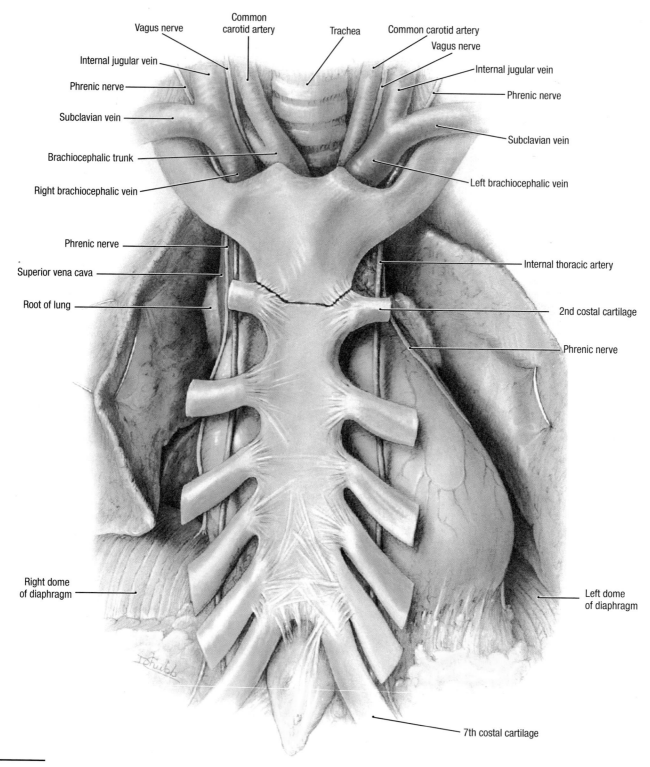

Common
carotid artery

Vagus nerve

Trachea

Common carotid artery

Vagus nerve

Internal jugular vein

Phrenic nerve

Internal jugular vein

Phrenic nerve

Subclavian vein

Subclavian vein

Brachiocephalic trunk

Left brachiocephalic vein

Right brachiocephalic vein

Phrenic nerve

Internal thoracic artery

Superior vena cava

Root of lung

2nd costal cartilage

Phrenic nerve

Right dome
of diaphragm

Left dome
of diaphragm

7th costal cartilage

1.44 Pericardial sac in relation to sternum, anterior view

To complete this dissection, the manubriosternal (sternomanubrial) joint was divided to enable the body of the sternum to be turned inferiorly.

Observe:
1. The pericardial sac lies posterior to the body of the sternum from just superior to the sternal angle to the level of the xiphisternal joint; approximately two thirds lies to the left of the median plane;

2. The heart lies between the sternum and the anterior mediastinum anteriorly and the vertebral column and the posterior mediastinum posteriorly. *In cardiac compression, the sternum is depressed 4 to 5 cm, forcing blood out of the heart and into the great vessels;*
3. Internal thoracic arteries lateral to the sternum;
4. Right and left phrenic nerves applied to the pericardial sac;
5. The relationship of the nerves and vessels at the thoracic inlet.

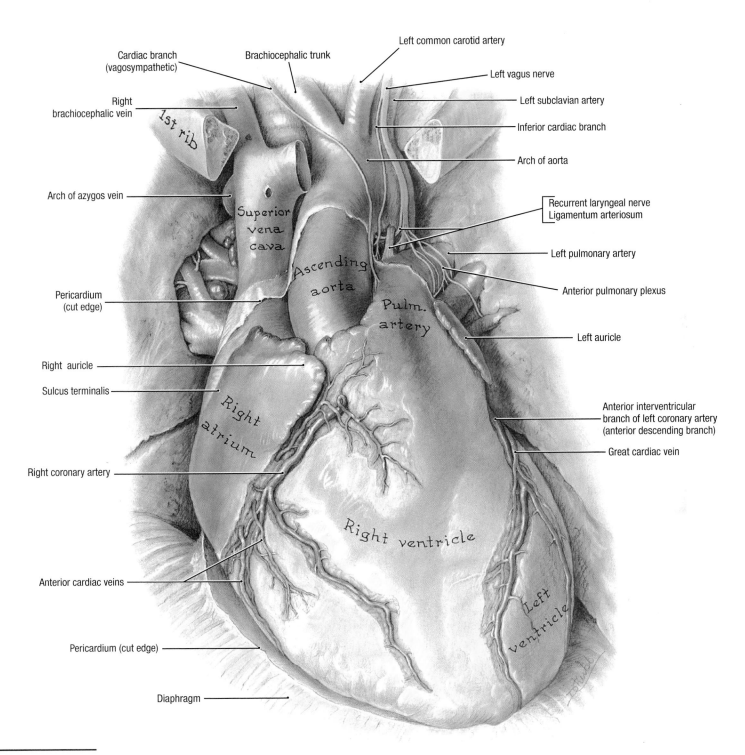

Left common carotid artery

Cardiac branch
(vagosympathetic)

Brachiocephalic trunk

Left vagus nerve

Right
brachiocephalic vein

Left subclavian artery

Inferior cardiac branch

Arch of aorta

Arch of azygos vein

Recurrent laryngeal nerve
Ligamentum arteriosum

Left pulmonary artery

Pericardium
(cut edge)

Anterior pulmonary plexus

Left auricle

Right auricle

Sulcus terminalis

Anterior interventricular
branch of left coronary artery
(anterior descending branch)

Great cardiac vein

Right coronary artery

Anterior cardiac veins

Pericardium (cut edge)

Diaphragm

1st rib

Superior vena cava

Ascending aorta

Pulm. artery

Right atrium

Right ventricle

Left ventricle

1.45 **Sternocostal (anterior) surface of heart and great vessels in situ**

OBSERVE:

1. The entire right auricle and much of the right atrium are visible anteriorly, but only a small portion of the left auricle is visible; the auricles, like two closing claws, grasp the pulmonary artery and ascending aorta from posterior;

2. The ligamentum arteriosum passes from the origin of the left pulmonary artery to the arch of the aorta;

3. The right coronary artery is in the anterior atrioventricular groove, and the anterior interventricular branch of left coronary artery (anterior descending branch) is in the anterior interventricular groove;

4. The left vagus nerve passes anterior to the aortic arch and then posterior to the root of the lung; the recurrent laryngeal nerve passes inferior to the aortic arch just lateral to the ligamentum arteriosum.

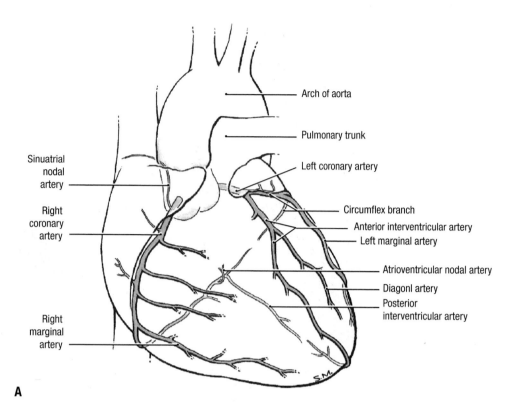

Arch of aorta

Pulmonary trunk

Left coronary artery

Sinuatrial
nodal
artery

Right
coronary
artery

Circumflex branch

Anterior interventricular artery

Left marginal artery

Atrioventricular nodal artery

Diagonl artery

Posterior
interventricular artery

Right
marginal
artery

A

1.46   Coronary arteries

A. Anterior view. **B.** Posteroinferior view.

OBSERVE:

1. The right coronary artery travels in the coronary
groove (sulcus) to reach the posterior surface of the
heart, where it anastomoses with the circumflex
branch of the left coronary artery. Early in its course, it
gives off the sinuatrial (SA) nodal artery that supplies
the right atrium and reaches the SA node; major
branches are a marginal branch supplying much of the
anterior wall of the right ventricle, an atrioventricular
(AV) nodal artery given off near the posterior border
of the interventricular septum, and a posterior interventricular artery in the interventricular groove that
anastomoses with the anterior interventricular artery,
a branch of the left coronary artery.
2. The left coronary artery divides into a circumflex
branch that passes posteriorly to anastomose with the
right coronary on the posterior aspect of the heart and
an anterior descending branch in the interventricular
groove; the origin of the SA nodal artery is variable
and may be a branch of the left coronary artery;
3. The interventricular septum receives its blood supply
from septal branches of the two descending branches:
the anterior two thirds from the left coronary, and the
posterior one third from the right.

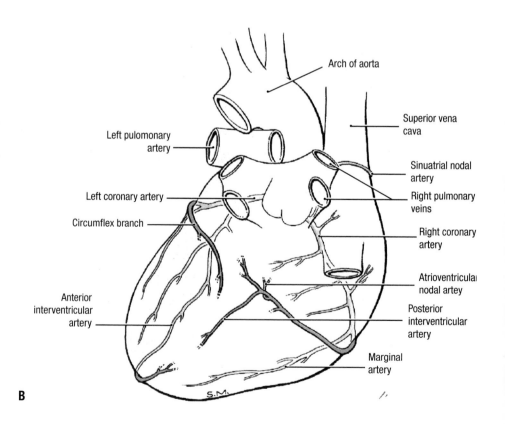

Arch of aorta

Left pulomonary
artery

Superior vena
cava

Sinuatrial nodal
artery

Left coronary artery

Right pulmonary
veins

Circumflex branch

Right coronary
artery

Atrioventricula
nodal artey

Anterior
interventricular
artery

Posterior
interventricular
artery

Marginal
artery

B

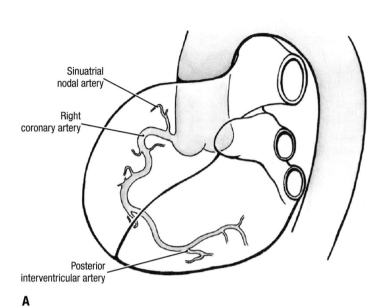

A

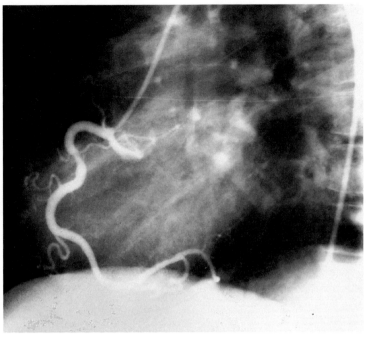

B

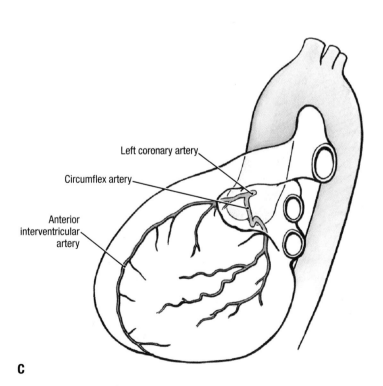

C

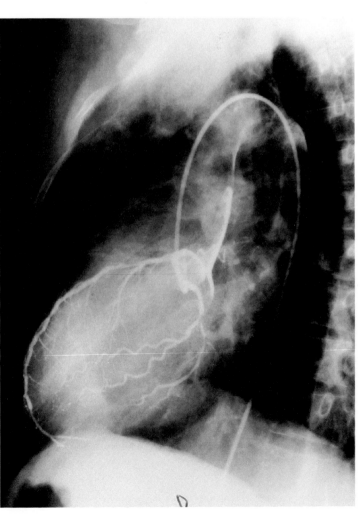

D

1.47　**Coronary arteriograms with orientation drawings**

The right (**A** and **B**) and left (**C** and **D**) coronary arteriograms are from a left anterior oblique, almost lateral, view.

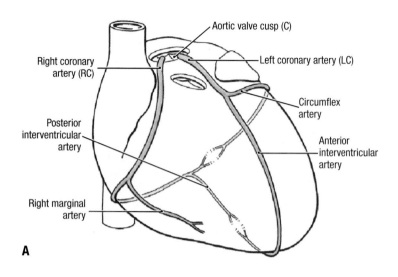

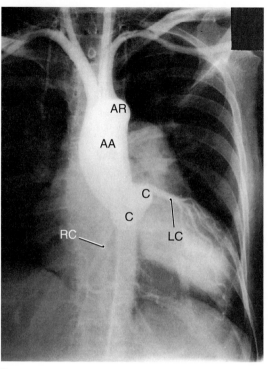

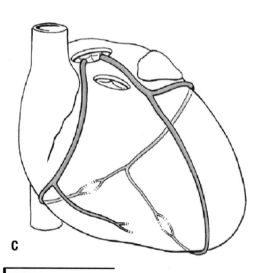

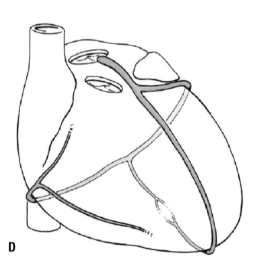

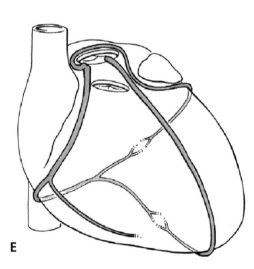

1.48   Coronary circulation, anterior views

A. Blood supply to heart. The coronary circulation is extremely variable in detail. In most cases, the right and left coronary arteries share equally in the blood supply to the heart. **B.** Aortic root angiogram. Observe the arch of aorta *(AR)*, ascending aorta *(AA)*, cusp of aortic valve *(C)*, left coronary artery *(LC)*, and right coronary artery *(RC)*.

C. Dominant left coronary artery. In approximately 15% of hearts, the left coronary artery is dominant in that the posterior interventricular branch comes off the circumflex branch. **D.** Single coronary artery. **E.** Circumflex branch emerging from right coronary sinus.

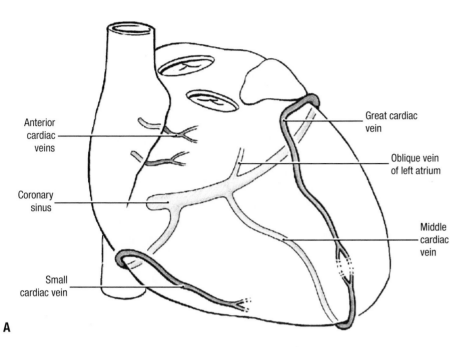

Anterior
cardiac
veins

Coronary
sinus

Small
cardiac vein

Great cardiac
vein

Oblique vein
of left atrium

Middle
cardiac
vein

A

1.49 Cardiac veins

A. Anterior view. **B.** Posteroinferior view.

OBSERVE:
1. The coronary sinus is the major venous drainage vessel of the heart; it is located posteriorly in the atrioventricular (coronary) groove and empties into the right atrium;
2. The great, middle, and small cardiac veins, the oblique vein of the left atrium, and the posterior vein of the left ventricle are the principal vessels draining into the coronary sinus; the anterior cardiac veins drain directly into the right atrium;
3. The cardiac veins accompany the coronary arteries and their branches, i.e., the great cardiac vein and the anterior interventricular artery, middle cardiac vein and posterior interventricular artery, etc.;
4. The smallest vessels, the venae cordis minimae, drain the myocardium directly into the atria and ventricles.

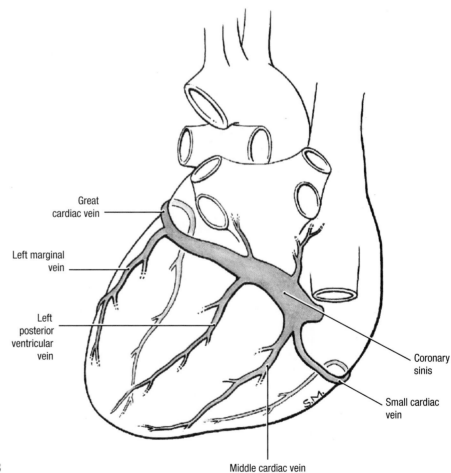

Great
cardiac vein

Left marginal
vein

Left
posterior
ventricular
vein

Coronary
sinis

Small cardiac
vein

Middle cardiac vein

B

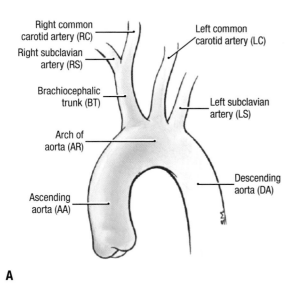

A

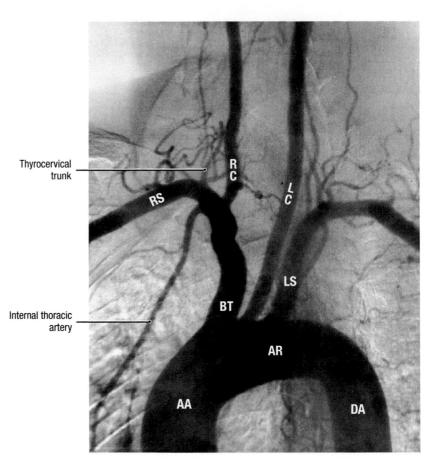

B

1.50   Branches of aortic arch, anterior view

A. Aortic arch. **B.** Aortic angiogram. Observe the ascending aorta *(AA)*, the arch of the aorta *(AR)*, the descending aorta *(DA)*, the brachiocephalic *(BT)* trunk (artery) branching into the right subclavian *(RS)* and right common carotid *(RC)* arteries, and the left subclavian *(LS)* and left common carotid *(LC)* arteries arising directly from the aorta.

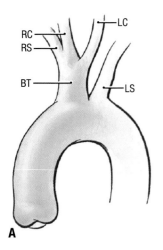

A

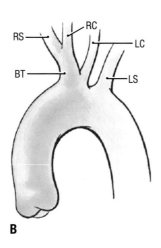

B

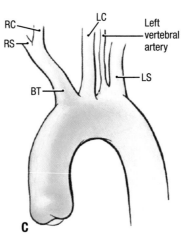

C

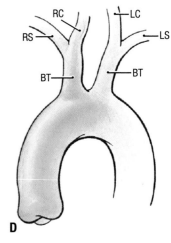

D

1.51   Variations in origins of branches of aortic arch, anterior view

The most common pattern (65%) is shown in Figure 1.50A. Less common variations include: **A** and **B.** Left common carotid artery originating from the brachiocephalic trunk (27%). **C.** Each of the four arteries originating independently from the arch of the aorta (2.5%). **D.** Right and left brachiocephalic trunks originate from the arch of the aorta (1.2%).

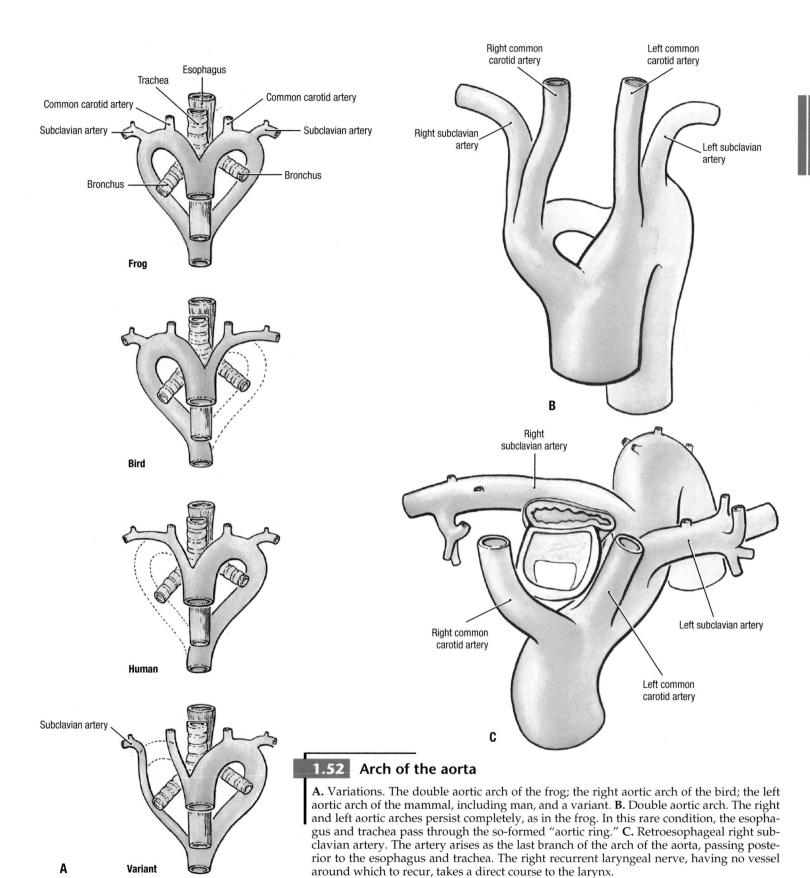

Frog

Bird

Human

Esophagus
Trachea
Common carotid artery
Subclavian artery
Bronchus
Common carotid artery
Subclavian artery
Bronchus

Subclavian artery

A   **Variant**

Right common carotid artery
Left common carotid artery
Right subclavian artery
Left subclavian artery

B

Right subclavian artery
Right common carotid artery
Left subclavian artery
Left common carotid artery

C

1.52 Arch of the aorta

A. Variations. The double aortic arch of the frog; the right aortic arch of the bird; the left aortic arch of the mammal, including man, and a variant. **B.** Double aortic arch. The right and left aortic arches persist completely, as in the frog. In this rare condition, the esophagus and trachea pass through the so-formed "aortic ring." **C.** Retroesophageal right subclavian artery. The artery arises as the last branch of the arch of the aorta, passing posterior to the esophagus and trachea. The right recurrent laryngeal nerve, having no vessel around which to recur, takes a direct course to the larynx.

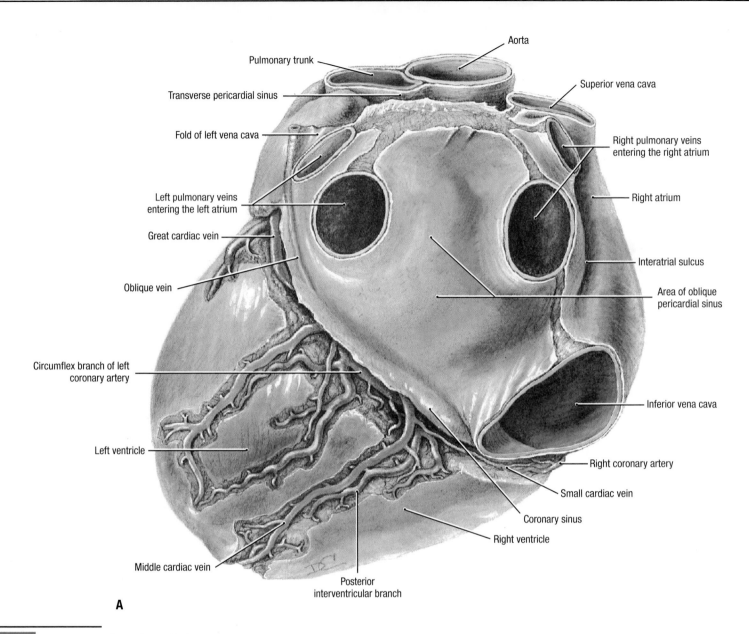

Aorta

Pulmonary trunk

Transverse pericardial sinus

Superior vena cava

Fold of left vena cava

Right pulmonary veins entering the right atrium

Left pulmonary veins entering the left atrium

Great cardiac vein

Right atrium

Oblique vein

Interatrial sulcus

Area of oblique pericardial sinus

Circumflex branch of left coronary artery

Inferior vena cava

Left ventricle

Right coronary artery

Small cardiac vein

Coronary sinus

Right ventricle

Middle cardiac vein

Posterior interventricular branch

A

1.53 Heart and pericardial sac

A. Heart, posteroinferior view. **B.** Interior of pericardial sac, anterior view. **C.** Coronal section. This heart was removed from the interior of the pericardial sac. The heart is covered by a visceral layer of serous pericardium and pericardial sac, and lined by a parietal layer of serous pericardium.

OBSERVE IN **A**:
1. The entire base, or posterior surface, and part of the diaphragmatic surface are in view;
2. The superior vena cava and larger inferior vena cava joining the upper and lower limits of the right atrium;
3. The left atrium forms the greater part of the posterior surface;
4. The coronary arteries in this specimen are irregular in that the left one supplies the posterior interventricular branch;
5. Branches of the cardiac veins, when crossing branches of the coronary arteries, mostly do so superficially;
6. The visceral layer of serous pericardium covers the heart and reflects onto the great vessels; from around the great vessels, the serous pericardium reflects to line the fibrous pericardium as the parietal layer of serous pericardium;

7. The cut edge of the reflections of serous pericardia around the arterial vessels (the pulmonary trunk and aorta) and venous vessels (the superior and inferior venae cavae and the pulmonary veins);

OBSERVE IN **B**:
8. Eight vessels are severed on excising the heart: two caval veins (superior and inferior venae cavae), four pulmonary veins, and two pulmonary arteries;
9. The oblique sinus is bounded anteriorly by the visceral layer of serous pericardium covering the left atrium **(A)**, posteriorly by the parietal layer of serous pericardium lining the fibrous pericardium, and superiorly and laterally by the reflection of serous pericardium around the four pulmonary veins and the superior and inferior venae cavae;
10. The transverse sinus is bounded anteriorly by the serous pericardium covering the posterior aspect of the pulmonary trunk and aorta, and posteriorly by the visceral pericardium covering the atria **(A)** (also see Fig. 1.58);
11. The peak of the pericardial sac is near the junction of the ascending aorta and arch of the aorta;

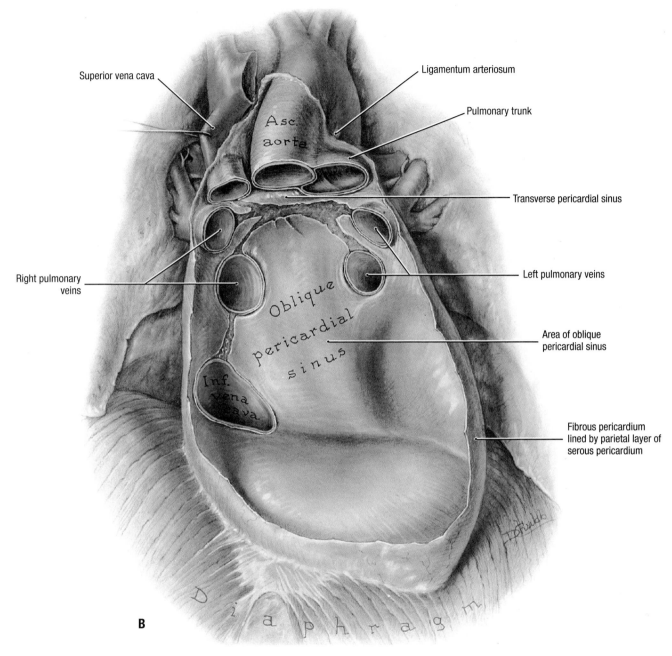

B

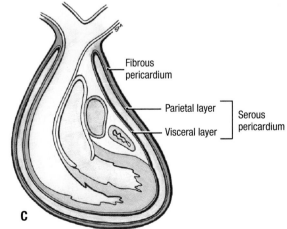

C

12. The superior vena cava is partly inside and partly outside the pericardium, and the ligamentum arteriosum is entirely outside.

Observe in **C:**

13. The fibrous pericardium is lined by a double-layered membranous sac, the serous pericardium;

14. The outer parietal layer lines the fibrous pericardium and is continuous with the inner visceral layer, or epicardium, that covers the heart and great vessels. A thin film of fluid between the visceral and parietal layers allows the heart to move within the sac.

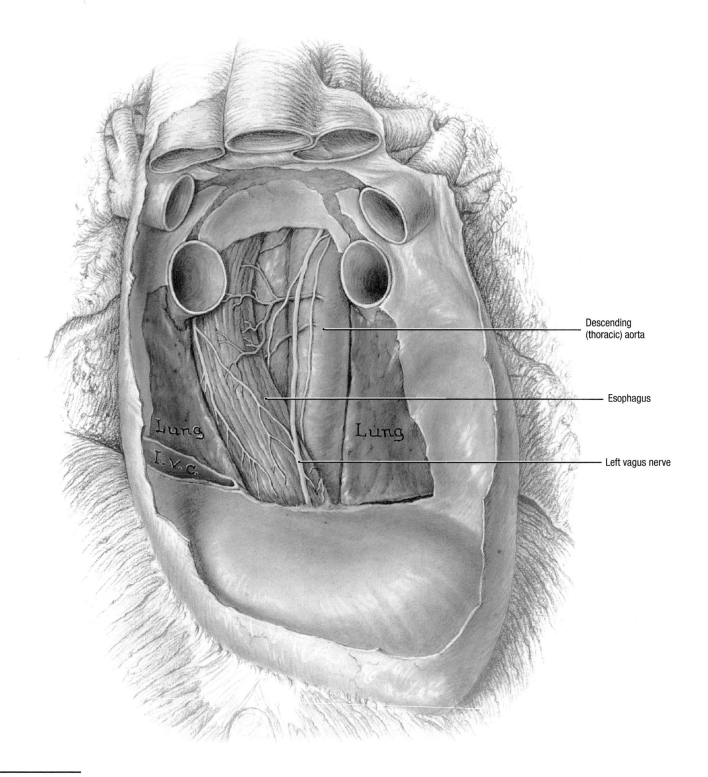

Descending (thoracic) aorta

Esophagus

Left vagus nerve

Lung

Lung

I.V.C.

1.54   Posterior relations of heart and pericardium, anterior view

The fibrous and parietal layers of serous pericardium have been removed from posterior and lateral to the oblique sinus.

OBSERVE:

1. The esophagus forms a groove in part of the right lung;

2. The aorta forms a groove in part of the left lung;
3. The vagus nerves form a plexus on the esophagus;
4. The esophagus in this specimen is unduly deflected to the right; it
usually lies in contact with the aorta.

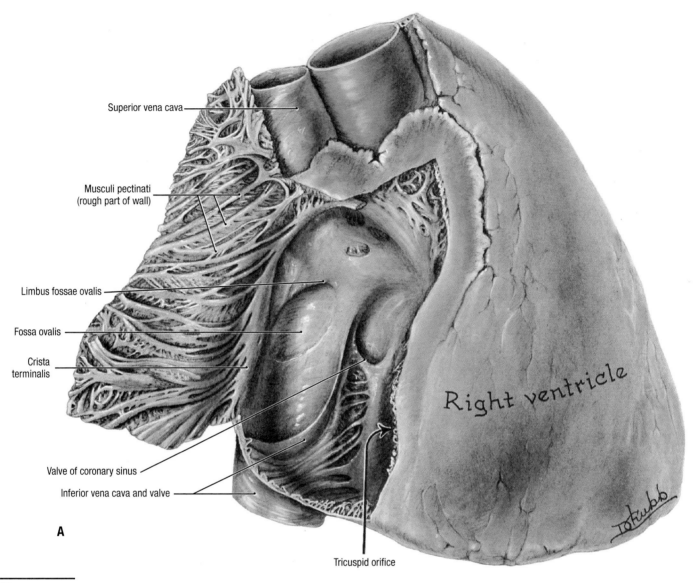

Superior vena cava

Musculi pectinati
(rough part of wall)

Limbus fossae ovalis

Fossa ovalis

Crista
terminalis

Right ventricle

Valve of coronary sinus

Inferior vena cava and valve

A

Tricuspid orifice

1.55   Right atrium, anterolateral view

A. Interior of right atrium. **B.** Inflow.

OBSERVE:
1. The smooth part of the atrial wall is formed by the absorption of the right horn of the sinus venosus, and the rough part is formed from the primitive atrium;
2. Crista terminalis, the valve of the inferior vena cava, and the valve of the coronary sinus separate the smooth part from the rough part;
3. The musculi pectinati passes anterior from the crista terminalis like teeth from the back of a comb; the crista underlies the sulcus terminalis (not shown), which is a groove visible externally on the posterolateral surface of the right atrium between the superior and inferior venae cavae;
4. The superior and inferior venae cavae and the coronary sinus open onto the smooth part of the right atrium; the anterior cardiac veins and venae cordis minimae (not shown) also open into the atrium;
5. The right atrioventricular, or tricuspid, orifice, is situated at the anterior aspect of the atrium;
6. In **B,** the inflow from the superior vena cava is directed toward the tricuspid orifice, whereas blood from the inferior vena cava is directed toward the fossa ovalis.

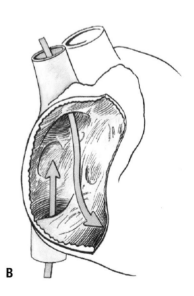

B

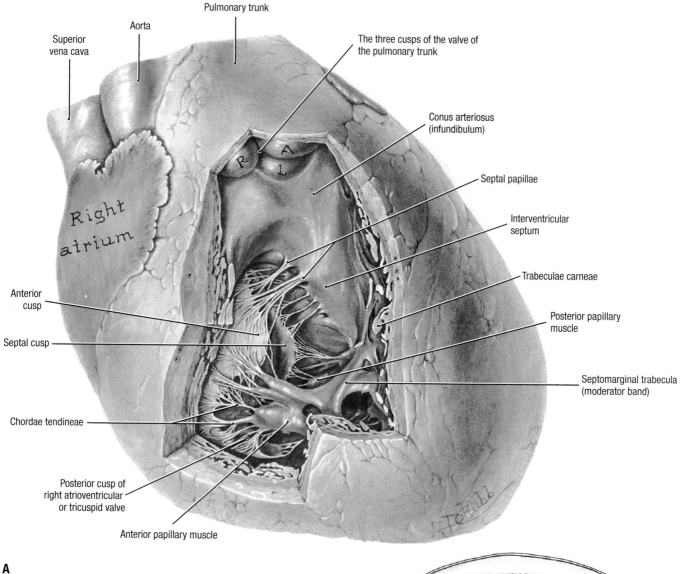

A

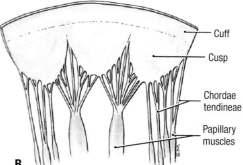

B

1.56 Right ventricle

A. Interior of right ventricle, anteroinferior view. **B.** Right atrioventricular, or tricuspid, valve spread out.

OBSERVE:

1. The entrance to this chamber, the right atrioventricular or tricuspid orifice, is situated posteriorly; the exit, the orifice of the pulmonary trunk, is superior;
2. The smooth, funnel-shaped wall (conus arteriosus) inferior to the pulmonary orifice; the remainder of the ventricle is rough with fleshy trabeculae;
3. Three types of trabeculae: mere ridges, bridges attached only at each end, and finger-like projections called papillary muscles. The anterior papillary muscle rises from the anterior wall, the posterior (not labeled) from the posterior wall, and a series of small septal papillae from the septal wall;

4. The septomarginal trabecula, here thick, extends from the septum to the base of the anterior papillary muscle;
5. The chordae tendineae pass from the tips of the papillary muscles to the free margins and ventricular surfaces of the three cusps of the tricuspid valve;
6. The three cusps of the pulmonary valve: right *(R)*, left *(L)*, and anterior *(A)*.
7. In **B,** each papillary muscle controls the adjacent sides of two cusps.

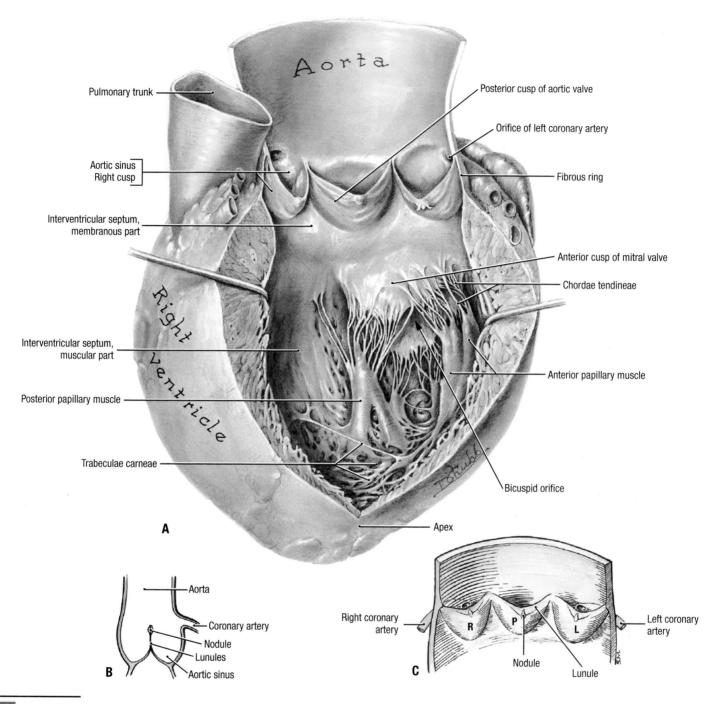

Pulmonary trunk

Aorta

Posterior cusp of aortic valve

Orifice of left coronary artery

Aortic sinus
Right cusp

Fibrous ring

Interventricular septum,
membranous part

Anterior cusp of mitral valve

Chordae tendineae

Right Ventricle

Interventricular septum,
muscular part

Anterior papillary muscle

Posterior papillary muscle

Trabeculae carneae

Bicuspid orifice

Apex

A

Aorta

Coronary artery

Nodule

Lunules

Aortic sinus

B

Right coronary
artery

R   P   L

Left coronary
artery

Nodule

Lunule

C

1.57 Left ventricle

A. Interior of left ventricle. **B.** Longitudinal section of closed aortic valve. **C.** Spread out aortic valve.

OBSERVE:

1. The conical shape of the left chamber;
2. The entrance (left atrioventricular, bicuspid, or mitral orifice) is situated posteriorly, and the exit (aortic orifice) is superior;
3. The wall is thin and muscular near the apex, thick and muscular above, and thin and fibrous (nonelastic) at the aortic orifice;
4. Trabeculae carneae, as in the right ventricle, form ridges, bridges, and papillary muscles;

5. Two large papillary muscles, the anterior from the anterior wall and the posterior from the posterior wall, control with chordae tendineae the adjacent halves of two cusps of the mitral valve;
6. The anterior cusp of the mitral valve intervenes between the inlet (mitral orifice) and the outlet (aortic orifice).
7. In **B** and **C,** the aortic valve, like that of the pulmonary trunk, has three semilunar cusps: right *(R)*, posterior *(P)*, and left *(L)*, each with a fibrous nodule at the midpoint of its free edge and a thin connective tissue area, the lunula, to each side of the nodule. When the valve is closed, the nodules and lunulae meet in the center.

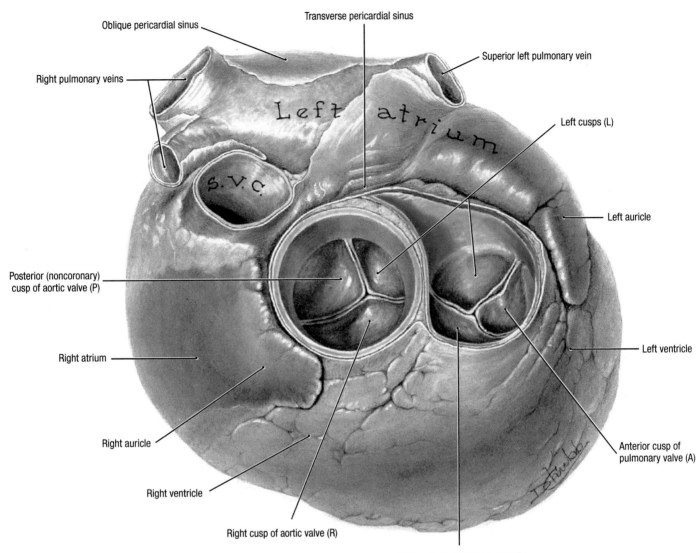

1.58   Excised heart, superior view

OBSERVE:
1. The anterior position of the ventricles, and the posterior position of the atria;
2. The stems of the aorta and pulmonary artery, which conduct blood from the ventricles, are placed anterior to the atria and their incoming blood vessels (the superior vena cava and pulmonary veins);
3. The aorta and pulmonary artery are enclosed within a common tube of serous pericardium and partly embraced by the auricles of the atria;
4. The transverse pericardial sinus curves posterior to the enclosed stems of the aorta and pulmonary trunk, and anterior to the superior vena cava and upper limits of the atria;
5. The three cusps of the aortic and pulmonary valves; the names of the cusps of the aortic and pulmonary valves have a developmental origin, as explained in Figure 1.59.

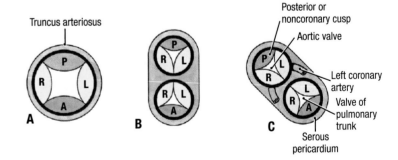

1.59   Pulmonary and aortic valve names

The names of these cusps have a developmental origin: the truncus arteriosus with four cusps (**A**) splits to form two valves, each with three cusps (**B**). The heart undergoes partial rotation to the left on its axis, resulting in the arrangement of cusps shown in **C**. *Inability of the valve to close completely is called insufficiency and results in regurgitation; fusion of the cusps produces stenosis.*

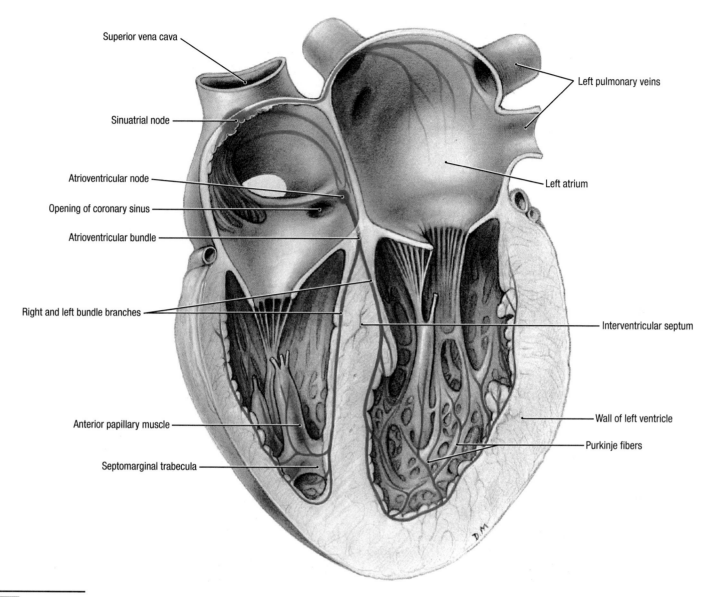

Superior vena cava

Sinuatrial node

Atrioventricular node

Opening of coronary sinus

Atrioventricular bundle

Right and left bundle branches

Anterior papillary muscle

Septomarginal trabecula

Left pulmonary veins

Left atrium

Interventricular septum

Wall of left ventricle

Purkinje fibers

1.60 Conduction system of heart, coronal section

OBSERVE:

1. The sinuatrial (SA) node in the wall of the right atrium near the superior end of the sulcus terminalis extends over the anterior aspect of the opening of the superior vena cava. The SA node is the "pacemaker" of the heart because it initiates muscle contraction and determines the heart rate. It is supplied by the sinuatrial nodal artery, usually a branch of the right coronary artery, but may be a branch of the left.

2. Contraction spreads through the atrial wall until it reaches the atrioventricular (AV) node in the interatrial septum just superior to the opening of the coronary sinus. The AV node is supplied by the atrioventricular nodal artery, usually arising from the right coronary artery posteriorly at the inferior margin of the interatrial septum;

3. The AV bundle, usually supplied by the right coronary artery, passes from the AV node in the membranous part of the interventricular septum, dividing into right and left bundle branches on either side of the muscular part of the interventricular septum;

4. The right bundle branch travels inferiorly in the interventricular septum to the anterior wall of the ventricle, then through the sep-

tomarginal trabecula to the anterior papillary muscle; excitation spreads throughout the right ventricular wall through a network of branches from the right bundle (Purkinje fibers);

5. The left bundle branch lies beneath the endocardium on the left side of the interventricular septum and branches to enter the anterior and posterior papillary muscles and the wall of the left ventricle; further branching into a plexus of Purkinje fibers allows the impulses to be conveyed throughout the left ventricular wall. The bundle branches are usually supplied by the left coronary, except the posterior limb of the left bundle branch, which is supplied by both coronary arteries;

6. *Damage to the cardiac conduction system (often by compromised blood supply as in coronary artery disease) leads to disturbances of muscle contraction. Damage to the AV node results in "heart block" because the atrial excitation wave does not reach the ventricles, which begin to contract independently at their own, slower rate. Damage to one of the branches results in "bundle branch block," in which excitation goes down the unaffected branch to cause systole of that ventricle; the impulse then spreads to the other ventricle, producing later, asynchronous contraction.*

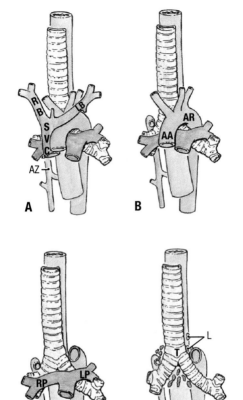

1.61 **Relations of great vessels and trachea, anterior view**

OBSERVE FROM SUPERFICIAL TO DEEP:
A. Brachiocephalic veins (*RB* and *LB*) forming the superior vena cava (*SVC*), and the arch of the azygos vein (*AZ*) entering it posteriorly. **B.** Ascending aorta (*AA*) and arch of the aorta (*AR*). **C.** Pulmonary arteries (*RP* and *LP*). **D.** Lymph nodes (*L*) at the tracheal bifurcation (*T*)

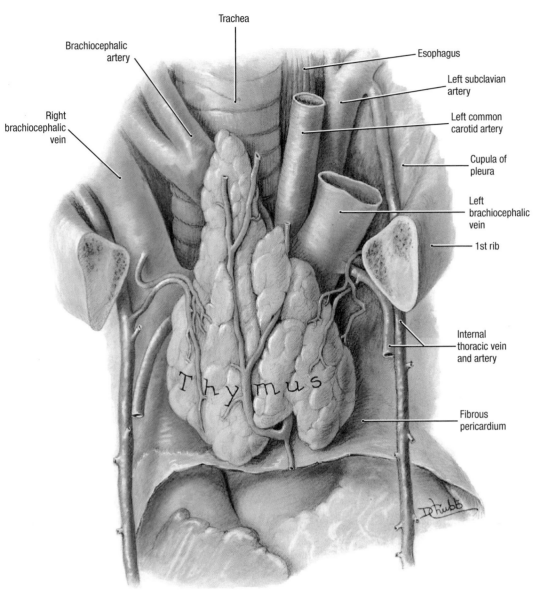

Trachea

Brachiocephalic artery

Esophagus

Right brachiocephalic vein

Left subclavian artery

Left common carotid artery

Cupula of pleura

Left brachiocephalic vein

1st rib

Internal thoracic vein and artery

Thymus

Fibrous pericardium

1.62 **Superior mediastinum-I: superficial dissection, anterior view**

The sternum and ribs have been excised and the pleurae removed. *It is unusual in an adult to see such a discrete thymus, which is impressive during puberty but subsequently regresses and is largely replaced by fat and fibrous tissue.*

OBSERVE:
1. The thymus lies in the superior mediastinum, overlapping the pericardial sac inferiorly and extending superiorly into the neck (in this specimen, farther than usual);
2. The longitudinal fissure divides the thymus into two asymmetrical lobes, a larger right and smaller left; these two developmentally separate parts are easily separated from each other by blunt dissection;
3. The blood supply to the thymus: arteries from the internal thoracic arteries, veins to the brachiocephalic and internal thoracic veins, and veins communicating superiorly with the inferior thyroid veins.

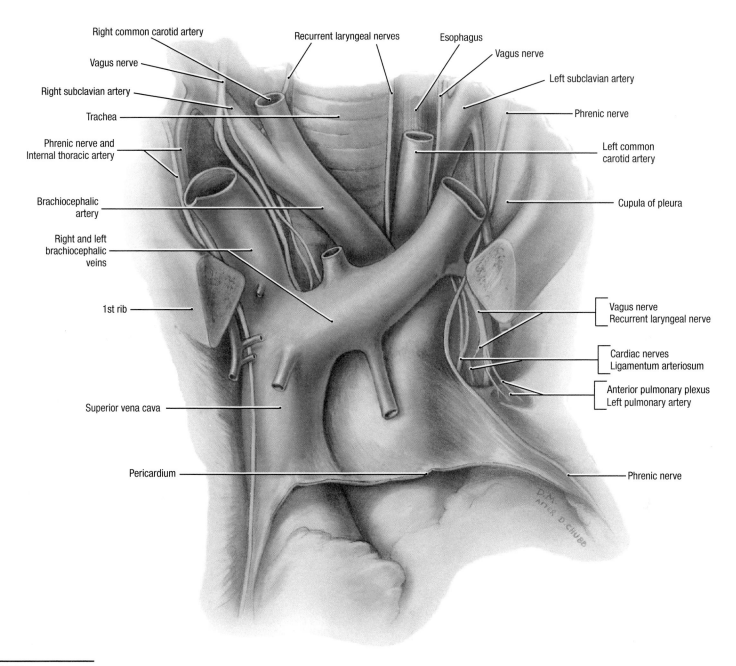

Right common carotid artery

Vagus nerve

Right subclavian artery

Trachea

Phrenic nerve and
Internal thoracic artery

Brachiocephalic
artery

Right and left
brachiocephalic
veins

1st rib

Superior vena cava

Pericardium

Recurrent laryngeal nerves

Esophagus

Vagus nerve

Left subclavian artery

Phrenic nerve

Left common
carotid artery

Cupula of pleura

Vagus nerve
Recurrent laryngeal nerve

Cardiac nerves
Ligamentum arteriosum

Anterior pulmonary plexus
Left pulmonary artery

Phrenic nerve

1.63 **Superior mediastinum-II: root of neck,
anterior view**

After removal of the thymus gland, observe:

1. The great veins are anterior to the great arteries;
2. The posterior direction of the arch of the aorta and the nerves crossing its left side;
3. The ligamentum arteriosum is outside the pericardial sac, with the left recurrent laryngeal nerve on its left side and the vagal and sympathetic branches of the superficial cardiac plexus on its right;
4. The right vagus nerve crosses anterior to the right subclavian artery, there giving off its recurrent branch and then passing medially to reach the trachea and esophagus;
5. The left vagus nerve crosses anterior to the arch of the aorta, there giving off its recurrent branch, which passes posterior to the arch of the aorta and then ascends between the trachea and esophagus to the larynx; the left vagus nerve then passes posterior to the root of the lung;
6. The left phrenic nerve crosses the path of the vagus nerve, but anterior to it.

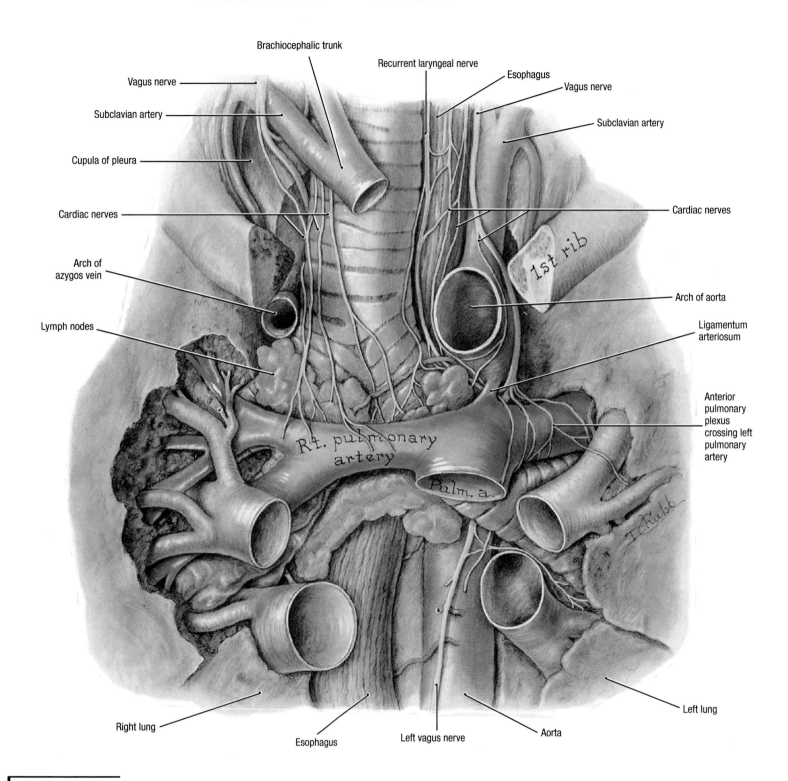

Brachiocephalic trunk
Vagus nerve
Subclavian artery
Cupula of pleura
Cardiac nerves
Arch of azygos vein
Lymph nodes
Right lung
Esophagus
Recurrent laryngeal nerve
Esophagus
Vagus nerve
Subclavian artery
Cardiac nerves
1st rib
Arch of aorta
Ligamentum arteriosum
Anterior pulmonary plexus crossing left pulmonary artery
Left lung
Left vagus nerve
Aorta
Rt. pulmonary artery
Pulm. a.

1.64   Superior mediastinum-III: pulmonary arteries, anterior view

OBSERVE:
1. The pulmonary trunk divides into right and left pulmonary arteries, the right crossing inferior to the bifurcation of the trachea and separated from the esophagus by lymph nodes.

2. Cardiac branches of the vagus and sympathetic nerves stream down the sides of the trachea and form cardiac plexuses.

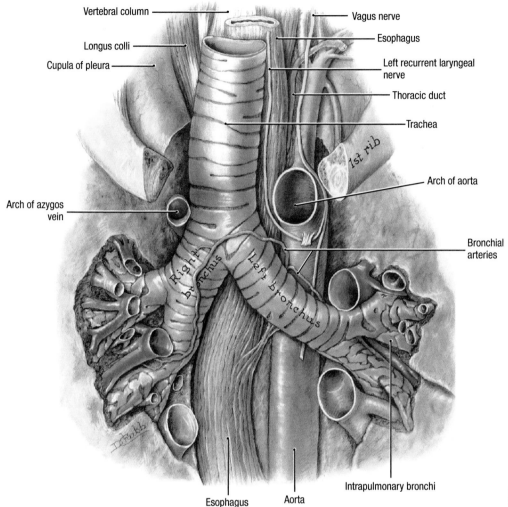

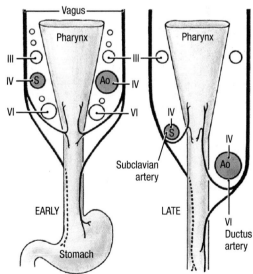

1.65 Superior mediastinum-IV: tracheal bifurcation and bronchi, anterior view

OBSERVE:

1. Four parallel structures: the trachea, esophagus, left recurrent laryngeal nerve, and thoracic duct. The esophagus bulges to the left of the trachea, the recurrent nerve lies in the angle between the trachea and esophagus, and the duct is at the left side of the esophagus;
2. The arch of the aorta passes posteriorly to the left of these four structures, and the arch of the azygos vein passes anteriorly to their right;
3. The trachea inclines slightly to the right; thus the right bronchus is more vertical than the left, and its stem is shorter and wider. The first right branch arises approximately 2.5 cm from the bifurcation, whereas the first left branch arises approximately 5 cm from the bifurcation;
4. The U-shaped rings of the trachea are commonly bifurcated; the ring at the bifurcation of the trachea is V shaped;
5. The bronchial arteries supply the trachea and follow the bronchial tree to supply the bronchi, lung tissue, and lymph nodes.

1.66 Great vessels and nerves

Scheme to explain the asymmetrical courses of the right and left recurrent laryngeal nerves. (III, IV, and VI are embryonic aortic arches.)

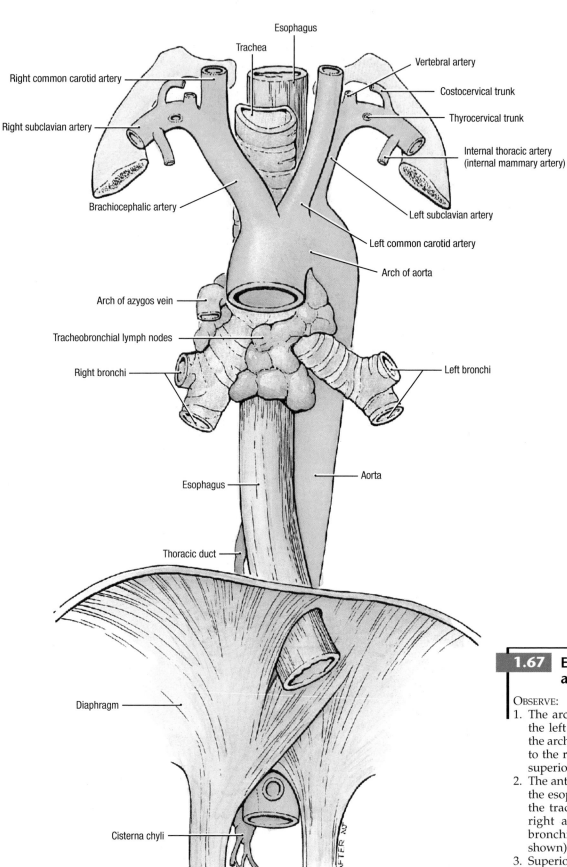

Right common carotid artery

Trachea

Esophagus

Vertebral artery

Costocervical trunk

Thyrocervical trunk

Right subclavian artery

Internal thoracic artery
(internal mammary artery)

Brachiocephalic artery

Left subclavian artery

Left common carotid artery

Arch of aorta

Arch of azygos vein

Tracheobronchial lymph nodes

Right bronchi

Left bronchi

Aorta

Esophagus

Thoracic duct

Diaphragm

Cisterna chyli

1.67 **Esophagus, trachea, and aorta, anterior view**

OBSERVE:

1. The arch of the aorta arches posteriorly to the left of the trachea and esophagus, and the arch of the azygos vein arches anteriorly to the right of these structures; each arches superior to the root of a lung;

2. The anterior relations of the thoracic part of the esophagus from superior to inferior are the trachea (throughout its entire length), right and left bronchi, inferior tracheobronchial lymph nodes, pericardium (not shown) and, finally, the diaphragm;

3. Superior to the level of the arch of the aorta, the esophagus bulges to the left beyond the trachea.

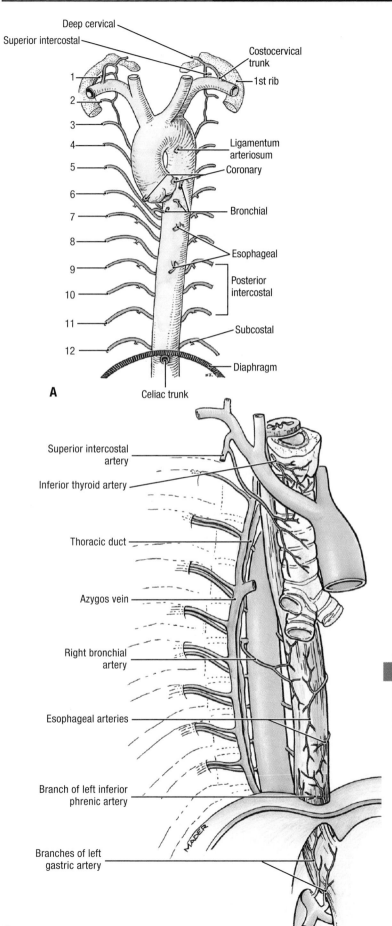

A

Deep cervical

Superior intercostal

Costocervical trunk

1st rib

1

2

3

4

Ligamentum arteriosum

Coronary

5

6

Bronchial

7

8

Esophageal

9

Posterior intercostal

10

11

Subcostal

12

Diaphragm

Celiac trunk

Superior intercostal artery

Inferior thyroid artery

Thoracic duct

Azygos vein

Right bronchial artery

Esophageal arteries

Branch of left inferior phrenic artery

Branches of left gastric artery

C

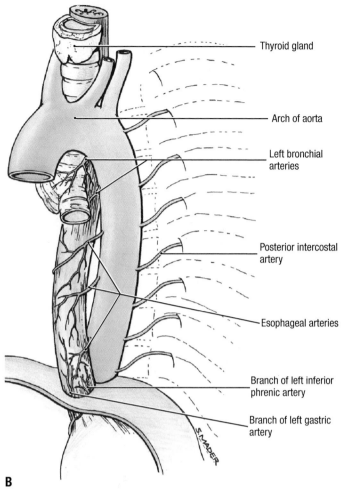

Thyroid gland

Arch of aorta

Left bronchial arteries

Posterior intercostal artery

Esophageal arteries

Branch of left inferior phrenic artery

Branch of left gastric artery

B

1.68 Arterial supply to trachea and esophagus

A. Branches of the thoracic aorta, anterior view. The superior phrenic branches arising from the inferior part of the thoracic aorta are not shown. These small vessels supply the posterosuperior aspect of the diaphragm. Note the superior intercostal arteries (1), posterior intercostal arteries (2–11), and subcostal arteries (12) are paired.
B. Left anterolateral view. **C.** Right anterolateral view.

OBSERVE:
1. The unpaired median bronchial and esophageal branches of the descending thoracic aorta supply the trachea, bronchi, and esophagus;
2. The continuous anastomotic chain of arteries on the esophagus are formed: (a) by branches of the right and left inferior thyroid and right superior intercostal arteries superiorly, (b) by the unpaired median aortic branches, and (c) by branches of the left gastric and left inferior phrenic arteries inferiorly;
3. The right bronchial artery usually arises from the upper left bronchial or 3rd right posterior intercostal artery (here the 5th) or from the aorta directly.

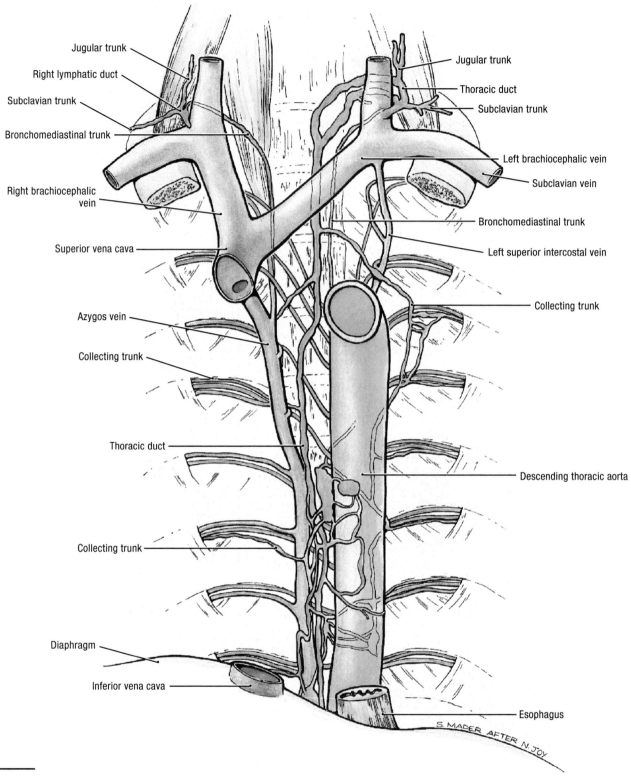

Jugular trunk

Right lymphatic duct

Subclavian trunk

Bronchomediastinal trunk

Right brachiocephalic vein

Superior vena cava

Azygos vein

Collecting trunk

Thoracic duct

Collecting trunk

Diaphragm

Inferior vena cava

Jugular trunk

Thoracic duct

Subclavian trunk

Left brachiocephalic vein

Subclavian vein

Bronchomediastinal trunk

Left superior intercostal vein

Collecting trunk

Descending thoracic aorta

Esophagus

S. MADER AFTER N. JOY

1.69   Thoracic duct, anterior view

The descending aorta is pulled slightly to the left, and the azygos vein slightly to the right.

OBSERVE:

1. The thoracic duct (a) ascends on the vertebral column between the azygos vein and the descending aorta and (b) at the junction of the posterior and superior mediastina, passes to the left and continues its ascent to the neck, where (c) it arches laterally to open near or at the angle of union of the internal jugular and subclavian veins;

2. The duct, here, is commonly (a) plexiform (resembling a network) in the posterior mediastinum and (b) splits and reunites in the neck;

3. The duct receives branches from the intercostal spaces on both sides through several collecting trunks, as well as branches from posterior mediastinal structures;

4. The duct arches laterally, receiving the jugular, subclavian, and bronchomediastinal trunks;

5. The right lymph duct is very short and formed by the union of the right jugular, subclavian, and bronchomediastinal trunks.

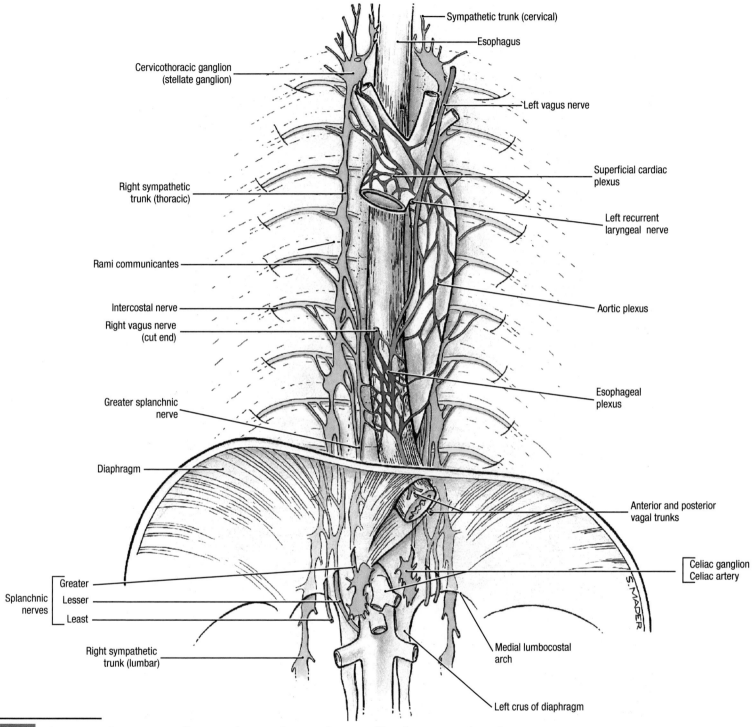

Sympathetic trunk (cervical)

Esophagus

Cervicothoracic ganglion
(stellate ganglion)

Left vagus nerve

Right sympathetic
trunk (thoracic)

Superficial cardiac
plexus

Left recurrent
laryngeal nerve

Rami communicantes

Intercostal nerve

Aortic plexus

Right vagus nerve
(cut end)

Esophageal
plexus

Greater splanchnic
nerve

Diaphragm

Anterior and posterior
vagal trunks

Greater

Celiac ganglion
Celiac artery

Splanchnic
nerves

Lesser

Least

Right sympathetic
trunk (lumbar)

Medial lumbocostal
arch

Left crus of diaphragm

1.70　Autonomic nerves of posterior and superior mediastina, anterior view

OBSERVE:
1. The right and left sympathetic trunks enter the abdomen by passing deep to the medial lumbocostal arches of the diaphragm;
2. The large cervicothoracic ganglion is formed by the fusion of the inferior cervical ganglion and the 1st thoracic ganglion;
3. The sympathetic nerve cell bodies are located in the lateral horn of gray matter of the spinal cord in segments T1 to L2 or L3; the fibers are conveyed through the ventral roots, spinal nerves, and rami communicantes to the thoracic sympathetic trunks. The thoracic sympathetic trunks are in continuity with the cervical and lumbar sympathetic trunks. Fibers are distributed to thoracic viscera by contributions to the plexuses (e.g., cardiac, esophageal) to abdominal ganglia (e.g., celiac) by the greater, lesser, and least splanchnic nerves, and to the intercostal nerves by the rami communicantes;
4. The left vagus and recurrent laryngeal nerves contribute parasympathetic fibers to the pulmonary, cardiac, and esophageal plexuses, and the cut end of the right vagus nerve, which also contributes fibers to these plexuses;
5. The vagus nerves passes through the esophageal opening of the diaphragm to become the anterior and posterior vagal trunks.

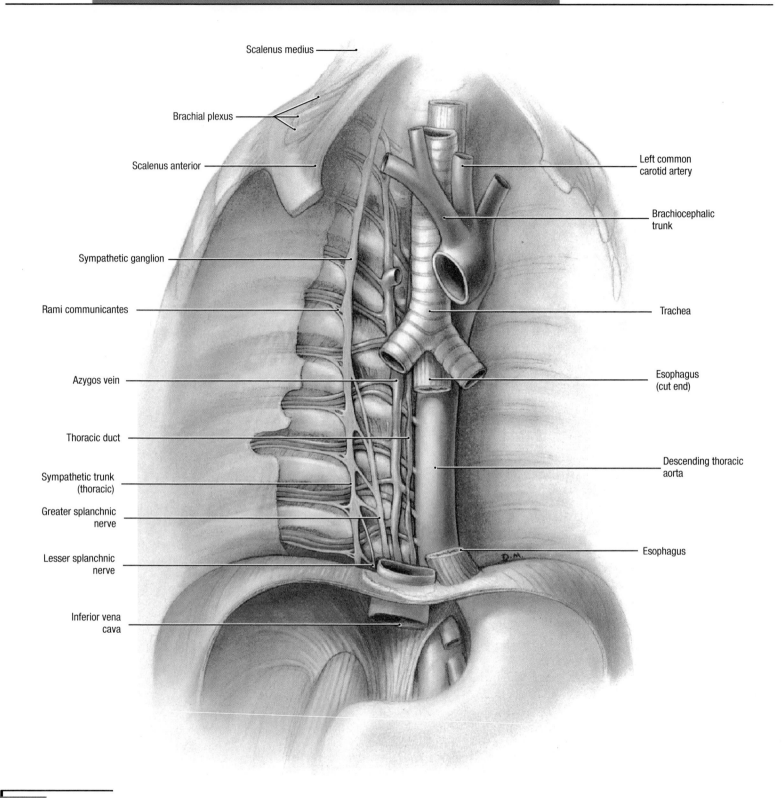

Scalenus medius

Brachial plexus

Scalenus anterior

Left common
carotid artery

Brachiocephalic
trunk

Sympathetic ganglion

Rami communicantes

Trachea

Azygos vein

Esophagus
(cut end)

Thoracic duct

Descending thoracic
aorta

Sympathetic trunk
(thoracic)

Greater splanchnic
nerve

Lesser splanchnic
nerve

Esophagus

Inferior vena
cava

1.71   Posterior mediastinum viewed from the right

In this specimen, the parietal pleura is intact on the left side and partially removed on the right side . A portion of the esophagus, between
the bifurcation of the trachea and the diaphragm, is also removed.

OBSERVE:
1. The thoracic sympathetic trunk lies against the heads of the ribs;
the sympathetic ganglia and the rami communicantes connect to
each intercostal nerve;

2. The greater splanchnic nerve is formed by fibers from the 5th to
10th thoracic ganglia, and the lesser splanchnic nerve receives
fibers from the 10th and 11th thoracic ganglia. Both nerves contain
preganglionic and visceral afferent fibers;
3. The azygos vein passes anterior to the intercostal vessels and to the
right of the thoracic duct and aorta.

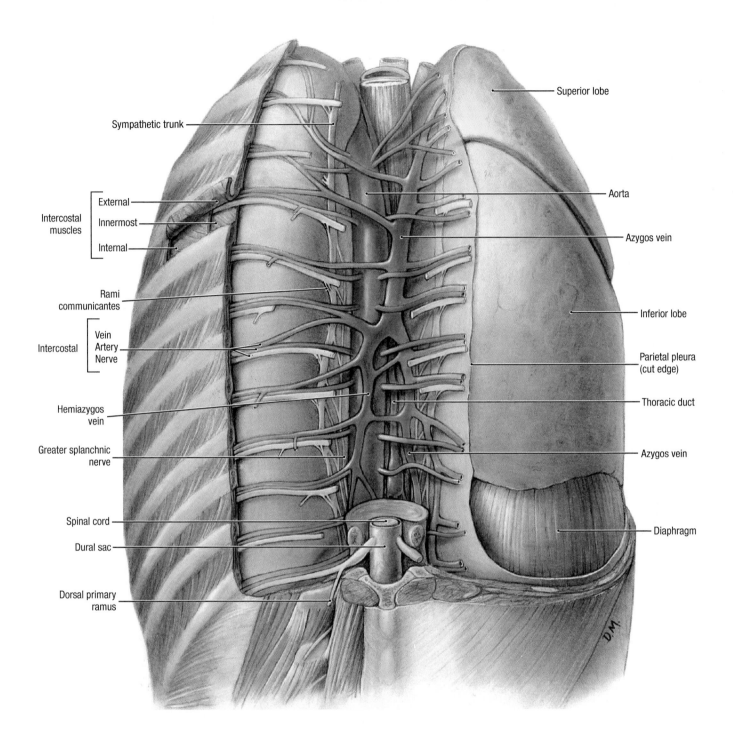

Sympathetic trunk

Intercostal muscles
- External
- Innermost
- Internal

Rami communicantes

Intercostal
- Vein
- Artery
- Nerve

Hemiazygos vein

Greater splanchnic nerve

Spinal cord

Dural sac

Dorsal primary ramus

Superior lobe

Aorta

Azygos vein

Inferior lobe

Parietal pleura (cut edge)

Thoracic duct

Azygos vein

Diaphragm

D.M.

1.72 Mediastinum and lungs, posterior view

The thoracic vertebral column and thoracic cage are removed on the right. On the left, the ribs and intercostal musculature are removed posteriorly as far laterally as the angles of the ribs. The parietal pleura is intact on the left side, but partially removed on the right to reveal the visceral pleura covering the right lung.

OBSERVE:
1. The azygos vein is on the right side, and the hemiazygos vein is on the left, crossing the midline (usually at T9, but higher in this specimen) to join the azygos vein. The accessory hemiazygos vein is absent; instead, three posterior intercostal veins drain directly into the azygos vein;
2. The thoracic aorta lies against the left lung, partially embedded in the parietal pleura.

1.73 Azygos system of veins, anterior view

WHILE CONSULTING FIGURE 1.74, OBSERVE:

1. The left renal vein is anterior to the aorta, and the left brachiocephalic vein is anterior to the three branches of the arch of the aorta; these two cross-channels conduct blood from the left side of the body to the right side and so into the right atrium;

2. The paired and approximately symmetrical longitudinal veins anterior to the vertebral column: the azygos vein on the right side, communicating inferiorly with the inferior vena cava, and the hemiazygos vein, on the left side, communicating with the left renal vein; each receives the respective right and left posterior intercostal veins;

3. In this specimen, the hemiazygos, accessory hemiazygos, and left superior intercostal veins are continuous, but commonly they are discontinuous, as in Figure 1.74;

4. The hemiazygos vein crosses the vertebral column at approximately T9, and the accessory hemiazygos vein crosses at T8 to enter the azygos vein; in this specimen, there are four cross- connecting channels between the azygos and hemiazygos systems;

5. The azygos vein arches superior to the root of the right lung at T4 to drain into the superior vena cava.

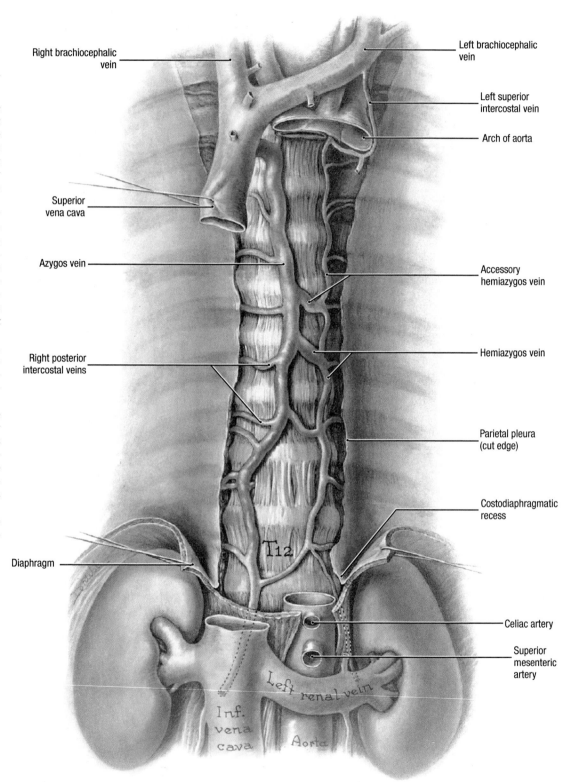

Right brachiocephalic vein

Left brachiocephalic vein

Left superior intercostal vein

Arch of aorta

Superior vena cava

Azygos vein

Accessory hemiazygos vein

Right posterior intercostal veins

Hemiazygos vein

Parietal pleura (cut edge)

Costodiaphragmatic recess

Diaphragm

T12

Celiac artery

Superior mesenteric artery

Left renal vein

Inf. vena cava

Aorta

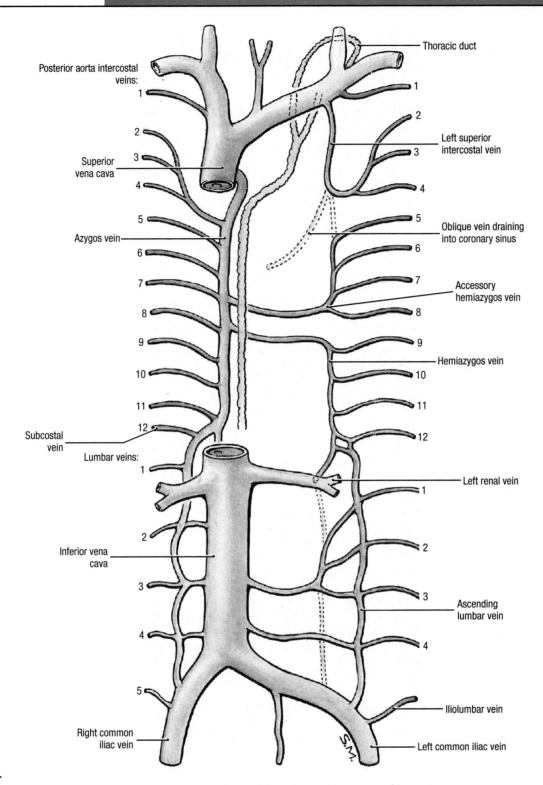

1.74   Azygos, hemiazygos, posterior intercostal, and lumbar veins, anterior view

OBSERVE:
1. *This system is of great importance in continued venous return to the heart if there is an obstruction of the venae cavae;*
2. The lumbar veins lie directly anterior to the vertebral bodies and drain blood from the posterior abdominal wall and from vertebral structures (vertebral column, spinal cord, meninges, etc.) into the inferior vena cava; branches of the lumbar veins also anastomose with the vertebral venous plexuses;
3. The ascending lumbar veins connect the common iliac veins to the

lumbar veins and join the subcostal veins to become the lateral roots of the azygos and hemiazygos veins;
4. The medial roots of the azygos and hemiazygos veins are usually from the inferior vena cava and left renal vein, if present;
5. The right posterior intercostal veins drain into the azygos and right superior intercostal veins; the left posterior intercostal veins draining into the hemiazygos, accessory hemiazygos, and left superior intercostal veins;

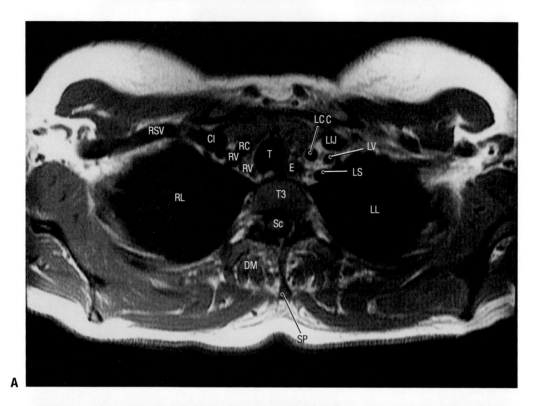

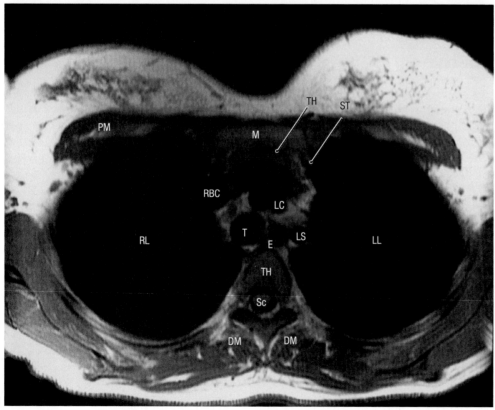

CI	Confluence of internal jugular vein
DM	Deep back muscles
E	Esophagus
LCC	Left common carotid artery
LIJ	Left internal jugular vein
LL	Left lung
LS	Left subclavian vein
LV	Left vertebral artery
M	Manubrium
PM	Pectoralis major
RBC	Right brachiocephalis vein
RC	Right common carotid artery
RCC	Right common carotid artery
RL	Right lung
RSV	Right subclavian vein
RV	Right vertebral artery
SC	Spinal cord
SP	Spinous process
ST	Sternoclavicular joint
T	Trachea
TH	Thymus
T3	Vertebral body (T3)
T4	Vertebral body (T4)

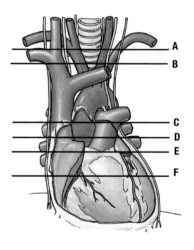

1.75   Transverse, or horizontal (axial), MRIs of the thorax (A–F).

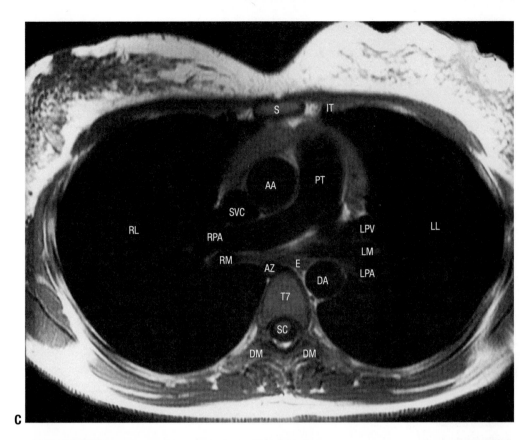

AA	Ascending aorta
AI	Anterior interventricular artery
AZ	Azygos vein
DA	Descending aorta
DM	Deep back muscles
E	Esophagus
IT	Internal thoracic vessels
LA	Left atrium
LC	Left coronary artery
LL	Left lung
LM	Left main bronchus
LPA	Left pulmonary vein
LPV	Left pulmonary vein
PT	Pulmonary trunk
RA	Right atrium
RL	Right lung
RM	Right middle bronchus
RPA	Right pulmonary artery
RPV	Right pulmonary vein
S	Sternum
SC	Spinal cord
SVC	Superior vena cava
T7	Vertebral body (T7)
T8	Vertebral body (T8)

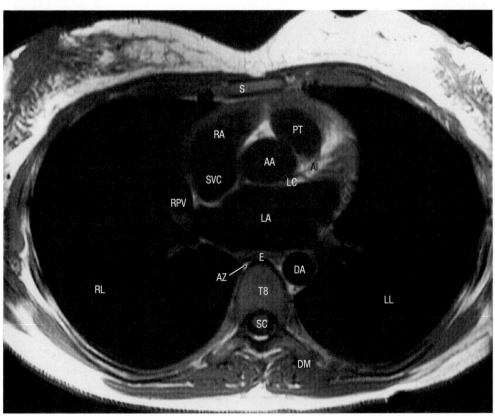

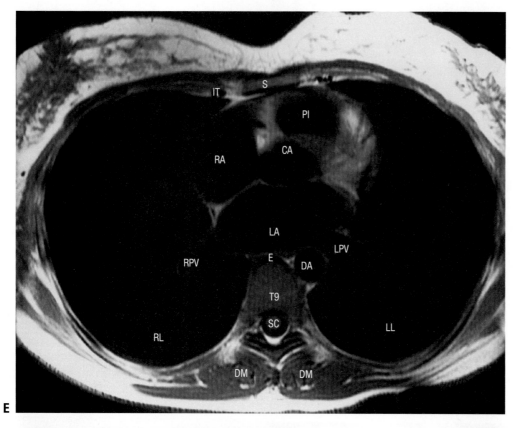

AZ	Azygos vein
CA	Cusp of aortic valve
DA	Descending aorta
DM	Deep back muscles
E	Esophagus
HR	Head of rib
HZ	Hemiazygos vein
IT	Internal thoracic vessels
IVS	Interventricular septum
LA	Left atrium
LL	Left lung
LV	Left ventricle
LPV	Left pulmonary vein
P	Pericardium
PI	Pulmonary infundibulum
PM	Papillary muscle
RA	Right atrium
RL	Right lung
RPV	Right pulmonary vein
RV	Right ventricle
S	Sternum
SC	Spinal cord
T9	Vertebral body (T9)
T10	Vertebral body (T10)

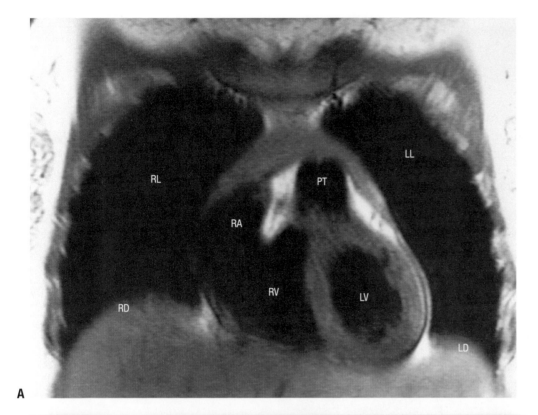

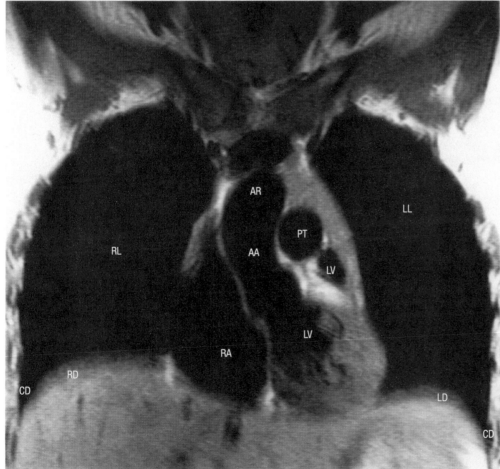

AA	Ascending aorta
AR	Arch of aorta
CD	Costodiphragmatic recess
LD	Left dome of diaphragm
LL	Left lung
LU	Left auricle
LV	Left ventricle
PT	Pulmonary trunk
RA	Right atrium
RL	Right lung
RV	Right ventricle

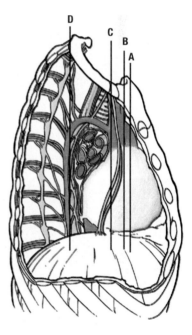

1.76 Coronal MRIs of the thorax (A–D).

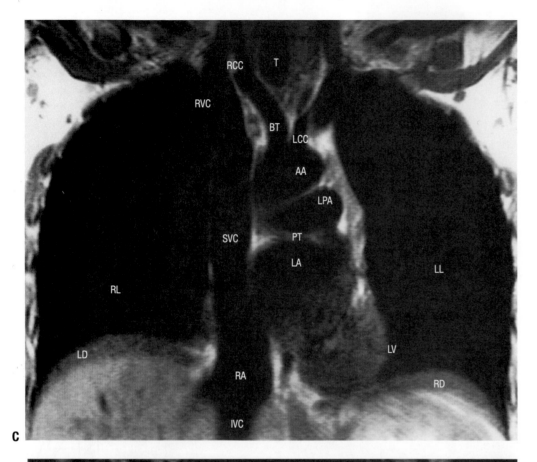

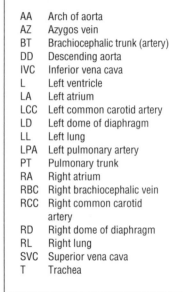

AA	Arch of aorta
AZ	Azygos vein
BT	Brachiocephalic trunk (artery)
DD	Descending aorta
IVC	Inferior vena cava
L	Left ventricle
LA	Left atrium
LCC	Left common carotid artery
LD	Left dome of diaphragm
LL	Left lung
LPA	Left pulmonary artery
PT	Pulmonary trunk
RA	Right atrium
RBC	Right brachiocephalic vein
RCC	Right common carotid artery
RD	Right dome of diaphragm
RL	Right lung
SVC	Superior vena cava
T	Trachea

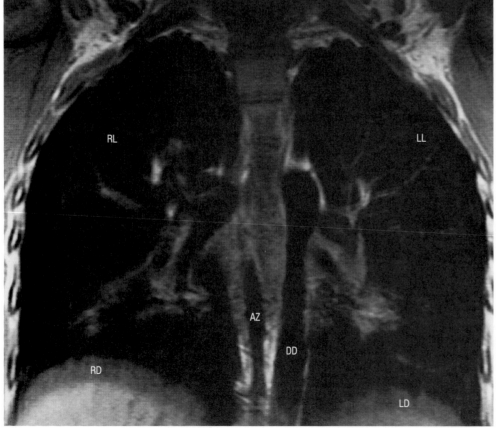

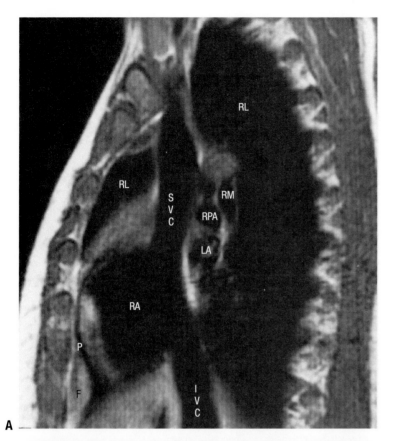

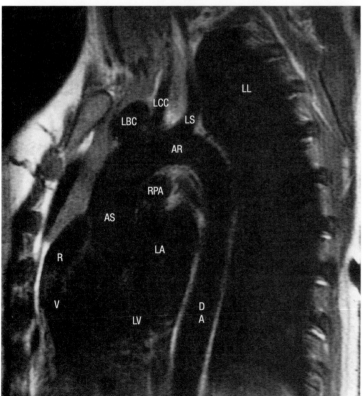

AA	Arch of aorta
AS	Ascending aorta
DA	Descending aorta
F	Fat
IVC	Inferior vena cava
LA	Left atrium
LBC	Left brachiocephalic vein
LCC	Left common carotid artery
LL	Left lung
LS	Left subclavian artery
LV	Left ventricle
P	Pericardium
RA	Right atrium
RL	Right lung
RM	Right main bronchus
RPA	Right pulmonary artery
RV	Right ventricle
SVC	Superior vena cava

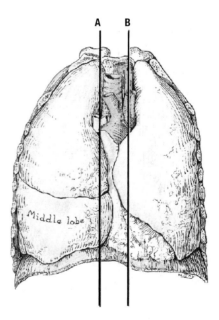

1.77   **Sagittal MRIs of the thorax.**

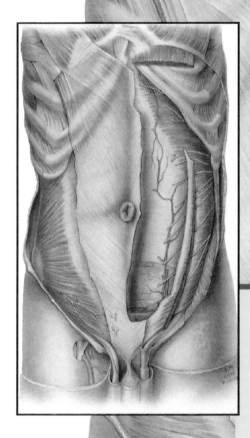

CHAPTER *Abdomen*

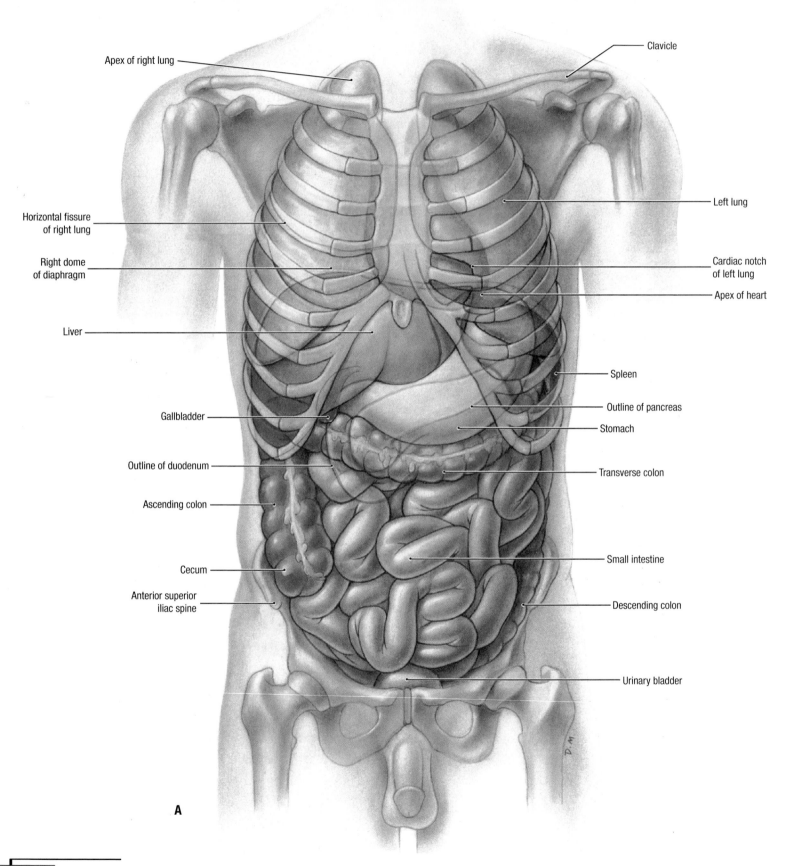

Apex of right lung

Clavicle

Horizontal fissure
of right lung

Left lung

Right dome
of diaphragm

Cardiac notch
of left lung

Apex of heart

Liver

Spleen

Outline of pancreas

Gallbladder

Stomach

Outline of duodenum

Transverse colon

Ascending colon

Cecum

Small intestine

Anterior superior
iliac spine

Descending colon

Urinary bladder

A

2.1   **Abdominal and thoracic viscera in situ**

A. Anterior view.

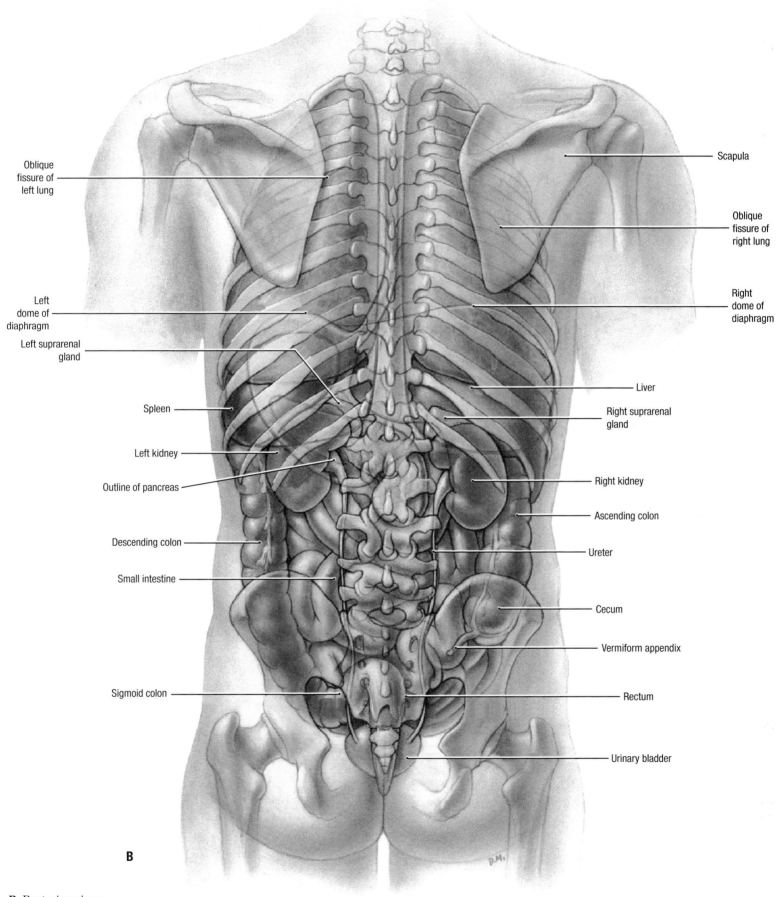

Oblique fissure of left lung

Scapula

Oblique fissure of right lung

Left dome of diaphragm

Right dome of diaphragm

Left suprarenal gland

Liver

Spleen

Right suprarenal gland

Left kidney

Right kidney

Outline of pancreas

Ascending colon

Descending colon

Ureter

Small intestine

Cecum

Vermiform appendix

Sigmoid colon

Rectum

Urinary bladder

B

D.M.

B. Posterior view.

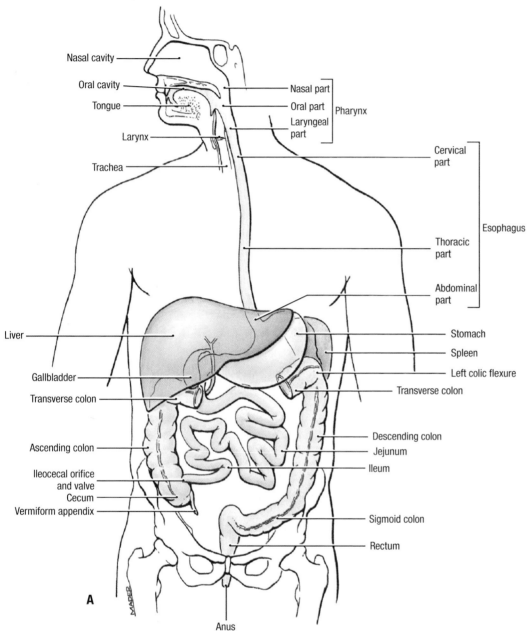

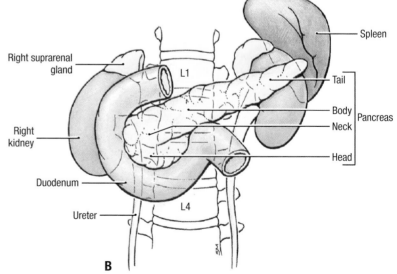

2.2   **Overview of abdomen and pelvis, anterior views**

A. The digestive system. The head is sagittally sectioned and turned laterally. The digestive system extends from the lips to the anus and consists of the oral cavity, pharynx, esophagus, stomach, small intestine (duodenum, jejunum, ileum), and large intestine (vermiform appendix; cecum; ascending, transverse, descending, and sigmoid colon; rectum; and anal canal). Associated organs include the liver, gallbladder, spleen, and pancreas. **B.** The spleen, pancreas, duodenum, and kidneys. These organs are revealed by the removal of the stomach, liver, transverse colon, peritoneum, and fat.

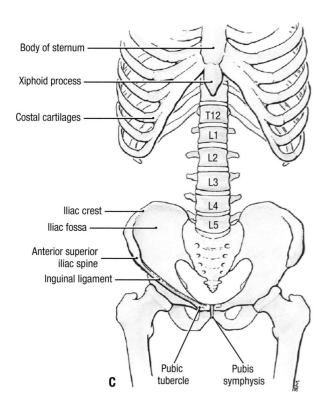

Body of sternum

Xiphoid process

Costal cartilages

T12
L1
L2
L3
L4
L5

Iliac crest

Iliac fossa

Anterior superior
iliac spine

Inguinal ligament

Pubic
tubercle

Pubis
symphysis

C

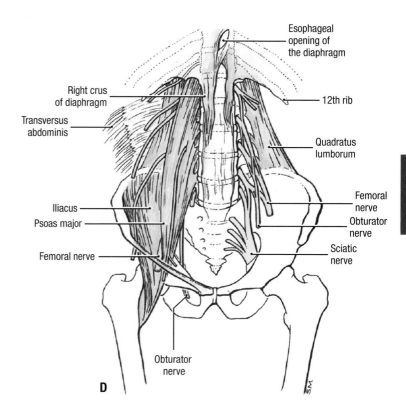

Esophageal
opening of
the diaphragm

Right crus
of diaphragm

12th rib

Transversus
abdominis

Quadratus
lumborum

Iliacus

Psoas major

Femoral
nerve

Obturator
nerve

Femoral nerve

Sciatic
nerve

Obturator
nerve

D

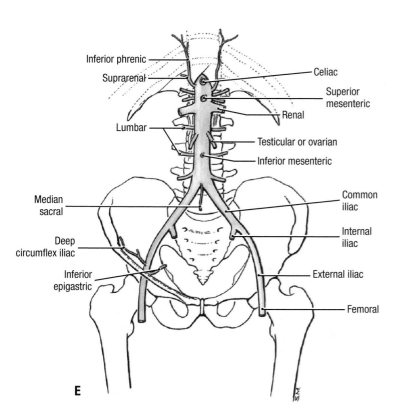

Inferior phrenic

Suprarenal

Celiac

Superior
mesenteric

Renal

Lumbar

Testicular or ovarian

Inferior mesenteric

Median
sacral

Common
iliac

Deep
circumflex iliac

Internal
iliac

Inferior
epigastric

External iliac

Femoral

E

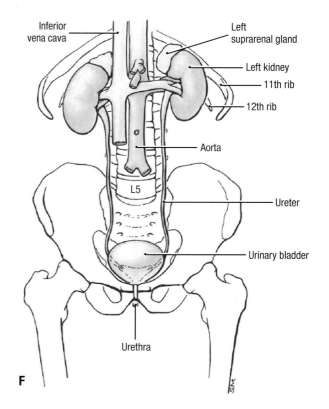

Inferior
vena cava

Left
suprarenal gland

Left kidney

11th rib

12th rib

Aorta

L5

Ureter

Urinary bladder

Urethra

F

C. Skeleton.   **D.** Musculature of posterior abdominal wall.
E. Lumbosacral plexus and abdominal aorta. **F.** Urinary apparatus.

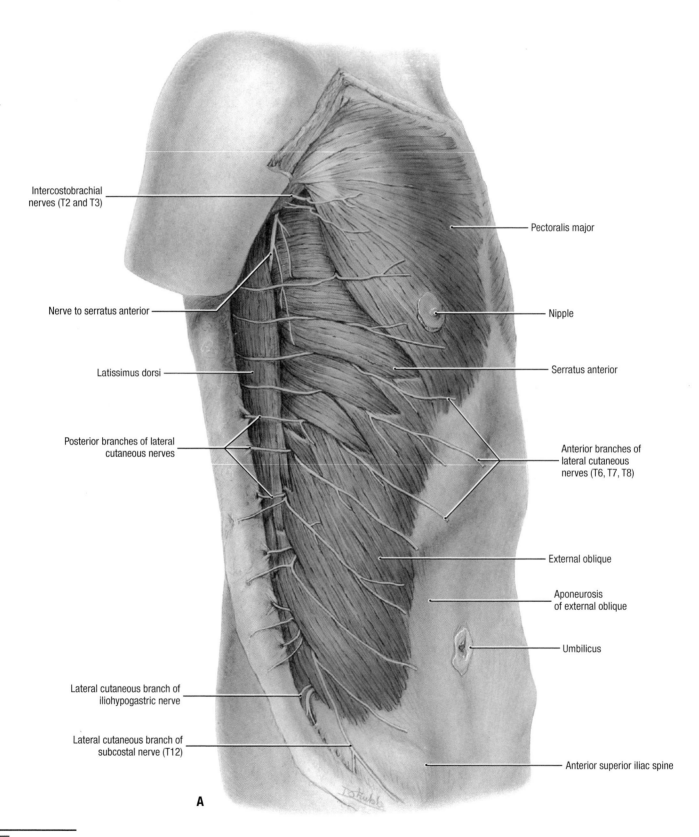

Intercostobrachial
nerves (T2 and T3)

Nerve to serratus anterior

Latissimus dorsi

Posterior branches of lateral
cutaneous nerves

Lateral cutaneous branch of
iliohypogastric nerve

Lateral cutaneous branch of
subcostal nerve (T12)

Pectoralis major

Nipple

Serratus anterior

Anterior branches of
lateral cutaneous
nerves (T6, T7, T8)

External oblique

Aponeurosis
of external oblique

Umbilicus

Anterior superior iliac spine

A

2.3 Trunk, lateral views

A. This superficial dissection shows the external oblique muscle and
lateral cutaneous nerves. Observe the interdigitations of the fibers of
the serratus anterior muscle with the external oblique muscle.

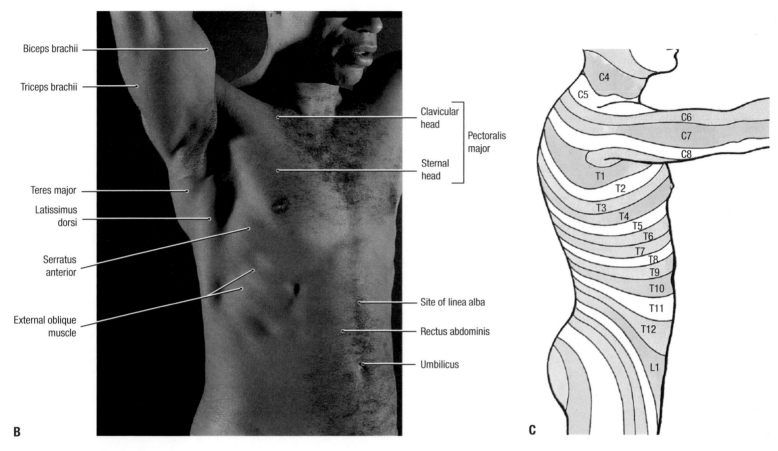

B. Surface anatomy. **C.** Dermatomes. A dermatome is the area of skin supplied by the sensory fibers of a single dorsal root. There is considerable overlapping of closely related dermatomes (e.g., T2, T3, and T4).

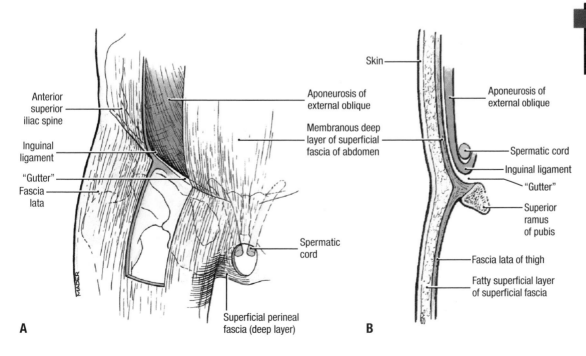

2.4 Membranous deep layer of superficial fascia

A. Anterior view, and **B.** Sagittal section.

OBSERVE:

1. The fascia blends with the fascia lata of the thigh, a finger breadth inferior to the inguinal ligament, forming a "gutter" that empties into the superficial perineal region;

2. The fascia follows along the penis and spermatic cord to the scrotum and continues posteriorly to blend with the deep layer of superficial fascia of the perineum.

3. The inguinal ligament lies between the anterior superior iliac spine and the pubic tubercle; this ligament is formed by the inferior margin of the aponeurosis of the external oblique muscle.

2.5 Surface anatomy of anterior abdominal wall, anterior view

OBSERVE:

1. The linea alba extends the full length of the anterior abdominal wall, from the xiphoid process to the symphysis pubis; the linea alba is formed by the interweaving of the aponeurotic fibers of the external, internal, and transversus abdominis muscles;
2. The right and left rectus abdominis muscles span from the pubic bone to the xiphoid process and costal cartilages of the 5th, 6th, and 7th ribs;
3. The linea semilunaris is located at the lateral border of the rectus abdominis muscle;
4. The transversely oriented tendinous intersections interrupt the continuity of the rectus abdominis muscle; these intersections are adherent to the anterior rectus sheath and seldom penetrate the full thickness of the muscle belly.

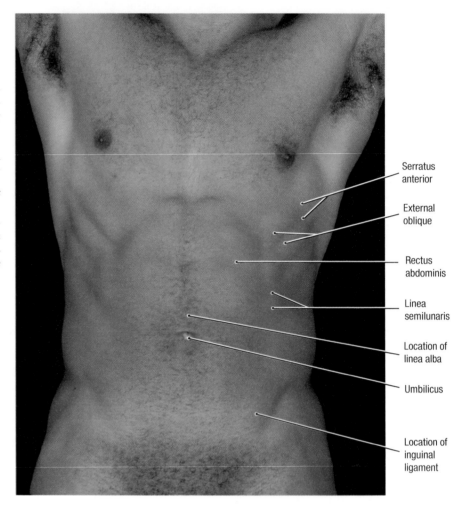

Serratus anterior

External oblique

Rectus abdominis

Linea semilunaris

Location of linea alba

Umbilicus

Location of inguinal ligament

Table 2.1 Principal Muscles of Anterolateral Abdominal Wall

Muscles	Origin	Insertion	Innervation	Action(s)
External oblique	External surfaces of 5th to 12th ribs	Linea alba, public tubercle, and anterior half of iliac crest	Inferior six thoracic nerves and subcostal nerve	Compress and support abdominal viscera; flex and rotate trunk
Internal oblique	Thoracolumbar fascia, anterior two-thirds of iliac crest, and lateral half of inguinal ligament	Inferior borders of 10th–12th ribs, linea alba, and pubis via conjoint tendon	Ventral rami of inferior six thoracic and first lumbar nerves	
Transverse abdominis	Internal surfaces of seventh to twelfth costal cartilages, thoracolumber fascia, iliac crest, and lateral third of inguinal ligament	Linea alba with aponeurosis of internal oblique, pubic crest, and pecten pubis via conjoint tendon		Compress and-supports abdominal viscera
Rectus abdominis	Pubic symphysis and pubic crest	Xiphoid process and fifth to seventh costal cartilages	Ventral rami of inferior six thoracic nerves	Flexes trunk and compresses abdominal viscera

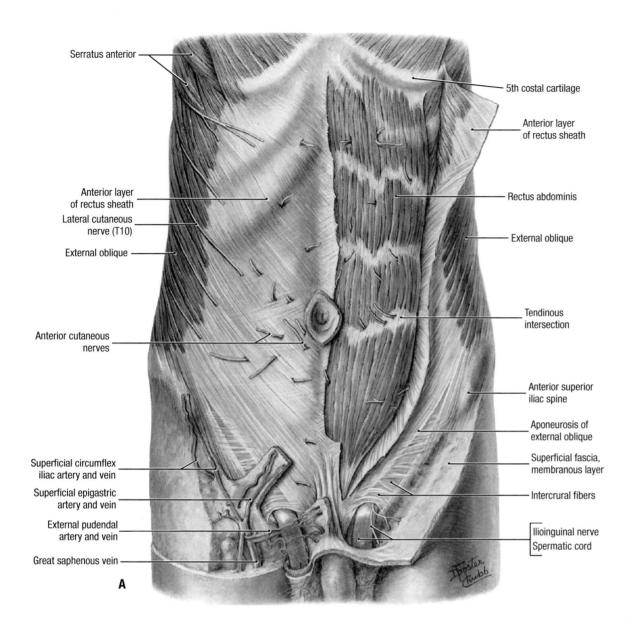

A

2.6　Anterior abdominal wall, superficial dissection, anterior view

A. Anterior abdominal wall. The anterior layer of rectus sheath is reflected on the left side. **B.** Superficial inguinal ring. The superficial inguinal ring is an oblique, triangular opening, 2 to 3 cm long; its central point is superior to the pubic tubercle.

OBSERVE IN **A**:
1. The anterior cutaneous nerves (T8 to T12) pierce the rectus abdominis muscle and anterior layer of its sheath; T10 supplies the region of the umbilicus;
2. In the fatty superficial layer of superficial fascia, the three superficial inguinal branches of the femoral artery (superficial circumflex iliac artery, superficial epigastric artery, and external pudendal artery) and the great (long) saphenous vein;
3. The spermatic cord and ilioinguinal nerve pass through the superficial inguinal ring.

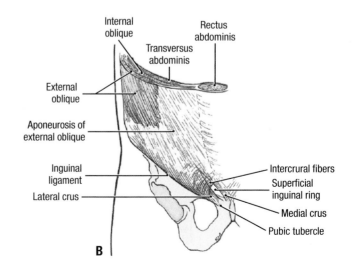

B

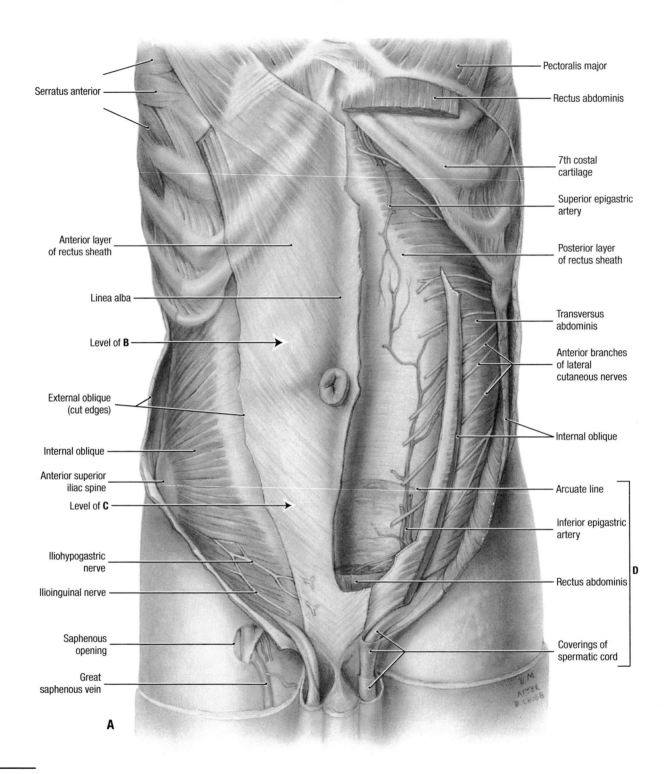

2.7   Anterior abdominal wall, deep dissection

A. Anterior view. On the right side, most of the external oblique muscle is excised. On the left, the rectus abdominis muscle is excised, and the internal oblique muscle is divided.

OBSERVE IN **A**:
1. The fibers of the internal oblique muscle run horizontally at the level of the anterior superior iliac spine, obliquely upward superior to this level, and obliquely downward inferior to it;
2. The arcuate line at the level of the anterior superior iliac spine;

3. The anastomosis between the superior and inferior epigastric arteries indirectly unites the arteries of the upper limb to those of the lower limb (subclavian to external iliac); *The anastomosis can become functionally patent because of slow occlusion of the aorta.*
4. The linea alba, usually indicated by a midline vertical skin groove, is a subcutaneous fibrous band extending from the sternum to the symphysis pubis.

B. Sheath of rectus abdominis (rectus sheath), transverse section superior to the umbilicus, as indicated in **A. C.** Sheath of rectus abdominis (rectus sheath), transverse section inferior to the umbilicus, as indicated in **A.**

OBSERVE IN **B** and **C**:

1. The aponeuroses of the external oblique, internal oblique, and transversus abdominis muscles are bilaminar;

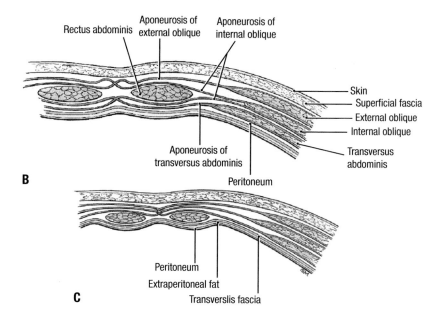

2. The decussation and interweaving of the aponeuroses, occurring at the linea alba, are from side to side and from superficial to deep;
3. Superior to the umbilicus, both anterior and posterior rectus sheaths are trilaminar. Anteriorly, there are the two layers of the aponeurosis of the external oblique muscle and the superficial layer of the aponeurosis of the internal oblique muscle. Posteriorly, there are the deep layer of the aponeurosis of the internal oblique muscle and two layers of the aponeurosis of the transversus abdominis muscle;
4. Approximately midway between the umbilicus and the symphysis pubis, all of the aponeuroses pass anterior to the rectus abdominis muscle; the posterior rectus sheath gradually ends at the arcuate line where the transversalis fascia comes into contact with the posterior aspect of the rectus abdominis muscle.

D. Posterior rectus sheath and inguinal canal, anterior view. The location of this dissection is indicated in **A.**

On the right: The external oblique and its aponeurosis are cut away to reveal the iliohypogastric and ilioinguinal nerves. The spermatic cord is pulled medially to reveal the genital branch of the genitofemoral nerve.

On the left: The internal oblique is divided and reflected, and a section of the spermatic cord is excised, revealing fibers of internal oblique and transversus abdominis, arching medially to form the aponeurotic conjoint tendon.

Coverings of the cord: (a) internal spermatic fascia, derived from fascia transversalis; (b) cremaster muscle and fascia, from internal oblique and transversus abdominis; (c) external spermatic fascia, from external oblique aponeurosis.

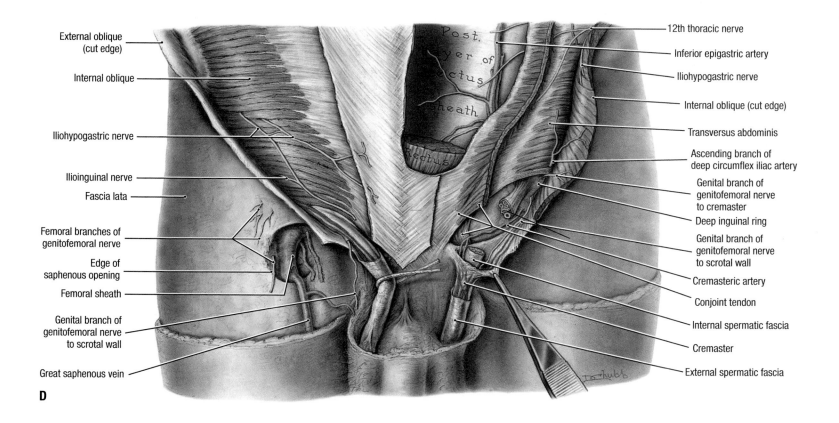

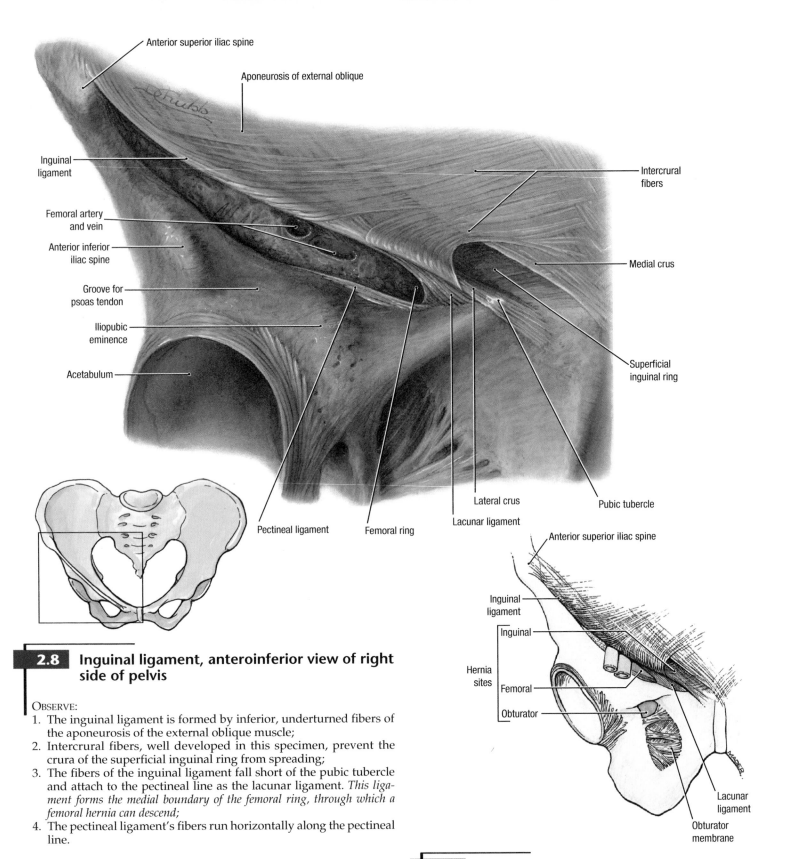

Anterior superior iliac spine

Aponeurosis of external oblique

Inguinal ligament

Femoral artery and vein

Anterior inferior iliac spine

Groove for psoas tendon

Iliopubic eminence

Acetabulum

Intercrural fibers

Medial crus

Superficial inguinal ring

Lateral crus

Pubic tubercle

Lacunar ligament

Pectineal ligament

Femoral ring

Anterior superior iliac spine

Inguinal ligament

Hernia sites

Inguinal

Femoral

Obturator

Lacunar ligament

Obturator membrane

2.8   **Inguinal ligament, anteroinferior view of right side of pelvis**

OBSERVE:
1. The inguinal ligament is formed by inferior, underturned fibers of the aponeurosis of the external oblique muscle;
2. Intercrural fibers, well developed in this specimen, prevent the crura of the superficial inguinal ring from spreading;
3. The fibers of the inguinal ligament fall short of the pubic tubercle and attach to the pectineal line as the lacunar ligament. *This ligament forms the medial boundary of the femoral ring, through which a femoral hernia can descend;*
4. The pectineal ligament's fibers run horizontally along the pectineal line.

2.9   **Three hernia sites, anteroinferior view**

Observe three hernial sites of clinical significance and the structures separating them. Relate this diagram to Figure 2.8.

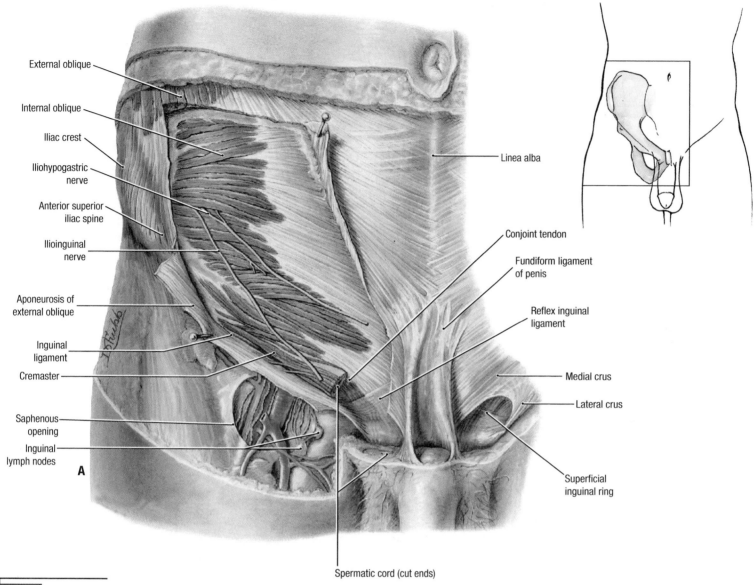

Labels (clockwise from top left): External oblique, Internal oblique, Iliac crest, Iliohypogastric nerve, Anterior superior iliac spine, Ilioinguinal nerve, Aponeurosis of external oblique, Inguinal ligament, Cremaster, Saphenous opening, Inguinal lymph nodes, **A**, Spermatic cord (cut ends), Linea alba, Conjoint tendon, Fundiform ligament of penis, Reflex inguinal ligament, Medial crus, Lateral crus, Superficial inguinal ring.

2.10 Inguinal region of male-I, anterior view

A. Male inguinal region. Part of the aponeurosis of the external oblique muscle is cut away, and the spermatic cord is cut short. **B.** Internal oblique and conjoint tendon. The inferior fibers of the internal oblique arch inferiorly to attach to the pubis, along with similarly arching fibers of the transversus abdominis, to form the conjoint tendon.

OBSERVE IN **A**:
1. The laminated, fundiform ligament of the penis descends to the junction of the fixed and mobile parts of the organ;
2. The reflex inguinal ligament, formed by aponeurotic fibers of the external oblique muscle, lies anterior to the conjoint tendon. The conjoint tendon is formed by the aponeurosis of the internal oblique and transversus abdominis muscles;
3. Only two structures course between the external and internal oblique muscles, namely, the iliohypogastric and ilioinguinal branches of the 1st lumbar nerve. They are sensory from this point to their terminations;
4. The fleshy fibers of the internal oblique muscle run horizontally at the level of the anterior superior iliac spine, pass superomedially from the iliac crest, and arch inferomedially from the inguinal ligament;
5. The cremaster muscle covers the spermatic cord and fills the arched space between conjoint tendon and inguinal ligament;
6. At the level of the umbilicus, the aponeurosis of the external oblique muscle blends with the aponeurosis of the internal oblique muscle near the lateral border of the rectus abdominis muscle; in the suprapubic region, it is free as far as the median plane.

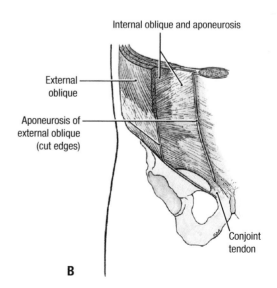

Labels: Internal oblique and aponeurosis, External oblique, Aponeurosis of external oblique (cut edges), Conjoint tendon, **B**

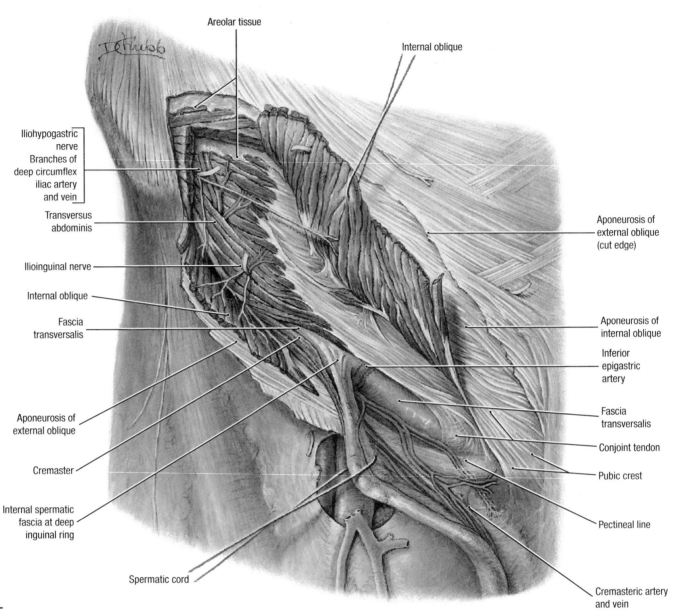

Areolar tissue

Internal oblique

Iliohypogastric nerve

Branches of deep circumflex iliac artery and vein

Transversus abdominis

Ilioinguinal nerve

Internal oblique

Fascia transversalis

Aponeurosis of external oblique

Cremaster

Internal spermatic fascia at deep inguinal ring

Spermatic cord

Aponeurosis of external oblique (cut edge)

Aponeurosis of internal oblique

Inferior epigastric artery

Fascia transversalis

Conjoint tendon

Pubic crest

Pectineal line

Cremasteric artery and vein

2.11   Inguinal region of male-II, anterior view

The internal oblique muscle is reflected, and the spermatic cord is retracted.

OBSERVE:
1. The transversus abdominis muscle in this region takes the same inferomedial direction as the fibers of the external oblique aponeurosis and internal oblique muscle;
2. The internal oblique portion of the conjoint tendon is attached to the pubic crest, and the transversus portion extends laterally along the pectineal line;
3. The conjoint tendon blends with the fascia transversalis;
4. The iliohypogastric and ilioinguinal nerves supply the fibers of the internal oblique and transversus abdominis muscles, which control the conjoint tendon;
5. The fascia transversalis is evaginated to form the tubular internal spermatic fascia. The mouth of the tube, called the deep inguinal ring, is situated lateral to the inferior epigastric vessels;
6. The cremasteric artery (a branch of the inferior epigastric artery) supplies the testes, along with the testicular artery and the artery of the deferent duct;

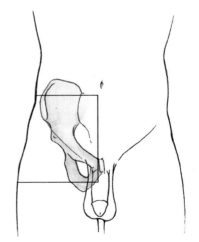

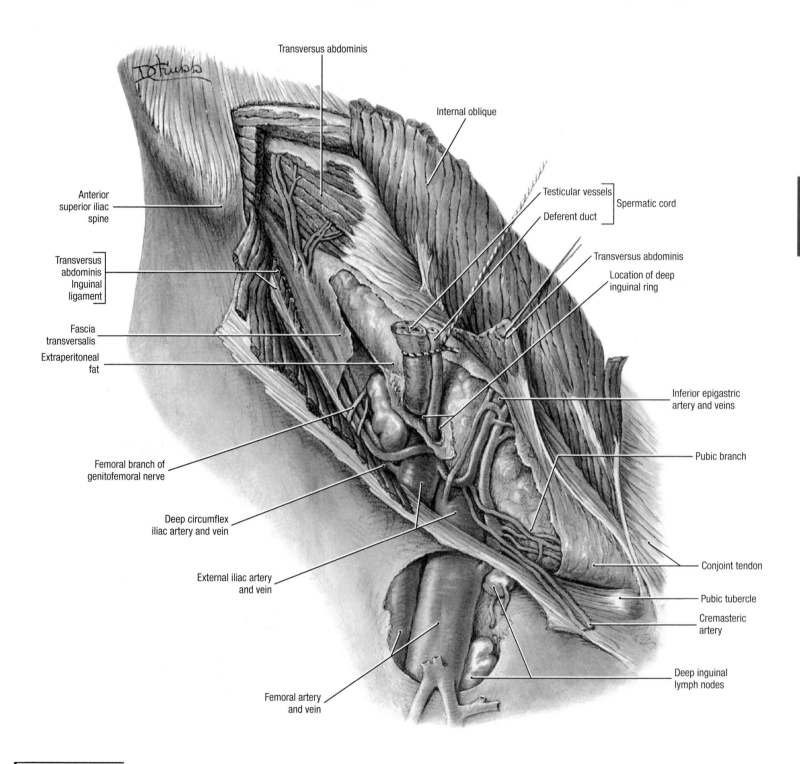

Transversus abdominis

Internal oblique

Anterior superior iliac spine

Transversus abdominis Inguinal ligament

Fascia transversalis

Extraperitoneal fat

Femoral branch of genitofemoral nerve

Deep circumflex iliac artery and vein

External iliac artery and vein

Femoral artery and vein

Testicular vessels ⎫ Spermatic cord
Deferent duct ⎭

Transversus abdominis

Location of deep inguinal ring

Inferior epigastric artery and veins

Pubic branch

Conjoint tendon

Pubic tubercle

Cremasteric artery

Deep inguinal lymph nodes

2.12 **Inguinal region of male-III, anterior view**

The inguinal part of the transversus abdominis muscle and fascia transversalis is partially cut away, and the spermatic cord is excised. For orientation of specimen, see drawing in Figure 2.11.

OBSERVE:
1. The inferior limit of the peritoneal sac, demarcated by the extraperitoneal fat, lies some distance superior to the inguinal ligament laterally but close to it medially;
2. The location of the deep inguinal ring, a finger breadth superior to

the inguinal ligament at the midpoint between the anterior superior iliac spine and pubic tubercle;
3. The testicular vessels and deferent duct (retracted) part company at the deep inguinal ring;
4. The proximity of the external iliac artery and vein to the inguinal canal;
5. The only two branches of the external iliac artery, are the deep circumflex iliac and inferior epigastric arteries. Note also the cremasteric and pubic branches of the latter.

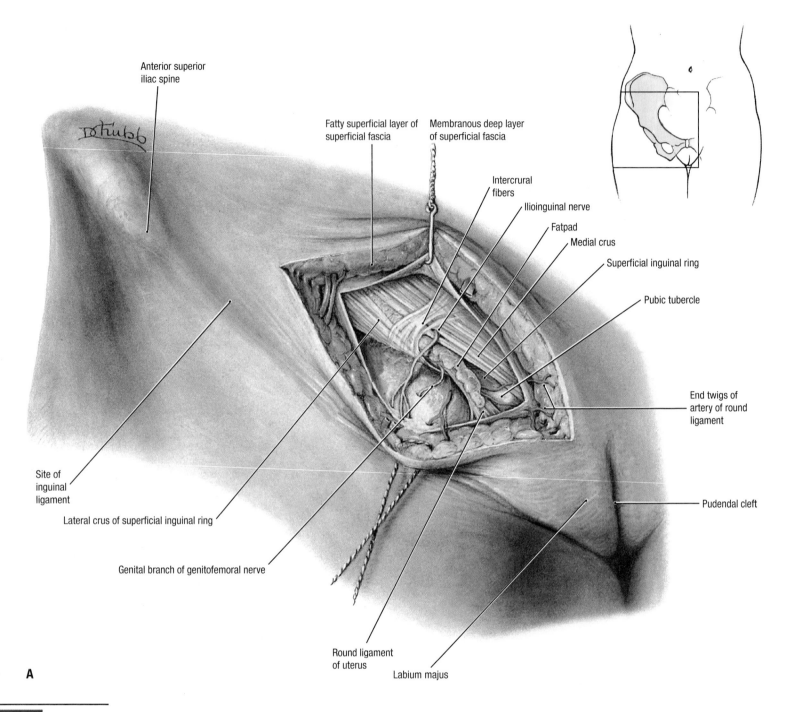

Anterior superior
iliac spine

Fatty superficial layer of
superficial fascia

Membranous deep layer
of superficial fascia

Intercrural
fibers

Ilioinguinal nerve

Fatpad

Medial crus

Superficial inguinal ring

Pubic tubercle

End twigs of
artery of round
ligament

Pudendal cleft

Site of
inguinal
ligament

Lateral crus of superficial inguinal ring

Genital branch of genitofemoral nerve

Round ligament
of uterus

Labium majus

A

2.13 Female inguinal canal

Progressive dissections of the female inguinal canal (**A–D**), anterior
views.

OBSERVE:

1. In **A,** the small superficial inguinal ring and its crura are prevented
from spreading by the intercrural fibers;
2. Passing through the superficial inguinal ring are: (a) the round ligament of the uterus, (b) a closely applied fatpad, (c) the genital
branch of the genitofemoral nerve, and (d) the artery of the round
ligament of the uterus;

3. The ilioinguinal nerve perforates the medial crus of the superficial
inguinal ring;
4. In **B,** the cremaster muscle does not extend beyond the superficial
inguinal ring **(A);**
5. In **C,** the round ligament breaks up into strands as it leaves the inguinal canal and approaches the labium majus;
6. In **D,** the close relationship of the external iliac artery and vein to
the inguinal canal.

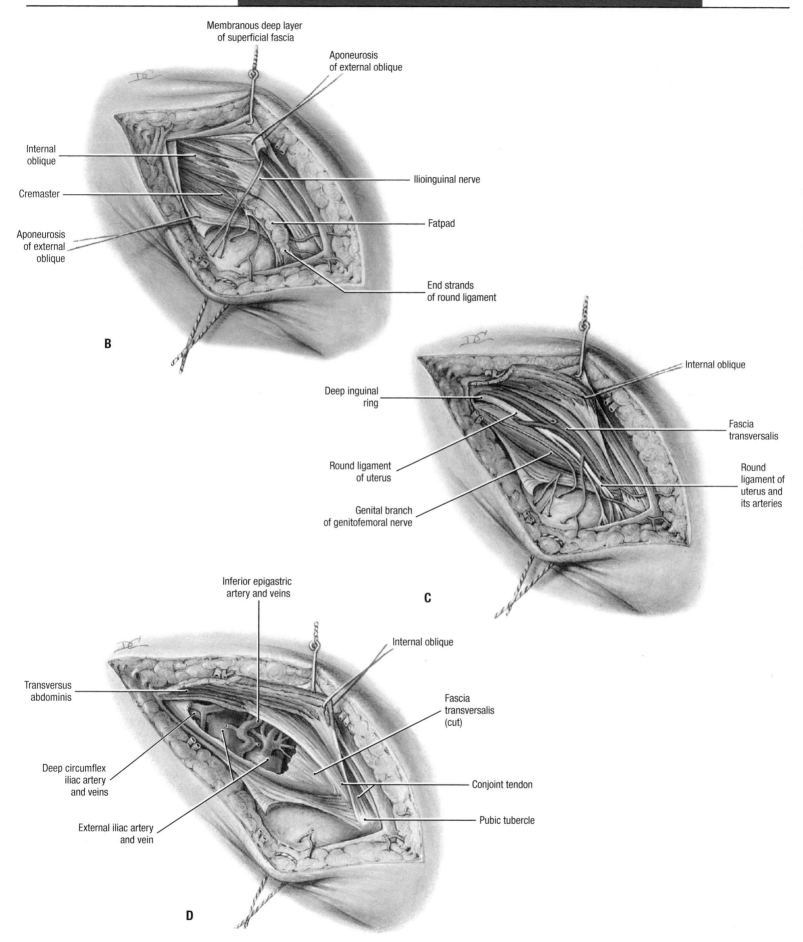

Membranous deep layer
of superficial fascia

Aponeurosis
of external oblique

Internal
oblique

Ilioinguinal nerve

Cremaster

Fatpad

Aponeurosis
of external
oblique

End strands
of round ligament

B

Internal oblique

Deep inguinal
ring

Fascia
transversalis

Round ligament
of uterus

Round
ligament of
uterus and
its arteries

Genital branch
of genitofemoral nerve

C

Inferior epigastric
artery and veins

Internal oblique

Transversus
abdominis

Fascia
transversalis
(cut)

Deep circumflex
iliac artery
and veins

Conjoint tendon

External iliac artery
and vein

Pubic tubercle

D

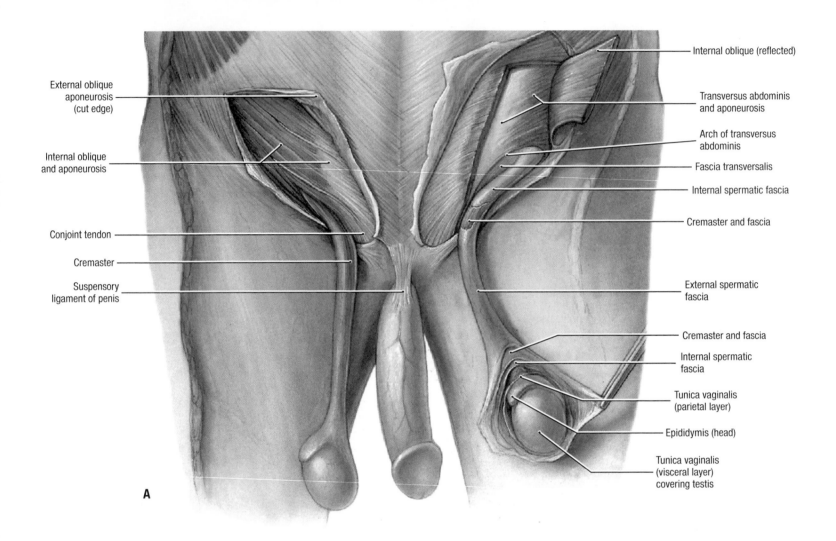

External oblique
aponeurosis
(cut edge)

Internal oblique
and aponeurosis

Conjoint tendon

Cremaster

Suspensory
ligament of penis

Internal oblique (reflected)

Transversus abdominis
and aponeurosis

Arch of transversus
abdominis

Fascia transversalis

Internal spermatic fascia

Cremaster and fascia

External spermatic
fascia

Cremaster and fascia

Internal spermatic
fascia

Tunica vaginalis
(parietal layer)

Epididymis (head)

Tunica vaginalis
(visceral layer)
covering testis

A

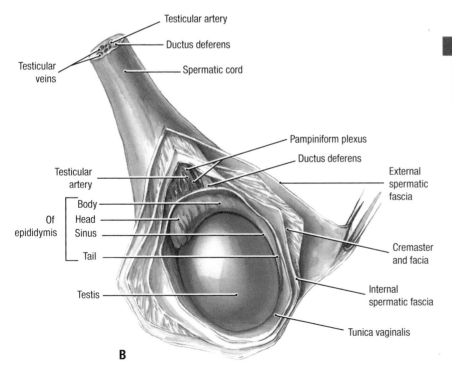

Testicular artery

Ductus deferens

Spermatic cord

Testicular
veins

Testicular
artery

Of
epididymis { Body / Head / Sinus / Tail }

Testis

Pampiniform plexus

Ductus deferens

External
spermatic
fascia

Cremaster
and facia

Internal
spermatic fascia

Tunica vaginalis

B

2.14 Coverings of spermatic cord and testis

A. Anterior view. **B.** Sequential dissection of coverings of
testis, anterior view.

OBSERVE IN **A** (ON THE LEFT SIDE OF THE BODY):
1. The aponeurosis of the external oblique muscle is incised
   and reflected, revealing the deeper internal oblique muscle; the external spermatic fascia is from the aponeurosis
   of the external oblique;
2. A window has been made by cutting and reflecting the internal oblique muscle laterally to expose the deeper
   transversus abdominis muscle and aponeurosis. The arch
   of the transversus abdominis muscle and aponeurosis, laterally, arch superior to the spermatic cord and, medially,
   terminate posterior to it;
3. The cremaster muscle and fascia are derived from the internal oblique and transversus abdominis;
4. The fascia transversalis is evaginated to form the tubular
   internal spermatic fascia;
5. All of the layers covering the testis have been cut open sequentially: the external spermatic fascia, the cremaster
   muscle and fascia, the internal spermatic fascia, and the
   visceral and parietal layers of the tunica vaginalis of the
   testis.

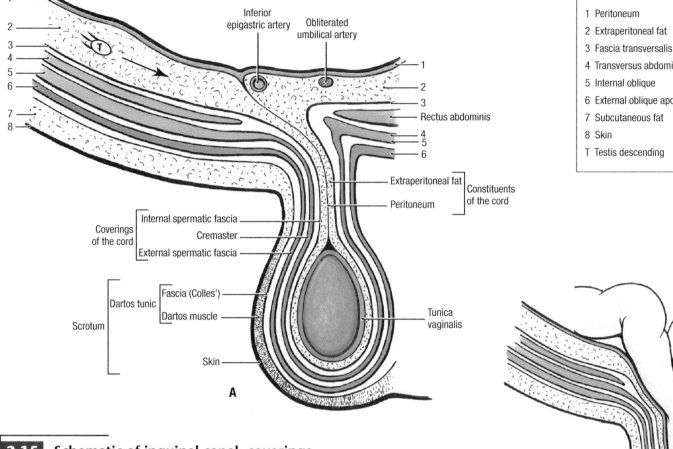

1 Peritoneum
2 Extraperitoneal fat
3 Fascia transversalis
4 Transversus abdominis
5 Internal oblique
6 External oblique aponearosis
7 Subcutaneous fat
8 Skin
T Testis descending

Inferior epigastric artery
Obliterated umbilical artery

Rectus abdominis

Extraperitoneal fat ⎫ Constituents
Peritoneum ⎭ of the cord

Coverings of the cord
Internal spermatic fascia
Cremaster
External spermatic fascia

Scrotum
Dartos tunic
Fascia (Colles')
Dartos muscle

Tunica vaginalis

Skin

A

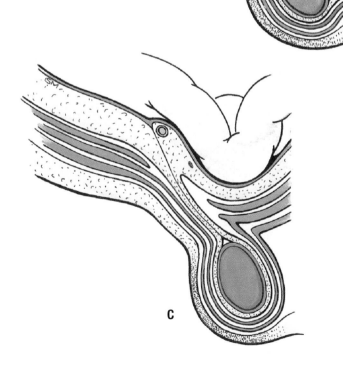

B

C

2.15 Schematic of inguinal canal, coverings of spermatic cord and testes, and inguinal hernias

A. Horizontal section. The scrotum and testis are assumed to have been raised to the level of the superficial inguinal ring. **B.** Indirect inguinal hernia. **C.** Direct inguinal hernia.

OBSERVE:

1. The eight layers of the abdominal wall and their three evaginations: scrotum, coverings of the spermatic cord, and constituents of the cord;
2. The external spermatic fascia is derived from the fascia of the external oblique muscle;
3. The cremaster muscle and fascia are derived from the internal oblique and transversus abdominis muscles;
4. The internal spermatic fascia is derived from transversalis fascia;
5. The tunica vaginalis is derived from peritoneum;
6. The dartos tunic consists of a) superficial (Colles') fascia that is continuous with the subcutaneous tissue of the abdomen, but lacks fat, and b) smooth muscle fibers of dartos muscle;
7. The deep inguinal ring is lateral to the inferior epigastric artery. *Indirect inguinal hernias pass through this ring, with the sac following the course of the spermatic cord* **(B)**. *Direct inguinal hernias bulge directly through the abdominal wall, medial to the inferior epigastric artery* **(C).**

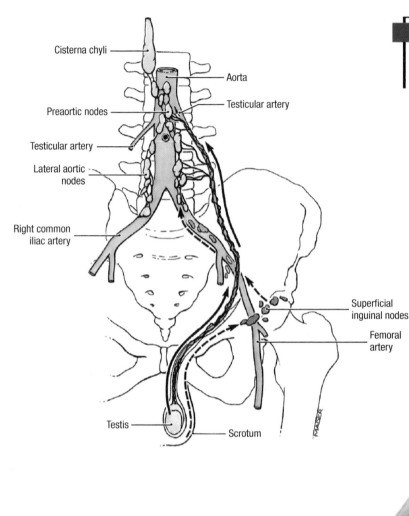

2.16 Lymphatic drainage of the testis and scrotum, schematic anterior view

Note the lymphatic drainage of the testis into the lateral and preaortic lymph nodes. The lymph vessels originate just deep to the tunica vaginalis and from within the testis, and then follow the spermatic cord and testicular vessels to the aorta. The scrotal lymphatics drain into the superficial inguinal nodes.

2.17 Testis and spermatic cord

A. Blood supply of the testis, posterior view. Note the anastomosis between the three arteries. There are three groups of longitudinal veins: (a) around the testicular artery, (b) medial to the ductus deferens with the artery of the ductus deferens, and (c) lateral to the ductus deferens. Observe the epididymis displaced slightly laterally and the ductus deferens lying posteromedial to the testis. **B.** Testis, lateral view. The tunica vaginalis testis has been incised longitudinally to expose its cavity, surrounding the testis anteriorly and laterally, and extending between the testis and epididymis at the sinus of the epididymis. Note the epididymis, lying posterolateral to the testis. It indicates to which side a testis belongs, for it is on the right side of the right testis, and the left side of the left testis. **C.** Coverings of the spermatic cord, lateral view. **D.** Epididymis, lateral view. Note the eight efferent ductules, uniting the epididymis to the superior pole of the testis. **E.** Structure of the epididymis and testis, schematic vertical section. Note the pyramidal compartments of the seminiferous tubules, shown semidiagrammatically; each of the 250 compartments contains two or three hair-like seminiferous tubules that join in the mediastinum testis to form a rete.

A

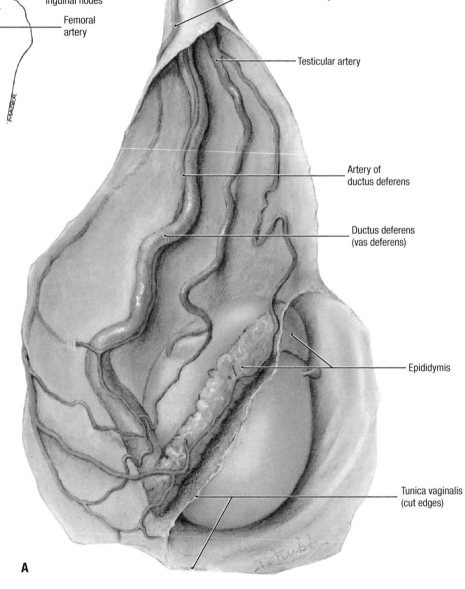

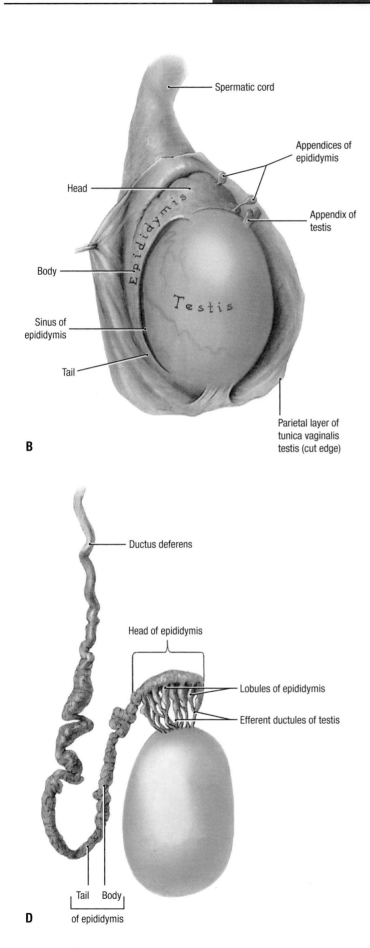

B

Spermatic cord

Appendices of
epididymis

Head

Appendix of
testis

Body

Sinus of
epididymis

Tail

Parietal layer of
tunica vaginalis
testis (cut edge)

Epididymis

Testis

Ductus deferens

Head of epididymis

Lobules of epididymis

Efferent ductules of testis

Tail   Body
of epididymis

D

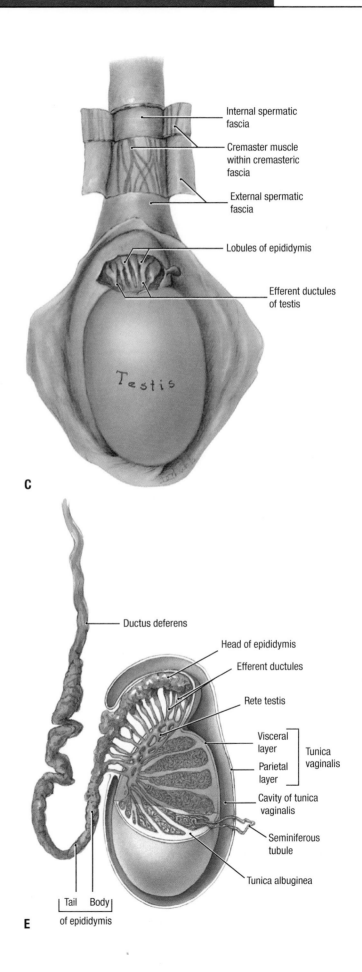

C

Internal spermatic
fascia

Cremaster muscle
within cremasteric
fascia

External spermatic
fascia

Lobules of epididymis

Efferent ductules
of testis

Testis

Ductus deferens

Head of epididymis

Efferent ductules

Rete testis

Visceral
layer

Parietal
layer

Tunica
vaginalis

Cavity of tunica
vaginalis

Seminiferous
tubule

Tunica albuginea

Tail   Body
of epididymis

E

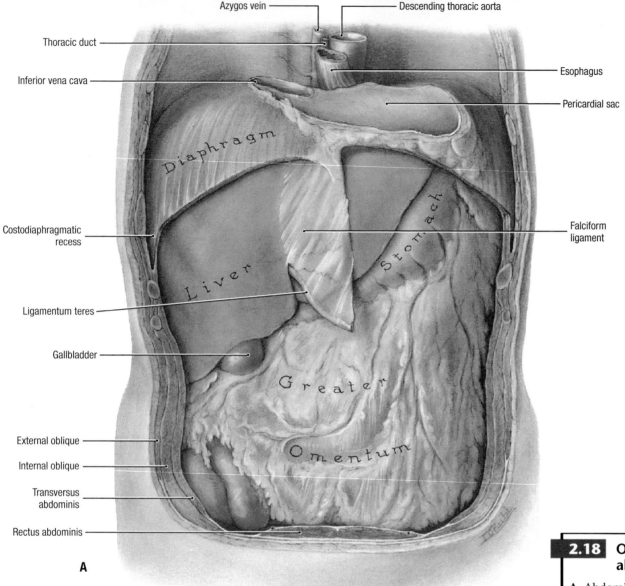

Azygos vein — Descending thoracic aorta
Thoracic duct —
Inferior vena cava —
— Esophagus
— Pericardial sac
Diaphragm
Costodiaphragmatic recess —
— Falciform ligament
Liver
Stomach
Ligamentum teres —
Gallbladder —
Greater
External oblique —
Internal oblique —
Omentum
Transversus abdominis —
Rectus abdominis —

A

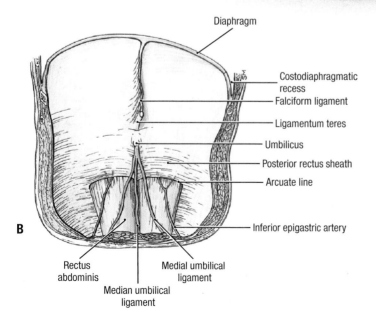

Diaphragm

Costodiaphragmatic recess
Falciform ligament
Ligamentum teres
Umbilicus
Posterior rectus sheath
Arcuate line

Inferior epigastric artery

Rectus abdominis
Medial umbilical ligament
Median umbilical ligament

B

2.18   Opening the abdominal cavity

A. Abdominal contents, undisturbed, anterior view. **B.** Posterior aspect of anterior abdominal wall, cut from **A.** Note the attachment of the falciform ligament and ligamentum teres to the abdominal wall; the ligamentum teres (the obliterated umbilical vein); the median umbilical ligament (the remnant of the urachus) the medial umbilical ligament (the obliterated umbilical artery); and the inferior epigastric artery (lateral umbilical ligament).

OBSERVE IN **A**:
1. The falciform ligament, with the ligamentum teres in its free edge, is severed at its attachment to the abdominal wall and diaphragm in the median plane. Its attachment to the liver is to the right of the median plane; it resists displacement of the liver to the right;
2. The gallbladder projects inferior to the sharp, inferior border of the liver;
3. The internal oblique muscle is the thickest of the three flat abdominal muscles;
4. The costodiaphragmatic recesses *(right and left)* of the pleural cavities separates the diaphragm and superior abdominal viscera from the body wall;
5. Two thirds of the pericardial sac lies to the left of the median plane; its apex, the lowest and leftmost point, overlies the stomach.

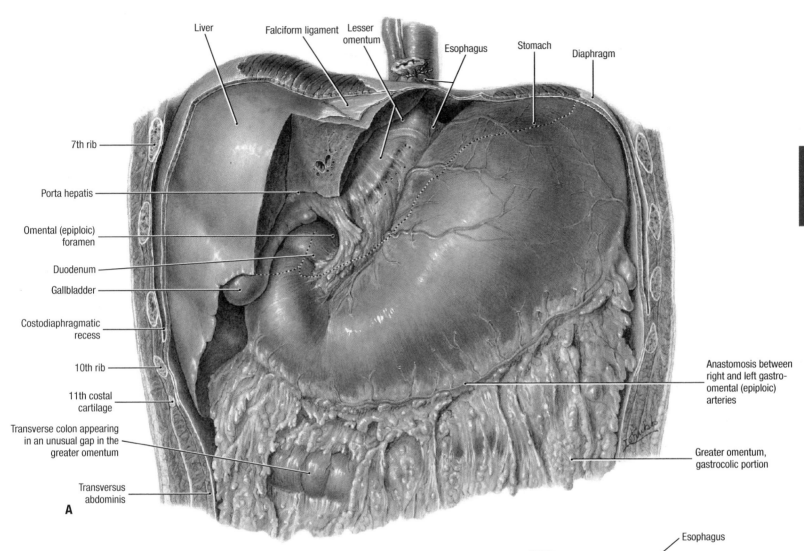

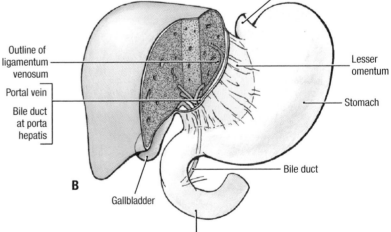

2.19　**Stomach and omenta**

A. The lesser and greater omenta, anterior view. The stomach is inflated with air, and the left part of the liver is cut away, but the outline of the liver is demarcated with a dotted line. **B.** The lesser omentum. Two sagittal cuts have been made through the liver: one at the fissure for the ligamentum venosum, and the other at the right limit of the porta hepatis. These two cuts have been joined by a coronal cut. Note that the lesser omentum may be regarded as the "mesentery" of the bile passages because they occupy its free edge.

OBSERVE IN **A**:

1. During development, the pyloric end of the stomach moved to the right, to lie inferoposterior to the gallbladder;
2. The first, or superior, part of the duodenum is posterior to the arrowhead, almost occluding the omental (epiploic) foremen (mouth of the lesser sac);
3. The gallbladder, followed superiorly, leads to the free margin of the lesser omentum, and serves as a guide to the epiploic foremen, which lies posterior to that free margin;
4. The lesser omentum passes from the lesser curvature of the stomach and first inch of the duodenum to the fissure for the ligamentum venosum **(B)** and porta hepatis.

5. This omentum, thickened at its free margin but thin elsewhere, is much perforated, and the caudate lobe of the liver is visible through it;
6. The greater omentum hangs from the greater curvature of the stomach;
7. The right dome of the diaphragm rises higher than the left dome.

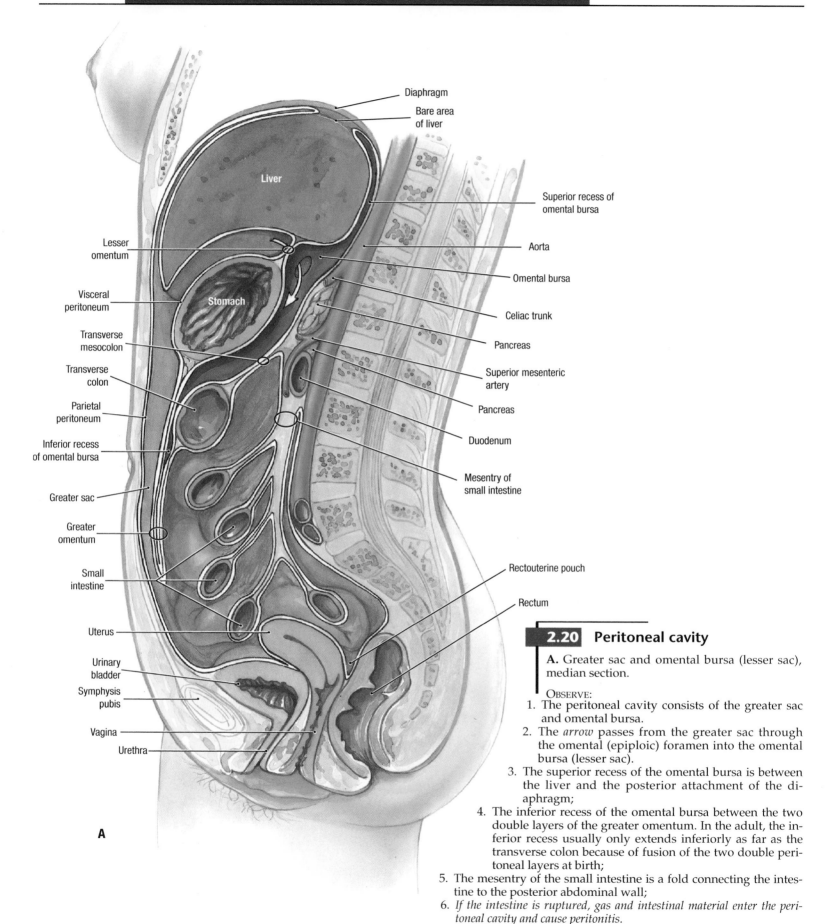

2.20   Peritoneal cavity

A. Greater sac and omental bursa (lesser sac), median section.

OBSERVE:

1. The peritoneal cavity consists of the greater sac and omental bursa.
2. The *arrow* passes from the greater sac through the omental (epiploic) foramen into the omental bursa (lesser sac).
3. The superior recess of the omental bursa is between the liver and the posterior attachment of the diaphragm;
4. The inferior recess of the omental bursa between the two double layers of the greater omentum. In the adult, the inferior recess usually only extends inferiorly as far as the transverse colon because of fusion of the two double peritoneal layers at birth;
5. The mesentery of the small intestine is a fold connecting the intestine to the posterior abdominal wall;
6. *If the intestine is ruptured, gas and intestinal material enter the peritoneal cavity and cause peritonitis.*

B. Omental bursa, median section.

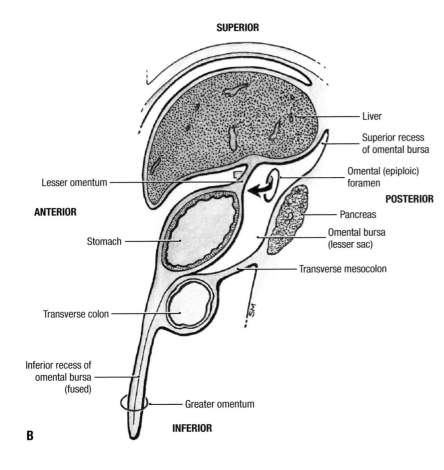

SUPERIOR

Liver

Superior recess
of omental bursa

Omental (epiploic)
foramen

POSTERIOR

Lesser omentum

ANTERIOR

Pancreas

Stomach

Omental bursa
(lesser sac)

Transverse mesocolon

Transverse colon

Inferior recess of
omental bursa
(fused)

Greater omentum

INFERIOR

B

2.21 Omental bursa, transverse section, inferior view

The *arrow* passes from the greater sac through the omental foramen into the omental bursa (lesser sac).

OBSERVE:

1. The gastrosplenic and splenorenal ligaments suspend the spleen between the stomach and the kidney; the ligaments form a pedicle (stalk), through which blood vessels run to and from the hilum of the spleen;
2. The gastrosplenic and splenorenal ligaments are double layers of peritoneum that form the left boundary of the omental bursa (lesser sac); the inner layer consists of peritoneum lining the omental bursa, and the outer layer consists of peritoneum lining the peritoneal cavity (greater sac).

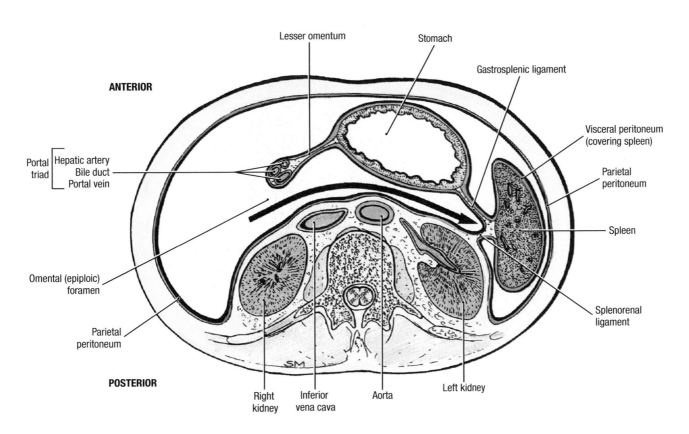

Lesser omentum

Stomach

Gastrosplenic ligament

ANTERIOR

Visceral peritoneum
(covering spleen)

Portal triad — Hepatic artery
Bile duct
Portal vein

Parietal
peritoneum

Spleen

Omental (epiploic)
foramen

Splenorenal
ligament

Parietal
peritoneum

POSTERIOR

Right
kidney

Inferior
vena cava

Aorta

Left kidney

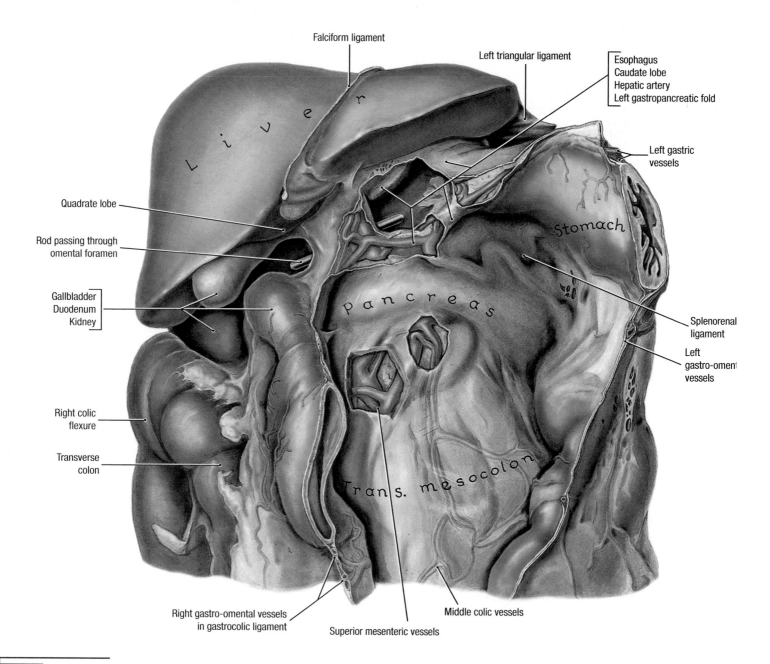

Falciform ligament

Left triangular ligament

Esophagus
Caudate lobe
Hepatic artery
Left gastropancreatic fold

Left gastric vessels

Quadrate lobe

Rod passing through omental foramen

Gallbladder
Duodenum
Kidney

Stomach

Pancreas

Splenorenal ligament

Left gastro-omental vessels

Right colic flexure

Transverse colon

Trans. mesocolon

Right gastro-omental vessels in gastrocolic ligament

Superior mesenteric vessels

Middle colic vessels

2.22 Omental bursa, opened, anterior view

The anterior wall of the bursa, consisting of the stomach with its two omenta and the vessels along its curvatures, has been sectioned sagittally; the two parts have been turned to the left and right.

OBSERVE:

1. The body of the stomach on the left side, and the pyloric part and the first part of the duodenum on the right;

2. The right kidney forms the posterior wall of the hepatorenal pouch; the rod passes through the omental foramen into the omental bursa;

3. The pancreas lies somewhat horizontally on the posterior wall of the bursa.

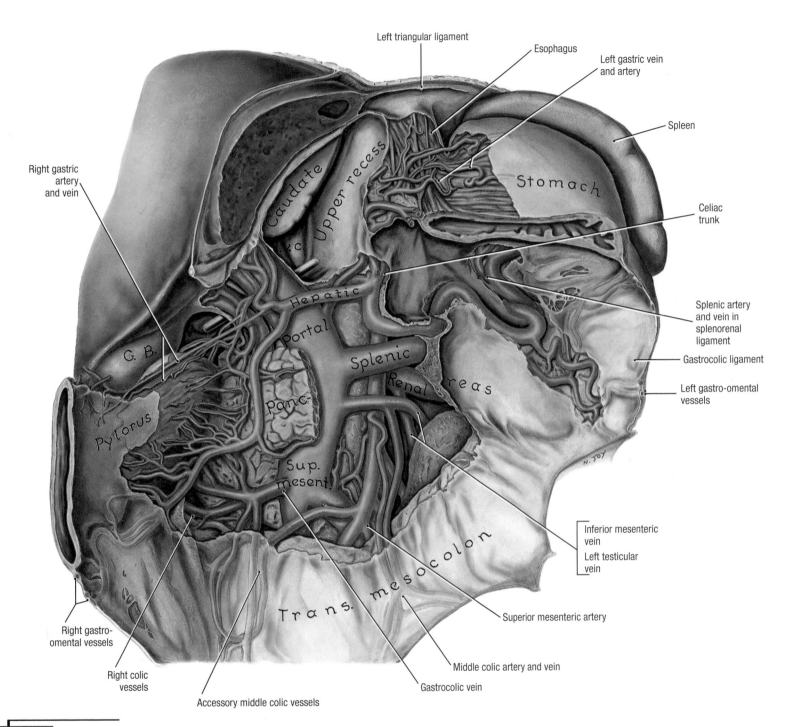

Left triangular ligament
Esophagus
Left gastric vein and artery
Spleen
Right gastric artery and vein
Caudate
Upper recess
Stomach
Celiac trunk
Hepatic
Portal
Splenic
Splenic artery and vein in splenorenal ligament
Renal
reas
Gastrocolic ligament
G. B.
Panc-
Left gastro-omental vessels
Pylorus
Sup. mesent.
Inferior mesenteric vein
Left testicular vein
Trans. mesocolon
N. JOY
Right gastro-omental vessels
Superior mesenteric artery
Middle colic artery and vein
Right colic vessels
Gastrocolic vein
Accessory middle colic vessels

2.23   Posterior wall of omental bursa, anterior view

The peritoneum of the posterior wall has mostly been removed, and a section of the pancreas has been excised.

OBSERVE:
1. The rod passes through the omental foramen;
2. The esophageal branches of the left gastric vessels, and the anterior and posterior vagal trunks applied to the esophagus;

3. The celiac trunk, from which the left gastric artery arches superiorly; the splenic artery runs tortuously to the left, and the hepatic artery runs to the right, passing anterior to the portal vein;
4. The portal vein, formed posterior to the neck of the pancreas by the union of the superior mesenteric and splenic veins, with the inferior mesenteric vein joining at or near the angle of union.

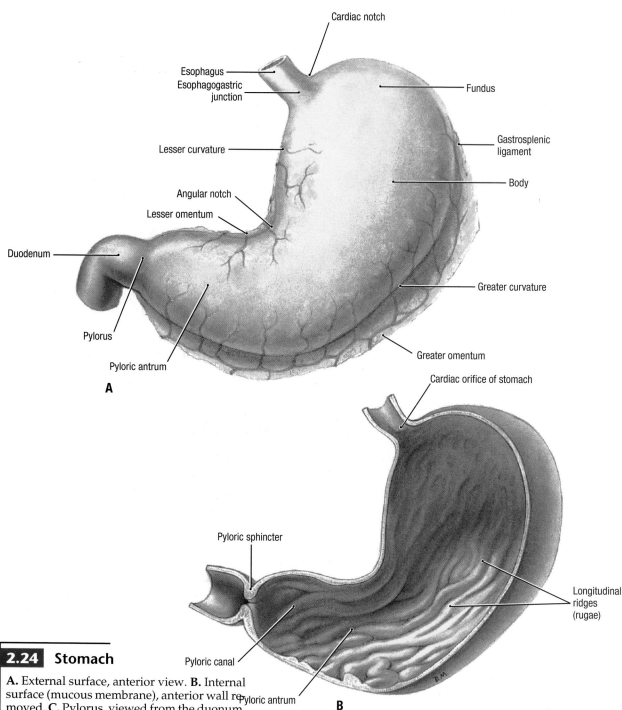

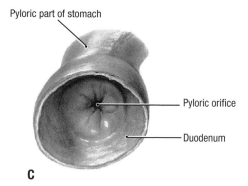

2.24 Stomach

A. External surface, anterior view. **B.** Internal surface (mucous membrane), anterior wall removed. **C.** Pylorus, viewed from the duonum.

OBSERVE:

1. The esophagogastric junction, usually located to the left of the midline, at the 11th thoracic vertebra, and the pylorus, usually located at the L1 vertebral level to the right of the midline at the transpyloric plane;
2. The angular notch separates the body from the pyloric region of the stomach; the pyloric sphincter is a ring of circular muscle at the junction of the stomach and duodenum;
3. The lesser omentum attaches to the lesser curvature of the stomach, and the continuous greater omentum and gastrosplenic ligament attaches to the greater curvature of the stomach;
4. Along the lesser curvature, several longitudinal ridges extend from the esophagus to the pylorus; elsewhere, the mucous membrane is wrinkled when the stomach is empty;
5. The pylorus projects into the 1st (superior) part of the duodenum. The first 4 cm of the duodenum have no plicae circulares (circular folds), but the mucous membrane may be ridged.

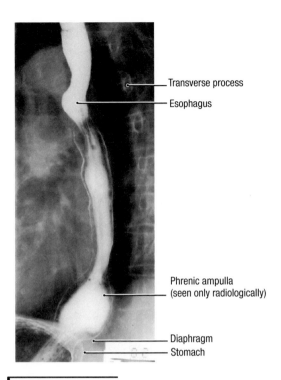

Transverse process
Esophagus

Phrenic ampulla
(seen only radiologically)

Diaphragm
Stomach

2.25 **Radiograph of esophagus, lateral view**

The esophagus seen after swallowing barium. The esophageal (phrenic) ampulla is the distensible portion of the esophagus seen only radiologically.

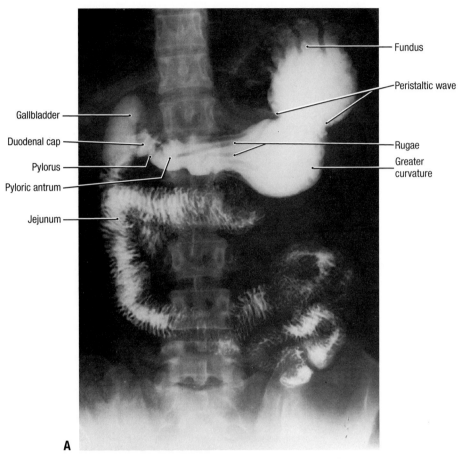

Gallbladder
Duodenal cap
Pylorus
Pyloric antrum
Jejunum

Fundus
Peristaltic wave
Rugae
Greater curvature

A

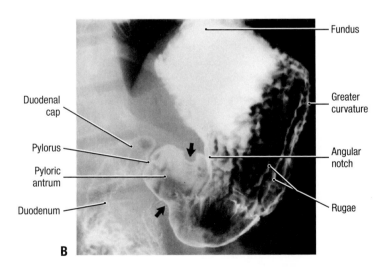

Duodenal cap
Pylorus
Pyloric antrum
Duodenum

Fundus
Greater curvature
Angular notch
Rugae

B

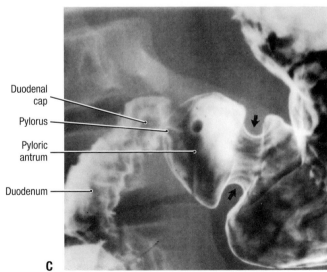

Duodenal cap
Pylorus
Pyloric antrum
Duodenum

C

2.26 **Radiographs of stomach, small intestine, and gallbladder**

A. The stomach, small intestine, and gallbladder, anterior view. **B.** Radiograph of the stomach and small intestine after barium ingestion, anterior view. Observe the longitudinal ridges of mucous membrane (rugae); the angular notch; a peristaltic wave (arrowheads); the pylorus; the duodenal cap; the feathery appearance of barium in the small intestine; and the relationship of the gallbladder to the first part of the duodenum. **C.** Radiograph of pyloric region of stomach and proximal duodenum, anterior view.

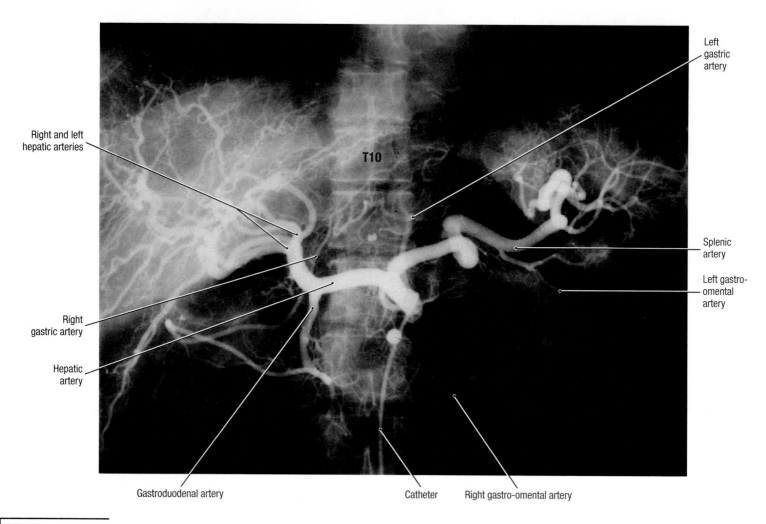

Left gastric artery

Right and left hepatic arteries

T10

Splenic artery

Left gastro-omental artery

Right gastric artery

Hepatic artery

Gastroduodenal artery   Catheter   Right gastro-omental artery

2.27   Celiac arteriogram, anterior view

Observe the hepatic artery; the right gastro-omental (gastroepiploic) artery following the greater curvature of the stomach; the tortuous splenic artery; and the left gastric artery. Consult Figures 2.28 and 2.29.

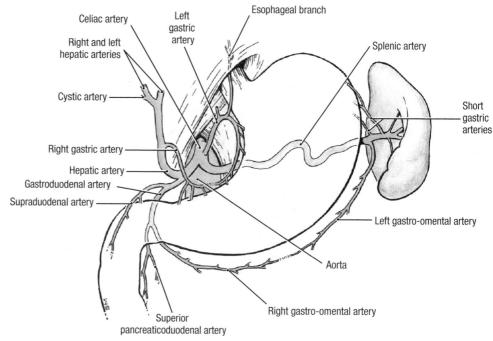

Celiac artery   Left gastric artery   Esophageal branch

Right and left hepatic arteries

Splenic artery

Cystic artery

Short gastric arteries

Right gastric artery

Hepatic artery

Gastroduodenal artery

Supraduodenal artery

Left gastro-omental artery

Aorta

Superior pancreaticoduodenal artery

Right gastro-omental artery

2.28   Branches of celiac artery, anterior view

The celiac artery is a branch of the abdominal aorta, arising from just inferior to the aortic hiatus of the diaphragm. The artery is usually 1 to 2 cm long and divides into the left gastric, hepatic, and splenic arteries. For descriptive purposes, the hepatic artery is often divided into the common hepatic artery from its origin to the gastroduodenal artery, with the remainder of the vessel called the hepatic artery proper.

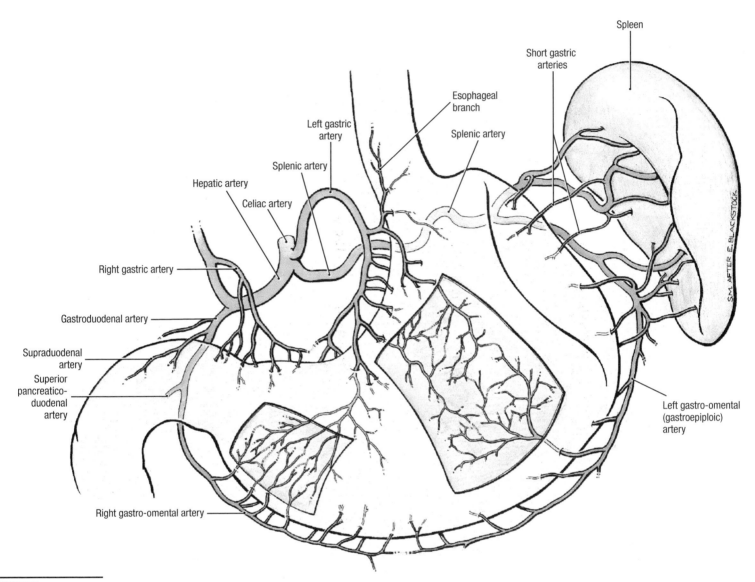

Spleen

Short gastric
arteries

Esophageal
branch

Left gastric
artery

Splenic artery

Splenic artery

Hepatic artery

Celiac artery

Right gastric artery

Gastroduodenal artery

Supraduodenal
artery

Superior
pancreatico-
duodenal
artery

Left gastro-omental
(gastroepiploic)
artery

Right gastro-omental artery

S.M. AFTER E. BLACKSTOCK

2.29 Arteries of stomach and spleen, anterior view

The serous and muscular coats are removed from two areas of the stomach, revealing the anastomotic networks in the submucous coat.

OBSERVE:
1. The arterial arch on the lesser curvature is formed by the larger left gastric artery and smaller right gastric artery;
2. The arterial arch on the greater curvature is formed equally by the right and the left gastro-omental (gastroepiploic) arteries; the anastomoses between their two trunks is attentuated, but it is usually absent;

3. The anastomoses between the branches of these arterial arches take place in the submucous coat two thirds of the distance from the lesser to greater curvature;
4. Four or five tenuous, short gastric arteries leave the terminal branches of the splenic artery close to the spleen. The left gastro-omental artery, belonging to the short gastric artery series, arises from within close to the hilum of the spleen.

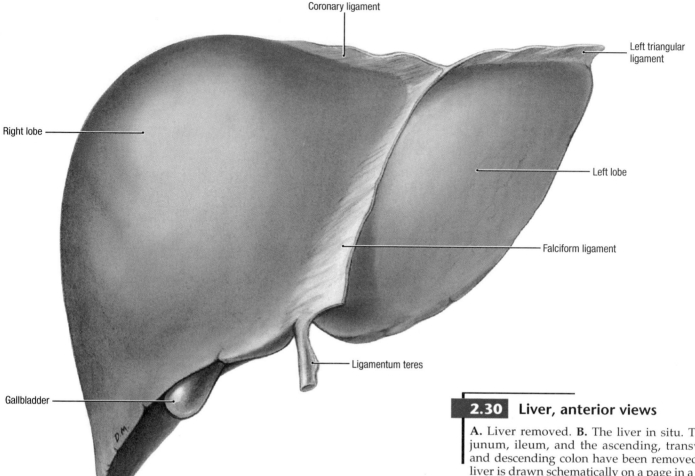

Coronary ligament

Left triangular ligament

Right lobe

Left lobe

Falciform ligament

Ligamentum teres

Gallbladder

A

2.30 Liver, anterior views

A. Liver removed. **B.** The liver in situ. The jejunum, ileum, and the ascending, transverse, and descending colon have been removed. The liver is drawn schematically on a page in a book, so, as the page is turned, the liver is reflected to the right to reveal its posterior and inferior surfaces (Fig. 2.31B).

OBSERVE IN **A:**
1. The right and left lobes of the liver and the falciform ligament;
2. The ligamentum teres lies enclosed in the free edge of the falciform ligament, which is the obliterated umbilical vein that carried oxygenated blood from the placenta to the liver before birth;
3. The falciform ligament has been severed from its attachment to the diaphragm and anterior abdominal wall. The two layers of peritoneum that form the falciform ligament separate over the superior aspect of the liver to form the superior layer of the coronary ligament on the right and the left triangular ligament on the left.
4. The fundus of the gallbladder lies visible at the inferior border of the liver.

Stomach

Right lobe of liver

Falciform ligament

Ligamentum teres

Gallbladder

Transverse mesocolon (cut edge)

Site where ascending colon removed

Mesentery of small intestine (cut edge)

Site where descending colon removed

B

MADER AFTER N.JOY

2.31　Inferior and posterior surfaces of liver

A: Liver, removed. **B.** Posterior relations of liver, anterior view. The peritoneal ligaments of the liver are cut, and the liver is turned to the right side of the cadaver as the page of the book is turned; the posterior and inferior aspects of the liver are shown on page 2, with its posterior relations on page 3 of this schematic illustration. The arrow indicates the site of the omental foramen.

OBSERVE IN **A**:
1. The visceral areas for: (a) esophagus, stomach, pylorus, and duodenum; (b) transverse colon (colic area); and (c) right kidney and right suprarenal gland. The gallbladder rests on the transverse colon and duodenum;
2. The posterior surface comprises (a) the bare area, occupied on its left by the inferior vena cava, (b) the caudate lobe, and (c) the groove for the esophagus;
3. The caudate lobe is separated from the quadrate lobe by the porta hepatis and joined to the right lobe by the caudate process;
4. The bare area is triangular; hence, the coronary ligament that surrounds it is three-sided; its left side, or base, is between the inferior vena cava and caudate lobe, and its apex is at the right triangular ligament, where the superior and inferior layers of the coronary ligament meet;

OBSERVE IN **B**:
5. The inferior layer of the coronary ligament is reflected from the liver onto the diaphragm, right kidney, and right suprarenal gland; *it is called the hepatorenal ligament by the surgeon;*
6. Followed medially, this layer crosses the inferior vena cava at the omental (epiploic) foramen and, turning superiorly, it becomes the left layer of the coronary ligament;
7. Followed to the left, this layer of peritoneum forms the superior limit of the superior recess of the omental bursa and then turns inferiorly as the posterior layer of the lesser omentum.

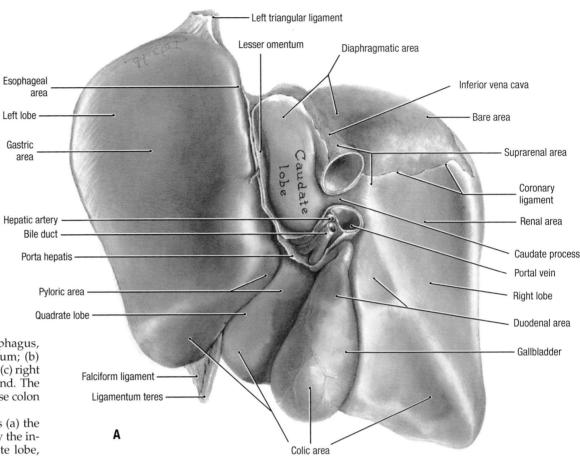

A

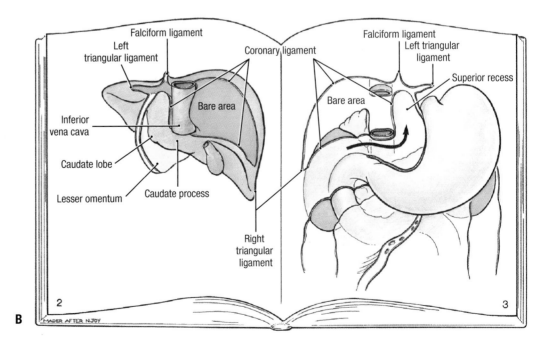

B

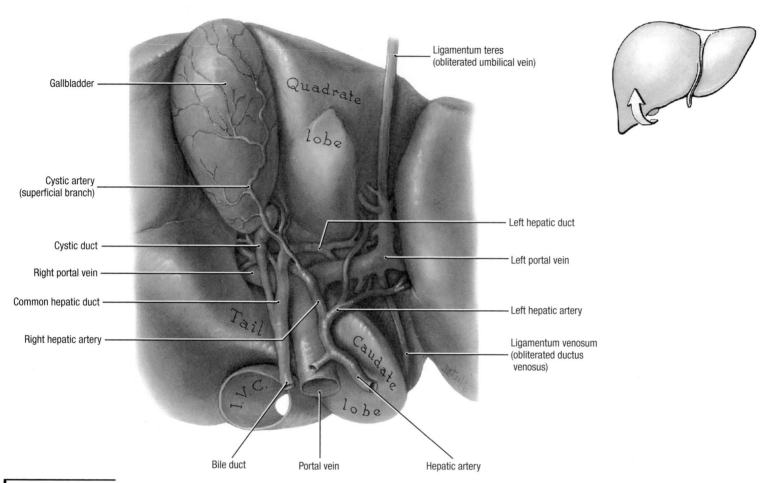

Gallbladder

Cystic artery
(superficial branch)

Cystic duct

Right portal vein

Common hepatic duct

Right hepatic artery

Quadrate lobe

Tail

I.V.C.

Caudate lobe

Ligamentum teres
(obliterated umbilical vein)

Left hepatic duct

Left portal vein

Left hepatic artery

Ligamentum venosum
(obliterated ductus
venosus)

Bile duct   Portal vein   Hepatic artery

2.32 Porta hepatis and cystic artery, posterior view

You are standing on the right side of the cadaver facing the head. The attachments of the liver are severed, and the inferior border of the liver is raised, as in the orientation drawing.

OBSERVE:
1. The caudate lobe forms the superior boundary of the omental (epiploic) foramen and lies between the portal vein and inferior vena cava;
2. The relation of structures as they ascend to the porta hepatis: duct to the right, artery to the left, and vein posterior;
3. The order of structures at the porta hepatis: duct, artery, and vein from anterior to posterior;
4. The left portal vein and left hepatic artery supply the quadrate and caudate lobes en route to the left lobe and are accompanied by tributaries of the left hepatic duct;
5. The ligamentum teres passes to the left portal vein, and the ligamentum venosum arises opposite it and ascends to the inferior vena cava;
6. The cystic artery springs from the right hepatic artery and divides into superficial and deep branches that arborize on the respective surfaces of the gallbladder;
7. The cystic duct is sinuous at its origin.

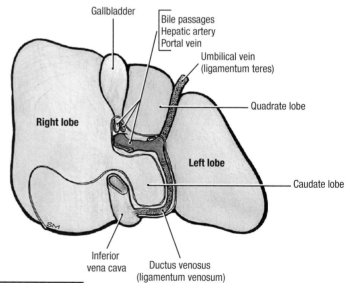

Gallbladder

Bile passages
Hepatic artery
Portal vein

Umbilical vein
(ligamentum teres)

Quadrate lobe

Right lobe

Left lobe

Caudate lobe

Inferior
vena cava

Ductus venosus
(ligamentum venosum)

2.33 Ligamentum teres and ligamentum venosum, posteroinferior surface of liver

The ligamentum teres is the obliterated remains of the umbilical vein that carried well-oxygenated blood from the placenta to the fetus. The ligamentum venosum is the fibrous remnant of the fetal ductus venosus that shunted blood from the umbilical vein to the inferior vena cava, short circuiting the liver.

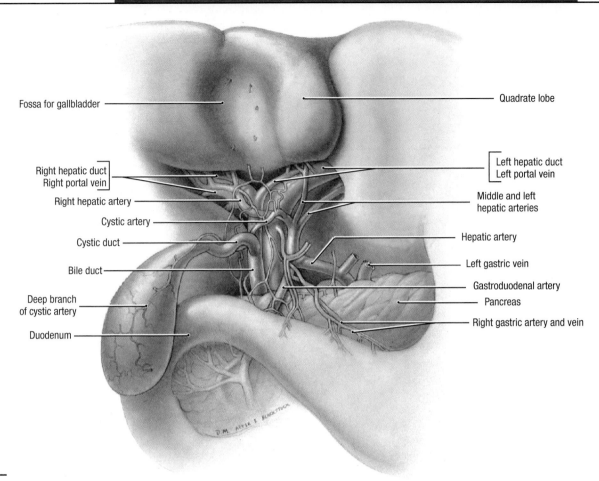

Fossa for gallbladder

Quadrate lobe

Right hepatic duct
Right portal vein

Left hepatic duct
Left portal vein

Right hepatic artery

Middle and left
hepatic arteries

Cystic artery

Cystic duct

Hepatic artery

Bile duct

Left gastric vein

Deep branch
of cystic artery

Gastroduodenal artery

Pancreas

Duodenum

Right gastric artery and vein

2.34 **Vessels in porta hepatis, deep anterior surface of gallbladder, and fossa for gallbladder, anterior view with liver reflected superiorly**

The gallbladder is freed from its bed, or fossa, and turned inferiorly and to the right.

OBSERVE:

1. The anastomoses seen in the porta hepatis involves various branches of the right hepatic artery;
2. The deep branch of the cystic artery on the deep, or attached, surface of the gallbladder anastomoses with branches of the superficial branch of the cystic artery and sends twigs into the bed of the gallbladder (the cut ends of the arterial and venous twigs can be seen);
3. The network of arteries on the gallbladder; most of the smaller arteries lie on a deeper plane than the larger arteries;
4. Many fine, sinuous arterial twigs supply the bile passages and spring from nearby arteries;
5. Several anastomotic arteries bring blood from various gastric and pancreatic arteries to the porta hepatis;
6. Veins (not all shown) accompany most arteries.

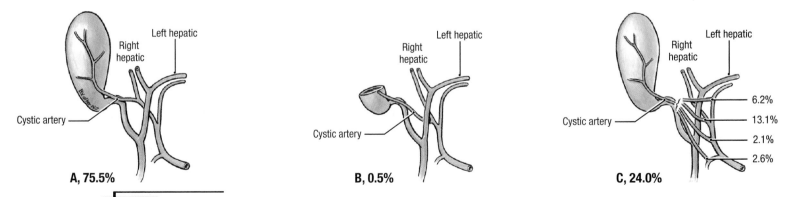

Left hepatic

Right
hepatic

Cystic artery

A, 75.5%

Left hepatic

Right
hepatic

Cystic artery

B, 0.5%

Left hepatic

Right
hepatic

Cystic artery

6.2%

13.1%

2.1%

2.6%

C, 24.0%

2.35 **Variations in origin and course of cystic artery**

The cystic artery usually arises from the right hepatic artery in the angle between the common hepatic duct and cystic duct, without crossing the common hepatic duct (**A** and **B**). However, when it arises on the left of the bile passages, it almost always crosses anterior to the passages (**C**).

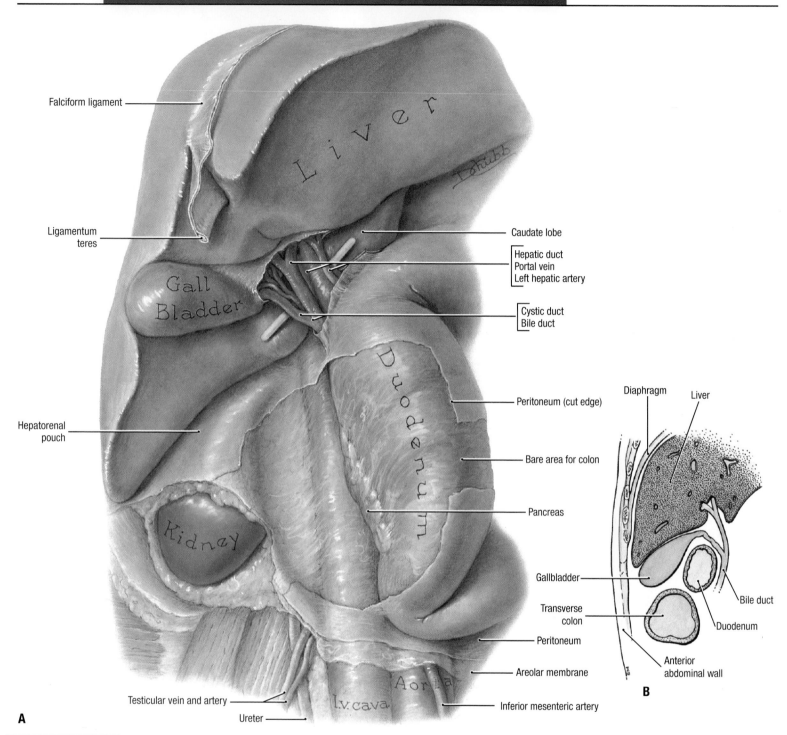

Falciform ligament

Ligamentum teres

Hepatorenal pouch

Testicular vein and artery

Ureter

A

Caudate lobe

Hepatic duct
Portal vein
Left hepatic artery

Cystic duct
Bile duct

Peritoneum (cut edge)

Bare area for colon

Pancreas

Peritoneum

Areolar membrane

Inferior mesenteric artery

Diaphragm   Liver

Gallbladder

Transverse colon

Bile duct

Duodenum

Anterior abdominal wall

B

2.36   Portal triad and gallbladder

A white rod is passed through the omental (epiploic) foramen. The lesser omentum and transverse colon are removed, and the peritoneum is cut along the right border of the duodenum; this part of the duodenum is swung anteriorly.
A: Exposure of anterior aspect of bile duct-I. **B.** Relations of gallbladder, schematic sagittal section.
Note the gallbladder contacts the visceral surface of the liver, the transverse colon, and the superior part of the duodenum.

OBSERVE IN **A:**
1. The space opened up reveals two smooth areolar membranes applied to each other; one membrane covers the posterior aspect of the second part of the duodenum and the head of the pancreas, and

the other covers the aorta, inferior vena cava, renal vessels, and perirenal fat;
2. To find the omental foramen, either: (a) follow the liver at the superior limit of the hepatorenal pouch medially to the caudate process, which forms the superior wall of the foremen, and the inferior vena cava, which forms the posterior wall, or (b) follow the gallbladder to the cystic duct, which occupies the free edge of the lesser omentum and forms the anterior wall of the foramen;
3. Of the three main structures in the anterior wall, the portal vein is posterior, the hepatic artery ascends from the left, and the bile passages descend to the right;
4. In this specimen, the right hepatic artery springs from the superior mesenteric artery, a common variant (Fig. 2.46).

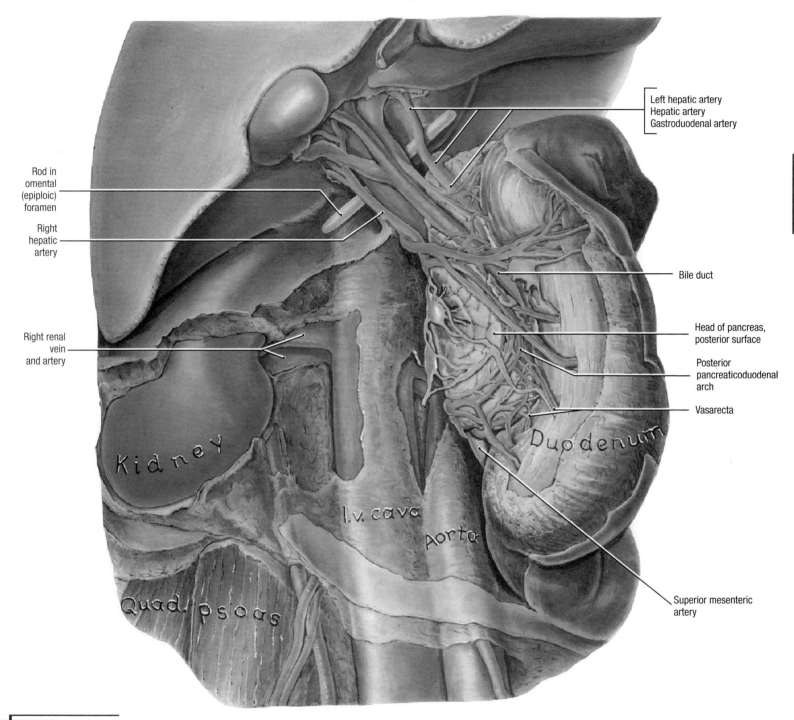

Left hepatic artery
Hepatic artery
Gastroduodenal artery

Rod in omental (epiploic) foramen

Right hepatic artery

Bile duct

Right renal vein and artery

Head of pancreas, posterior surface

Posterior pancreaticoduodenal arch

Vasarecta

Kidney

I.v. cava

Aorta

Duodenum

Quad. psoas

Superior mesenteric artery

2.37 Exposure of posterior aspect of bile duct-II

In this further dissection of Figure 2.36, the duodenum is swung still further anteriorly and to the left, taking the head of the pancreas with it. In effect, the omental foramen has been enlarged inferiorly; the areolar membrane covering the pancreas and duodenum is largely removed, and that covering the great vessels is in part removed.

OBSERVE:

1. The bile duct descends in a groove on the posterior aspect of the head of the pancreas;
2. The bile duct ends at the level of the hilum of the kidney;
3. The close relationship of the inferior vena cava to the portal vein; they are separated by the omental foramen. *A portacaval shunt to di-*

vert the portal circulation into the caval system may be done here by an end-to-side anastomosis;

4. The vasa recta, accompanied by veins and lymph vessels, passes from the posterior pancreaticoduodenal arch to the duodenum;
5. Of the two posterior pancreaticoduodenal arteries that form the posterior arch, the inferior arises from the superior mesenteric artery, and, in this specimen, the superior from the right hepatic artery; usually the superior arises from the gastroduodenal artery;
6. The posterior superior pancreaticoduodenal vein ends in the portal vein;
7. The right renal vein is short, whereas the right renal artery is long, passing posterior to the inferior vena cava to the hilus of the kidney.

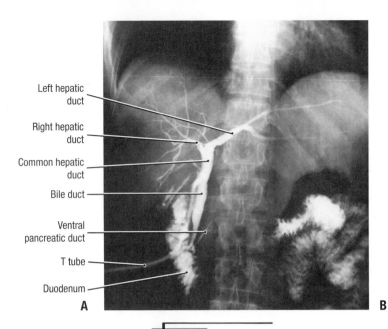

Left hepatic duct

Right hepatic duct

Common hepatic duct

Bile duct

Ventral pancreatic duct

T tube

Duodenum

A

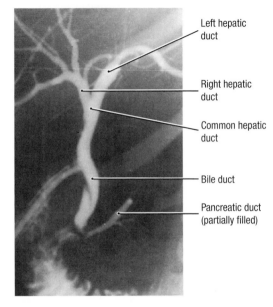

Left hepatic duct

Right hepatic duct

Common hepatic duct

Bile duct

Pancreatic duct (partially filled)

B

2.38   Radiographs of biliary passages, anterior views

After a cholecystectomy (removal of the gallbladder), contrast medium has been injected with a T tube inserted into the bile passages. The biliary passages are visualized in the superior abdomen in **A** and are more localized in **B**.

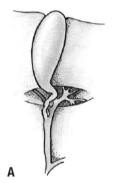

A   **B**

2.39   Accessory hepatic ducts

Accessory hepatic ducts are common and in positions of surgical danger. Of 95 gallbladders and bile passages studied, seven had accessory ducts. Of these: four joined the common hepatic duct near the cystic duct **(A)**, two joined the cystic duct **(B)**, and one was an anastomosing duct connecting the cystic with the common hepatic duct.

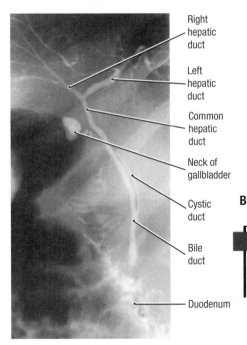

Right hepatic duct

Left hepatic duct

Common hepatic duct

Neck of gallbladder

Cystic duct

Bile duct

Duodenum

A

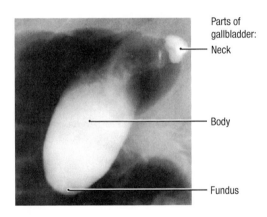

Parts of gallbladder:

Neck

Body

Fundus

B

2.40   Endoscopic retrograde cholangiography of gallbladder and biliary passages

A. The cystic duct. The cystic duct usually lies on the right of the common hepatic duct and joins it just superior to the first part of the duodenum. The course and length of the cystic duct is variable. **B.** Parts of the gallbladder.

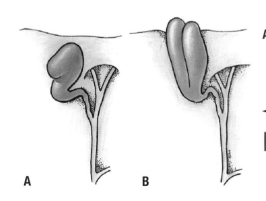

A   **B**

2.41   Folded and double gallbladders

A. Folded gallbladder. **B.** Double gallbladder.

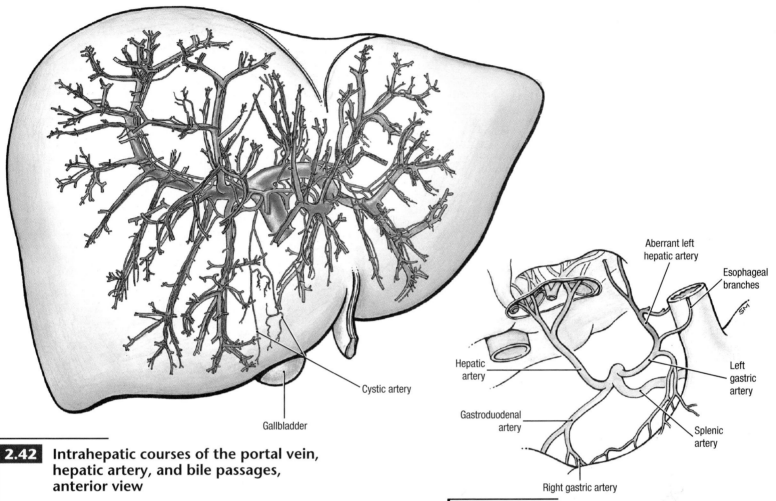

Cystic artery

Gallbladder

Aberrant left
hepatic artery

Esophageal
branches

Hepatic
artery

Left
gastric
artery

Gastroduodenal
artery

Splenic
artery

Right gastric artery

2.42 **Intrahepatic courses of the portal vein, hepatic artery, and bile passages, anterior view**

It is simplest to regard the portal vein, hepatic artery, and bile passages as branching and rebranching dichotomously, although the left portal vein differs slightly in its branching pattern. Note the segmental distribution of these vessels. The branches of the cystic artery are not intrahepatic, but lie on the surface of the gallbladder and cystic duct.

2.43 **Aberrant left hepatic artery, anterior view**

In some cases, the left hepatic artery is entirely replaced by a branch of the left gastric artery; in others, it is partially replaced.

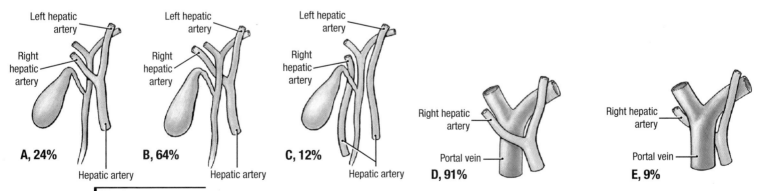

Left hepatic artery

Right hepatic artery

Hepatic artery

A, 24%

Left hepatic artery

Right hepatic artery

Hepatic artery

B, 64%

Left hepatic artery

Right hepatic artery

Hepatic artery

C, 12%

Right hepatic artery

Portal vein

D, 91%

Right hepatic artery

Portal vein

E, 9%

2.44 **Variations in hepatic arteries, anterior view**

In a study of 165 cadavers, five patterns were seen: **A.** Right hepatic artery crossed ventral to bile passages, 24%; **B.** Right hepatic artery crossed dorsal to bile passages, 64%; **C.** Aberrant artery arose from the superior mesenteric artery, 12%. The artery crossed ventral (**D**) to the portal vein in 91%, and dorsal (**E**) in 9%.

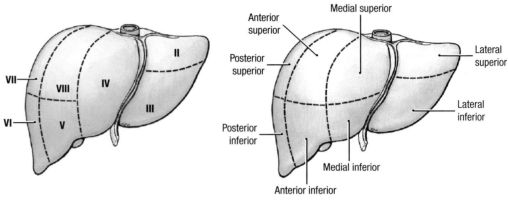

2.45   Segments of liver

A. Anterior view. **B.** Posteroinferior view. The liver is divisible functionally into almost equal halves, "the right and left portal lobes," served by right and left portal veins, hepatic arteries, and bile passages. The two lobes are demarcated by a plane passing through the gallbladder fossa and the fossa for the inferior vena cava. Each of the lobes is subdivided into segments that can be numerically identified, as in **A,** or named, as in **B.** Segment 1 can only be seen in the posteroinferior view of A.

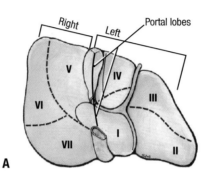

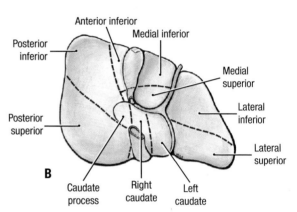

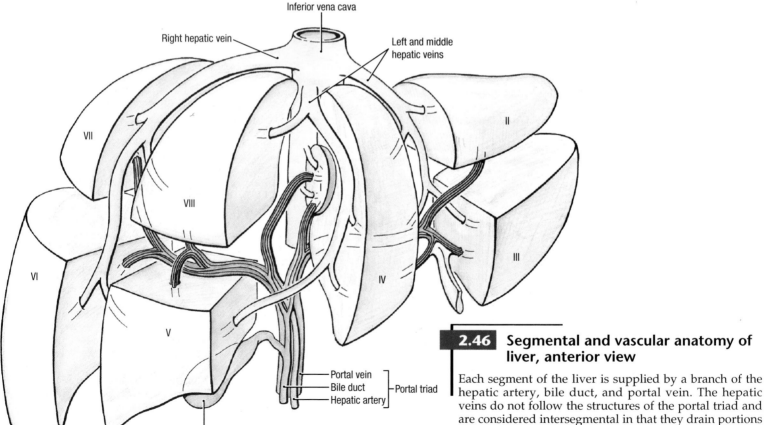

2.46   Segmental and vascular anatomy of liver, anterior view

Each segment of the liver is supplied by a branch of the hepatic artery, bile duct, and portal vein. The hepatic veins do not follow the structures of the portal triad and are considered intersegmental in that they drain portions of adjacent segments.

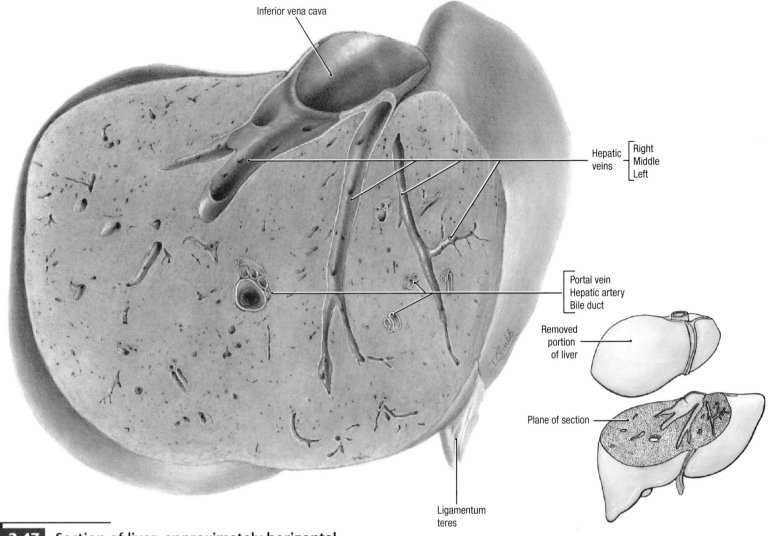

Inferior vena cava

Hepatic veins { Right Middle Left

Portal vein Hepatic artery Bile duct

Removed portion of liver

Plane of section

Ligamentum teres

2.47 **Section of liver, approximately horizontal**

OBSERVE:
1. Perivascular fibrous capsules, each containing a branch (or branches) of the portal vein, hepatic artery, bile ductules, and lymph vessels cut across throughout the section;
2. Interdigitating with these are branches of the three main hepatic veins, which, unaccompanied and having no capsules, converge fanwise on the inferior vena cava.

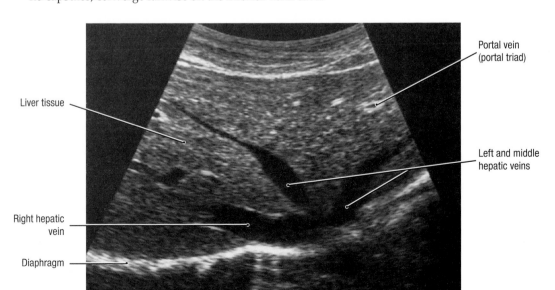

Liver tissue

Right hepatic vein

Diaphragm

Portal vein (portal triad)

Left and middle hepatic veins

2.48 **Ultrasound scan of hepatic veins**

Compare the scan to the drawing of the section of the liver (Figure 2.47). The transducer was placed under the costal margin, angled toward the diaphragm.

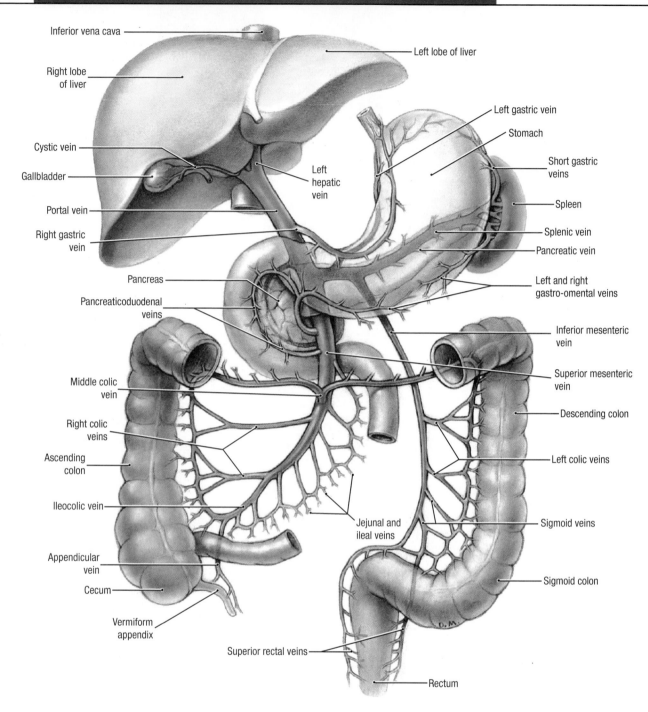

Inferior vena cava

Right lobe of liver

Cystic vein

Gallbladder

Portal vein

Right gastric vein

Pancreas

Pancreaticoduodenal veins

Middle colic vein

Right colic veins

Ascending colon

Ileocolic vein

Appendicular vein

Cecum

Vermiform appendix

Superior rectal veins

Left lobe of liver

Left gastric vein

Stomach

Short gastric veins

Spleen

Splenic vein

Pancreatic vein

Left and right gastro-omental veins

Inferior mesenteric vein

Superior mesenteric vein

Descending colon

Left colic veins

Sigmoid veins

Sigmoid colon

Rectum

Left hepatic vein

Jejunal and ileal veins

2.49   Portal venous system, anterior view

OBSERVE:
1. The portal vein drains venous blood from the gastrointestinal tract, spleen, pancreas, and gallbladder to the sinusoids of the liver; from here, the blood is conveyed to the systemic venous system by the hepatic veins that drain directly into the inferior vena cava;
2. The portal vein forms posterior to the neck of the pancreas by the union of the superior mesenteric and splenic veins, with the inferior mesenteric vein joining at or near the angle of union. Here, the left gastric vein joins the portal vein; usually, it is also joined by the right gastric vein, cystic vein, and one or two small duodenal or pancreatic veins;
3. The splenic vein drains blood from the inferior mesenteric, left gastro-omental (epiploic), short gastric, and pancreatic veins;

4. The right gastro-omental (epiploic), pancreaticoduodenal, jejunal, ileal, right, and middle colic veins drain into the superior mesenteric vein;
5. The inferior mesenteric vein commences in the rectal plexus as the superior rectal vein and, after crossing the common iliac vessels, becomes the inferior mesenteric vein; branches include the sigmoid and left colic veins;
6. The portal vein divides into right and left branches at the porta hepatis; the left hepatic vein carries mainly, but not exclusively, blood from the inferior mesenteric, gastric, and splenic veins, and the right hepatic vein carries blood from the superior mesenteric vein.

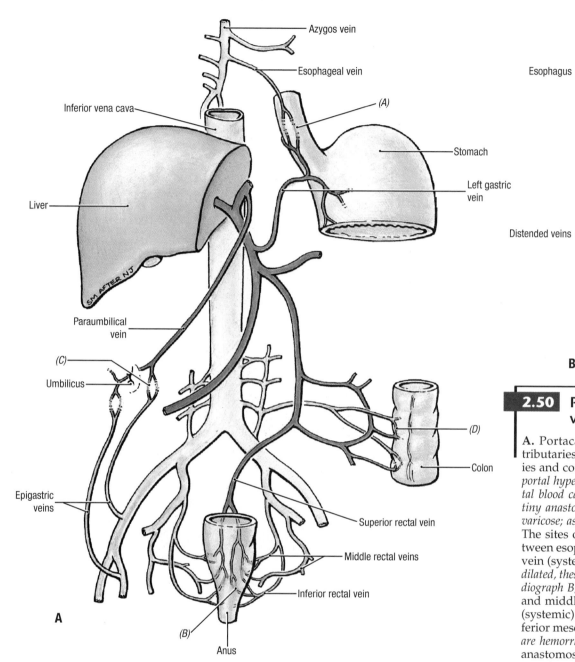

Azygos vein

Esophageal vein

Inferior vena cava

(A)

Stomach

Liver

Left gastric vein

Paraumbilical vein

(C)

Umbilicus

(D)

Colon

Epigastric veins

Superior rectal vein

Middle rectal veins

Inferior rectal vein

A

(B)

Anus

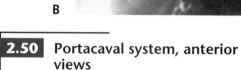

Esophagus

Distended veins

B

2.50 Portacaval system, anterior views

A. Portacaval system. In this diagram, portal tributaries are a dark blue, and systemic tributeries and communicating veins are a light blue. *In portal hypertension (as in hepatic cirrhosis), the portal blood cannot drain freely into the liver, and the tiny anastomotic veins become engorged, dilated, or varicose; as a consequence, these veins may rupture.* The sites of the anastomosis shown are: *(A)* Between esophageal veins draining into the azygos vein (systemic) or left gastric vein (portal). *When dilated, these are esophageal varices, also shown in radiograph B; (B)* Between rectal veins, the inferior and middle draining into the inferior vena cava (systemic) and the superior continuing as the inferior mesenteric vein (portal). *When dilated, these are hemorrhoids; (C)* Paraumbilical veins (portal) anastomosing with small epigastric veins of the anterior abdominal wall (systemic). *These may produce the "caput medusae," so named because of their resemblance to the serpents on the head of Medusa, a character in Greek mythology; (D)* Twigs of colic veins (portal) anastomosing with systemic retroperitoneal veins. **B.** Esophageal varices. Note the distended veins of the esophagus.

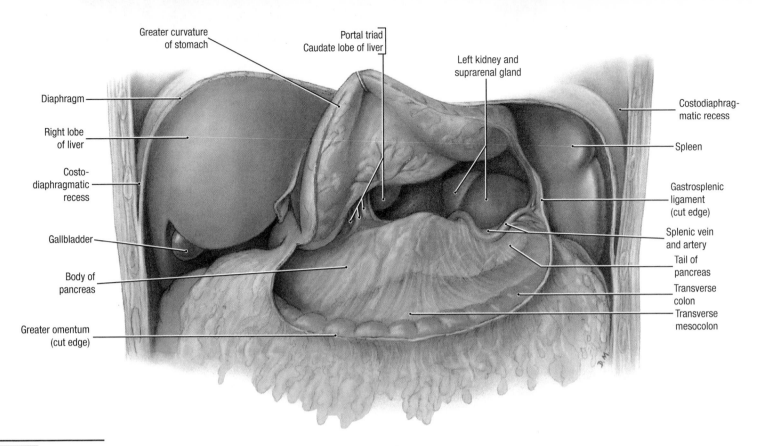

Greater curvature of stomach

Portal triad
Caudate lobe of liver

Left kidney and suprarenal gland

Diaphragm

Costodiaphragmatic recess

Right lobe of liver

Spleen

Costo-diaphragmatic recess

Gastrosplenic ligament (cut edge)

Gallbladder

Splenic vein and artery

Body of pancreas

Tail of pancreas

Transverse colon

Greater omentum (cut edge)

Transverse mesocolon

2.51 **Posterior relationships of omental bursa, anterior view**

The greater omentum and gastrosplenic ligament have been cut along the greater curvature of the stomach, and the stomach is reflected superiorly.

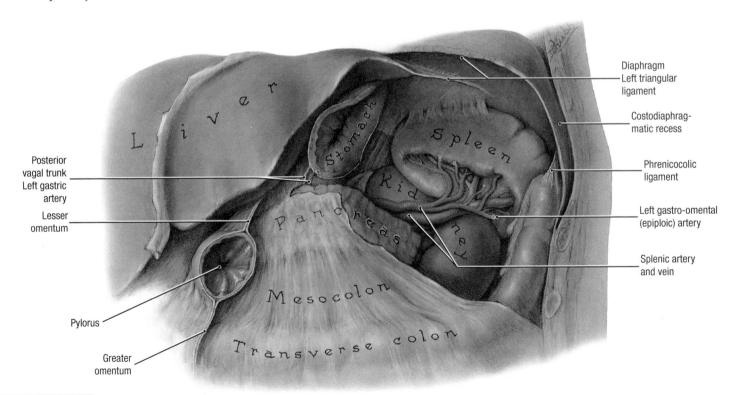

Diaphragm
Left triangular ligament

Costodiaphragmatic recess

Posterior vagal trunk
Left gastric artery

Phrenicocolic ligament

Lesser omentum

Left gastro-omental (epiploic) artery

Splenic artery and vein

Pylorus

Greater omentum

Liver *Stomach* *Spleen* *Kidney* *Pancreas* *Mesocolon* *Transverse colon*

2.52 **Stomach bed, anterior view**

The stomach is excised. The peritoneum of the omental bursa covering the stomach bed is largely removed, as is the peritoneum of the greater sac covering the inferior part of the kidney and pancreas. The pancreas is unusually short, and the adhesions binding the spleen to diaphragm are pathological, but not unusual.

2.53 Exposure of the left kidney and suprarenal gland, anterior view

The spleen and splenorenal ligament are turned anteriorly, taking the splenic vessels and tail of the pancreas with them. Part of the fatty capsule of the kidney is cut away.

OBSERVE:

1. The exposed left kidney, renal vessels, ureter, and left suprarenal gland, which is separated from the kidney by a thin layer of fat.
2. *The proximity of the splenic vein and left renal vein, a relationship used in the surgical relief of portal hypertension through a splenorenal shunt.*

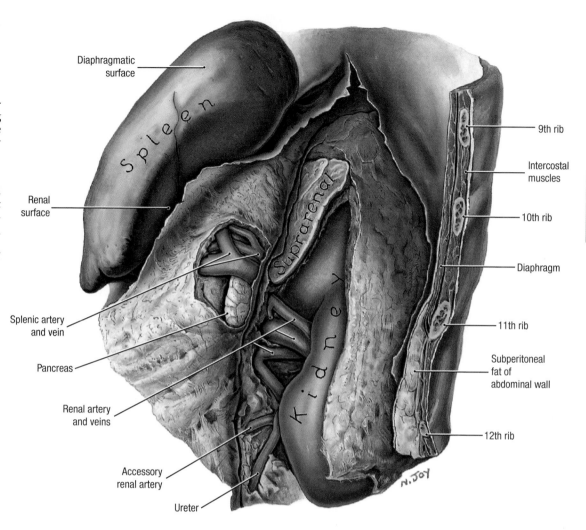

Diaphragmatic surface

Renal surface

Splenic artery and vein

Pancreas

Renal artery and veins

Accessory renal artery

Ureter

9th rib

Intercostal muscles

10th rib

Diaphragm

11th rib

Subperitoneal fat of abdominal wall

12th rib

2.54 Spleen, visceral surface

OBSERVE:

1. A "circumferential border" comprising the inferior, superior, and anterior borders, and separating the visceral surface from the diaphragmatic surface;
2. The notches characteristic of the superior border;
3. The left limit of the omental bursa at the hilum of the spleen, between the splenorenal and gastrosplenic ligaments;
4. The impressions of the structures in contact with the spleen;
5. The long axis of the spleen lying parallel to the 9th, 10th, and 11th ribs. *The spleen is not usually palpable inferior to the costal margin, unless it is enlarged* (Figs 2.1A and B).

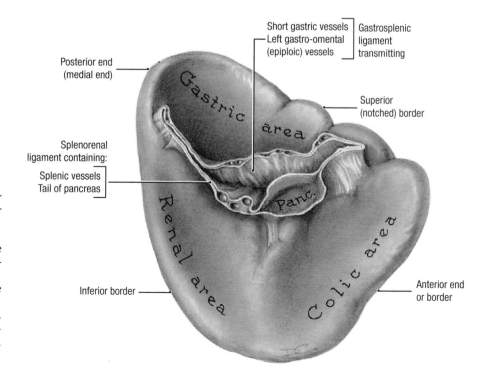

Short gastric vessels

Left gastro-omental (epiploic) vessels

Gastrosplenic ligament transmitting

Posterior end (medial end)

Splenorenal ligament containing:

Splenic vessels
Tail of pancreas

Superior (notched) border

Inferior border

Anterior end or border

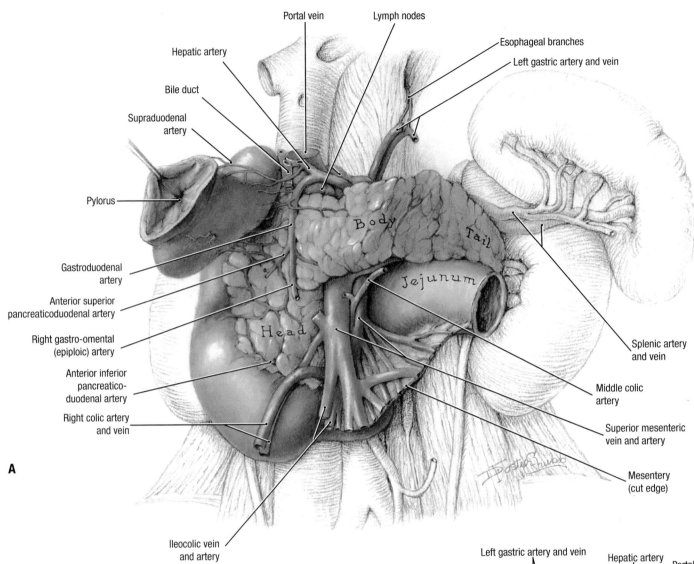

A

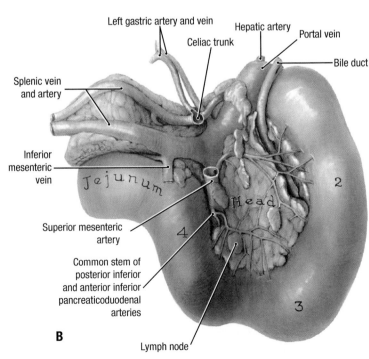

B

2.55   Duodenum and pancreas

A, Anterior view. **B,** Posterior view.

OBSERVE:

1. The duodenum is molded around the head of the pancreas; its 1st, or superior, part (retracted) passes posteriorly, superiorly, and to the right. The remaining parts (2nd, 3rd, and 4th) overlap by the pancreas; near the junction of its 3rd and 4th parts, the duodenum is crossed by the superior mesenteric vessels, which descend anterior to the uncinate process and enter the root of the mesentery. *By constricting the duodenum, the superior mesenteric vessels can cause its 1st, 2nd, and 3rd parts to be dilated;*
2. The tail of the pancreas, here short, usually abuts on the spleen;
3. The celiac trunk, which lies posterior to the superior border of the pancreas, sends (a) the left gastric artery superiorly toward the cardiac orifice of the stomach to enter the lesser omentum, (b) the splenic artery to the left, and (c) the hepatic artery to the right, giving off the gastroduodenal artery;
4. In **B,** only the end of the 1st part of the duodenum is in view; the bile duct descends in a fissure (opened up) in the posterior part of the head of the pancreas.

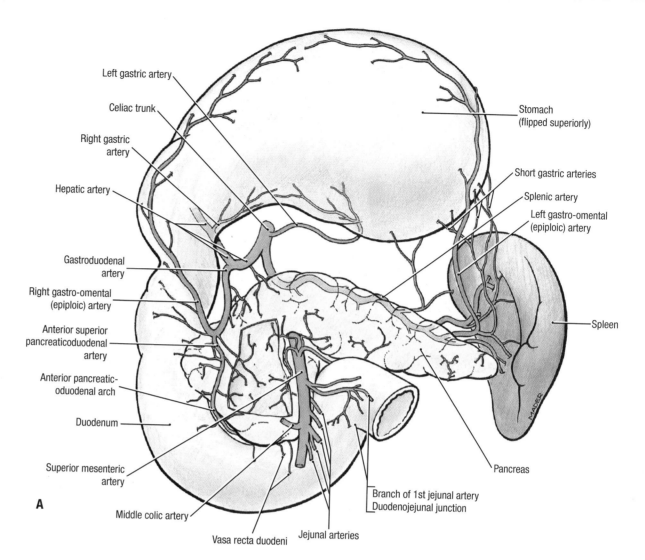

Left gastric artery

Celiac trunk

Right gastric artery

Hepatic artery

Gastroduodenal artery

Right gastro-omental (epiploic) artery

Anterior superior pancreaticoduodenal artery

Anterior pancreaticoduodenal arch

Duodenum

Superior mesenteric artery

Middle colic artery

Vasa recta duodeni

Jejunal arteries

Stomach (flipped superiorly)

Short gastric arteries

Splenic artery

Left gastro-omental (epiploic) artery

Spleen

Pancreas

Branch of 1st jejunal artery

Duodenojejunal junction

A

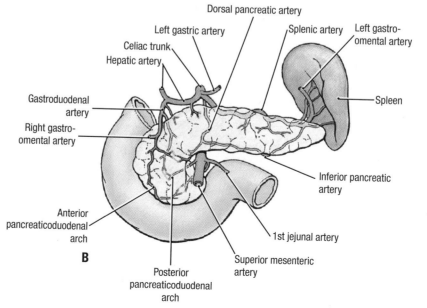

Dorsal pancreatic artery

Left gastric artery

Splenic artery

Left gastro-omental artery

Celiac trunk

Hepatic artery

Gastroduodenal artery

Right gastro-omental artery

Spleen

Anterior pancreaticoduodenal arch

Inferior pancreatic artery

1st jejunal artery

B

Posterior pancreaticoduodenal arch

Superior mesenteric artery

2.56 Blood supply to the pancreas, duodenum, and spleen, anterior views

A. Celiac trunk and superior mesenteric artery. **B.** Pancreatic and pancreaticoduodenal arteries.

OBSERVE:

1. This territory is supplied by the hepatic, splenic, and superior mesenteric arteries;
2. Several retroduodenal branches from the right gastro-omental (epiploic) artery;
3. The anterior superior pancreaticoduodenal branch of the gastroduodenal artery and the anterior inferior pancreaticoduodenal branch of the superior mesenteric artery form the anterior pancreaticoduodenal arch anterior to the head of the pancreas. The posterior superior and posterior inferior branches of the same two arteries form the posterior pancreaticoduodenal arch posterior to the pancreas. The anterior and posterior inferior arteries spring from a common stem;
4. From each arch straight vessels, called vasa recta duodeni, that pass to the anterior and posterior surfaces, respectively, of the 2nd, 3rd, and 4th parts of the duodenum;
5. The fine network of arteries supplying the pancreas are derived from the common hepatic artery, gastroduodenal artery, pancreaticoduodenal arches, splenic artery, and superior mesenteric artery.

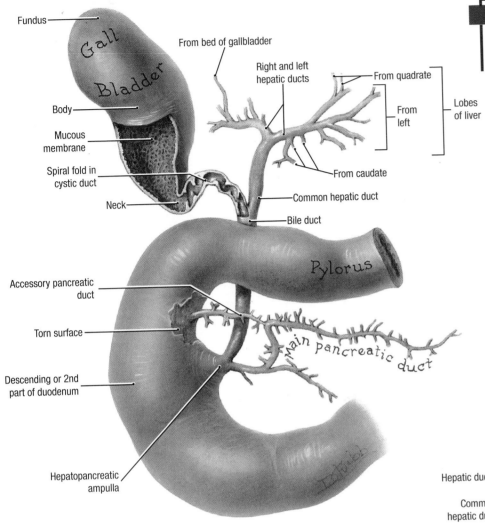

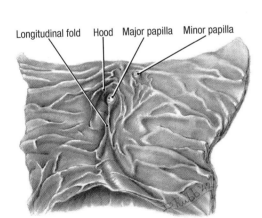

2.58 Duodenal papilla, interior of 2nd part of duodenum

Observe the larger duodenal papilla, projecting into the duodenum approximately 9 cm from the pylorus; a hood is over the larger papilla, a longitudinal fold descends from it, and the small duodenal papilla of the accessory pancreatic duct lies just anterosuperior to it. The plicae circulares are pronounced.

2.57 Extrahepatic bile passages and pancreatic ducts, anterior view

OBSERVE:

1. The mucous membrane of the gallbladder has a low, honeycomb surface, whereas the cystic duct is sinuous, with its mucous membrane forming a spiral fold (spiral valve);
2. The right and left hepatic ducts collect bile from the liver; the common hepatic duct unites with the cystic duct just superior to the duodenum to form the bile duct;
3. The bile duct, after descending posterior to the 1st part of the duodenum and the accessory pancreatic duct, is joined by the main pancreatic duct; these open on the duodenal papilla (Figure 2.58);
4. The accessory pancreatic duct retains its anastomosis with the main duct; the pancreas invades the duodenal wall around the accessory duct and cannot be removed without lacerating the duodenum. In a small percentage of cases, the bile and pancreatic ducts open separately on the duodenal papilla.

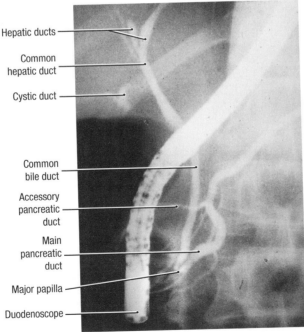

2.59 Endoscopic retrograde cholangiography and pancreatography (ERCP) of the bile and pancreatic ducts

Note the course of the dorsal and ventral pancreatic ducts.

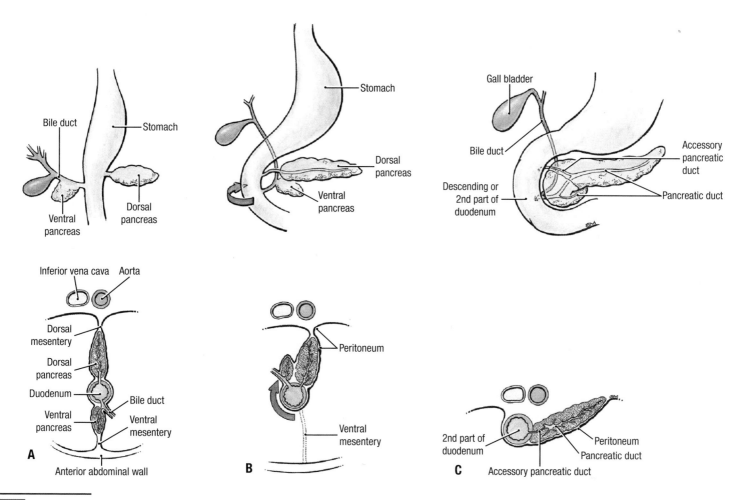

2.60   Development of pancreatic ducts

Examine the anterior views (top) and transverse sections (bottom) of the stages in the development of the pancreas to understand the variability of pancreatic ducts. **A**. A smaller, primitive ventral bud arises in common with the bile duct, and a larger, primitive dorsal bud arises independently from the duodenum. **B.** The 2nd, or descending, part of the duodenum rotates on its long axis, which brings the ventral bud and bile duct posterior to the dorsal bud. **C.** A connecting segment unites the dorsal duct to the ventral duct, whereupon the duodenal end of the dorsal duct atrophies, and the direction of flow within it is reversed.

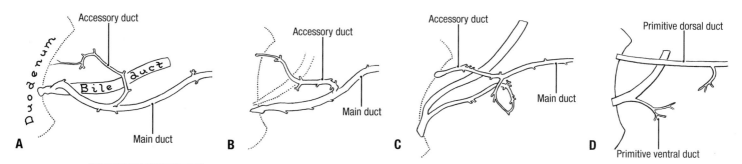

2.61   Variability of pancreatic duct

Some of the more common variations include: **(A)** an acessory duct that has lost its connection with the duodenum; **(B)** an accessory duct that is large enough to relieve an obstructed main duct; **(C)** an accessory duct that could probably substitute for the main duct; **(D)** a persisting primitive dorsal duct unconnected to the primitive ventral duct.

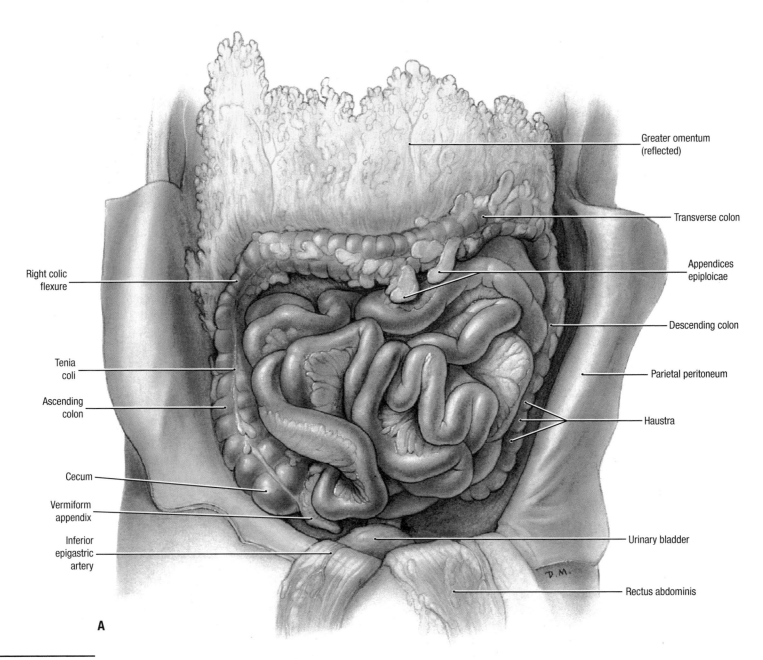

Greater omentum
(reflected)

Transverse colon

Appendices
epiploicae

Right colic
flexure

Descending colon

Tenia
coli

Parietal peritoneum

Ascending
colon

Haustra

Cecum

Vermiform
appendix

Urinary bladder

Inferior
epigastric
artery

Rectus abdominis

A

2.62   Small and large intestine, anterior views

A. Intestines in situ, greater omentum reflected. **B.** Descending and
sigmoid colon and mesentery of small intestine.

OBSERVE IN **A:**
1. The extensive coiling of the jejunum and ileum of the small intestine (together approximately 6 m in length);
2. The small intestine is continuous with the large intestine at the cecum;
3. The ileum is reflected to expose the vermiform appendix in the lower
   right quadrant; the vermiform appendix usually lies posterior to the
   cecum (retrocecal) or, as in this case, projects over the pelvic brim;
4. The distinguishing features of the large intestine: (a) its position
   around the small intestine; (b) the teniae coli, or longitudinal muscle bands; (c) the sacculations, or haustra; and (d) the appendices
   epiploicae.

OBSERVE IN **B:**
5. The duodenojejunal junction is situated to the left of the median
   plane;
6. The root of the mesentery of the small intestine fans extensively to
   accommodate the jejunum and ileum;
7. The descending colon, the narrowest part of the large intestine,
   spans from the left colic flexure to the pelvic brim, where it is continuous with the sigmoid colon;
8. The descending colon is retroperitoneal, but the sigmoid colon has
   a mesentery, the sigmoid mesocolon; the sigmoid colon is continuous with the rectum at the point at which the sigmoid mesocolon is
   no longer present.

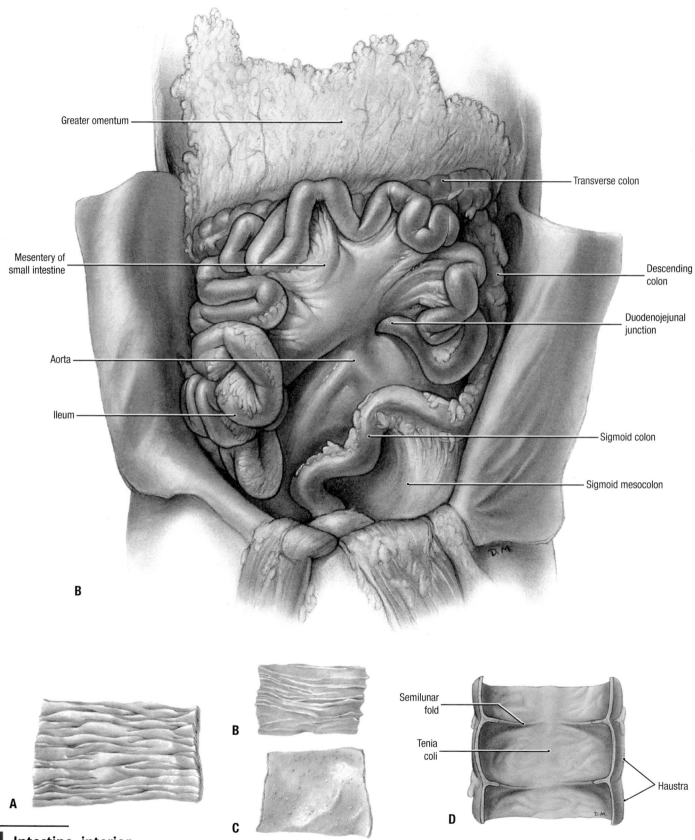

Greater omentum

Mesentery of
small intestine

Aorta

Ileum

Transverse colon

Descending
colon

Duodenojejunal
junction

Sigmoid colon

Sigmoid mesocolon

B

A

B

C

Semilunar
fold

Tenia
coli

Haustra

D

2.63 | Intestine, interior

A. Jejunum, proximal part. The plicae circulares are tall, closely packed, and commonly branched. **B.** Ileum, proximal part. The plicae circulares are low and becoming sparse. The caliber of the gut is reduced, and the wall is thinner. **C.** Ileum, distal part. Plicae circulares are now absent. Solitary lymph nodules stud the wall. **D.** Transverse colon. The semilunar folds and teniae coli form prominent features on the smooth-surfaced wall.

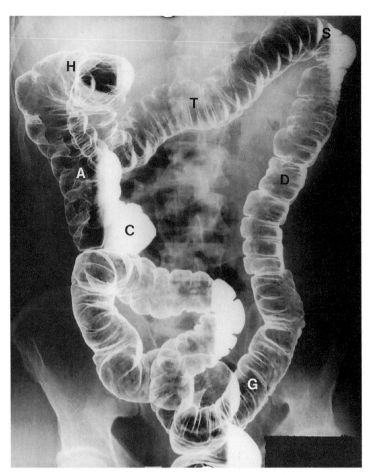

A

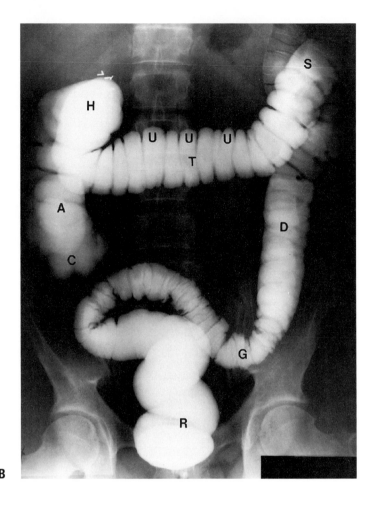

B

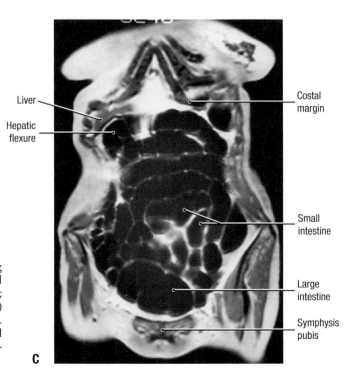

C

2.64   Barium enema of the colon

A. Anteroposterior double contrast study. Barium can be seen coating the walls of the colon, which is distended with air, providing a vivid view of the mucosal relief and haustra. *C*, cecum; *A*, ascending colon; *H*, hepatic (right colic) flexure; *T*, transverse colon; *S*, splenic (left colic) flexure; *D*, descending colon; *G*, sigmoid colon; *R*, rectum; *U*, haustra. **B.** Anteroposterior single contrast study. A barium enema has filled the colon. Observe the relative levels of the hepatic and splenic flexures. **C.** Coronal magnetic resonance images (MRI) of abdomen.

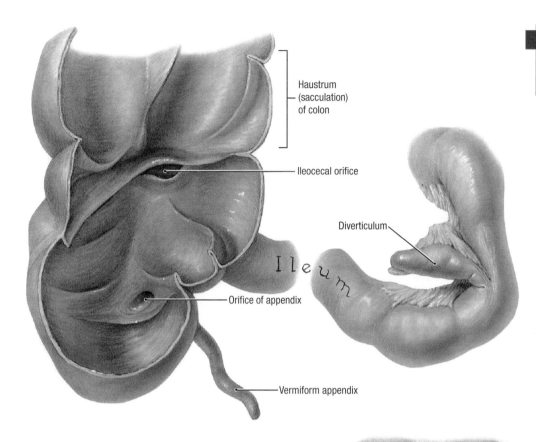

Haustrum (sacculation) of colon

Ileocecal orifice

Diverticulum

Ileum

Orifice of appendix

Vermiform appendix

2.65 Interior of a dried cecum and diverticulum ilei (Meckel's diverticulum), anterior view

This cecum was filled with air until dry, opened, and varnished.

OBSERVE:

1. The ileocecal valve guards the ileocecal orifice; its "pouting" upper lip overhangs the lower lip, and the folds run horizontally from the corners of the lips;
2. A slight fold closes the superior part of the orifice of the appendix;
3. *Ileal (Meckel's) diverticulum is a congenital anomaly that occurs in 1 to 2% of people. It is a pouchlike remnant (3–6 cm long) of the proximal part of the yolk stalk, typically within 50 cm of the ileocecal junction. It sometimes becomes inflamed and produces pain that may mimic that produced by appendicitis.*

2.66 Blood supply of ileocecal region, anterior view

OBSERVE:

1. The appendix in one free border of the mesoappendix, with the artery in the other;
2. *The anterior tenia coli, leading to the appendix, is a guide for the surgeon;*
3. The inferior ileocecal (bloodless) fold extends from ileum to mesoappendix;
4. The vascular cecal fold is the official name for the superior ileocecal fold.

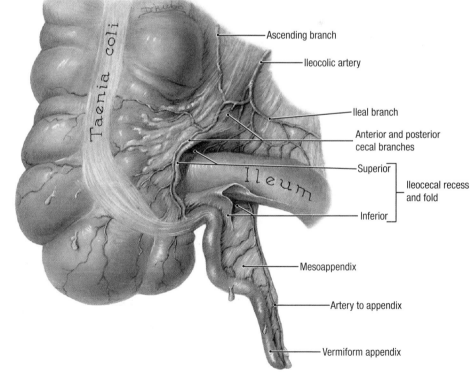

Taenia coli

Ileum

Ascending branch

Ileocolic artery

Ileal branch

Anterior and posterior cecal branches

Superior

Ileocecal recess and fold

Inferior

Mesoappendix

Artery to appendix

Vermiform appendix

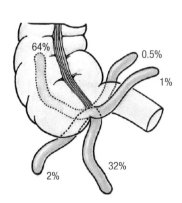

64%

0.5%

1%

32%

2%

2.67 Vermiform appendix, anterior view

This diagram shows the approximate incidence of various locations of the appendix. *Like the hands of a clock, the appendix can be long or short, and it can occupy any position consistent with its length.*

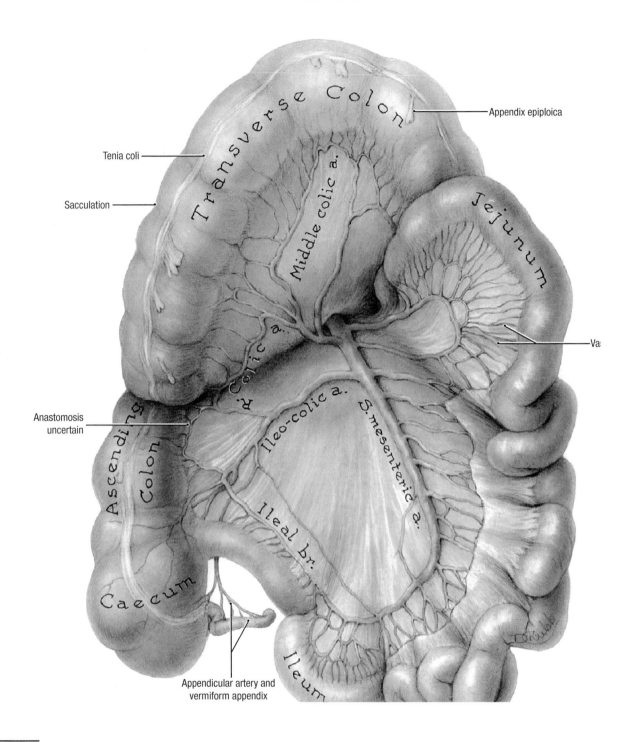

2.68 Superior mesenteric artery, anterior view

The peritoneum is partially stripped off.

OBSERVE:

1. The superior mesenteric artery ends by anastomosing with one of its own branches, the ileal branch of the ileocolic artery;
2. Its branches: (a) from its left side, 12 or more jejunal and ileal branches; these anastomose to form arcades from which vasta recta pass to the small intestine; (b) from its right side, the middle colic, ileocolic, and commonly, but not here, an independent right colic artery; these anastomose to form a marginal artery from which vasa recta pass to the large intestine; (c) the two inferior pancreatico-duodenal arteries arise from the main artery, either directly or in conjunction with the first jejunal branch;
3. Teniae coli, sacculations, and appendices epiploicae, which distinguish the large intestine from the smooth-walled small intestine.

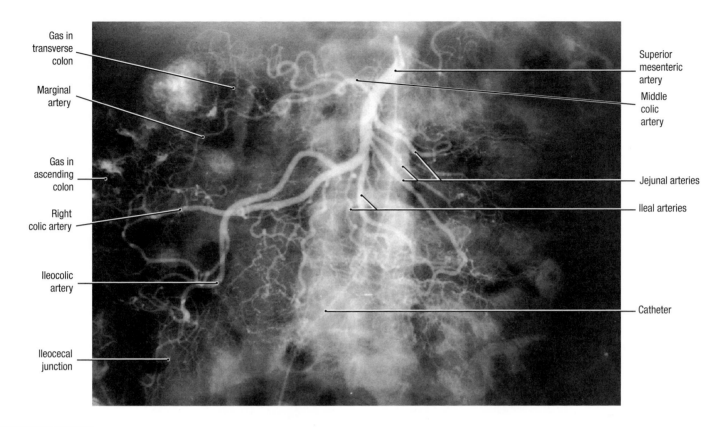

Gas in transverse colon

Marginal artery

Gas in ascending colon

Right colic artery

Ileocolic artery

Ileocecal junction

Superior mesenteric artery

Middle colic artery

Jejunal arteries

Ileal arteries

Catheter

2.69 **Anteroposterior superior mesenteric arteriogram**

Consult Figure 2.68 to identify the branches of the superior mesenteric artery. Observe, in particular, examples of anastomotic loops.

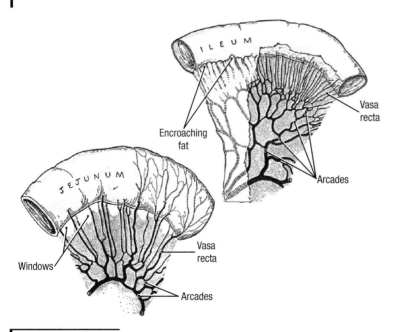

ILEUM

Vasa recta

Encroaching fat

Arcades

JEJUNUM

Windows

Vasa recta

Arcades

2.70 **Jejunum and ileum, external characteristics**

Compare diameter, thickness of wall, number of arterial arcades, long or short vasa recta, presence of translucent (fat free) areas at the mesenteric border, and fat encroaching on the wall of the gut.

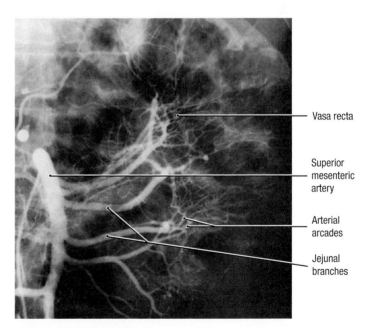

Vasa recta

Superior mesenteric artery

Arterial arcades

Jejunal branches

2.71 **Anteroposterior superior mesenteric arteriogram showing jejunal branches, arterial arcades, and vasa recta**

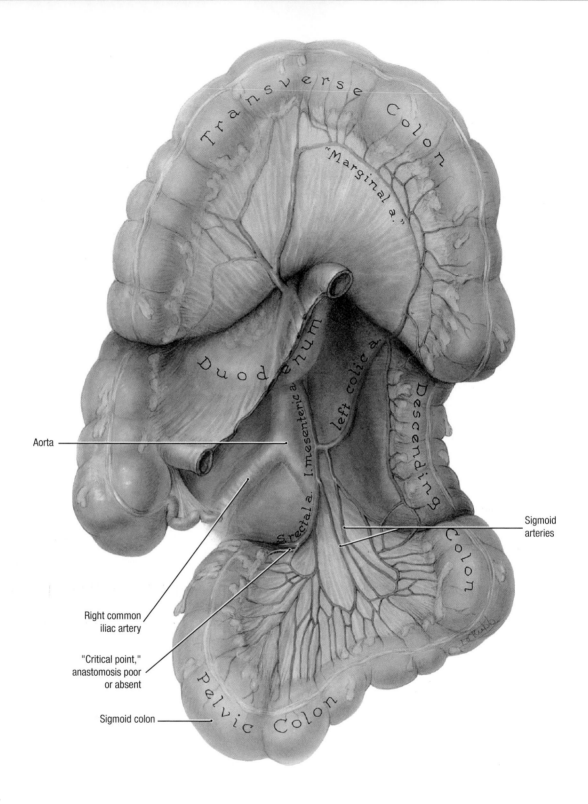

2.72   Inferior mesenteric artery

The mesentery of the small intestine has been cut at its root and discarded with the jejunum and ileum.

OBSERVE

1. The inferior mesenteric artery arises posterior to the duodenum, 4 cm superior to the bifurcation of the aorta; on crossing the left common iliac artery, it becomes the superior rectal artery;

2. The branches of the inferior mesenteric artery include the left colic artery and several sigmoid arteries; the inferior two sigmoid arteries branch from the superior rectal artery.

3. *The point at which the last artery to the colon branches from the superior rectal artery is known as the "critical point"; this branch has poor or no anastomotic connections with the superior rectal artery.*

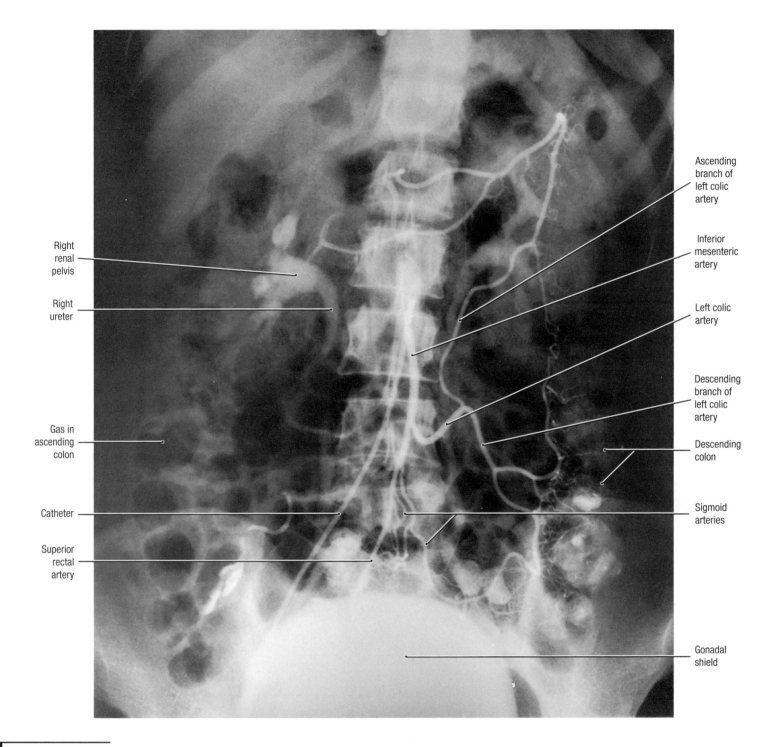

Right renal pelvis

Right ureter

Gas in ascending colon

Catheter

Superior rectal artery

Ascending branch of left colic artery

Inferior mesenteric artery

Left colic artery

Descending branch of left colic artery

Descending colon

Sigmoid arteries

Gonadal shield

2.73 **Anteroposterior inferior mesenteric arteriogram**

Consult Figure 2.72.

OBSERVE:

1. The left colic artery courses to the left toward the descending colon and splits into ascending and descending branches;
2. The sigmoid arteries, two to four in number, supply the sigmoid colon;
3. The superior rectal artery, which is the continuation of the inferior mesenteric artery, supplying the rectum; the latter anastomoses with branches of the middle and inferior rectal arteries (from the internal iliac artery). See Figure 2.53.

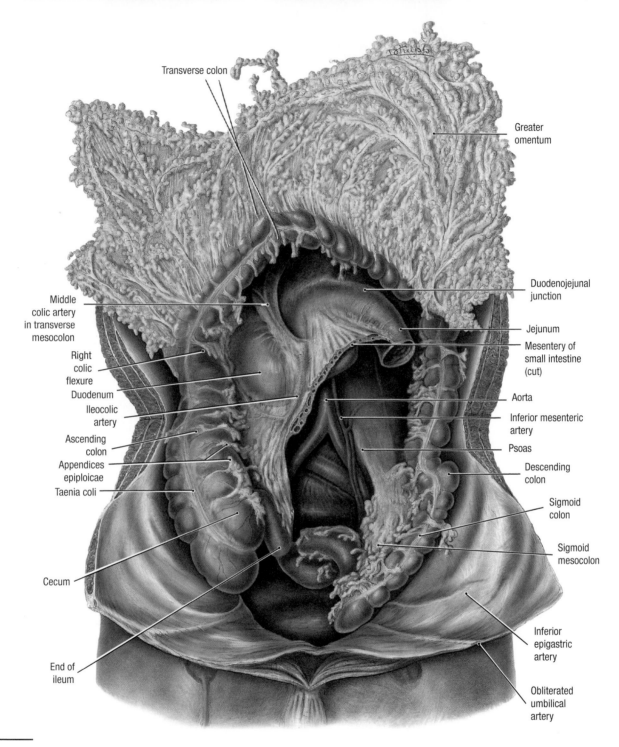

2.74   **Peritoneum of posterior abdomen, anterior view**

The greater omentum is turned superiorly, taking with it the transverse colon and transverse mesocolon. Examine in conjunction with Figure 2.75.

OBSERVE:

1. The duodenojejunal junction is situated to the left of the median plane and directly inferior to the root of the transverse mesocolon;
2. The first few centimeters of the jejunum descends inferiorly and to the left, anterior to the left kidney. The last few centimeters of the ileum ascend superiorly and to the right out of the pelvic cavity;

3. The root of the mesentery of the small intestine, approximately 15 to 20 cm in length, extending between the duodenojejunal junction and ileocecal junction. The mesentery fans extensively to accommodate the jejunum and ileum, approximately 6 m in length;
4. The large intestine forms $3\frac{1}{2}$ sides of a square "picture frame" around the jejunum and ileum. On the right side are the cecum and ascending colon; the transverse colon is superior. On the left are the descending colon and sigmoid colon;
5. The vermiform appendix had been surgically removed.

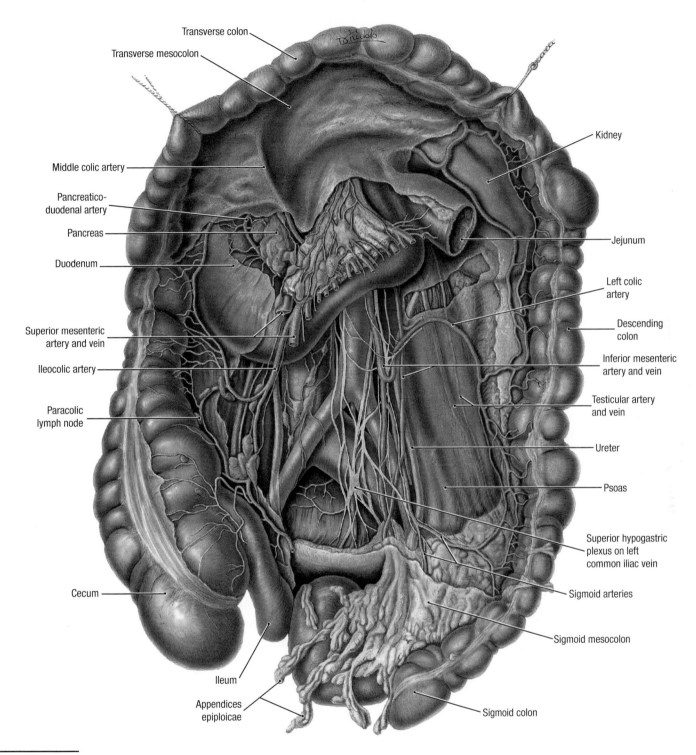

Transverse colon

Transverse mesocolon

Middle colic artery

Pancreatico-
duodenal artery

Pancreas

Duodenum

Superior mesenteric
artery and vein

Ileocolic artery

Paracolic
lymph node

Cecum

Ileum

Appendices
epiploicae

Kidney

Jejunum

Left colic
artery

Descending
colon

Inferior mesenteric
artery and vein

Testicular artery
and vein

Ureter

Psoas

Superior hypogastric
plexus on left
common iliac vein

Sigmoid arteries

Sigmoid mesocolon

Sigmoid colon

2.75 **Posterior abdomen with peritoneum removed, anterior view**

This is the same specimen as in Figure 2.74.

OBSERVE:
1. The duodenum is large in diameter before crossing the superior mesenteric vessels, and narrow beyond;
2. The jejunal and ileal branches (cut) pass from the left side of the superior mesenteric artery; the right colic artery here is a branch of the ileocolic artery;

3. On the right side, there are lymph nodes on the colon; paracolic nodes beside the colon; and nodes along the ileocolic artery, which drain into nodes ventral to the pancreas;
4. The intestines and intestinal vessels lie on a plane anterior to that of the testicular vessels; these in turn lie anterior to the plane of the kidney, its vessels and the ureter.
5. The superior hypogastric plexus lie within the bifurcation of the aorta and ventral to the left common iliac vein, the body of the 5th lumbar vertebra, and the 5th intervertebral disc.

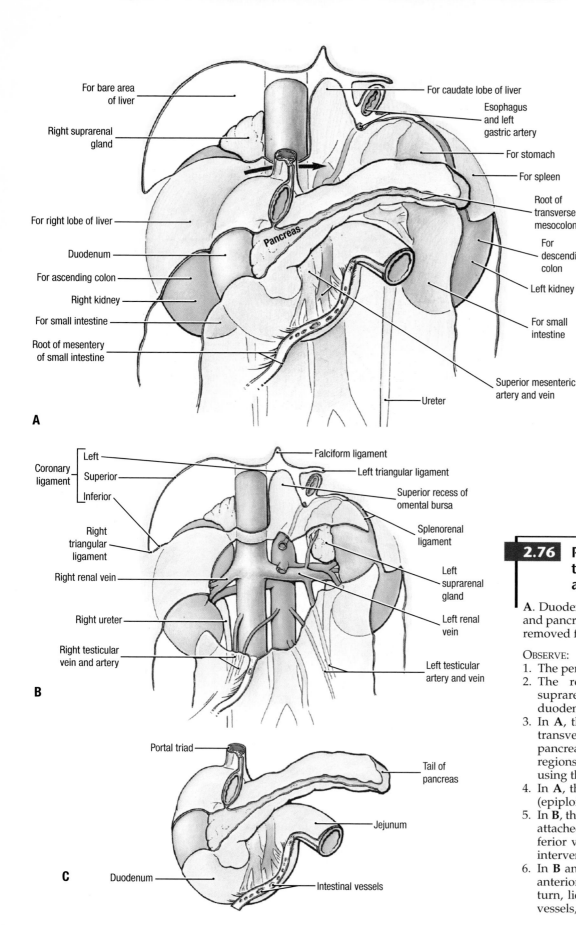

A

For bare area of liver

Right suprarenal gland

For right lobe of liver

Duodenum

For ascending colon

Right kidney

For small intestine

Root of mesentery of small intestine

Pancreas

For caudate lobe of liver

Esophagus and left gastric artery

For stomach

For spleen

Root of transverse mesocolon

For descending colon

Left kidney

For small intestine

Superior mesenteric artery and vein

Ureter

B

Coronary ligament
- Left
- Superior
- Inferior

Right triangular ligament

Right renal vein

Right ureter

Right testicular vein and artery

Falciform ligament

Left triangular ligament

Superior recess of omental bursa

Splenorenal ligament

Left suprarenal gland

Left renal vein

Left testicular artery and vein

C

Portal triad

Tail of pancreas

Jejunum

Duodenum

Intestinal vessels

2.76   **Posterior abdominal viscera and their anterior relations, anterior views**

A. Duodenum and pancreas in situ. **B.** Duodenum and pancreas removed. **C.** Pancreas and duodenum removed from (**A**).

OBSERVE:
1. The peritoneal coverings (yellow);
2. The relationships of the kidneys to the suprarenal glands, bare area of the liver, colon, duodenum, stomach, pancreas, and spleen.
3. In **A**, the line of attachment of the root of the transverse mesocolon to the body and tail of the pancreas; the viscera that lie adjacent to specific regions of the right and left kidneys are indicated using the term "for";
4. In **A**, the right suprarenal gland at the omental (epiploic) foramen is indicated by an arrow;
5. In **B**, the three parts of the coronary ligament are attached to the diaphragm, except where the inferior vena cava, suprarenal gland, and kidney intervene;
6. In **B** and **C**, the intestinal vessels lie on a plane anterior to that of the testicular vessels; these, in turn, lie anterior to the plane of the kidney, its vessels, and the ureter;

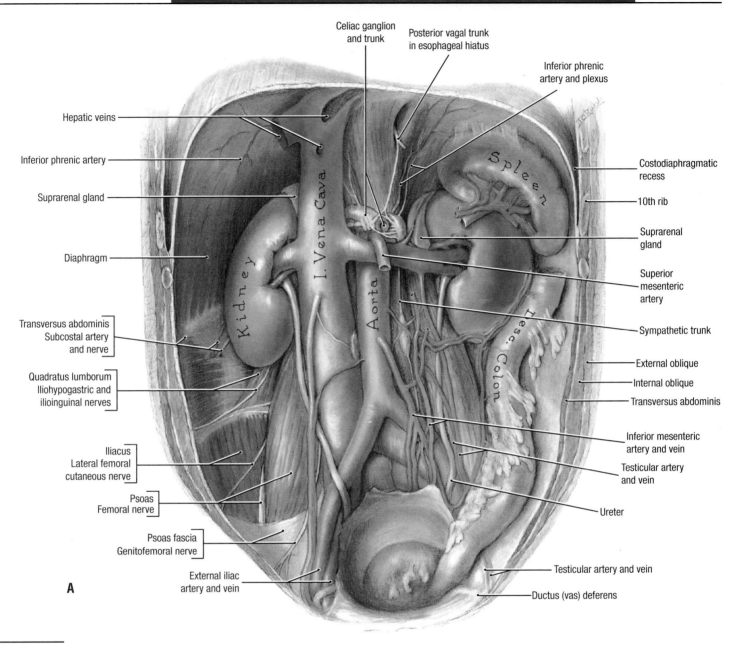

A

Labels (clockwise from top):
Celiac ganglion and trunk — Posterior vagal trunk in esophageal hiatus — Inferior phrenic artery and plexus — Costodiaphragmatic recess — 10th rib — Suprarenal gland — Superior mesenteric artery — Sympathetic trunk — External oblique — Internal oblique — Transversus abdominis — Inferior mesenteric artery and vein — Testicular artery and vein — Ureter — Testicular artery and vein — Ductus (vas) deferens — External iliac artery and vein — Psoas fascia / Genitofemoral nerve — Psoas / Femoral nerve — Iliacus / Lateral femoral cutaneous nerve — Quadratus lumborum / Iliohypogastric and ilioinguinal nerves — Transversus abdominis / Subcostal artery and nerve — Diaphragm — Suprarenal gland — Inferior phrenic artery — Hepatic veins

Inner labels: Kidney — I. Vena Cava — Aorta — Spleen — Desc. Colon

---

2.77   Viscera and vessels of posterior abdominal wall

A. Great vessels, kidneys, and suprarenal glands, anterior view. **B**. Relationships of left renal vein and third part of duodenum to aorta and superior mesenteric artery, lateral view.

OBSERVE:

1. The abdominal aorta is shorter and smaller in caliber than the inferior vena cava;
2. The celiac trunk is surrounded by the celiac plexus and celiac ganglia; the ganglia receive a branch of the posterior gastric nerve;
3. The superior mesenteric artery arises just inferior to the celiac trunk;
4. In B, the left renal vein and duodenum are compressed between the aorta posteriorly and the superior mesenteric artery, anteriorly, like nuts in a nutcracker;
5. The inferior mesenteric artery arises 4 cm superior to the aortic bifurcation and crosses the left common iliac vessels to become the superior rectal artery;
6. The kidneys lie anterior to the diaphragm, transversus abdominis aponeurosis, quadratus lumborum, and psoas muscles. The left renal vein drains the left testis, left suprarenal gland, and left kidney; the renal arteries are posterior to the renal veins;
7. The ureter crosses the external iliac artery just beyond the common iliac bifurcation; the blood supply to the ureter comes from three main sources: (a) the renal artery superiorly, (b) a vesical artery inferiorly, and (c) either the common iliac artery or the aorta;
8. The testicular vessels cross anterior to the ureter and join the ductus deferens at the deep inguinal ring.

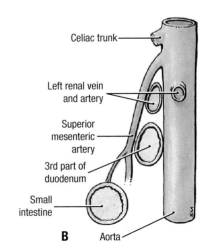

Celiac trunk — Left renal vein and artery — Superior mesenteric artery — 3rd part of duodenum — Small intestine — Aorta

B

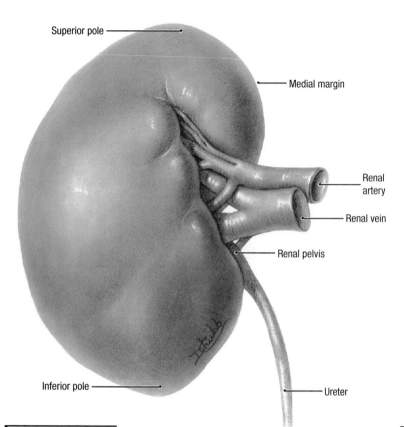

Superior pole

Medial margin

Renal artery

Renal vein

Renal pelvis

Inferior pole

Ureter

2.78   Right kidney, anterior view

OBSERVE:
1. The order of structures at the hilum (entrance to the renal sinus) from anterior to posterior: vein, artery, renal pelvis, or ureter;
2. Often, a branch of the artery passes posterior to the renal pelvis;
3. The superior pole of the kidney is usually wider than the inferior pole and closer to the median plane.

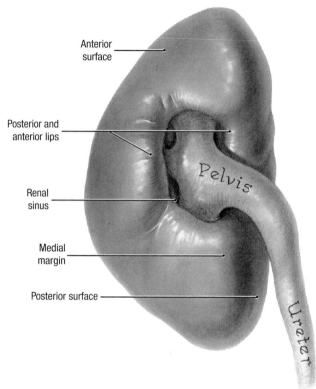

Anterior surface

Posterior and anterior lips

Renal sinus

Medial margin

Posterior surface

Pelvis

Ureter

2.79   Sinus of kidney, anteromedial view

The renal sinus is a vertical "pocket" on the medial side of the kidney. Tucked into the pocket are the renal pelvis and renal vessels.

2.80   Kidney, coronal section

OBSERVE:
1. The conical renal pyramids radiate from the renal sinus toward the surface of the kidney; their blunted apex, the renal papilla, "pouts" into a minor calix into which the renal papilla discharges urine. The pyramids, which appear striated, form the medulla of the kidney and contain loops of Henle and collecting tubules;
2. The renal cortex, forming the outer one third of the renal substance and extending between pyramids as renal columns, appears granular and contains glomeruli and convoluted tubules; interlobar arteries travel in the renal columns;
3. The ureter drains the renal pelvis; the renal pelvis receives two or three major calices. Each kidney has 7 to 14 minor calices, which drain into the major calices.

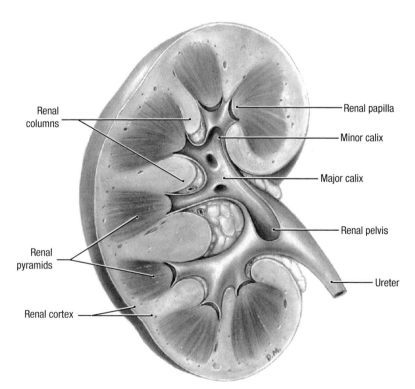

Renal columns

Renal papilla

Minor calix

Major calix

Renal pelvis

Renal pyramids

Ureter

Renal cortex

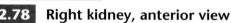

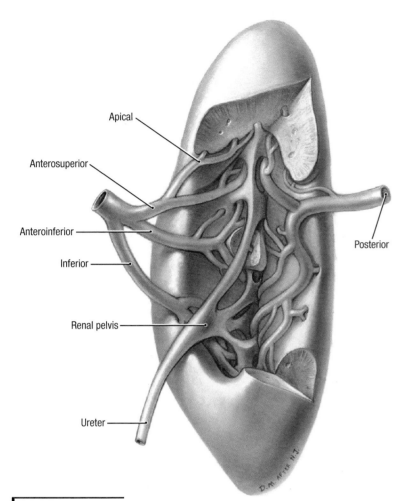

2.81　**Branches of renal artery within renal sinus, medial view**

Approximately 25% of kidneys may have a 2nd, 3rd, and even 4th renal artery branching from the aorta. These multiple vessels enter through the renal sinus or at the superior or inferior pole.

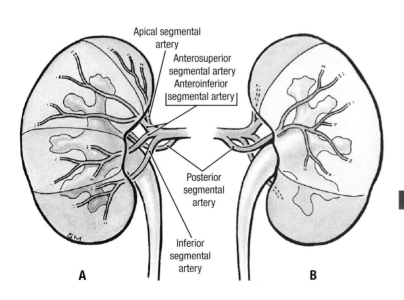

2.82　**Segmental arteries**

A. Anterior view. **B.** Posterior view.
Typically, the renal artery divides into five branches, each supplying a segment of the kidney; only the apical and inferior arteries supply the whole thickness of the kidney. The posterior artery crosses superior to the renal pelvis to reach its segment.

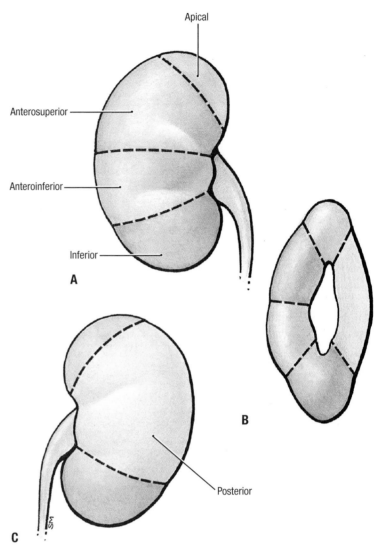

2.83　**Segments of the kidney**

A. Anterior view. **B.** Medial view. **C.** Posterior view. With regard to its arterial supply, the kidney has five segments: apical, anterosuperior (upper anterior), anteroinferior (middle anterior), inferior (lower), and posterior.

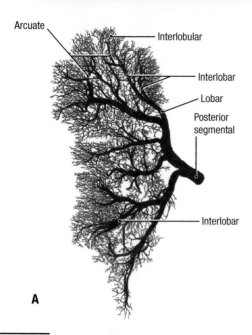

Arcuate

Interlobular

Interlobar

Lobar

Posterior segmental

Interlobar

A

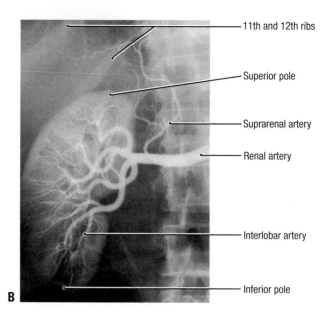

11th and 12th ribs

Superior pole

Suprarenal artery

Renal artery

Interlobar artery

Inferior pole

B

2.84   Branching of segmental arteries

A. Corrosion cast of posterior segmental artery of the kidney. **B.** Anteroposterior renal arteriogram.

OBSERVE:

1. A segmental artery provides a lobar artery to each pyramid; these divide to provide two or three interlobar arteries.

2. Near the junction of the medulla and cortex, arcuate arteries are given off at right angles to the parent stem; these do not anastomose; segmental arteries are end arteries.

3. From the arcuate arteries (and some from the interlobar arteries), interlobular arteries pass into the cortex.

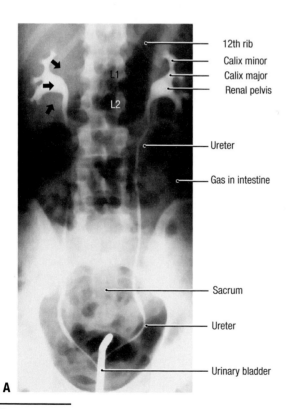

12th rib

Calix minor

Calix major

Renal pelvis

L1

L2

Ureter

Gas in intestine

Sacrum

Ureter

Urinary bladder

A

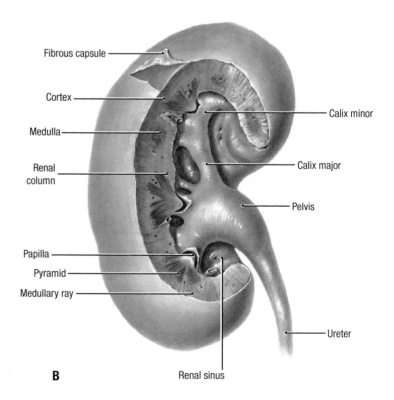

Fibrous capsule

Cortex

Medulla

Renal column

Papilla

Pyramid

Medullary ray

Calix minor

Calix major

Pelvis

Ureter

Renal sinus

B

2.85   Renal calices

A. Pyelogram. Radiopaque material outlines the cavities conducting urine. Note the papillae (indicated with arrows) bulging into the minor calices, which empty into a major calix; this opens into the renal pelvis, which drains into the ureter. The ureter travels inferiorly toward the urinary bladder along the transverse processes of the lumbar vertebrae. **B.** Anterior view. The anterior lip of the renal sinus has been cut away to expose the renal pelvis and the calices.

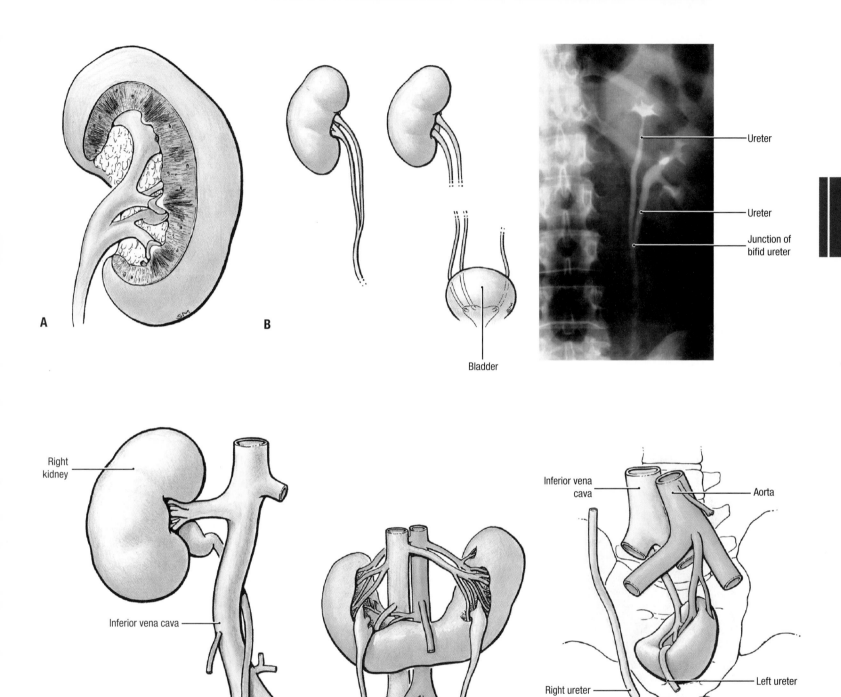

Ureter

Ureter

Junction of
bifid ureter

Bladder

Right
kidney

Inferior vena cava

Right ureter

C

Inferior vena
cava

Aorta

Right ureter

Left ureter

E

2.86　**Anomalies of kidney and ureter,
anterior views**

A. Bifid pelves. The pelves are almost replaced by two long major calices, which lie partly within and partly outside the sinus. **B.** Duplicated,
or bifid, ureters. These can be unilateral or bilateral, and complete or incomplete. **C.** Retrocaval ureter. The ureter courses posterior and then

anterior to the inferior vena cava. **D.** Horseshoe kidney. The right and
left kidneys are fused in the midline. **E.** Ectopic pelvic kidney. Pelvic
kidneys have no fatty capsule and can be unilateral or bilateral. During
childbirth, they may cause obstruction and suffer injury.

2.87   Posterior abdominal wall-I, posterolateral view

Latissimus dorsi is partially reflected.

OBSERVE:

1. The external oblique muscle has an oblique, free posterior border that extends from the tip of the 12th rib to the midpoint of the iliac crest;
2. The internal oblique muscle extends posterior to the external oblique muscle;
3. The lumbar triangle lies between the internal oblique and serratus posterior and inferior muscles.

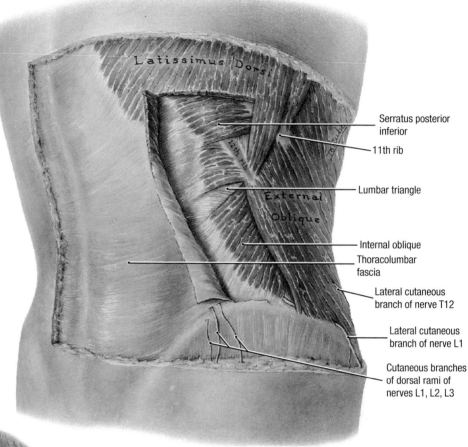

Serratus posterior inferior

11th rib

Lumbar triangle

Internal oblique

Thoracolumbar fascia

Lateral cutaneous branch of nerve T12

Lateral cutaneous branch of nerve L1

Cutaneous branches of dorsal rami of nerves L1, L2, L3

Serratus posterior inferior

11th rib

Subcostal nerve (nerve T12)

External oblique

Internal oblique

Transversus abdominis and its aponeurosis

Iliohypogastric nerve (nerve L1)

2.88   Posterior abdominal wall-II, posterolateral view

The external oblique muscle is incised and turned laterally, and the internal oblique muscle is incised and turned medially; the transversus abdominis muscle and its posterior aponeurosis are exposed where pierced by the subcostal (T12) and iliohypogastric (L1) nerves. These nerves give off motor twigs and lateral cutaneous branches, and continue anteriorly between the internal oblique and transversus abdominis muscles.

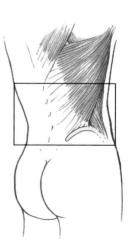

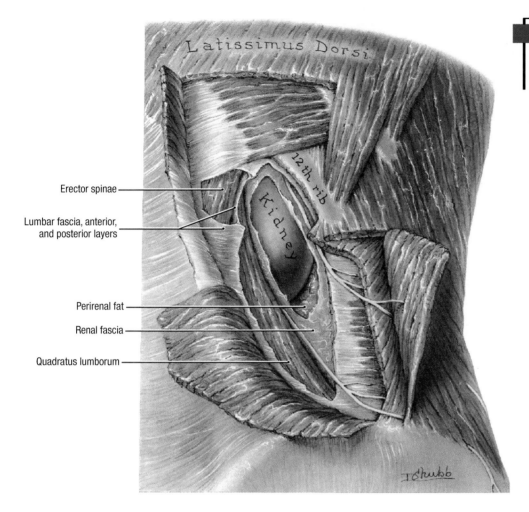

Erector spinae

Lumbar fascia, anterior, and posterior layers

Perirenal fat

Renal fascia

Quadratus lumborum

2.89 Posterior abdominal wall–III, posterolateral view

The posterior aponeurosis of the transversus abdominis is divided between the subcostal and iliohypogastric nerves and lateral to the oblique lateral border of the quadratus lumborum muscle; the retroperitoneal fat surrounding the kidney is exposed. The renal fascia is within this fat; the portion of fat inside the renal fascia is termed fatty renal capsule (perirenal fat), and the fat outside is pararenal fat.

2.90 Posterior abdominal wall and kidney, transverse section

OBSERVE:
1. The renal fascia is separated from the fibrous capsule of the kidney by perirenal fat, which is continuous at the hilum of the kidney with fat in the renal sinus;
2. External to the renal fascia is pararenal fat; renal fascia also envelopes the suprarenal glands;
3. The psoas fascia covers the psoas major and blends with the quadratus lumborum fascia;
4. The quadratus lumborum fascia is continuous laterally with the anterior layer of thoracolumbar fascia;
5. The thoracolumbar fascia has anterior and posterior layers, and covers the deep muscles of the back.

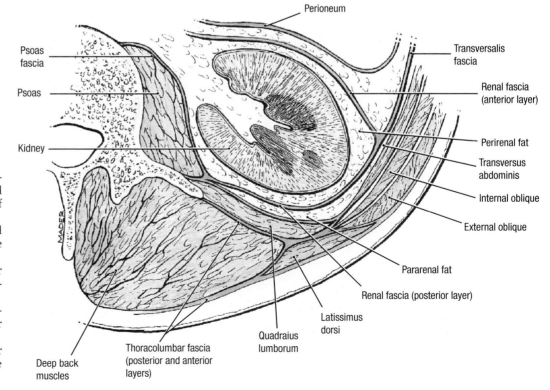

Perioneum

Psoas fascia

Psoas

Kidney

Transversalis fascia

Renal fascia (anterior layer)

Perirenal fat

Transversus abdominis

Internal oblique

External oblique

Pararenal fat

Renal fascia (posterior layer)

Latissimus dorsi

Quadraius lumborum

Thoracolumbar fascia (posterior and anterior layers)

Deep back muscles

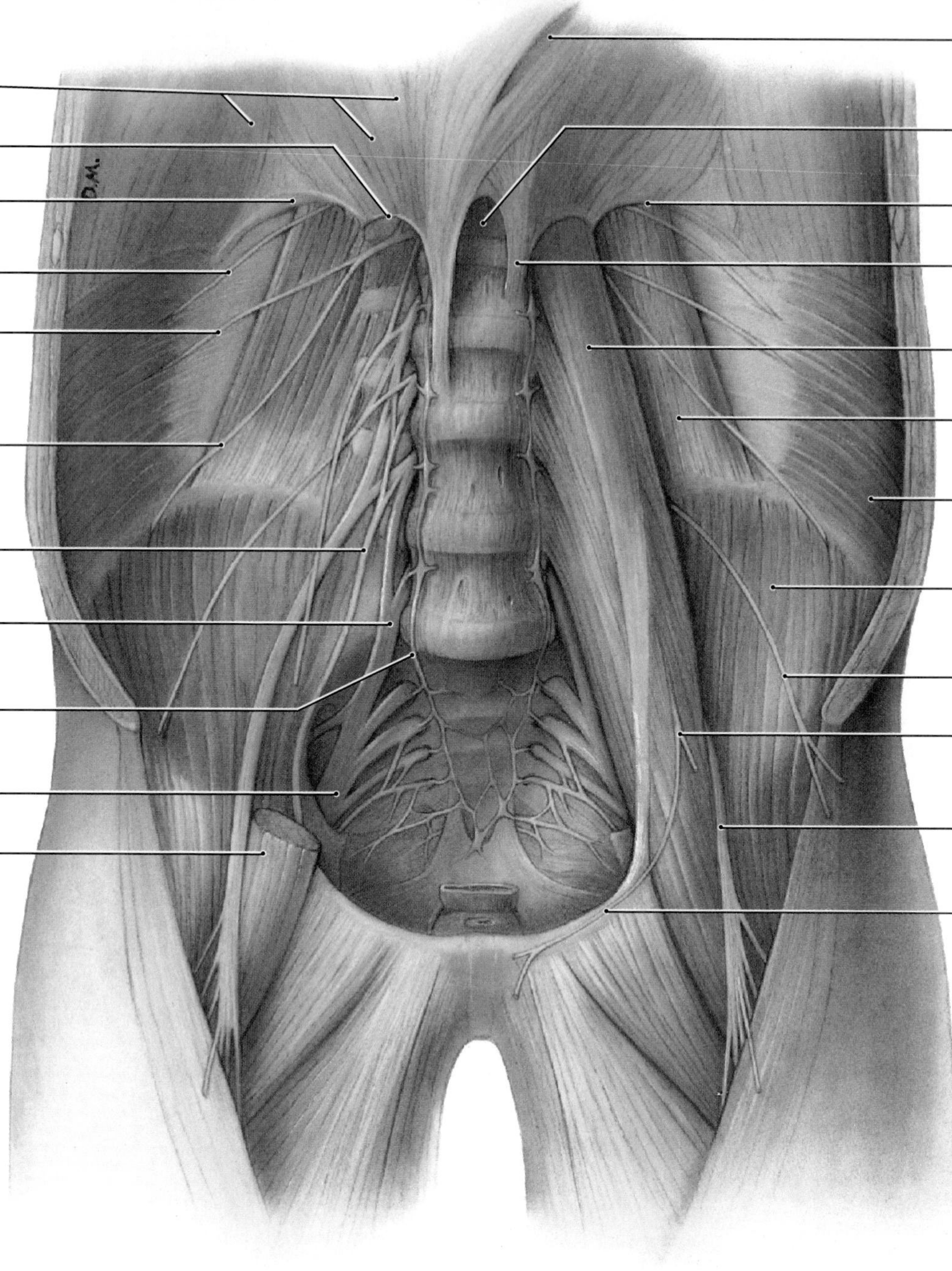

Esophageal opening
Diaphragm
Aortic opening
Medial arcuate ligament
12th rib
Lateral arcuate ligament
Subcostal nerve
Left crus
Iliohypogastric nerve
Psoas
Quadratus lumborum
Ilioinguinal nerve
Transversalis abdominis
Obturator nerve
Iliacus
Lumbosacral trunk
Lateral femoral cutaneous nerve
Sympathetic trunk
Genitofemoral nerve
Sciatic nerve
Femoral nerve
Psoas (cut end)
Genital branch

2.91 Lumbar plexus and vertebral attachment of diaphragm, anterior view

OBSERVE THE MUSCLES:

1. The transversus abdominis becomes aponeurotic on a line dropped from the tip of the 12th rib;
2. The quadratus lumborum has an oblique lateral border; its fascia is thickened to form the lateral arcuate ligament superiorly and the iliolumbar ligament inferiorly;
3. The iliacus lies inferior to the iliac crest;
4. The psoas major rises superior to the crest and extends superior to the medial arcuate ligament, which is thickened psoas fascia;

OBSERVE THE NERVES:

5. The subcostal nerve (T12) passes posterior to the lateral arcuate ligament and runs inferior to the 12th rib (with its artery);
6. The next four nerves appear at the lateral border of psoas. Of these, the iliohypogastric takes the characteristic course shown here; the ilioinguinal and lateral femoral cutaneous nerves (lateral cutaneous of the thigh) are variable; the femoral descends in the angle between iliacus and psoas;
7. The genitofemoral nerve pierces the psoas and its fascia anteriorly.
8. The obturator nerve, and a branch of L4 that joins with L5 to form the lumbosacral trunk, appear at the medial border of psoas and, crossing the ala of the sacrum, enter the pelvis;
9. The sympathetic trunk enters the abdomen with psoas major posterior to the medial arcuate ligament. It descends on vertebral bodies and intervertebral discs, following closely the attached border of psoas to enter the pelvis. Its rami communicantes run dorsally with, or near, the lumbar arteries to join the lumbar nerves.

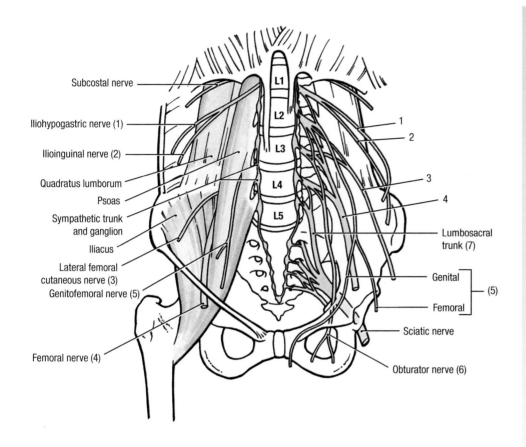

Table 2.2 Nerves of Lumbar Plexus

1 and 2. The ilioinguinal and iliohypogastric nerves (L1) arise from the ventral ramus of L1 and enter the abdomen posterior to the medial arcuate ligaments and pass inferolaterally, anterior to the quadratus lumborum muscle; they pierce the transversus abdominis muscle near the anterior superior iliac spine and pass through the internal and external oblique muscles to supply the skin of the suprapubic and inguinal regions

3. The lateral femoral cutaneous nerve (L2, L3) runs inferolaterally on the iliacus muscle and enters the thigh posterior to the inguinal ligament, just medial to the anterior superior iliac spine; it suplies the skin on the anterolateral surface of the thigh

4. The femoral nerve (L2–L4) emerges from the lateral border of the psoas and innervates the iliacus muscle and the extensor muscles of the knee

5. The genitofemoral nerve (L1, L2) pierces the anterior surface of the psoas major muscle and runs inferiorly on it deep to the psoas fascia; it divides lateral to the common and external iliac arties into femoral and genital branches

6. The obturator nerve (L2–L4) emerges from the medial border of the psoas to supply the adductor muscles of the thigh

7. The lumbosacral trunk (L4, L5) passes over the ala (wing) of the sacrum and decends into the pelvis to take part in the formation of the sacral plexus along with the ventral rami of S1–S4 nerves

Table 2.3 Principal Muscles of Posterior Abdominal Wall

Muscle	Superior Attachments	Inferior Attachment(s)	Innervation	Actions
Psoas major[a]	Transverse processes of lumbar vertebrae; sides of bodies of T12–L5 vertebrae and intervening intervertebral discs	By a strong tendon to lesser trochanter of femur	Lumbar plexus via ventral branches of L2–L4 nerves	Acting superiorly with iliacus, it flexes thigh; acting inferiorly it flexes vertebral column laterally; it is used to balance the trunk when sitting; acting inferiorly with iliacus; it flexes trunk
Iliacus[a]	Superior two-thirds of iliac fossa, ala of sacrum; and anterior sacrolliac ligaments	Lesser trochanter of femur and shalt inferior to it, and to psoas major tendon	Femoral nerve (L2–L4)	Flexes thigh and stabilizes hip joint; acts with psoas major
Quadratus lumborum	Medial half of inferior border of 127th rib and tips of lumbar transverse processes	Iliolumbar ligament and internal lip of iliac crest	Ventral branches of T12 and L1–L4 nerves.	Extends and laterally flexes vertebral column; fixes 12th rib during inspiration

[a] Psoas major and iliacus muscles are often described together as the iliopsoas muscle when flexion of the thigh is discussed. The iliopsoas is the chief flexor of the thigh, and when thigh is fixed, it is a strong flexor of the trunk (e.g., during situps).

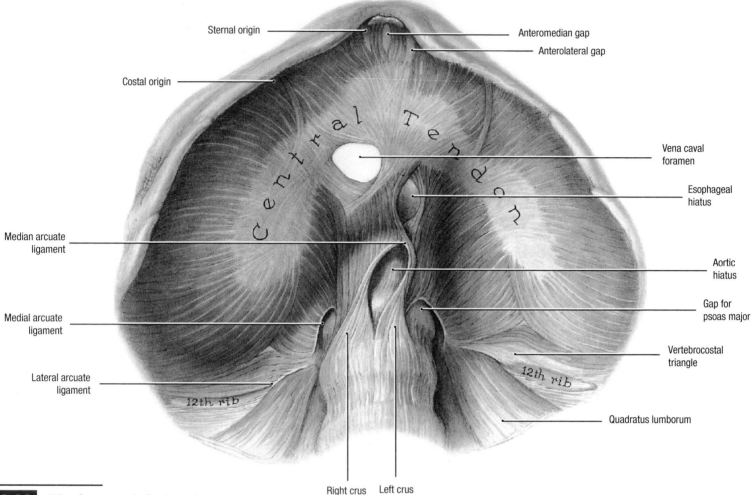

2.92 Diaphragm, inferior view

OBSERVE:

1. The clover-shaped central tendon is the aponeurotic insertion of the muscle;
2. The fleshy origins: anteriorly from the inner surface of the xiphoid process, circumferentially from the lower six costal cartilages, and posteriorly from the superior three lumbar vertebral bodies; the latter is with right and left crura that unite anterior to the aortic hiatus

to form the median arcuate ligament. Thickening of the psoas and quadratus lumborum fascia (the medial and lateral arcuate ligaments) also provides origin to the diaphragm;

3. The diaphragm, in this specimen, fails to arise from the left lateral arcuate ligament; hence, the vertebrocostal triangle, through which a herniation of abdominal contents into the pleural cavity can occur.

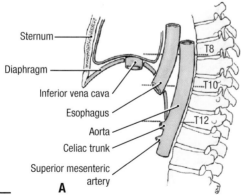

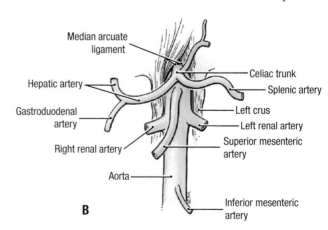

2.93 Lateral view

A. Openings of the diaphragm. There are three large openings through which major structures pass from the thorax into the abdomen: (a) the opening for the inferior vena cava, most anterior, at the T8 level to the right of the midline; (b) the esophageal opening, inter-

mediate, at T10 and to the left; (c) the opening for the aorta, which allows the aorta to pass posterior to the vertebral attachment of the diaphragm in the midline at T12. **B.** Median arcuate ligament and branches of the aorta, anterior view.

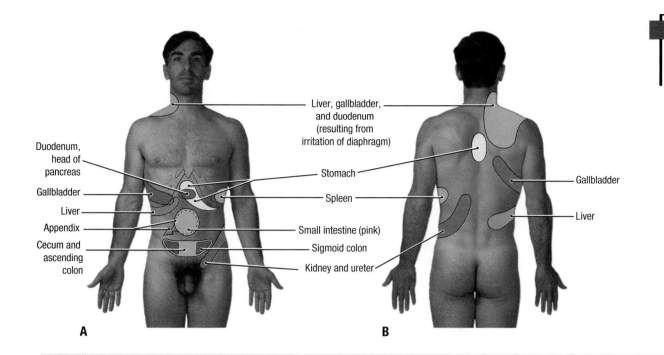

2.94 Surface projections of visceral pain

A. Anterior view. **B.** Posterior view. *Pain arising from a viscus (organ) varies from dull to severe, but is poorly localized. It radiates to the part of the body supplied by somatic sensory fibers associated with the same segment of the spinal cord that receives visceral sensory (autonomic) fibers from the viscus concerned. The pain is interpreted by the brain as though the irritation occurred in the area of skin supplied by the dorsal roots of the affected segments. This is called visceral referred pain.*

Labels (Anterior view A): Duodenum, head of pancreas; Gallbladder; Liver; Appendix; Cecum and ascending colon; Liver, gallbladder, and duodenum (resulting from irritation of diaphragm); Stomach; Spleen; Small intestine (pink); Sigmoid colon; Kidney and ureter

Labels (Posterior view B): Gallbladder; Liver

Table 2.4 Referred Pain

Organ	Nerve Supply	Spinal Cord	Referred Site and Clinical Example
Stomach	Anterior	T6–T9 or T10	Epigastric and left hypochondriac regions (e.g., gastric peptic ulcer)
Duodenum	Vagus nerves. Presynaptic sympathetic fibers reach celiac and superior mesenteric ganglia through greater splanchnic nerves.	T5–T9 or T10	Epigastric region (e.g., duodenal peptic ulcer) Right shoulder if ulcer perforates
Pancreatic head	Vagus and thoracic splanchnic nerves.	T8–T9	Inferior part of epigastric region (e.g., pancreatitis)
Small intestine (jejunum and ileum)	Posterior vagal trunks. Presynaptic sympathetic fibers reach celiac ganglion through greater splanchnic nerves.	T5–T9	Periumbilical region (e.g., acute intestinal obstruction)
Colon	Vagus nerves. Presynaptic sympathetic fibers reach celiac, superior mesenteric, and inferior mesenteric ganglia through greater splanchnic nerves.	T10–T12 (proximal colon)	Hypogastric region (e.g., ulcerative colitis)
	Parasympathetic supply to distal colon is derived from pelvic splanchnic nerves through hypogastric nerves and inferior hypogastric plexus.	L1–L3 (distal colon)	Left lower quadrant (e.g., sigmoiditis)
Spleen	Celiac plexus, especially from greater splanchnic nerve.	T6–T8	Left hypochondriac region (e.g., splenic infarct)
Appendix	Sympathetic and parasympathetic nerves from superior mesenteric plexus. Afferent nerve fibers accompany sympathetic nerves to T10 segment of spinal cord.	T10	Periumbilical region and later to right lower quadrant (e.g., appendicitis)
Gallbladder and liver	Nerves are derived from celiac plexus (sympathetic), vagus nerve (parasympathetic), and right phrenic nerve (sensory).	T6–T9	Epigastric region and later to right hypochondriac region; may cause pain on posterior thoracic wall or right shoulder owing to diaphragmatic irritation
Kidneys/ureters	Nerves arise from the renal plexus and consist of sympathetic, parasympathetic, and visceral afferent fibers from thoracic and lumbar splanchnics and the vagus nerve.	T11–T12	Small of back, flank (lumbar quadrant), extending to groin (inguinal region) and genitals (e.g., renal or ureteric calculi)

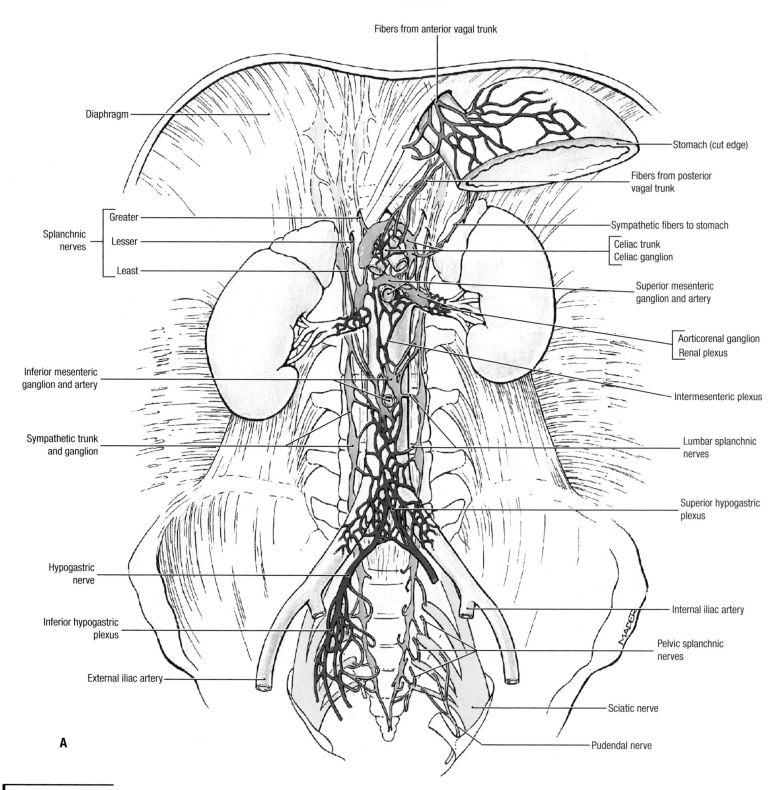

Fibers from anterior vagal trunk

Diaphragm

Stomach (cut edge)

Fibers from posterior vagal trunk

Splanchnic nerves
— Greater
— Lesser
— Least

Sympathetic fibers to stomach

Celiac trunk
Celiac ganglion

Superior mesenteric ganglion and artery

Aorticorenal ganglion
Renal plexus

Inferior mesenteric ganglion and artery

Intermesenteric plexus

Sympathetic trunk and ganglion

Lumbar splanchnic nerves

Superior hypogastric plexus

Hypogastric nerve

Internal iliac artery

Inferior hypogastric plexus

Pelvic splanchnic nerves

External iliac artery

Sciatic nerve

Pudendal nerve

A

2.95 Autonomic nerve supply of the abdomen

A. Abdominopelvic nerve plexuses and ganglia, anterior view.
B. Simplified diagram of abdominal nerve plexuses and ganglia, anterior view. Sympathetic and parasympathetic nerves mingle in the tangle of nerve plexuses anterior to the aorta; both types of fibers reach their destinations by "piggybacking" on the walls of branches of the abdominal aorta; this network is variable and difficult to dissect.

OBSERVE:
1. The interconnected plexuses on the abdominal aorta; the stems of the celiac, superior mesenteric, and inferior mesenteric arteries, and the areas between these vessels, are surrounded by networks of nerve fibers, e.g., the celiac, superior mesenteric, intermesenteric, and inferior mesenteric plexuses. The plexuses follow the

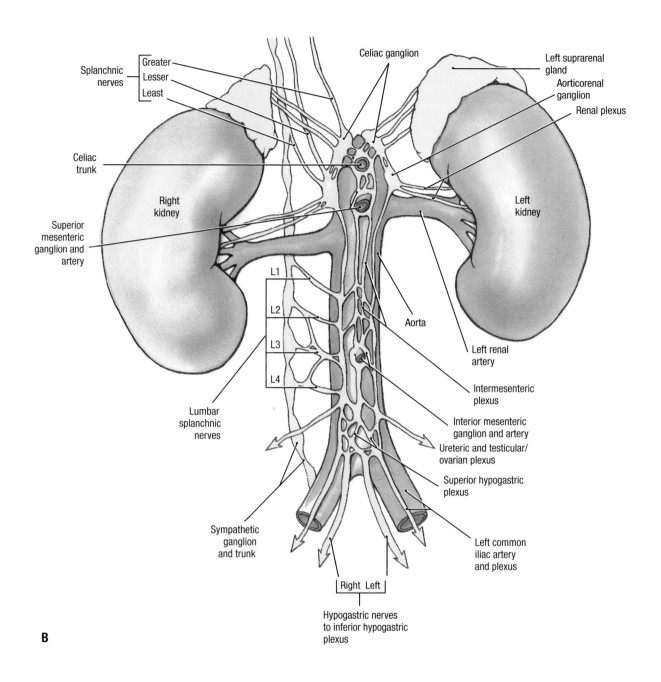

Splanchnic nerves
Greater
Lesser
Least

Celiac ganglion

Left suprarenal gland

Aorticorenal ganglion

Renal plexus

Celiac trunk

Right kidney

Left kidney

Superior mesenteric ganglion and artery

L1

L2

Aorta

L3

Left renal artery

L4

Intermesenteric plexus

Lumbar splanchnic nerves

Interior mesenteric ganglion and artery

Ureteric and testicular/ovarian plexus

Superior hypogastric plexus

Sympathetic ganglion and trunk

Left common iliac artery and plexus

Right Left

Hypogastric nerves to inferior hypogastric plexus

B

branches of these arteries to the viscera and are named according to which vessels they follow, e.g., the renal, testicular, ovarian, gastric, and cystic plexuses. The superior hypogastric plexus, at the bifurcation of the aorta, is connected by the hypogastric nerves to the inferior hypogastric plexus;

2. Sympathetic input is through preganglionic fibers (splanchnic nerves) from the right and left sympathetic trunks: greater, lesser, and least splanchnic nerves from the thorax, and lumbar splanchnic nerves from the abdomen. The greater splanchnic nerve is from thoracic ganglia 5 to 9, the lesser is from thoracic ganglia 10 and 11, the least is from thoracic ganglion 12, and the lumbar splanchnics are from the four lumbar ganglia.

3. The sympathetic splanchnic nerves synapse in preaortic ganglia, e.g., the greater splanchnic nerve ends in the celiac ganglion; the lesser splanchnic nerve ends in the renal plexus (aorticorenal gan-

glion); and the lumbar splanchnics in the intermesenteric and superior hypogastric plexuses. Usually, the greater splanchnic nerve pierces the crus at the level of the celiac trunk; the lesser nerve inferolateral to this, and the sympathetic trunk enters with the psoas major;

4. The sympathetic trunk lies on the vertebral bodies and descends along the anterior border of the psoas major; the trunk is slender where it enters the abdomen, its ganglia are ill defined, and approximately six lumbar splanchnic nerves leave it anteromedially;

5. Parasympathetic fibers through the posterior and anterior vagal trunks (formerly right and left vagus nerves) are distributed to the foregut and midgut; pelvic splanchnic nerves from branches of the anterior primary rami of sacral spinal nerves 2, 3, and 4 supply parasympathetic fibers to the hindgut and pelvic viscera.

A. Anterior and posterior. B. Vagal trunks, anterior view. Celiac plexus and ganglia, and suprarenal glands, anterosuperior view.

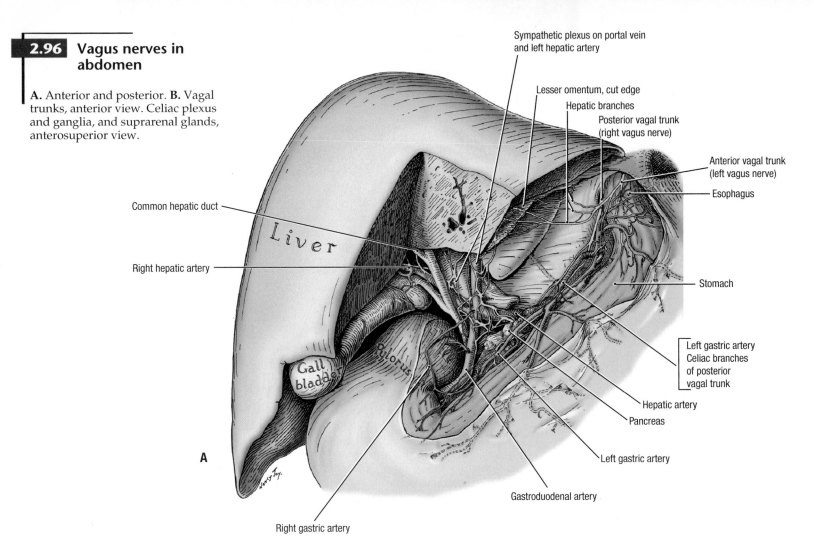

Sympathetic plexus on portal vein and left hepatic artery

Lesser omentum, cut edge

Hepatic branches

Posterior vagal trunk (right vagus nerve)

Anterior vagal trunk (left vagus nerve)

Esophagus

Stomach

Left gastric artery
Celiac branches of posterior vagal trunk

Hepatic artery

Pancreas

Left gastric artery

Gastroduodenal artery

Right gastric artery

Right hepatic artery

Common hepatic duct

Liver

Gall bladder

Pylorus

A

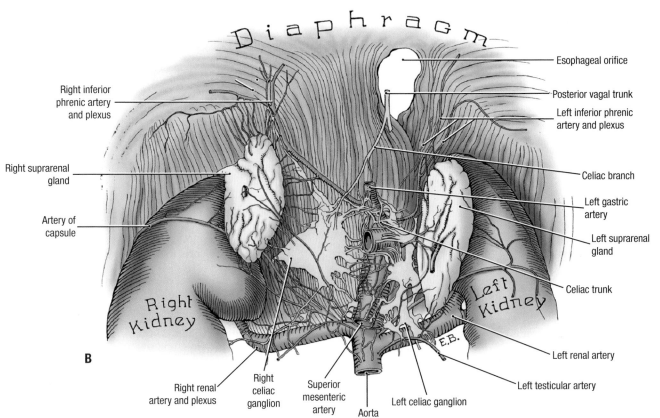

Diaphragm

Esophageal orifice

Posterior vagal trunk

Left inferior phrenic artery and plexus

Right inferior phrenic artery and plexus

Celiac branch

Left gastric artery

Left suprarenal gland

Celiac trunk

Left renal artery

Left testicular artery

Right suprarenal gland

Artery of capsule

Right Kidney

Left Kidney

E.B.

Right renal artery and plexus

Right celiac ganglion

Superior mesenteric artery

Aorta

Left celiac ganglion

B

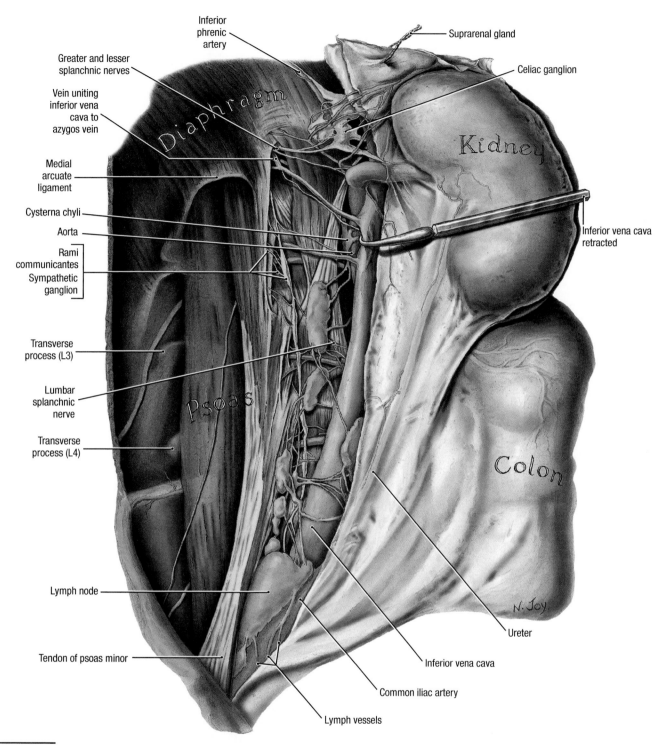

Inferior phrenic artery

Greater and lesser splanchnic nerves

Vein uniting inferior vena cava to azygos vein

Medial arcuate ligament

Cysterna chyli

Aorta

Rami communicantes

Sympathetic ganglion

Transverse process (L3)

Lumbar splanchnic nerve

Transverse process (L4)

Lymph node

Tendon of psoas minor

Suprarenal gland

Celiac ganglion

Kidney

Inferior vena cava retracted

Diaphragm

Psoas

Colon

N. Joy.

Ureter

Inferior vena cava

Common iliac artery

Lymph vessels

2.97 Splanchnic nerves, celiac ganglion, and sympathetic trunk

The right suprarenal gland, kidney, ureter, and colon are reflected; the inferior vena cava is pulled medially, and the third and fourth lumbar veins are removed. Recall that the splanchnic nerves are preganglionic fibers arising from the sympathetic trunk in the thoracic region. The greater splanchnic nerve is from ganglia 5 to 9, and the lesser from ganglia 10 to 11.

OBSERVE:
1. Both splanchnic nerves, the sympathetic trunk, and a communicating vein pass through an unusually wide cleft in the right crus;

2. The greater splanchnic nerve pierces the crus at the level of the celiac trunk and ends in the celiac ganglion; the lesser splanchnic nerve, inferolateral to the greater splanchnic nerve and ending in the aorticorenal ganglion;

3. The sympathetic trunk lies on the vertebral bodies; its ganglia are ill-defined. Numerous rami communicantes join it posterolaterally, and the lumbar splanchnic nerves leave it anteromedially;

4. The right lumbar lymph nodes and vessels drain into the cisterna chyli.

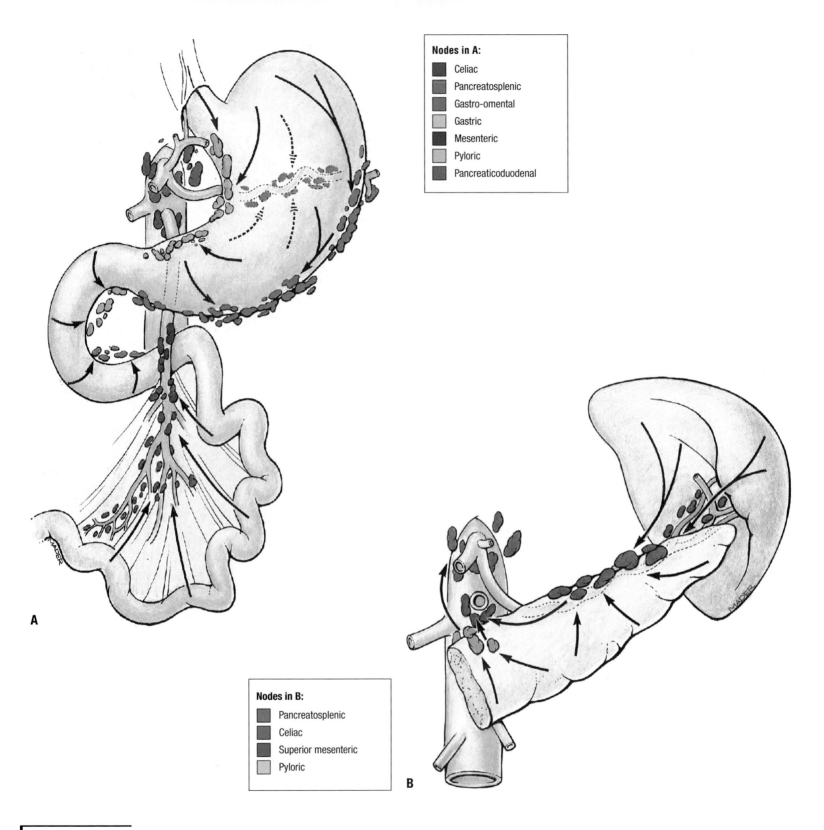

Nodes in A:

■ Celiac
■ Pancreatosplenic
■ Gastro-omental
■ Gastric
■ Mesenteric
■ Pyloric
■ Pancreaticoduodenal

Nodes in B:

■ Pancreatosplenic
■ Celiac
■ Superior mesenteric
■ Pyloric

2.98 **Lymphatic drainage, anterior views**

A. Stomach and small intestine. **B.** Spleen and pancreas. **C.** Large intestine. **D.** Liver and kidney. The *arrows* indicate the direction of lymph flow; each group of lymph nodes is color coded. Lymph from the abdominal nodes drains into the cisterna chyli, a sac at the inferior end of the thoracic duct. The thoracic duct receives all lymph that forms inferior to the diaphragm and empties into the junction of the left subclavian and left internal jugular veins (see Fig. 1.69).

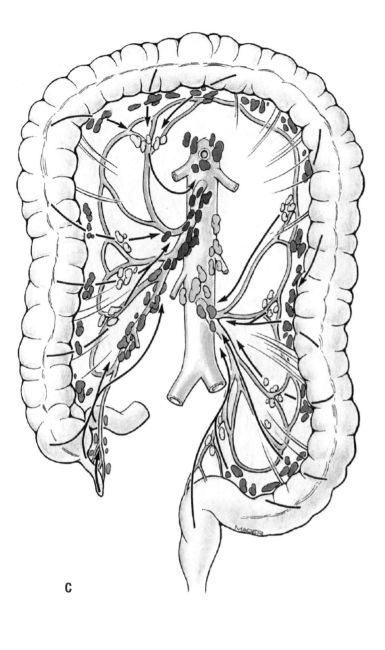

C

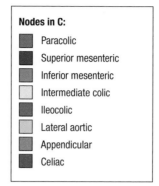

Nodes in C:

  Paracolic

  Superior mesenteric

  Inferior mesenteric

  Intermediate colic

  Ileocolic

  Lateral aortic

  Appendicular

  Celiac

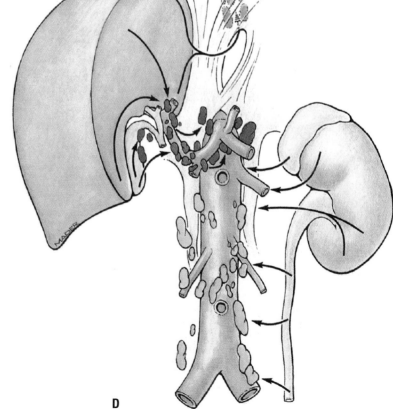

D

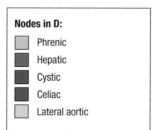

Nodes in D:

  Phrenic

  Hepatic

  Cystic

  Celiac

  Lateral aortic

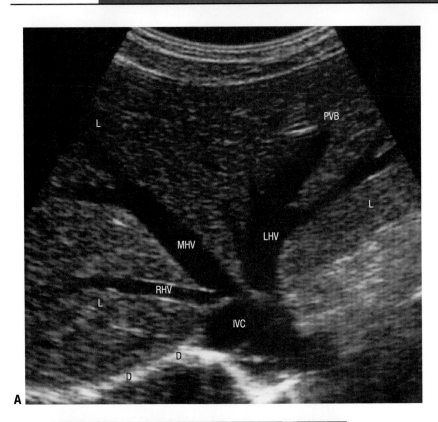

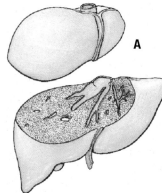

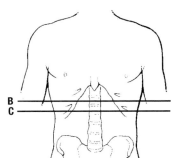

Ao	Aorta
CA	Celiac artery
D	Diaphragm
H	Hilum of kidney
IVC	Inferior vena cava
K	Kidney
L	Liver
LHV	Left hepatic vein
LPV	Left portal vein
LRA	Left renal artery
LRV	Left renal vein
MHV	Middle hepatic vein
P	Pancreas
PC	Portal confluence
PV	Portal vein
PVB	Branch of portal vein (portal triad)
RHV	Right hepatic vein
RPV	Right portal vein
SMA	Superior mesenteric artery
SV	Splenic vein
V	Vertebra

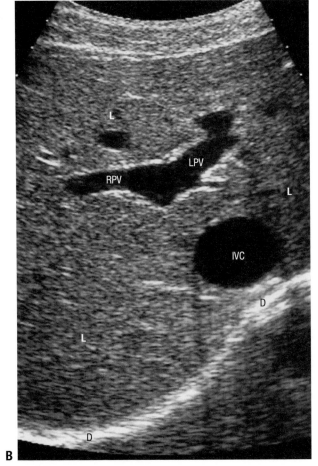

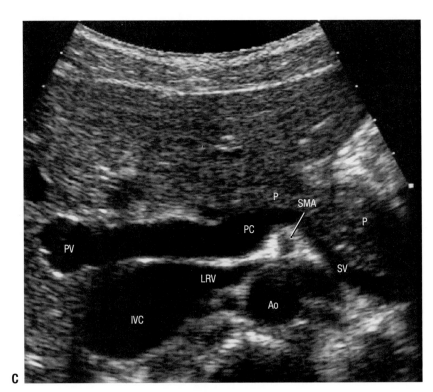

2.99 Ultrasound scans of the abdomen

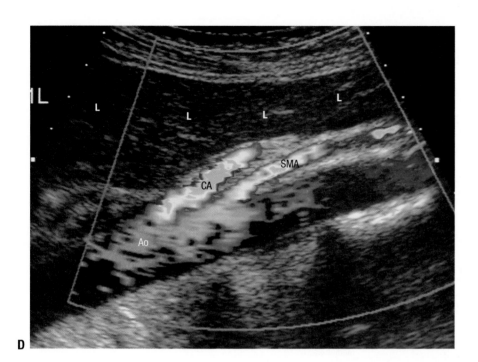

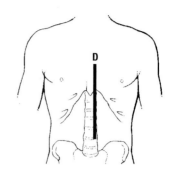

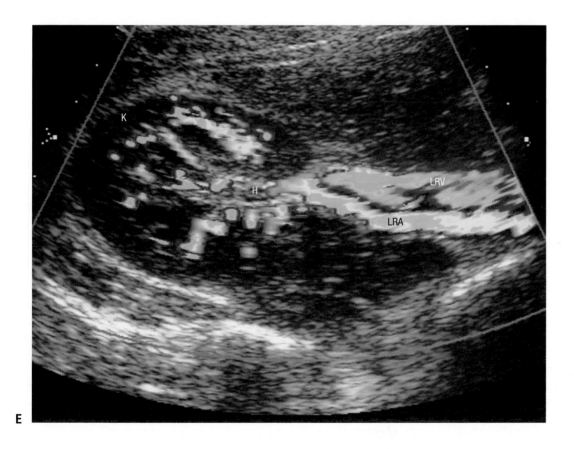

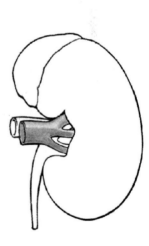

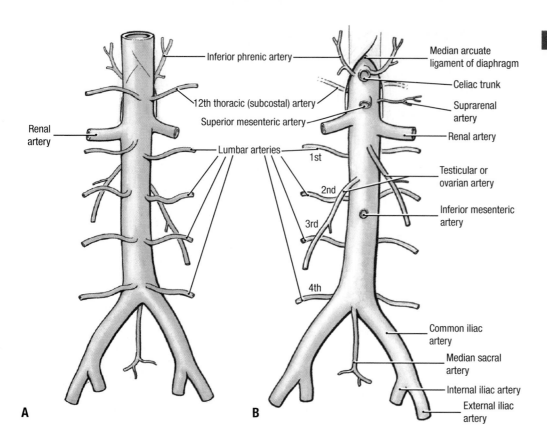

2.100 Abdominal aorta and its branches

A. Posterior view. **B**. Anterior view.

OBSERVE:

1. The unpaired visceral branches: celiac trunk (T12), superior mesenteric artery (L1), inferior mesenteric artery (L3);
2. The paired visceral branches: suprarenal arteries (L1), renal arteries (L1), gonadal arteries (ovarian or testicular, L2);
3. The paired parietal branches: subcostal arteries (T12), inferior phrenic arteries (T12), lumbar arteries (L1–L4);
4. The unpaired parietal branch, the median sacral artery, arises from the aorta at its bifurcation.

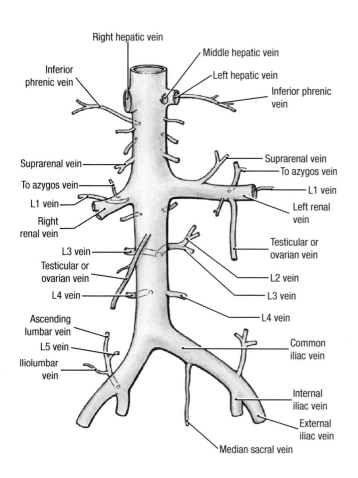

Key for Figure 2.102   ⟶

Ao	Aorta	PH	Head of pancreas
BAo	Bifurcation of aorta	PT	Tail of pancreas
CA	Celiac artery	PU	Uncinate process of
D	Diaphragm		pancreas
DB	Bulb of duodenum	Py	Pylorus of stomach
Dc	Descending colon	RC	Right crus
Do	Duodenum	RIL	Inferior lobe of right
DMB	Deep back muscles		lung
GE	Gastroesophageal	RL	Right lobe of liver
	junction	RRA	Right renal artery
IVC	Inferior vena cava	SA	Splenic artery
LIL	Inferior lobe of left	SI	Small intestine
	lung	SMA	Superior mesenteric
LK	Left kidney		artery
LL	Left lobe of liver	SMV	Superior mesenteric
LRV	Left renal vein		vein
MHV	Middle hepatic vein	Sp	Spleen
P	Pancreas	St	Stomach
Pa	Pyloric antrum	SV	Splenic vein
PC	Portal confluence	Tc	Transverse colon

2.101 Inferior vena cava and its tributaries, anterior view

Tributaries of the inferior vena cava correspond to branches of the aorta. Observe the common iliac veins, lumbar veins, right testicular or ovarian vein, renal veins, azygos vein, right suprarenal vein, inferior phrenic veins, and hepatic veins.

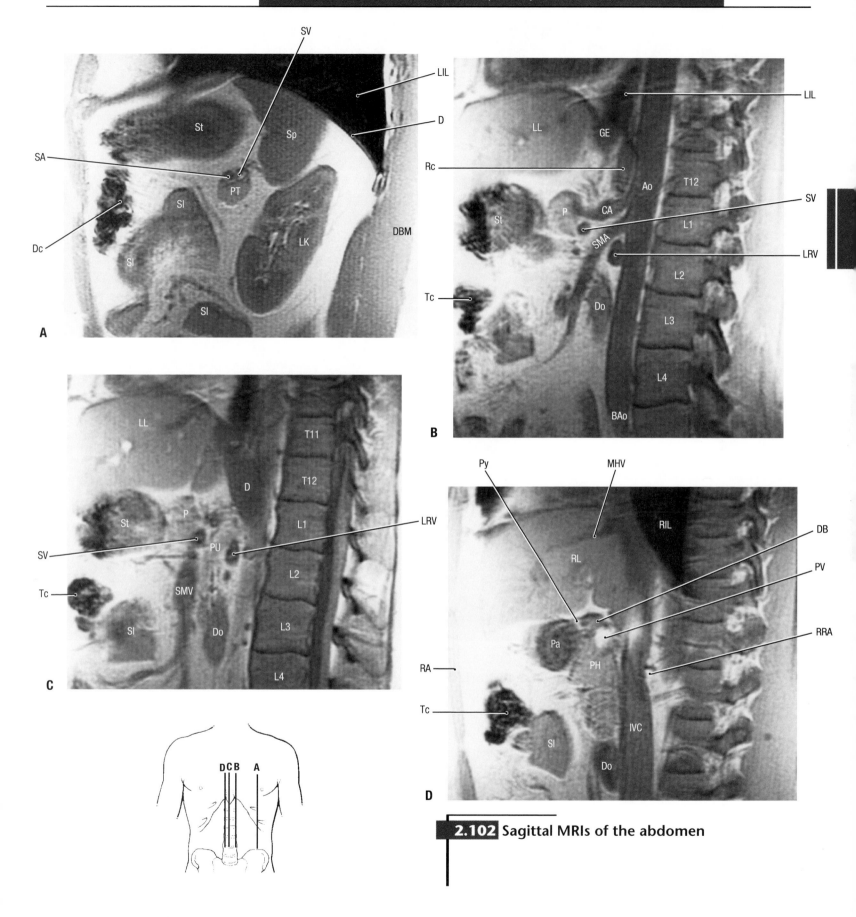

2.102 Sagittal MRIs of the abdomen

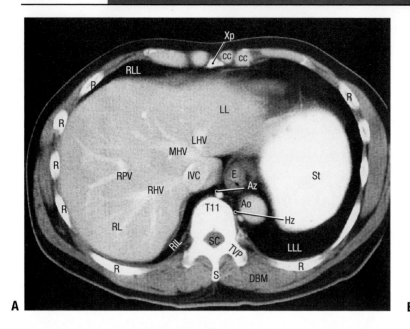

A

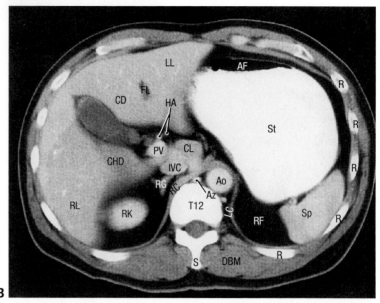

B

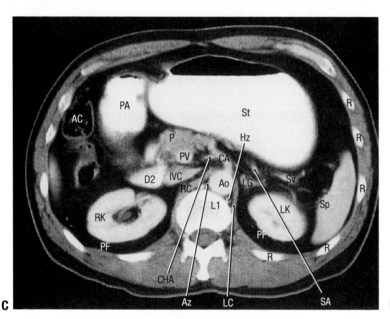

C

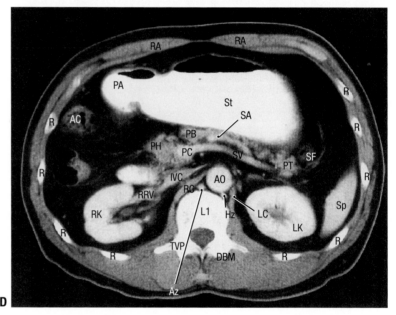

D

2.103 Transverse or horizontal (axial) MRIs of the abdomen

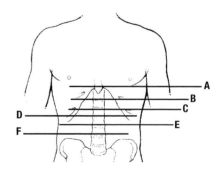

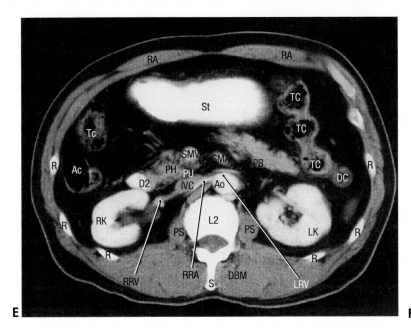

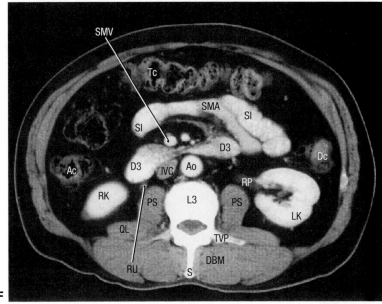

E   F

Ac	Ascending colon	PH	Head of pancreas
AF	Air-fluid level of stomach	PS	Psoas muscle
		PT	Tail of pancreas
Ao	Aorta	PU	Uncinate process of pancreas
Az	Azygos vein		
CA	Celiac artery	PV(R)	Branches of right portal vein
CC	Costal cartilage		
CD	Cystic duct	QL	Quadratus lumborum
CHA	Common hepatic artery	R	Rib
		RA	Rectus abdominis
CHD	Common hepatic duct	RC	Right crus of diaphragm
CL	Caudate lobe of liver		
DBM	Deep back muscles	RF	Retroperitoneal fat
Dc	Descending colon	RG	Right suprarenal gland
D2	2nd part of duodenum	RIL	Right inferior lobe of lung
D3	3rd part of duodenum		
E	Esophagus	RP	Renal pelvis
FL	Falciform ligament	RPV	Portal vein
GB	Gallbladder	RRA	Right renal artery
HA	Hepatic artery	RRV	Right renal vein
Hz	Hemiazygos vein	RU	Right ureter
IVC	Inferior vena cava	S	Spinous process
LC	Left crus of diaphragm	SA	Splenic artery
LG	Left suprarenal gland	SC	Spinal cord
LHV	Left hepatic vein	SF	Splenic flexure
LIL	Left inferior lobe of lung	SI	Small intestine
		SMA	Superior mesenteric artery
LL	Left lobe of liver		
LR	Right lobe of liver	SMV	Superior mesenteric vein
LRV	Left renal vein		
MHV	Middle hepatic vein	Sp	Spleen
P	Pancreas	St	Stomach
PA	Pyloric antrum of stomach	SV	Splenic vein
		Tc	Transverse colon
PB	Body of pancreas	TVP	Transverse process
PC	Portal confluence	XP	Xiphoid process
PF	Perirenal fat		

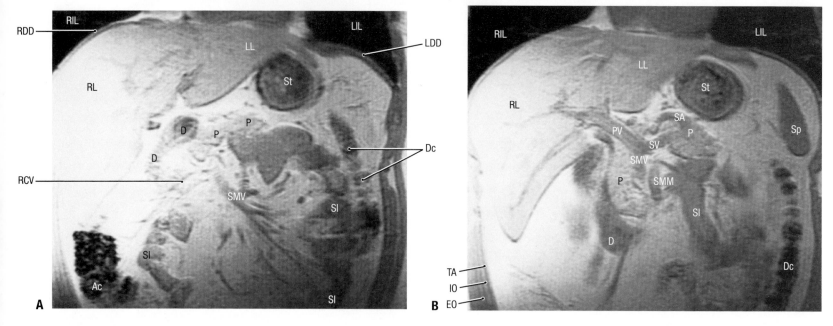

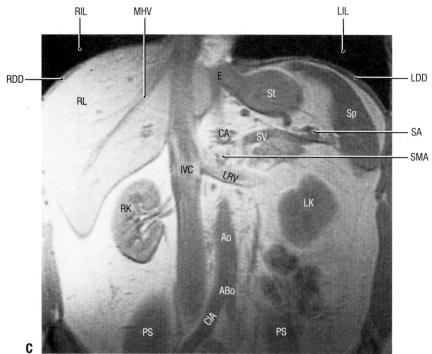

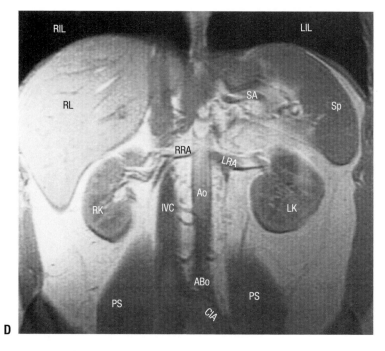

RIL	Right lung (inferior lobe)	SI	Small intestine	SA	Splenic artery	RRA	Right renal artery
LIL	Left lung (inferior lobe)	CA	Celiac artery	SV	Splenic vein	LRA	Left renal artery
RDD	Right dome of diaphragm	SMV	Superior mesenteric vein	D	Duodenum	RK	Right kidney
LDD	Left dome of diaphragm	SMA	Superior mesenteric artery	TA	Transversus abdominis	LK	Left kidney
RL	Right lobe of liver	RCV	Right colic vein	IO	Internal oblique	Ao	Aorta
LL	Left lobe of liver	Ac	Ascending colon	EO	External oblique	ABo	Aortic bifurcation
St	Stomach	Dc	Descending colon	MHV	Middle hepatic vein	CIA	Common iliac artery
Sp	Spleen	PV	Portal vein	IVC	Inferior vena cava	PS	Psoas
		P	Pancreas	LRV	Left renal vein		

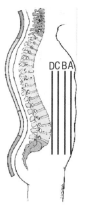

2.104 **Coronal MRIs of the abdomen**

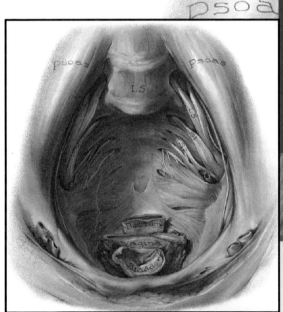

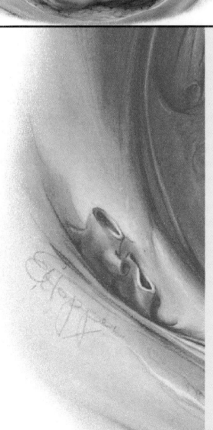

CHAPTER 3

Pelvis and Perineum

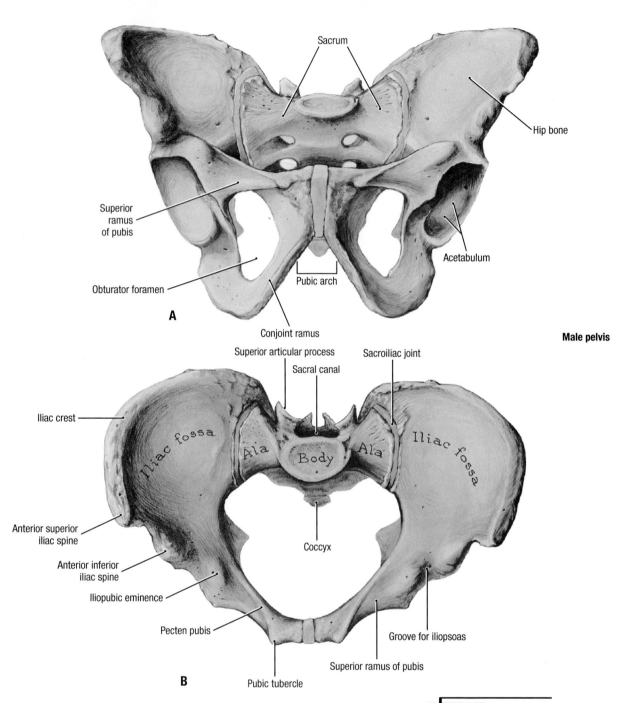

Male pelvis

A. Male pelvis, inferior view. **B.** Male pelvis, anterosuperior view.

3.1   Male and Female Pelves

Table 3.1. Differences Between Male and Female Pelves

Bony Pelvis	Male	Female
General structure	Thick and heavy	Thin and light
Greater pelvis (pelvis major)	Deep	Shallow
Lesser pelvis (pelvis minor)	Narrow and deep	Wide and shallow
Pelvic inlet (superior pelvic aperture)	Heart-shaped	Oval or rounded
Pelvis outlet (inferior pelvic aperture)	Comparatively small	Comparatively large
Pubic arch and subpubic angle	Narrow	Wide
Obturator foramen	Round	Oval
Acetabulum	Large	Small

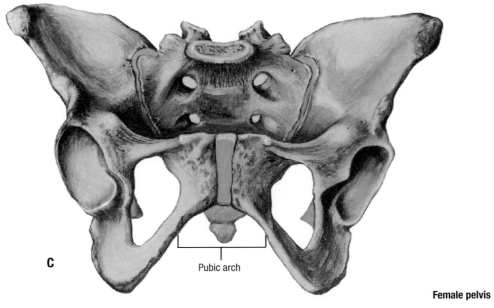

C

Pubic arch

Female pelvis

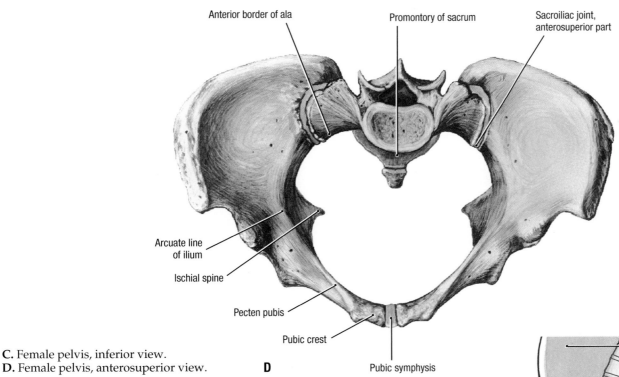

Anterior border of ala

Promontory of sacrum

Sacroiliac joint,
anterosuperior part

Arcuate line
of ilium

Ischial spine

Pecten pubis

Pubic crest

Pubic symphysis

C. Female pelvis, inferior view.
D. Female pelvis, anterosuperior view.   D

3.2   Pelvis major and pelvis minor, sagittal section

The pelvis major, or false pelvis (*green*), is formed by the iliac fossae and alae
of the sacrum. The pelvis minor, or true pelvis (*red*), is formed by the inner surface of the hip bone, sacrum, and coccyx. The superior broken line is the plane
of the pelvic brim surrounding the superior pelvic aperture; the inferior broken line is the plane of the inferior pelvic aperture. In the anatomic position,
the anterior superior iliac spine and anterior aspect of the pubic symphysis lie
in the same vertical plane.

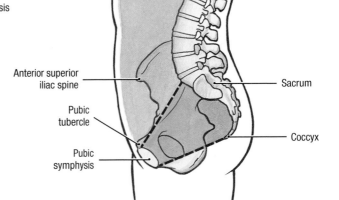

Abdominopelvic
cavity

Anterior superior
iliac spine

Sacrum

Pubic
tubercle

Coccyx

Pubic
symphysis

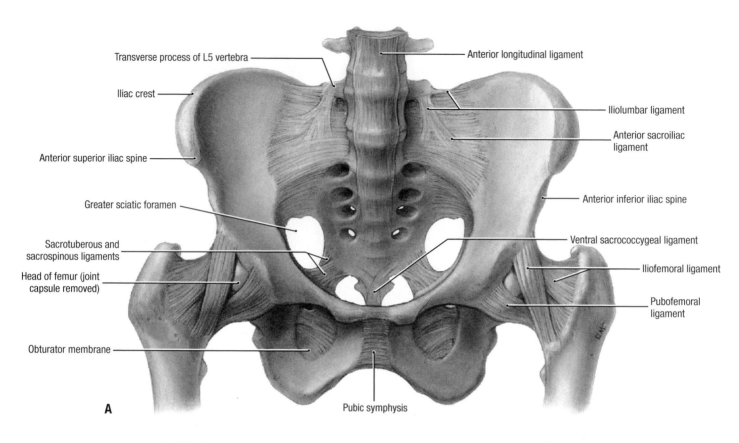

Transverse process of L5 vertebra

Iliac crest

Anterior superior iliac spine

Greater sciatic foramen

Sacrotuberous and sacrospinous ligaments

Head of femur (joint capsule removed)

Obturator membrane

Anterior longitudinal ligament

Iliolumbar ligament

Anterior sacroiliac ligament

Anterior inferior iliac spine

Ventral sacrococcygeal ligament

Iliofemoral ligament

Pubofemoral ligament

Pubic symphysis

A

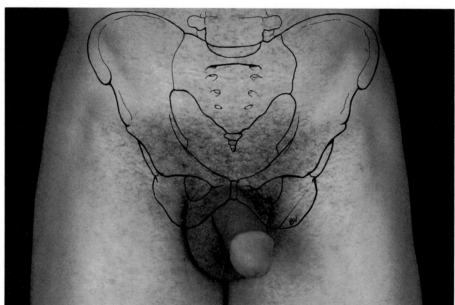

B

3.3   **Pelvis and pelvic ligaments**

A. Ligaments of pelvis, anterior view. **B.** Pelvis in situ, anterior view.

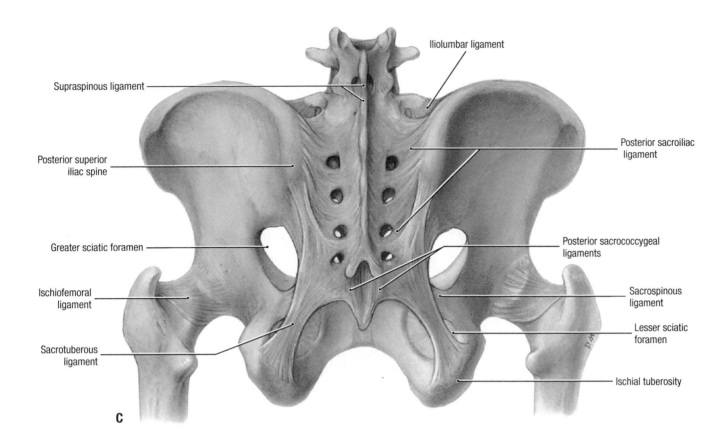

Iliolumbar ligament

Supraspinous ligament

Posterior sacroiliac ligament

Posterior superior iliac spine

Greater sciatic foramen

Posterior sacrococcygeal ligaments

Ischiofemoral ligament

Sacrospinous ligament

Lesser sciatic foramen

Sacrotuberous ligament

Ischial tuberosity

C

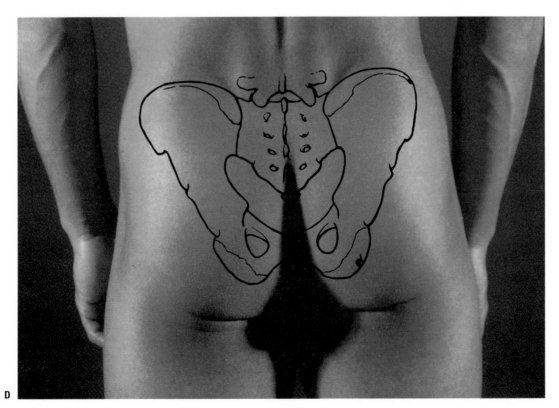

D

C. Ligaments of pelvis, posterior view. **D.** Pelvis in situ, posterior view.

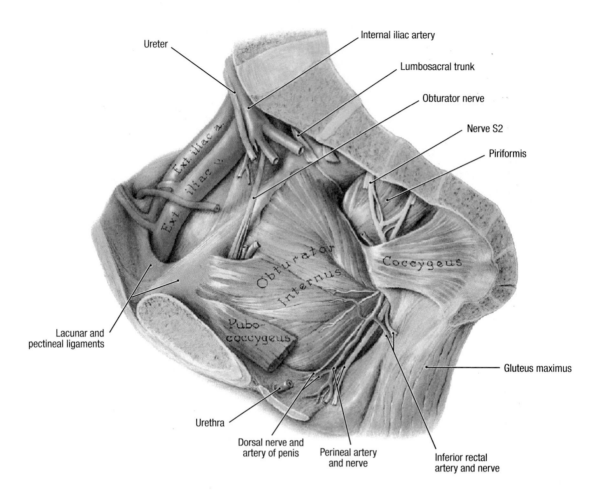

Ureter

Internal iliac artery

Lumbosacral trunk

Obturator nerve

Nerve S2

Piriformis

Ext. iliac a.

Ext. iliac v.

Obturator internus

Coccygeus

Pubo-coccygeus

Lacunar and pectineal ligaments

Gluteus maximus

Urethra

Dorsal nerve and artery of penis

Perineal artery and nerve

Inferior rectal artery and nerve

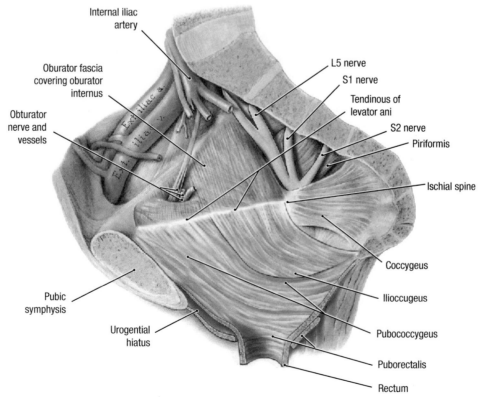

Internal iliac artery

Oburator fascia covering oburator internus

Obturator nerve and vessels

Ext. iliac a.

Ext. iliac v.

L5 nerve

S1 nerve

Tendinous of levator ani

S2 nerve

Piriformis

Ischial spine

Coccygeus

Ilioccugeus

Pubic symphysis

Urogential hiatus

Pubococcygeus

Puborectalis

Rectum

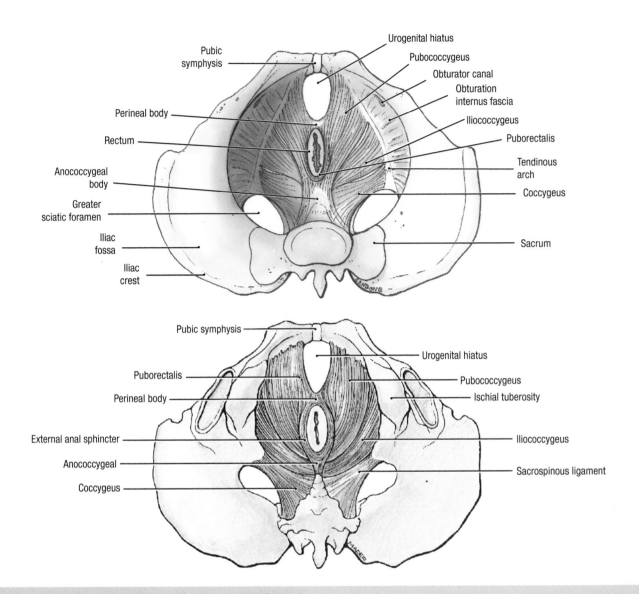

Table 3.2. Muscles of Pelvic Walls and Floor[a]

Muscle	Proximal Attachment	Distal Attachment	Innervation	Main Action
Obturator internus	Pelvic surfaces of ilium and ischium; obturator membrane		Nerve to obturator internus (L5, S1, and S2)	Rotates thigh laterally; assists in holding head of femur in acetabulum
Piriformis	Pelvic surface of second to fourth sacral segments: superior margin of greater sciatic notch, and sacrotuberous ligament	Greater trochanter of femur	Ventral rami of S1 and S2	Rotates thigh laterally; abducts thigh; assists in holding head of femur in acetabulum
Levator ani (pubococcygeus, puborectalis, and iliococcygeus)	Body of pubis, tendinous arch of obturator fascia, and ischial spine	Perineal body, coccyx, anococcygeal ligament, walls of prostate or vagina, rectum, and anal canal	Branches of S4 and pudendal	Form pelvic diaphragm; Help to support the pelvic viscera and resists increases in intraabdominal pressure
Coccygeus (ischiococcygeus)	Ischial spine	Inferior end of sacrum	Branches of S4 and S5	

[a]See Figures 3.20, 3.21, 3.22.

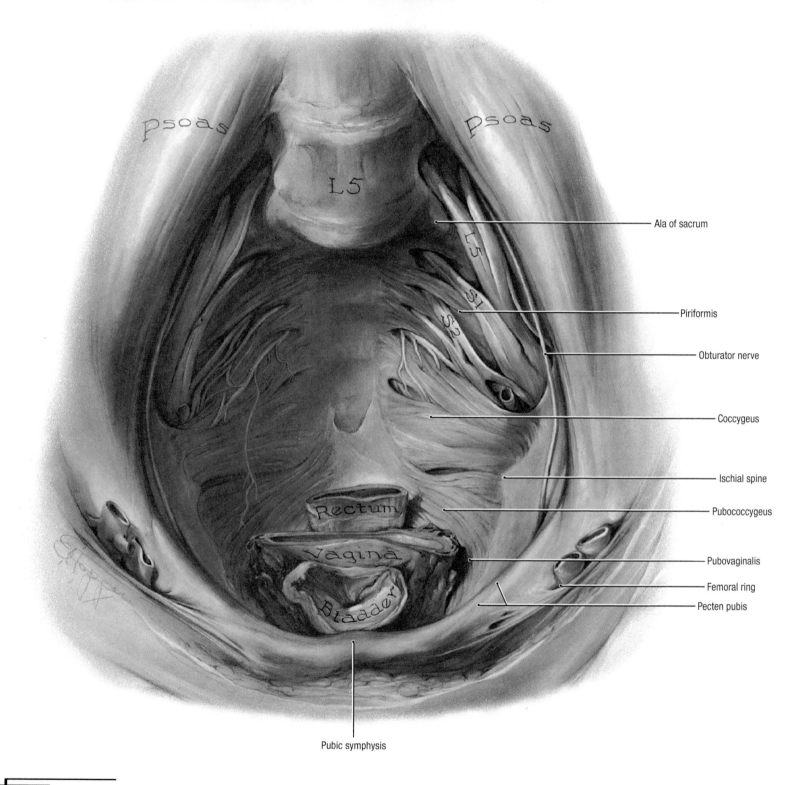

- Psoas
- Psoas
- L5
- Ala of sacrum
- L5
- S1
- S2
- Piriformis
- Obturator nerve
- Coccygeus
- Ischial spine
- Rectum
- Pubococcygeus
- Vagina
- Pubovaginalis
- Bladder
- Femoral ring
- Pecten pubis
- Pubic symphysis

3.4   Floor of female pelvis, superior view

The pelvic viscera are removed to reveal the levator ani and coccygeus muscles.

OBSERVE:

1. The muscles of the pelvic floor;
2. The relative positions of the bladder, vagina, and rectum;
3. The obturator nerve runs along the lateral wall of the pelvis and enters the thigh through the obturator foramen;

4. The femoral ring is the "doorway" into the femoral canal (see Fig. 5.12). *The femoral ring is a weak area in the anterior abdominal wall that is the common site of femoral hernias, protrusions of abdominal viscera (often the small intestine) through the femoral ring into the femoral canal.*

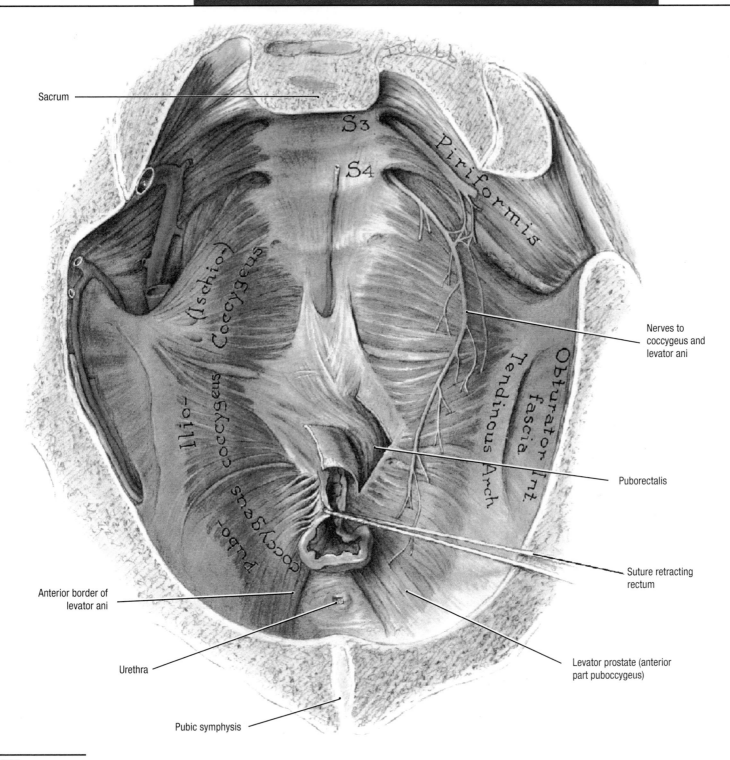

Sacrum

S3

S4

Piriformis

(Ischio-) Coccygeus

Ilio- coccygeus

Pubo- coccygeus

Obturator Int. fascia Tendinous Arch

Nerves to coccygeus and levator ani

Puborectalis

Suture retracting rectum

Anterior border of levator ani

Urethra

Levator prostate (anterior part puboccygeus)

Pubic symphysis

3.5   **Floor of male pelvis, superior view**

The pelvic viscera are removed, and the bony pelvis is sawed through transversely to reveal the levator ani and coccygeus muscles.

OBSERVE:

1. The pubococcygeus muscle arises mainly from the pubic bone, the ischiococcygeus muscle from the ischial spine, and the iliococcygeus muscle from the tendinous arch. The pubococcygeus muscle is strong, and the iliococcygeus muscle is weak; the ischiococcygeus muscle is part of the sacrospinous ligament;

2. The anterior free border of the pubococcygeus muscle and the posterior free border of the ischiococcygeus muscle; the clefts at the borders of the iliococcygeus muscle are closed by membranes;

3. In the male, the anterior part of the pubococcygeus muscle that lies adjacent to the prostate is called the levator prostatae; in the female, the part that lies adjacent to the vagina is called the pubovaginalis;

4. The urethra passes between the anterior borders and the rectum, perforating the pubococcygei muscles; the sphincter urethrae surrounds the urethra, and the deep transverse perineal is visible between the anterior borders of the pubococcygei muscles;

5. Branches of S3 and S4 nerves supply the levator ani and coccygeus muscles; the pudendal nerve, through its perineal branch, also supplies the levator ani muscle (see Fig. 3.22A).

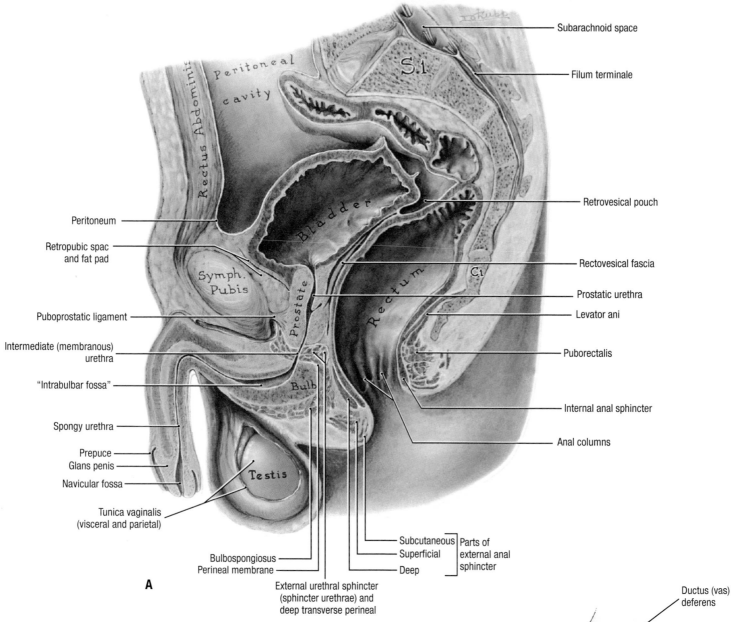

Peritoneum

Retropubic spac
and fat pad

Puboprostatic ligament

Intermediate (membranous)
urethra

"Intrabulbar fossa"

Spongy urethra

Prepuce
Glans penis
Navicular fossa

Tunica vaginalis
(visceral and parietal)

Bulbospongiosus
Perineal membrane

Subarachnoid space

Filum terminale

Retrovesical pouch

Rectovesical fascia

Prostatic urethra

Levator ani

Puborectalis

Internal anal sphincter

Anal columns

Subcutaneous ⎱ Parts of
Superficial ⎰ external anal
Deep   sphincter

A

External urethral sphincter
(sphincter urethrae) and
deep transverse perineal

3.6   Male pelvis

A. Median section. **B.** Overview of urogenital system, median section.

OBSERVE:

1. The urinary bladder is slightly distended and rests on the rectum. The prostatic urethra descends vertically through an elongated prostate, and the short intermediate (membranous) urethra passes through the perineal membrane. The spongy urethra has a low-lying dilation in the bulb, the intrabulbar fossa, and the navicular fossa in the glans penis. By contracting, the bulbospongiosus muscle empties the urethra;
2. The involuntary internal anal sphincter does not descend as far as the voluntary external anal sphincter, and is separated from it by a fascial layer;
3. There are two layers of rectovesical fascia in the median plane between the bladder and rectum; on each side the fascia contains the

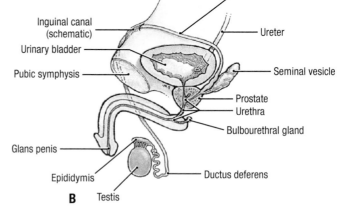

Inguinal canal
(schematic)
Urinary bladder
Pubic symphysis

Glans penis

Epididymis

B   Testis

Ductus (vas)
deferens

Ureter

Seminal vesicle

Prostate
Urethra
Bulbourethral gland

Ductus deferens

deferent duct (vas deferens), seminal vesicle, and vesical vessels (see Fig. 3.14B);
4. The tunica vaginalis is opened to expose the testis.

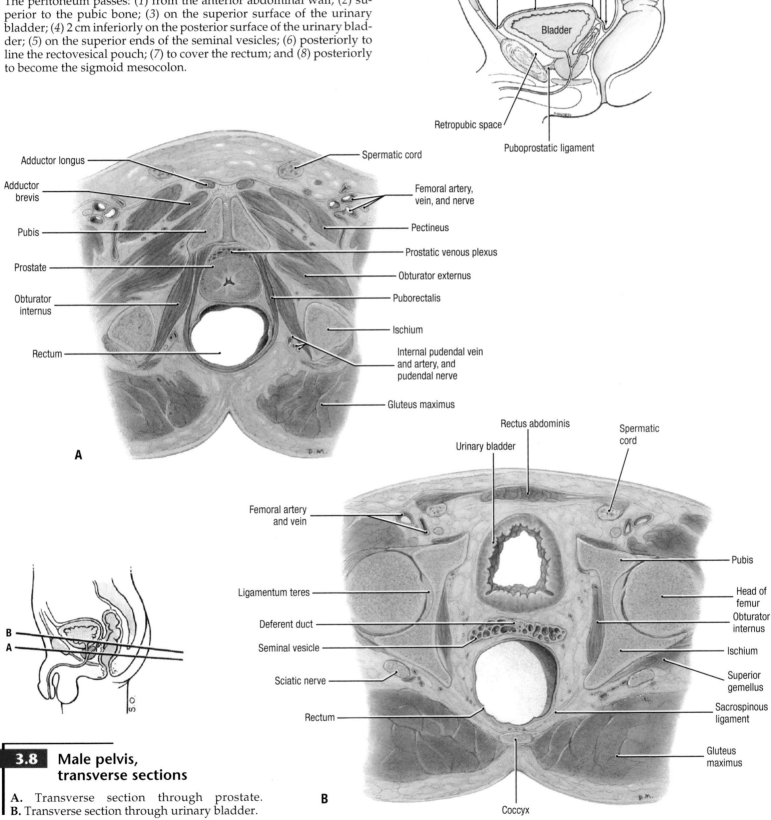

3.7   Peritoneum covering male pelvic organs, median section

The peritoneum passes: (*1*) from the anterior abdominal wall; (*2*) superior to the pubic bone; (*3*) on the superior surface of the urinary bladder; (*4*) 2 cm inferiorly on the posterior surface of the urinary bladder; (*5*) on the superior ends of the seminal vesicles; (*6*) posteriorly to line the rectovesical pouch; (*7*) to cover the rectum; and (*8*) posteriorly to become the sigmoid mesocolon.

Labels (top diagram): Bladder; Retropubic space; Puboprostatic ligament

Labels (section A): Adductor longus; Adductor brevis; Pubis; Prostate; Obturator internus; Rectum; Spermatic cord; Femoral artery, vein, and nerve; Pectineus; Prostatic venous plexus; Obturator externus; Puborectalis; Ischium; Internal pudendal vein and artery, and pudendal nerve; Gluteus maximus

A

Labels (section B): Rectus abdominis; Spermatic cord; Urinary bladder; Femoral artery and vein; Ligamentum teres; Deferent duct; Seminal vesicle; Sciatic nerve; Rectum; Pubis; Head of femur; Obturator internus; Ischium; Superior gemellus; Sacrospinous ligament; Gluteus maximus; Coccyx

B

3.8   Male pelvis, transverse sections

A. Transverse section through prostate.
B. Transverse section through urinary bladder.

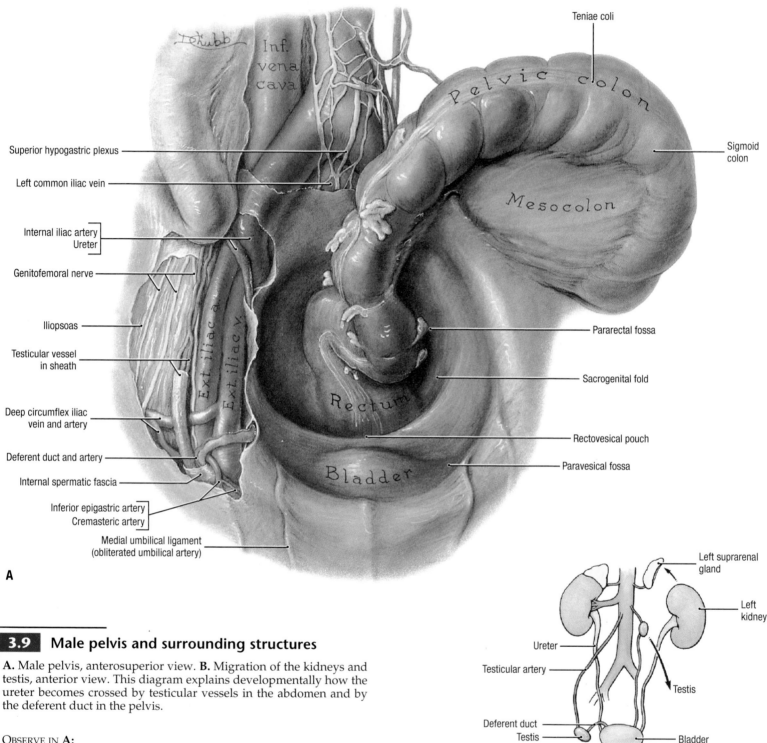

A. Male pelvis, anterosuperior view. **B.** Migration of the kidneys and testis, anterior view. This diagram explains developmentally how the ureter becomes crossed by testicular vessels in the abdomen and by the deferent duct in the pelvis.

3.9   Male pelvis and surrounding structures

OBSERVE IN **A**:
1. The sigmoid colon begins at the left pelvic brim and becomes the rectum anterior to the third sacral segment in the midline;
2. The inverted, V-shaped mesentery of the sigmoid colon, the sigmoid mesocolon, attaches the sigmoid colon to the pelvic wall;
3. The teniae coli form two wide bands: one anterior to the rectum, the other posterior;
4. The superior hypogastric plexus lies at the bifurcation of the aorta and anterior to the left common iliac vein;
5. The ureter adheres to the peritoneum, crosses the external iliac vessels, and descends anterior to the internal iliac artery. The deferent duct and its artery also adhere to the peritoneum, cross the external iliac vessels, and then hook around the inferior epigastric artery to join the other components of the spermatic cord;
6. The genitofemoral nerve lies on the psoas fascia; its two lateral (femoral) branches become cutaneous, and its medial (genital) branch supplies the cremaster muscle and becomes cutaneous.

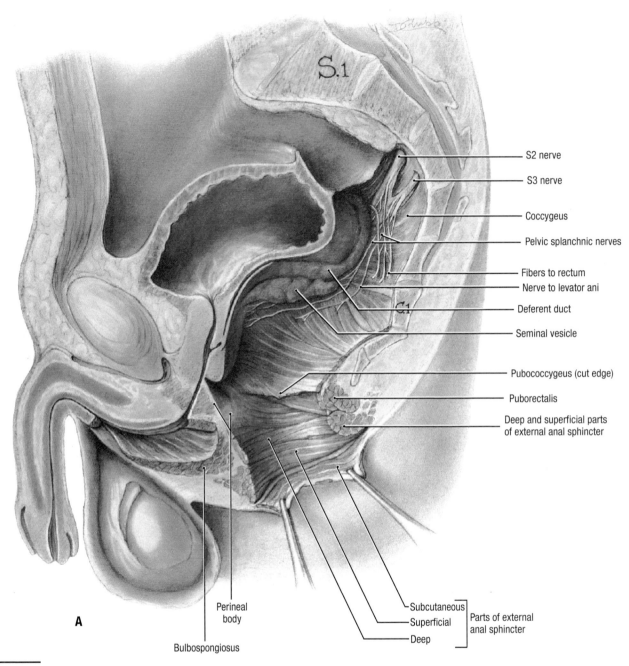

S2 nerve

S3 nerve

Coccygeus

Pelvic splanchnic nerves

Fibers to rectum

Nerve to levator ani

Deferent duct

Seminal vesicle

Pubococcygeus (cut edge)

Puborectalis

Deep and superficial parts
of external anal sphincter

Perineal
body

A

Bulbospongiosus

Subcutaneous
Superficial   Parts of external
                   anal sphincter
Deep

3.10 Levator ani

A. Levator ani, median section. The rectum, anal canal, and bulb of the penis are removed from the specimen in Figure 3.6A. The subcutaneous fibers of the external anal sphincter are reflected with forceps. **B.** Puborectalis, lateral view. The puborectalis muscle forms a U-shaped muscular "sling" around the anorectal junction, which maintains the anorectal flexure.

OBSERVE IN **A**:

1. The superficial fibers of the external anal sphincter mingle posteriorly with deep fibers, and the deep fibers mingle posteriorly with the puborectalis muscle, which forms a sling that occupies the angle between the rectum and anal canal;
2. The pubococcygeus muscle is divided to remove the anal canal, to which it is, in part, attached;
3. The deferent duct and seminal vesicle curve to fit the cyclindrical rectum.

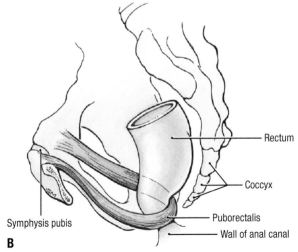

Rectum

Coccyx

Symphysis pubis

Puborectalis

Wall of anal canal

B

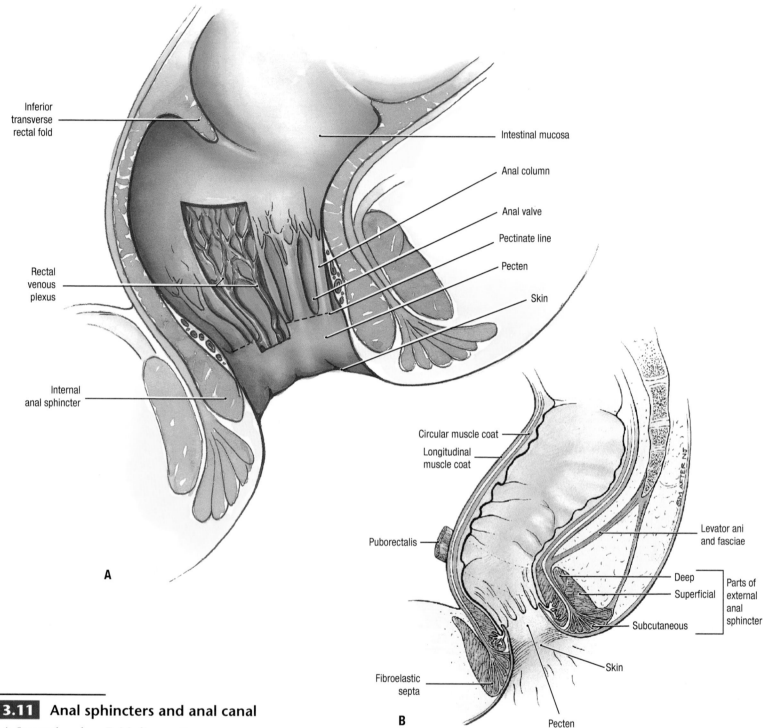

Inferior transverse rectal fold

Intestinal mucosa

Anal column

Anal valve

Pectinate line

Pecten

Rectal venous plexus

Skin

Internal anal sphincter

A

Circular muscle coat

Longitudinal muscle coat

Puborectalis

Levator ani and fasciae

Deep — Parts of external anal sphincter
Superficial
Subcutaneous

Skin

Fibroelastic septa

B

Pecten

3.11   Anal sphincters and anal canal

A. Internal surface. **B.** Median section.

OBSERVE:

1. The internal anal sphincter is a thickening of the inner, circular, muscular coat of the anal canal;
2. There are three parts of the external anal sphincter: deep, superficial, and subcutaneous; the deep part intermingles with the puborectalis muscle posteriorly;
3. The longitudinal muscle layer of the rectum separates the internal and external anal sphincters and terminates in the subcutaneous tissue and skin around the anus;
4. The anal columns are 5 to 10 vertical folds of mucosa separated by anal valves; they contain the rectal venous plexus;

5. The pecten is a smooth area of simple stratified epithelium that lies between the anal valves superiorly and the inferior border of the internal sphincter inferiorly. There is a transitional zone between the intestinal mucosa superiorly and skin with dermal papillae inferiorly;
6. The pecinate line is an irregular line at the base of the anal valves where the intestinal mucosa is continuous with the pecten; afferent innervation is visceral proximally to the line and somatic distally. Lymphatic drainage is to the pararectal nodes proximally and to the superficial inguinal nodes distally.

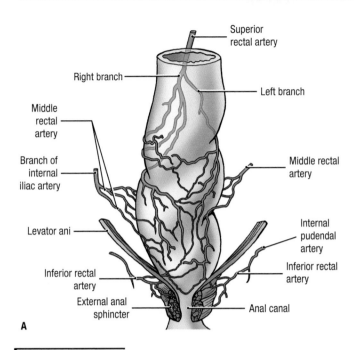

A

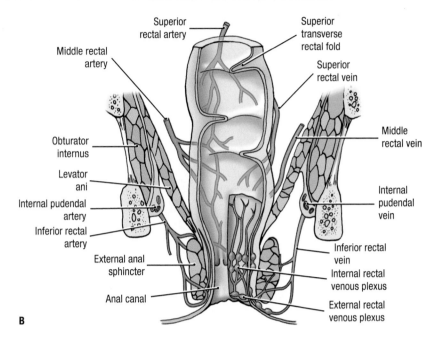

B

3.12 Rectum and anal canal

A. Arteries, anterior view. **B.** Venous drainage, coronal section. **C.** Innervation of rectum, anterior view.

OBSERVE IN **A**:
1. The branches of the right and left divisions of the superior rectal artery obliquely encircle the rectum;
2. The middle rectal arteries (branches of the internal iliac arteries) are usually small; in this specimen, the right artery is small, but the left one is large;
3. The inferior rectal arteries branch from the internal pudendal arteries;

OBSERVE IN **B**:
4. The venous drainage is through superior, middle, and inferior rectal veins; there are anastomoses between all three veins;
5. The rectal venous plexus surrounds the rectum and consists of an internal rectal plexus deep to the epithelium of the rectum and an external rectal plexus external to the muscular coats of the wall of the rectum;
6. The superior rectal vein drains into the portal system, and the middle and inferior veins drain into the systemic system; thus, this is an important area of portal caval anastomosis. *Varicosity of the internal rectal plexus can result in internal hemorrhoids; external hemorrhoids involve the external rectal plexus.*

OBSERVE IN **C**:
7. On the right side of the figure: The voluntary external anal sphincter and skin around the anus are innervated by the inferior rectal nerve, a branch of the pudendal nerve (S2, S3, and S4);
8. On the left: The autonomic innervation from the parasympathetic pelvic splanchnic nerves (S2, S3, and S4), sympathetic hypogastric nerves (from the superior hypogastric plexus), and visceral (sacral) splanchnic nerves (from the 2nd and 3rd sacral sympathetic ganglia). The sympathetic and parasympathetic fibers become intermingled in the inferior hypogastric plexus, located on the lateral wall of the rectum; the fibers are conveyed from the plexus to the wall of the rectum and the involuntary internal anal sphincter.

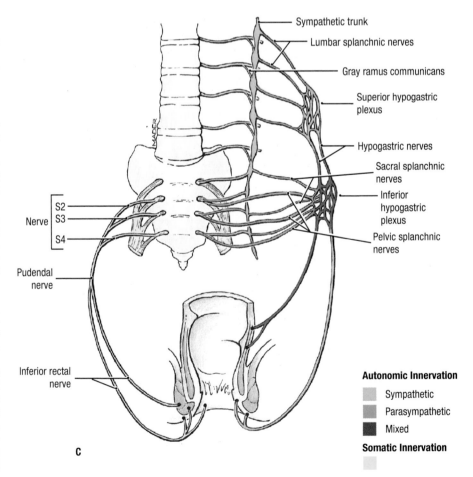

C

Autonomic Innervation
- Sympathetic
- Parasympathetic
- Mixed

Somatic Innervation

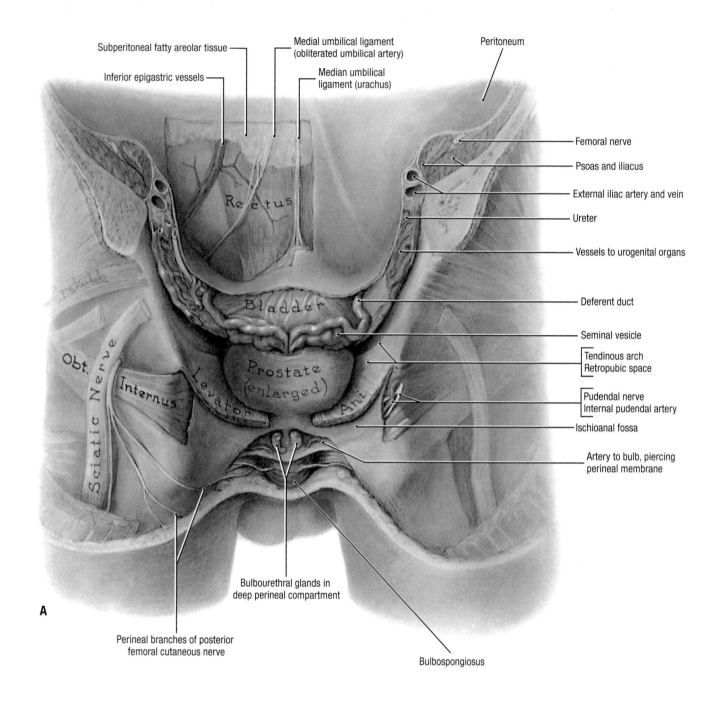

Subperitoneal fatty areolar tissue

Inferior epigastric vessels

Medial umbilical ligament
(obliterated umbilical artery)

Median umbilical
ligament (urachus)

Peritoneum

Femoral nerve

Psoas and iliacus

External iliac artery and vein

Ureter

Vessels to urogenital organs

Deferent duct

Seminal vesicle

Tendinous arch
Retropubic space

Pudendal nerve
Internal pudendal artery

Ischioanal fossa

Artery to bulb, piercing
perineal membrane

Bulbourethral glands in
deep perineal compartment

Bulbospongiosus

Perineal branches of posterior
femoral cutaneous nerve

Rectus · Ischium · Obt. Nerve · Sciatic Nerve · Internus · Levator · Ani · Bladder · Prostate (enlarged)

A

3.13   Male pelvis, coronal sections through pelvis anterior to rectum

A. Dissection, view of anterior portion from behind.

OBSERVE IN **A:**

1. The inferior epigastric artery and venae comitantes enter the rectus sheath to form the lateral umbilical ligament; the medial umbilical ligament formed by the obliterated umbilical artery and the median umbilical ligament formed by the urachus;
2. The femoral nerve lies between the psoas and iliacus muscles outside the psoas fascia, which is attached to the pelvic brim; the external iliac artery and vein lie inside the psoas fascia;

3. The deferent duct and ureter are subperitoneal; near the bladder, the ureter accompanies a "leash" of vesical vessels enclosed in the rectovesical fascia;
4. The levator ani muscle and its fascial coverings separate the retropubic space from the ischioanal fossa; note the free anterior borders of the levator ani;
5. The bulbourethral glands and the artery to the bulb lie superior to the perineal membrane;
6. The obturator internus muscle makes a right-angled "turn" as it leaves its osseofascial pocket.

B. Umbilical ligaments, posterior view.

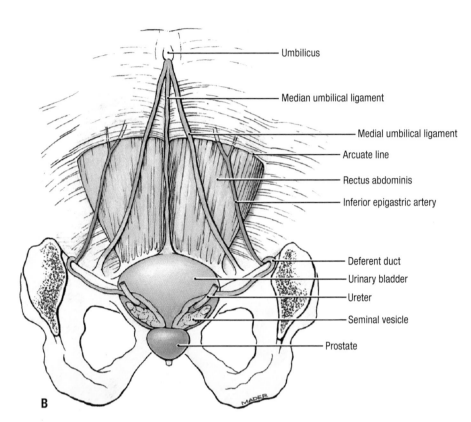

- Umbilicus
- Median umbilical ligament
- Medial umbilical ligament
- Arcuate line
- Rectus abdominis
- Inferior epigastric artery
- Deferent duct
- Urinary bladder
- Ureter
- Seminal vesicle
- Prostate

B

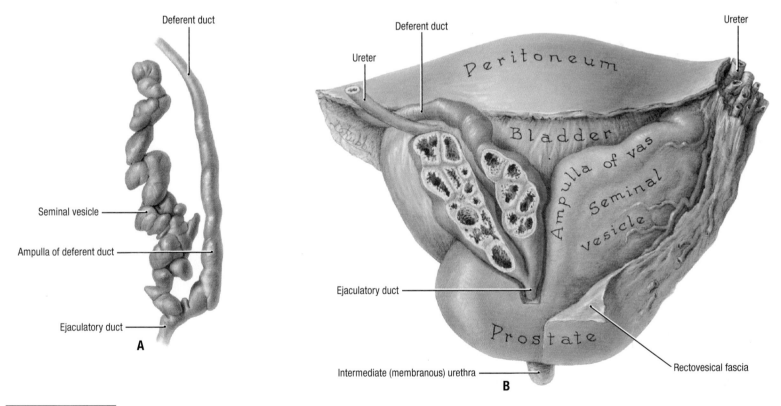

Deferent duct

Seminal vesicle

Ampulla of deferent duct

Ejaculatory duct

A

Deferent duct

Ureter

Ureter

Peritoneum

Bladder

Ampulla of vas

Seminal vesicle

Ejaculatory duct

Rectovesical fascia

Prostate

Intermediate (membranous) urethra

B

3.14 Seminal vesicles and prostate

A. Seminal vesicle, unraveled. The vesicle is a tortuous tube with numerous outpouchings. The ampulla of the deferent duct (vas deferens) has similar outpouchings. **B.** Bladder, deferent ducts, seminal vesicles, and prostate, posterior view. The left seminal vesicle and ampulla of the deferent duct are dissected free and sliced open; part of the prostate is cut away to expose the ejaculatory duct.

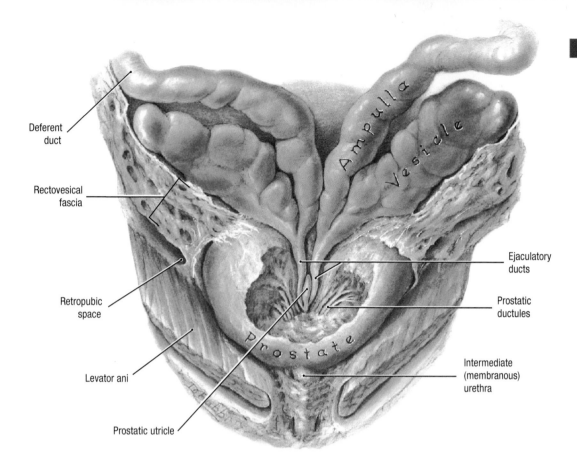

Deferent duct

Rectovesical fascia

Retropubic space

Levator ani

Prostatic utricle

Ampulla

Vesicle

Prostate

Ejaculatory ducts

Prostatic ductules

Intermediate (membranous) urethra

3.15   Prostate, posterior view

OBSERVE:
1. The right and left ejaculatory ducts are each formed where the duct of a seminal vesicle joins the ampullary end of a deferent duct;
2. The prostatic utricle lies between the ends of the two ejaculatory ducts; all three open into the prostatic urethra;
3. The prostatic ductules mostly open onto the prostatic sinus.

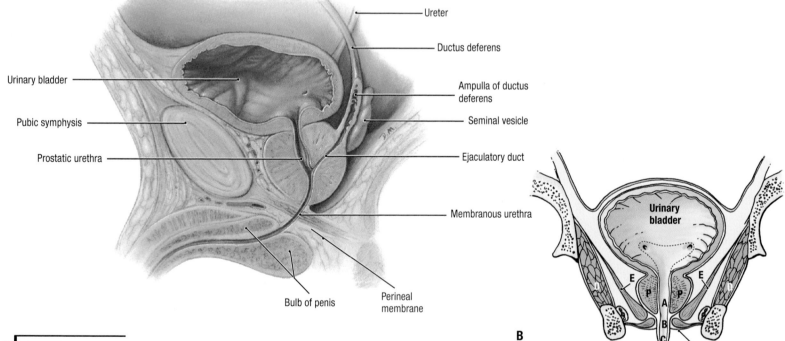

Ureter

Ductus deferens

Urinary bladder

Pubic symphysis

Prostatic urethra

Ampulla of ductus deferens

Seminal vesicle

Ejaculatory duct

Membranous urethra

Bulb of penis

Perineal membrane

Urinary bladder

A

B

3.16   Bladder, prostate, and deferent duct

A. Sagittal section. The ejaculatory duct (approximately 2 cm in length) is formed by the union of the deferent duct and duct of the seminal vesicle; it passes anteriorly and inferiorly through the substance of the prostate to enter the prostatic urethra on the seminal col-

liculus. **B.** Coronal section. Observe the parts of the urethra: prostatic (*A*), intermediate (membranous) (*B*), and spongy (*C*), the obturator internus (*D*) and levator ani (*E*) muscles, the perineal membrane (*F*), and the prostate (*P*).

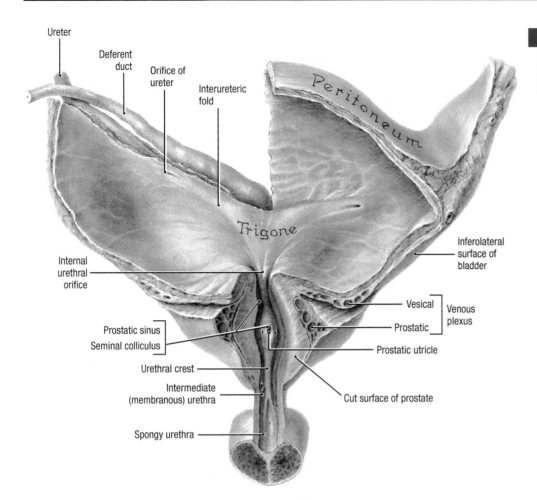

Ureter

Deferent duct

Orifice of ureter

Interureteric fold

Peritoneum

Trigone

Internal urethral orifice

Inferolateral surface of bladder

Prostatic sinus

Seminal colliculus

Urethral crest

Intermediate (membranous) urethra

Spongy urethra

Vesical

Prostatic

Venous plexus

Prostatic utricle

Cut surface of prostate

3.17 Interior of male urinary bladder and prostatic urethra, anterior view

The anterior walls of the bladder, prostate, and urethra were cut away. The knife was then carried through the posterior wall of the bladder at the right ureter and interureteric fold, which unites the two ureters along the superior limit of the smooth trigone.

OBSERVE:
1. The right ureter does not join the bladder wall, but traverses the wall obliquely to the wall's slit-like orifice, which is situated 2 to 4 cm from the left orifice;
2. The mucous membrane is smooth over the trigone, but rugose (folded) elsewhere, especially when the bladder is empty;
3. The mouth of the prostatic utricle is at the summit of the seminal colliculus on the urethral crest; there is an orifice of an ejaculatory duct on each side of the prostatic utricle;
4. In this specimen, the urethral crest extends more superior than usual and bifurcates more inferior than usual;
5. The prostatic fascia encloses a venous plexus.

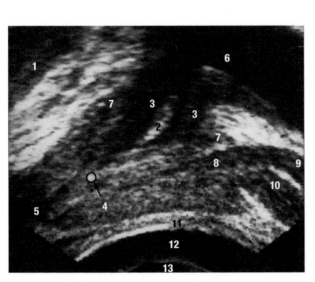

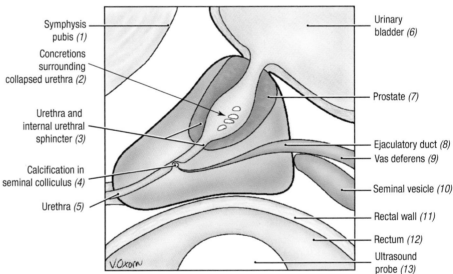

Symphysis pubis (1)

Concretions surrounding collapsed urethra (2)

Urethra and internal urethral sphincter (3)

Calcification in seminal colliculus (4)

Urethra (5)

V. Oxorn

Urinary bladder (6)

Prostate (7)

Ejaculatory duct (8)

Vas deferens (9)

Seminal vesicle (10)

Rectal wall (11)

Rectum (12)

Ultrasound probe (13)

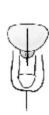

3.18 Transverse section and ultrasound of male pelvis

In this transverse (transrectal) ultrasound scan, the probe was inserted into the rectum to scan the anteriorly located prostate. The ducts of the glands in the peripheral zone open into the prostatic sinuses, whereas the ducts of the glands in the central (internal) zone open into the prostatic sinuses and seminal colliculus. *The large peripheral zone is the common site for carcinomas. The central zone is the site of enlargement in cases of benign prostate hypertrophy.*

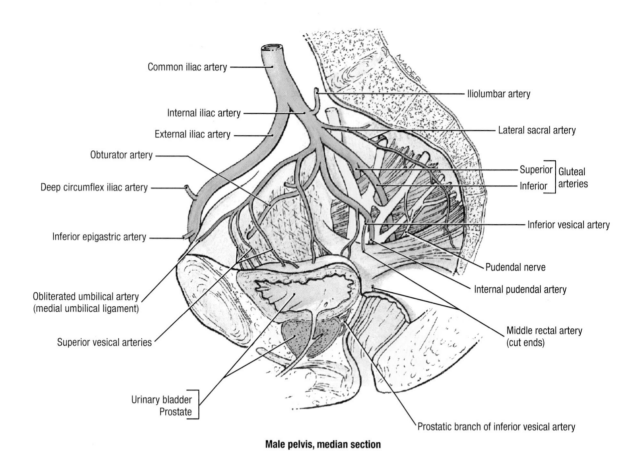

Common iliac artery

Internal iliac artery

External iliac artery

Obturator artery

Deep circumflex iliac artery

Inferior epigastric artery

Obliterated umbilical artery
(medial umbilical ligament)

Superior vesical arteries

Urinary bladder
Prostate

Iliolumbar artery

Lateral sacral artery

Superior | Gluteal
Inferior | arteries

Inferior vesical artery

Pudendal nerve

Internal pudendal artery

Middle rectal artery
(cut ends)

Prostatic branch of inferior vesical artery

Male pelvis, median section

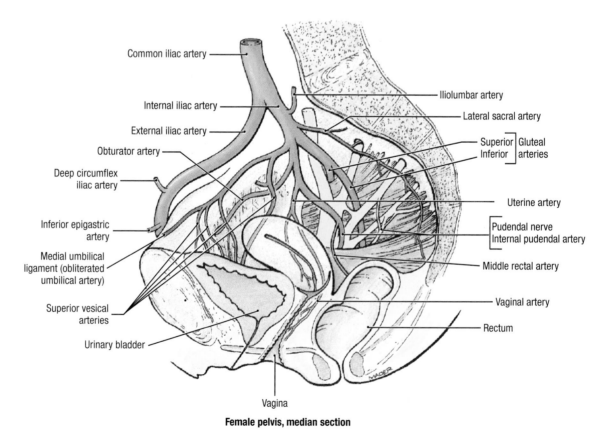

Common iliac artery

Internal iliac artery

External iliac artery

Obturator artery

Deep circumflex
iliac artery

Inferior epigastric
artery

Medial umbilical
ligament (obliterated
umbilical artery)

Superior vesical
arteries

Urinary bladder

Vagina

Iliolumbar artery

Lateral sacral artery

Superior | Gluteal
Inferior | arteries

Uterine artery

Pudendal nerve
Internal pudendal artery

Middle rectal artery

Vaginal artery

Rectum

Female pelvis, median section

Table 3.3. Arteries of Pelvis[a]

Artery	Origin	Course	Distribution
Internal iliac	Common iliac artery	Passes over brim of pelvis to reach pelvic cavity	Main blood supply to pelvic organs, gluteal muscles, and perineum
Anterior division of internal iliac artery	Internal iliac artery	Passes anteriorly and divides into visceral branches and obturator artery	Pelvic viscera and muscles in medial compartment of thigh
Umbilical	Anterior division of internal iliac artery	Short pelvic course and ends as superior vesical artery in females	Superior aspect of urinary bladder in females; deferent duct in males
Obturator	Anterior division of internal iliac artery	Runs anteroinferiorly on lateral pelvic wall	Pelvic muscles, nutrient artery to ilium, and head of femur
Superior vesical	Remnant of proximal part of umbilical artery	Passes to superior aspect of urinary bladder	Superior aspect of urinary bladder
Artery to deferent duct	Inferior vesical artery	Runs retroperitoneally to deferent duct	Deferent duct
Inferior vesical	Anterior division of internal iliac artery	Passes retroperitoneally to inferior portion of urinary bladder in males	Urinary bladder, seminal vesicle, and prostate
Middle rectal	Anterior division of internal iliac artery	Descends in pelvis to rectum	Seminal vesicle, prostate, and rectum
Internal pudendal	Anterior division of internal iliac artery	Leaves pelvis through greater sciatic foramen and enters perineum by passing through lesser sciatic foramen	Piriformis, coccygeus, levator ani, and gluteal muscles
Uterine	Anterior division of internal iliac artery	Runs medially on levator ani; crosses ureter to reach base of broad ligament	Uterus, ligament of uterus, uterine tube, and vagina
Vaginal	Uterine artery	At junction of body and cervix of uterus, it descends to vagina	Vagina and branches to inferior part of urinary bladder
Gonadal (testicular and ovarian)	Abdominal aorta	Descends retroperitoneally; testicular artery passes into deep inguinal ring; ovarian artery crosses brim of pelvis and runs medially in suspensory ligament to ovary	Testis and ovary, respectively
Posterior division of internal iliac artery	Internal iliac artery	Passes posteriorly and gives rise to parietal branches	Pelvic wall and gluteal region
Iliolumbar	Posterior division of internal iliac artery	Ascends anterior to sacroiliac joint and posterior to common iliac vessels and psoas major	Iliacus, psoas major, quadratus lumborum muscles, and cauda equina in vertebral canal
Lateral sacral (superior and inferior)	Posterior division of internal iliac artery	Run on superificial aspect of piriformis	Piriformis and vertebral canal

[a]See figures on opposite page.

3.19 Iliac arteriogram, anteroposterior view

Injection was made into the aorta in the lumbar region.

OBSERVE:

1. The aorta bifurcates into the right and left common iliac arteries (anterior to L4);
2. The common iliac arteries bifurcate into the internal and external iliac arteries, opposite the sacroiliac joint at the level of the lumbosacral disc;
3. *The oval on the arteriogram indicates a site of narrowing (stenosis) of the right common iliac artery.*

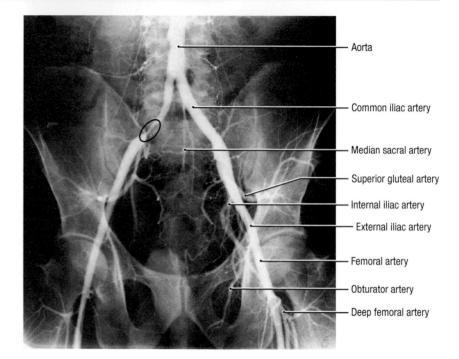

- Aorta
- Common iliac artery
- Median sacral artery
- Superior gluteal artery
- Internal iliac artery
- External iliac artery
- Femoral artery
- Obturator artery
- Deep femoral artery

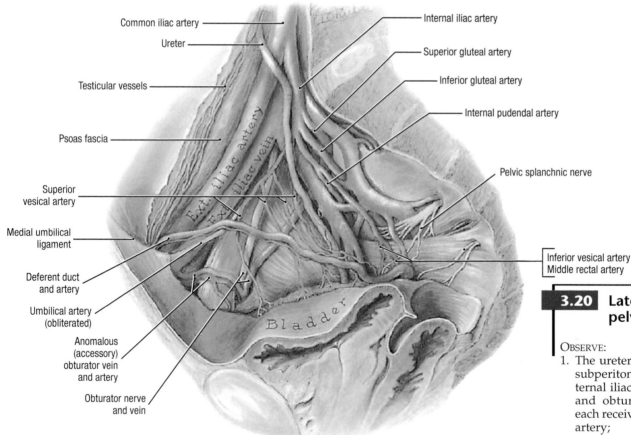

Common iliac artery
Ureter
Testicular vessels
Psoas fascia
Superior vesical artery
Medial umbilical ligament
Deferent duct and artery
Umbilical artery (obliterated)
Anomalous (accessory) obturator vein and artery
Obturator nerve and vein

Ext. iliac artery
Ext. iliac vein
Bladder

Internal iliac artery
Superior gluteal artery
Inferior gluteal artery
Internal pudendal artery
Pelvic splanchnic nerve
Inferior vesical artery
Middle rectal artery

3.20 Lateral wall of male pelvis, sagittal sections

OBSERVE:

1. The ureter and deferent duct take a subperitoneal course across the external iliac vessels, umbilical artery, and obturator nerve and vessels; each receives a branch from a vesical artery;
2. The ureter crosses the external iliac artery at its origin (common iliac bifurcation), and the deferent duct crosses the external iliac artery at its termination (deep inguinal ring);
3. In this specimen, an anomalous obturator artery branches from the inferior epigastric artery; there are normal and anomalous obturator veins.

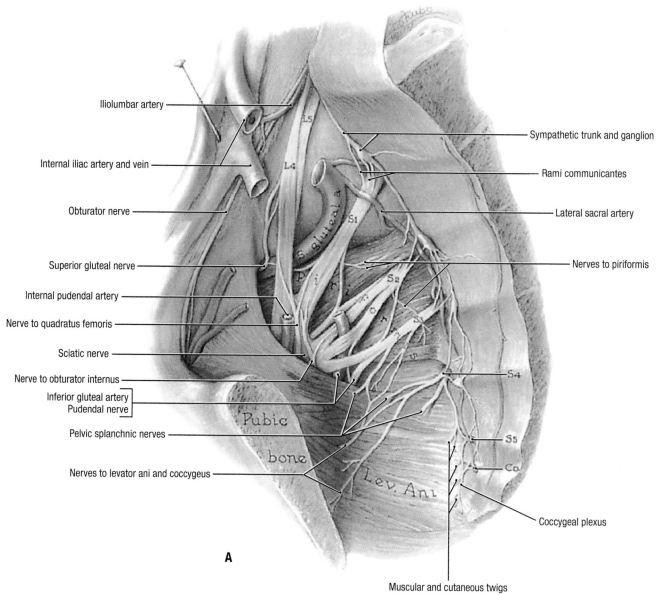

Iliolumbar artery

Internal iliac artery and vein

Obturator nerve

Superior gluteal nerve

Internal pudendal artery

Nerve to quadratus femoris

Sciatic nerve

Nerve to obturator internus

Inferior gluteal artery
Pudendal nerve

Pelvic splanchnic nerves

Nerves to levator ani and coccygeus

Sympathetic trunk and ganglion

Rami communicantes

Lateral sacral artery

Nerves to piriformis

Coccygeal plexus

Muscular and cutaneous twigs

A

3.21   Sacral and coccygeal nerve plexuses

A. Sagittal section. **B.** Anterior view.

OBSERVE:

1. The sympathetic trunk or its ganglia sends gray rami communicantes to each sacral nerve and the coccygeal nerve;
2. The branch from L4 joins L5 to form the lumbosacral trunk;
3. The roots of S1 and S2 supply the piriformis muscle; S3 and S4 supply the coccygeus and levator ani muscles, and S2, S3, and S4 each contributes a branch to the formation of the pelvic splanchnic nerves;
4. The sciatic nerve springs from segments L4, L5, S1, S2, and S3; the pudendal nerve from S2, S3, and S4; and the coccygeal plexus from S4, S5, and coccygeal segments;
5. The iliolumbar artery accompanies the L5 nerve, and the branches of the lateral sacral artery accompany the sacral nerves. The superior gluteal artery passes posteriorly between L5 and S1; its position is not constant.
6. In **B,** the sacral plexus is pierced by the superior and inferior gluteal arteries, which turn posteriorly; the internal pudendal artery continues anteroinferiorly toward the ischial spine.

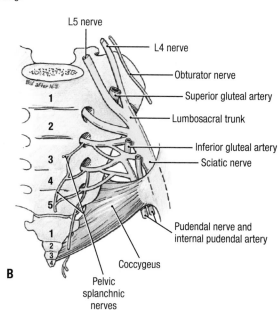

L5 nerve

L4 nerve

Obturator nerve

Superior gluteal artery

Lumbosacral trunk

Inferior gluteal artery

Sciatic nerve

Pudendal nerve and
internal pudendal artery

Coccygeus

Pelvic
splanchnic
nerves

B

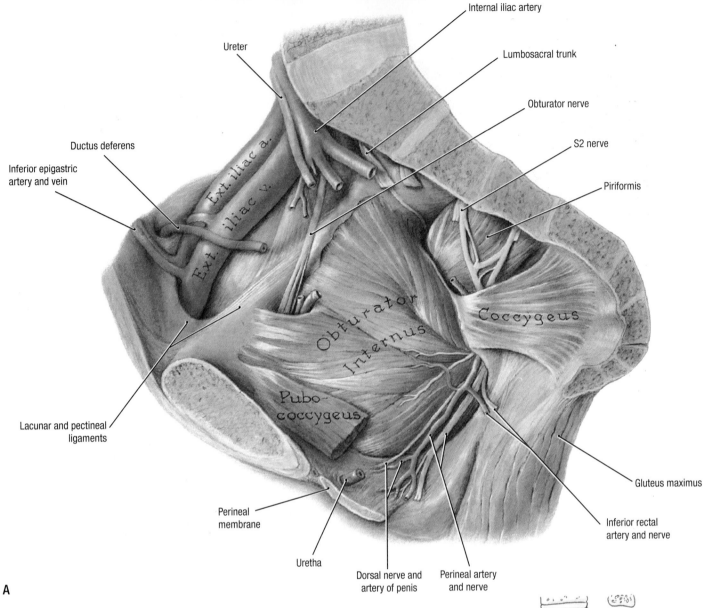

A

3.22 Walls of pelvis minor, sagittal sections

A. Muscles and branches of pudendal nerve. **B.** Ligaments and obturator nerve. **C.** Pudendal nerve, lateral view.

OBSERVE IN **A**:
1. The obturator internus muscle pads the lateral wall of the pelvis and leaves the pelvis minor through the lesser sciatic foramen, and the piriformis muscle pads the posterior wall and leaves through the greater sciatic foramen. The coccygeus muscle conceals the sacrospinous ligament. The pubococcygeus muscle, the chief and strongest part of the levator ani muscle, springs from the body of the pubis;
2. The obturator nerve, artery, and vein leave the pelvis minor through the obturator foramen. The internal pudendal artery and the pudendal nerve exit through the greater sciatic foramen, and reenter through the lesser sciatic foramen; they then take an anterior course (in the pudendal canal) within the obturator internus fascia.

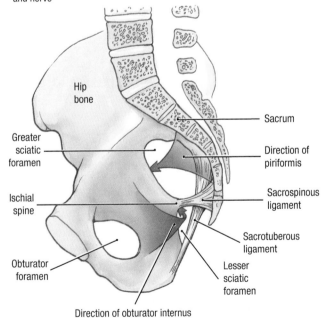

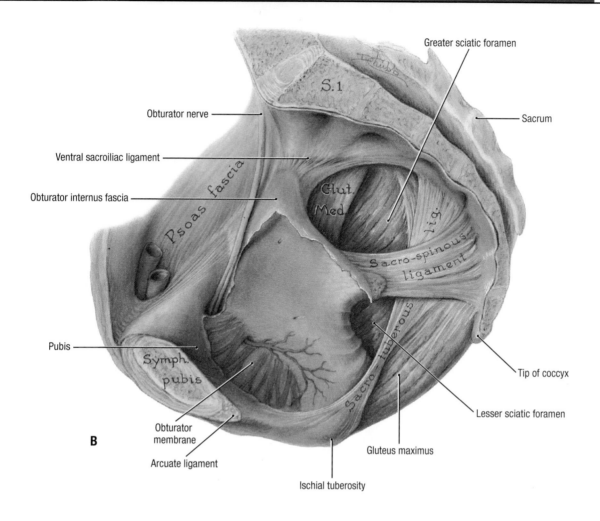

B

OBSERVE IN B:

3. Posterolaterally, the coccyx and inferior part of the sacrum are fastened to the ischial tuberosity by the sacrotuberous ligament and to the ischial spine by the sacrospinous ligament; the superior part of the sacrum is joined to the ilium by the ventral sacroiliac ligament;

4. The greater and lesser sciatic foramina are anterosuperior to the sacrotuberous ligament; the greater sciatic foramen is superior, and the lesser sciatic foramen is inferior to the sacrospinous ligament;

5. Anterolaterally, the fascia covering the obturator internus muscle was snipped away, and the obturator internus muscle was removed from its osseofascial pocket, thereby exposing the ischium and obturator membrane. The mouth of this pocket is the lesser sciatic foramen; through it, the obturator internus muscle leaves the pelvis, and the grooves made by its tendon are conspicuous;

6. The obturator internus fascia is attached along the line of the obturator nerve superiorly, to the sacrotuberous ligament inferiorly, and to the posterior border of the body of the ischium posteriorly.

OBSERVE IN C:

7. The five regions in which the pudendal nerve runs: pelvis, gluteal, pudendal canal, perineal membrane, and dorsum of penis.

8. The three divisions of the pudendal nerve: inferior rectal nerve, perineal nerve, and dorsal nerve of penis.

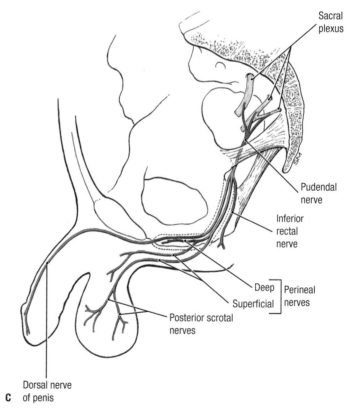

C

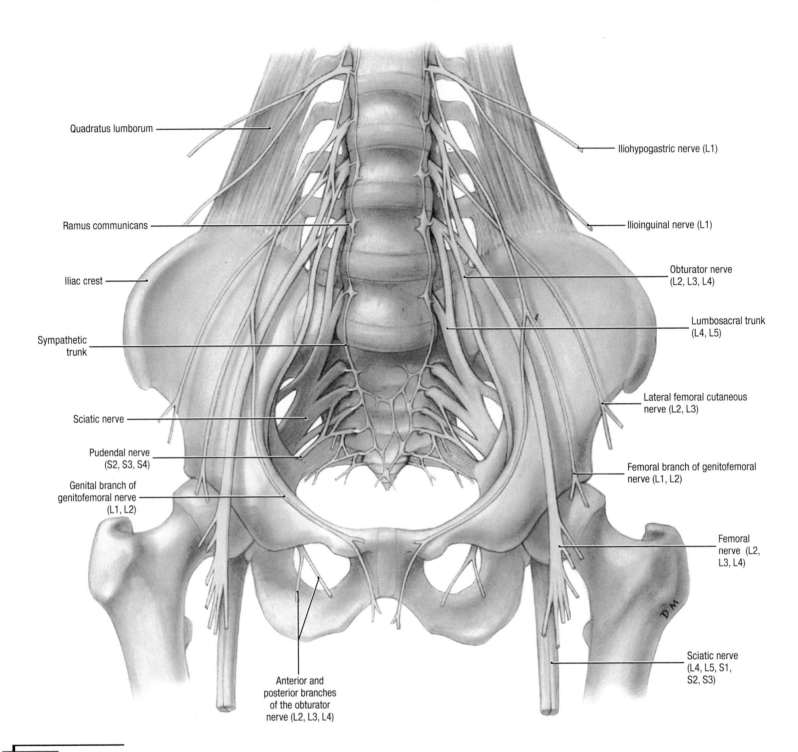

Quadratus lumborum

Ramus communicans

Iliac crest

Sympathetic trunk

Sciatic nerve

Pudendal nerve (S2, S3, S4)

Genital branch of genitofemoral nerve (L1, L2)

Iliohypogastric nerve (L1)

Ilioinguinal nerve (L1)

Obturator nerve (L2, L3, L4)

Lumbosacral trunk (L4, L5)

Lateral femoral cutaneous nerve (L2, L3)

Femoral branch of genitofemoral nerve (L1, L2)

Femoral nerve (L2, L3, L4)

Sciatic nerve (L4, L5, S1, S2, S3)

Anterior and posterior branches of the obturator nerve (L2, L3, L4)

3.23   Overview of lumbosacral plexus, anterior view

OBSERVE:
1. The lumbosacral trunk provides continuity for the lumbar and sacral plexuses;
2. The ventral primary rami of (T12), L1, L2, L3, and L4 form the lumbar plexus, and the ventral primary rami of L4, L5, S1, S2, and S3 form the sacral plexus;
3. The sciatic nerve passes posteriorly through the greater sciatic foramen to the gluteal region;

4. The femoral nerve splits into many branches in the femoral triangle just distal to the inguinal ligament;
5. The obturator nerve passes through the obturator foramen with the obturator artery and vein to supply the medial aspect of the thigh;
6. The rami communicantes connect the sympathetic trunk and ganglia with the ventral primary rami of the lumbosacral plexus.

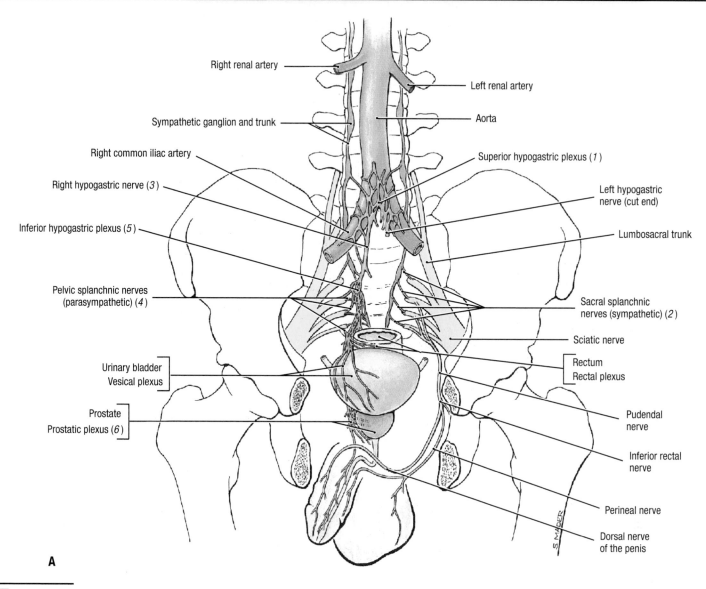

Right renal artery

Left renal artery

Sympathetic ganglion and trunk

Aorta

Right common iliac artery

Superior hypogastric plexus (*1*)

Right hypogastric nerve (*3*)

Left hypogastric nerve (cut end)

Inferior hypogastric plexus (*5*)

Lumbosacral trunk

Pelvic splanchnic nerves (parasympathetic) (*4*)

Sacral splanchnic nerves (sympathetic) (*2*)

Sciatic nerve

Urinary bladder
Vesical plexus

Rectum
Rectal plexus

Prostate
Prostatic plexus (*6*)

Pudendal nerve

Inferior rectal nerve

Perineal nerve

Dorsal nerve of the penis

A

3.24 Innervation of male pelvis and genitalia, anterior views

A. Autonomic and somatic innervation. **B.** Autonomic innervation of testis, deferent duct, prostate, and seminal vesicles.

OBSERVE:

1. The autonomic pelvic plexuses include the inferior hypogastric, vesical, middle rectal, and prostatic. The pelvic plexuses consist of sympathetic and parasympathetic fibers. The right and left hypogastric nerves join the superior hypogastric plexus to the inferior hypogastric plexus;
2. The right and left inferior hypogastric plexuses continue as the vesical plexus, supplying the urinary bladder, seminal vesicles, and deferent duct; as the middle rectal plexus, supplying the rectum; and as the prostatic plexus, supplying the prostate, seminal vesicles, corpus spongiosum, corpora cavernosum, and urethra;
3. The parasympathetic pelvic splanchnic nerves arise from the ventral primary rami of S2, S3, and S4 and supply motor fibers to the descending colon, sigmoid colon, rectum, pelvic organs, and the vasodilator fibers to the erectile tissue of the penis;
4. The sympathetic sacral splanchnic nerves arise from the sympathetic trunk and join the inferior hypogastric plexuses; vasoconstrictor fibers innervate the male genital organs and play an important role in ejaculation;

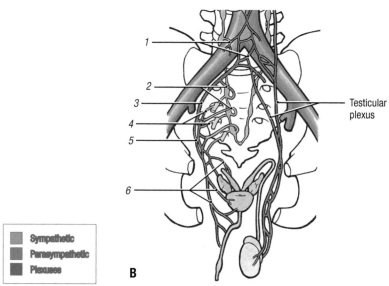

Testicular plexus

Sympathetic
Parasympathetic
Plexuses

B

5. The pudendal nerve, a branch of the sacral plexus, arises from the ventral primary rami of S2, S3, and S4; this nerve is part of the voluntary somatic nervous system and innervates the perineal region.

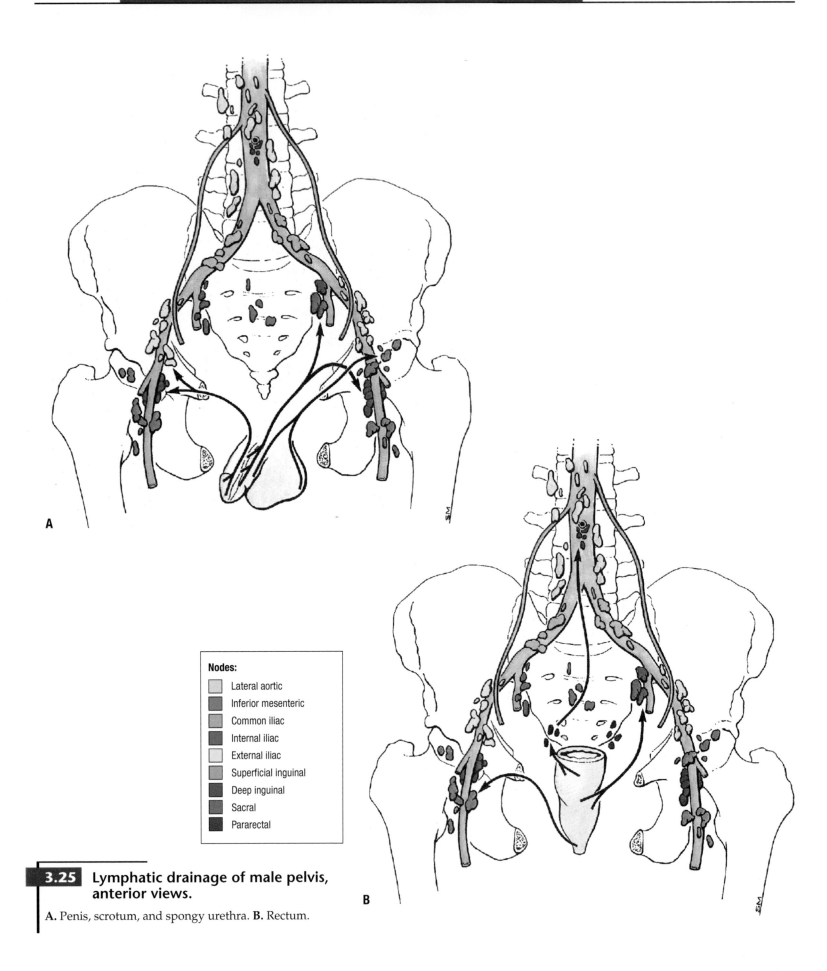

Nodes:

- Lateral aortic
- Inferior mesenteric
- Common iliac
- Internal iliac
- External iliac
- Superficial inguinal
- Deep inguinal
- Sacral
- Pararectal

3.25 Lymphatic drainage of male pelvis, anterior views.

A. Penis, scrotum, and spongy urethra. **B.** Rectum.

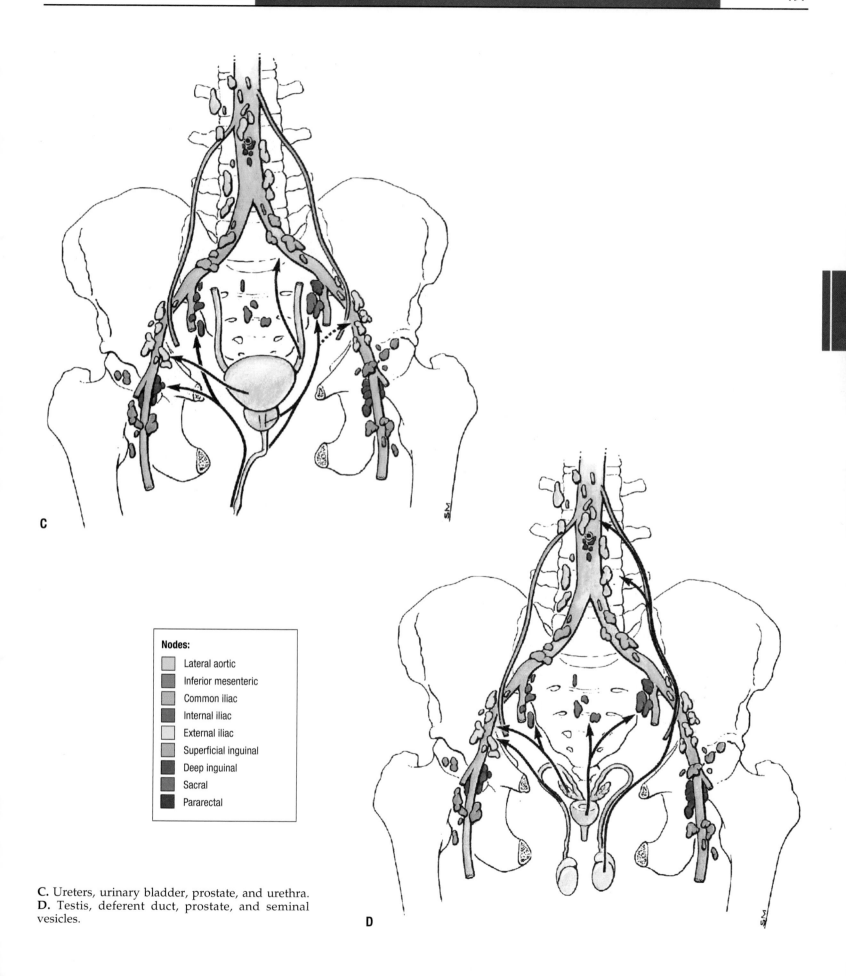

Nodes:

- Lateral aortic
- Inferior mesenteric
- Common iliac
- Internal iliac
- External iliac
- Superficial inguinal
- Deep inguinal
- Sacral
- Pararectal

C. Ureters, urinary bladder, prostate, and urethra.
D. Testis, deferent duct, prostate, and seminal vesicles.

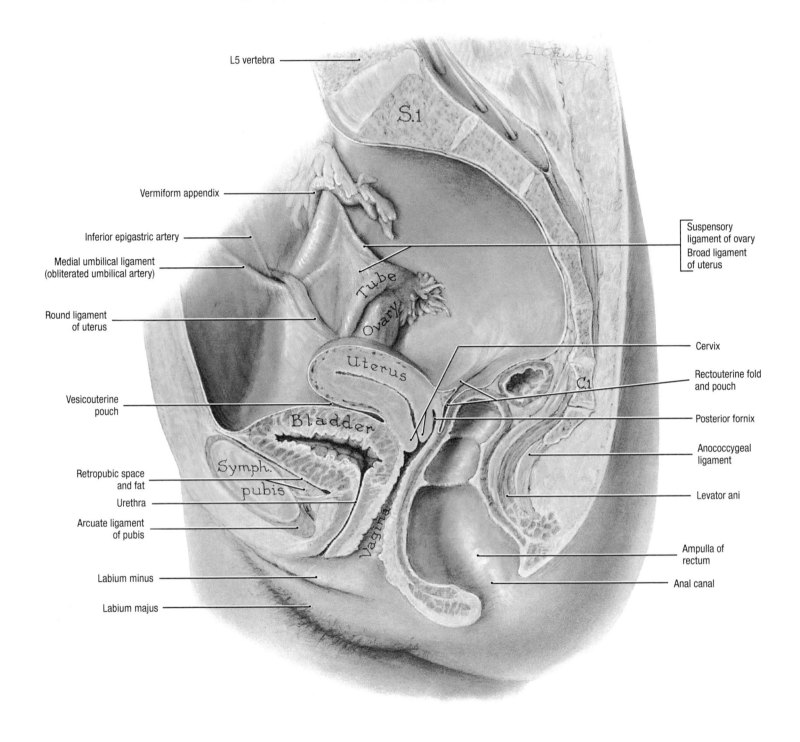

L5 vertebra

S.1

Vermiform appendix

Inferior epigastric artery

Medial umbilical ligament
(obliterated umbilical artery)

Round ligament
of uterus

Vesicouterine
pouch

Retropubic space
and fat

Urethra

Arcuate ligament
of pubis

Labium minus

Labium majus

Tube

Ovary

Uterus

Bladder

Symph.

pubis

Vagina

Suspensory
ligament of ovary
Broad ligament
of uterus

Cervix

Rectouterine fold
and pouch

Posterior fornix

Anococcygeal
ligament

Levator ani

Ampulla of
rectum

Anal canal

C.1

3.26   Female pelvis, median section

The uterus was sectioned in its own median plane and depicted as though this coincided with the median plane of the body, which is seldom the case.

OBSERVE:

1. The uterine tube and the ovary are on the lateral wall of the pelvis;
2. The uterus is bent on itself at the junction of its body and the cervix; the cervix, opening on the anterior wall of the vagina, has a short, round, anterior lip and a long, thin, posterior lip;

3. The external ostium (external os) of the uterus (see Fig. 3.33D) is at the level of the superior aspect of the symphysis pubis;
4. The anterior fornix of the vagina is 1 cm or more from the rectouterine pouch; the posterior fornix is covered with 1 cm or more of the rectouterine pouch when the subject is erect;
5. The urethra (3 cm long), the vagina, and the rectum are parallel to one another and to the pelvic brim; the uterus is nearly at right angles to these structures when the bladder is empty.

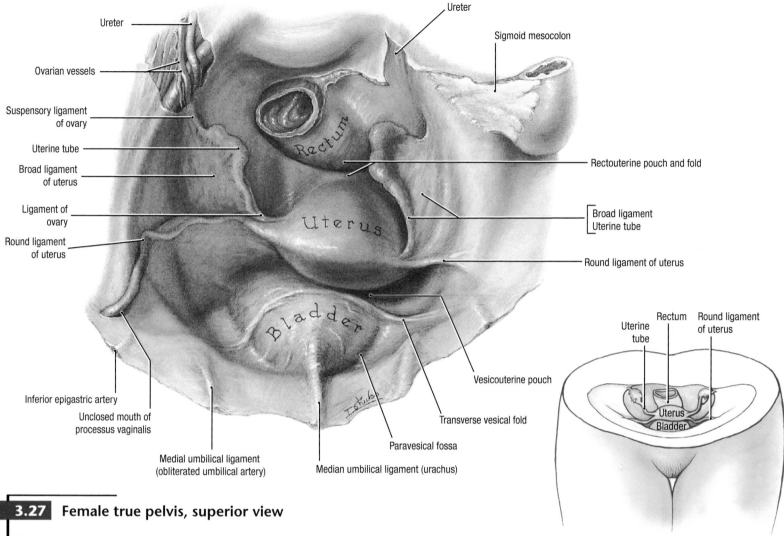

3.27 **Female true pelvis, superior view**

OBSERVE:
1. The pear-shaped uterus is asymmetrically placed; in this specimen, it leans to the left;
2. The right round ligament of the uterus in this specimen is longer than the left; the round ligament of the female takes the same subperitoneal course as the deferent duct of the male;
3. The free edge of the medial four-fifths of the broad ligament is occupied by the uterine tube (fallopian tube); the lateral one-fifth, occupied by the ovarian vessels, is the suspensory ligament of the ovary;
4. The ovarian vessels cross the external iliac vessels close to the ureter.

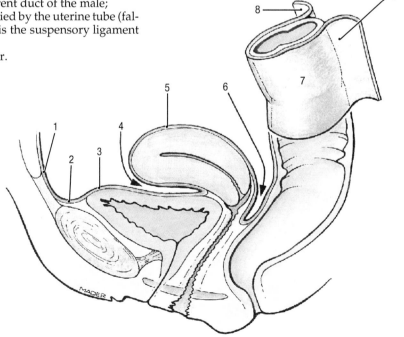

3.28 **Peritoneum covering female pelvic organs, median section**

The peritoneum passes: 1) from the anterior abdominal wall; 2) superior to the pubic bone; 3) on the superior surface of the urinary bladder; 4) from the bladder to the uterus (vesicouterine pouch); 5) on the fundus and body of the uterus, the posterior fornix, and the wall of the vagina; 6) between the rectum and uterus (rectouterine pouch); 7) on the anterior and lateral sides of the rectum; and 8) posteriorly to become the sigmoid mesocolon.

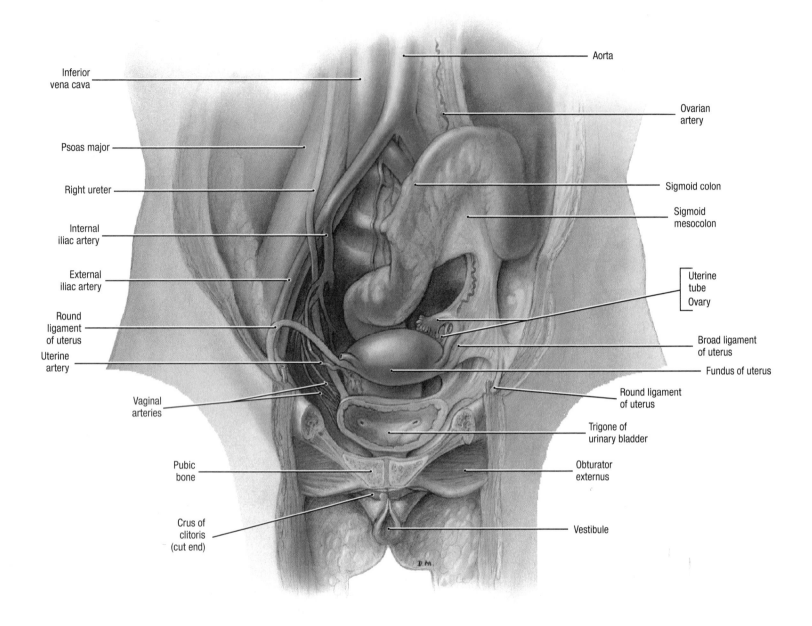

Aorta

Inferior vena cava

Ovarian artery

Psoas major

Right ureter

Sigmoid colon

Sigmoid mesocolon

Internal iliac artery

External iliac artery

Uterine tube
Ovary

Round ligament of uterus

Broad ligament of uterus

Uterine artery

Fundus of uterus

Vaginal arteries

Round ligament of uterus

Trigone of urinary bladder

Pubic bone

Obturator externus

Crus of clitoris (cut end)

Vestibule

3.29 Female genital organs, anterosuperior view

Part of the pubic bones, the anterior aspect of the bladder, and, on the specimen's right side, the uterine tube, ovary, broad ligament, and peritoneum covering the lateral wall of the pelvis have been removed.

OBSERVE:
1. The uterine artery is located in the base of the broad ligament and runs superiorly along the lateral margin of the uterus;
2. The vaginal arteries branching from the uterine artery supply the cervix and anterior surface of the vagina; the vaginal arteries arising from the internal iliac artery supply the posterior surface of the vagina;
3. The right ureter crosses the external iliac artery at the bifurcation of the common iliac artery; note the close proximity of the right ureter to the cervix of the uterus and lateral fornix of the vagina, where it is crossed by the uterine artery.

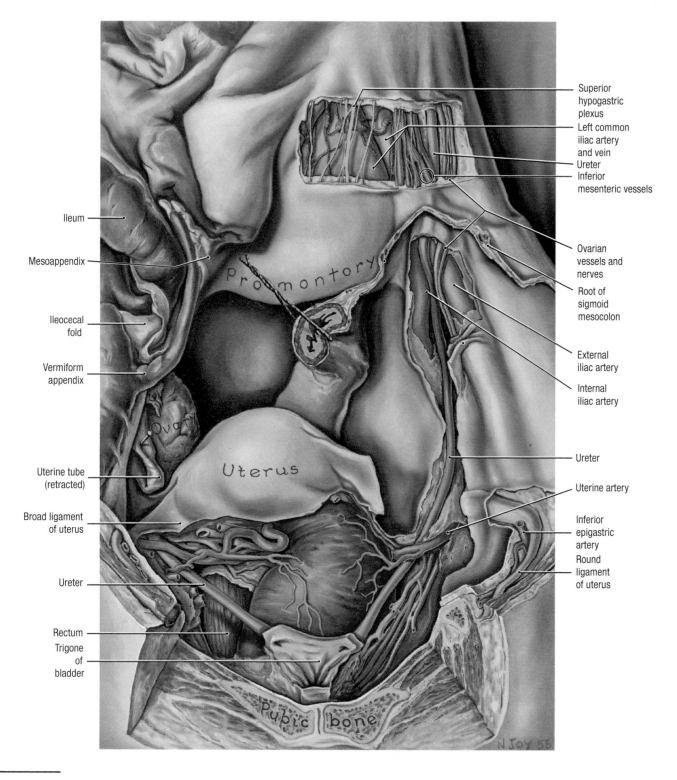

Superior hypogastric plexus

Left common iliac artery and vein

Ureter

Inferior mesenteric vessels

Ovarian vessels and nerves

Root of sigmoid mesocolon

External iliac artery

Internal iliac artery

Ureter

Uterine artery

Inferior epigastric artery

Round ligament of uterus

Ileum

Mesoappendix

Ileocecal fold

Vermiform appendix

Uterine tube (retracted)

Broad ligament of uterus

Ureter

Rectum

Trigone of bladder

Promontory

Ovary

Uterus

Pubic bone

N. Joy 55

3.30   Female ureter in pelvis, anterosuperior view

OBSERVE:

1. The left ureter is crossed by the ovarian vessels and nerves; the apex of the inverted V-shaped root of the sigmoid mesocolon is situated anterior to the left ureter and acts as a guide to it;

2. The left ureter crosses the external iliac artery at the bifurcation of the common iliac artery and then descends anterior to the internal iliac artery; its course is subperitoneal from where it enters the pelvis to where it passes deep to the broad ligament and is crossed by the uterine artery;

3. The superior hypogastric plexus and some lymph vessels anterior to the left common iliac vein;

4. The vermiform appendix is postileal.

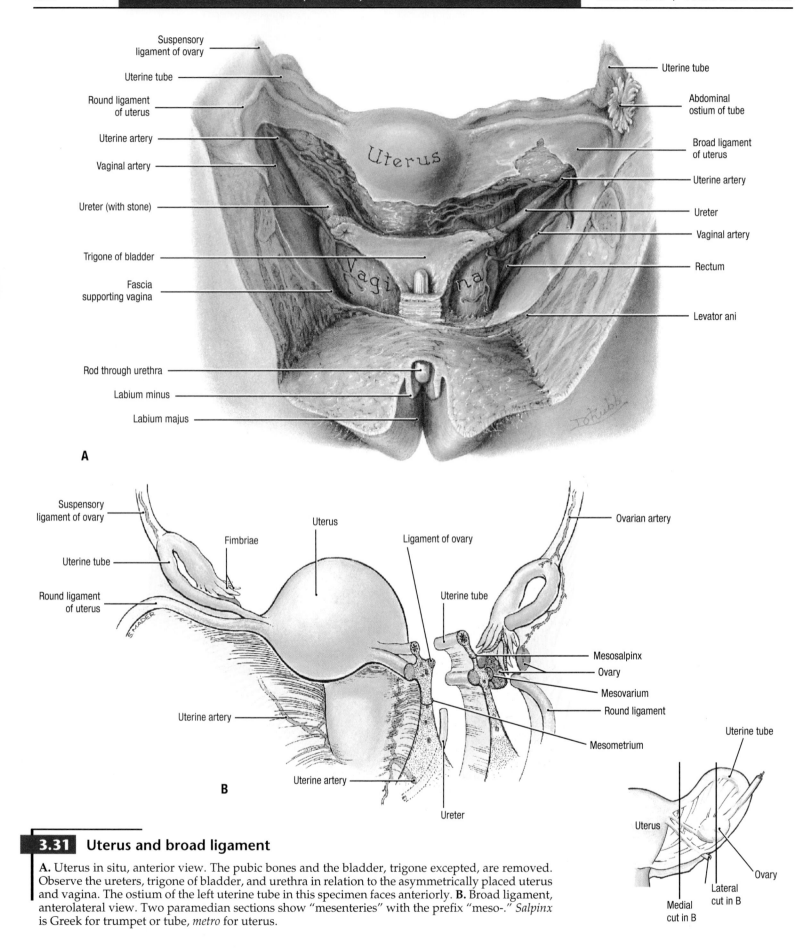

3.31   Uterus and broad ligament

A. Uterus in situ, anterior view. The pubic bones and the bladder, trigone excepted, are removed. Observe the ureters, trigone of bladder, and urethra in relation to the asymmetrically placed uterus and vagina. The ostium of the left uterine tube in this specimen faces anteriorly. **B.** Broad ligament, anterolateral view. Two paramedian sections show "mesenteries" with the prefix "meso-." *Salpinx* is Greek for trumpet or tube, *metro* for uterus.

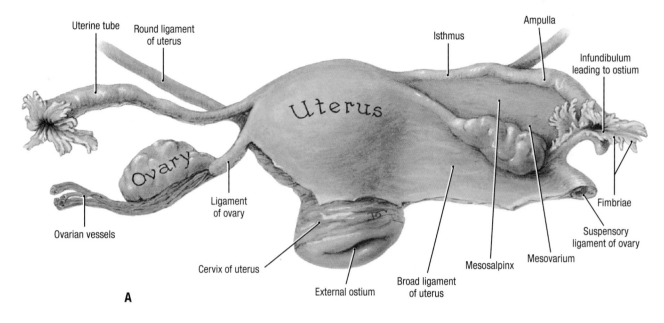

Uterine tube   Round ligament of uterus   Isthmus   Ampulla   Infundibulum leading to ostium

Uterus

Ovary

Ovarian vessels

Ligament of ovary

Cervix of uterus

External ostium

Broad ligament of uterus

Mesosalpinx   Mesovarium

Suspensory ligament of ovary

Fimbriae

A

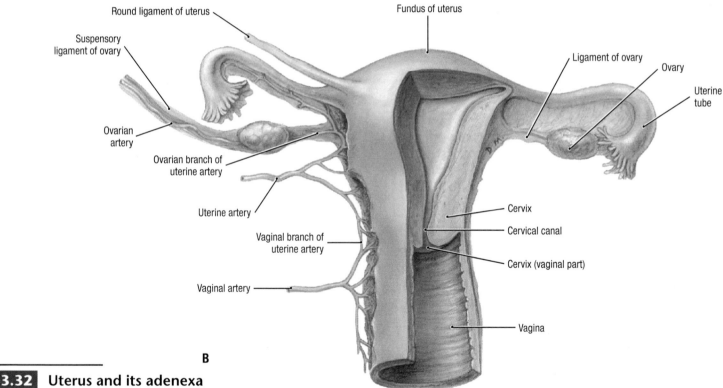

Round ligament of uterus   Fundus of uterus

Suspensory ligament of ovary

Ligament of ovary

Ovary

Uterine tube

Ovarian artery

Ovarian branch of uterine artery

Uterine artery

Vaginal branch of uterine artery

Vaginal artery

Cervix

Cervical canal

Cervix (vaginal part)

Vagina

B

3.32   Uterus and its adenexa

A. Posterior view. **B.** Blood supply, anterior view.

OBSERVE IN **A**:
1. On the specimen's left: The broad ligament of the uterus is removed, thereby setting free the uterine tube, round ligament of uterus, and ligament of ovary; these three structures are attached, close together, to the lateral wall of the uterus at the junction of its fundus and body.
2. On the specimen's right: The mesentery of the uterus and tube is called the broad ligament; the ovary is attached (a) to the broad ligament by a mesentery of its own, called the mesovarium; (b) to the uterus by the ligament of the ovary; and (c) near the pelvic brim, by the suspensory ligament of the ovary containing the ovarian vessels. The part of the broad ligament superior to the level of the mesovarium is called the mesosalpinx.

OBSERVE IN **B**:
3. On the specimen's left side: Part of the uterine wall with the round ligament and the vaginal wall have been cut away to expose the cervix, slit-like uterine cavity, and thick muscular wall of the uterus, the myometrium;
4. On the specimen's right side: the ovarian artery (from the aorta) and uterine artery (from the internal iliac) supply the ovary, uterine tube, and uterus, and anastomose in the broad ligament along the lateral aspect of the uterus. The uterine artery sends a uterine branch to supply the uterine body and fundus and a vaginal branch to supply the cervix and vagina. The vaginal artery anastomoses with the vaginal branch of the uterine artery.

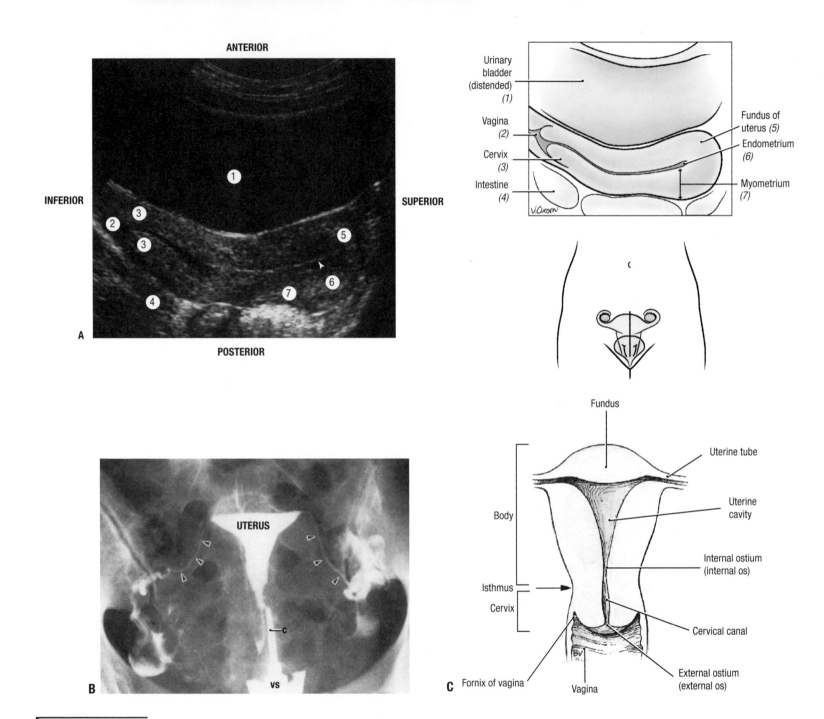

3.33   Female pelvis: ultrasound and hysterosalpingogram

A. Sagittal ultrasound scan and orientation drawing. The red line indicates the site of the scan. The numbers in parentheses correspond to labels on the ultrasound scan. **B.** Hysterosalpingogram. Radiopaque contrast medium was injected via a cannula (*C*) into the uterus through the external ostium; *VS*, vaginal speculum in vagina. The triangular uterine cavity is clearly outlined. Contrast medium has traveled through the uterine tubes (*arrowheads*) to the infundibulum and leaked into the peritoneal cavity on both sides. **C.** Parts of uterus, coronal section.

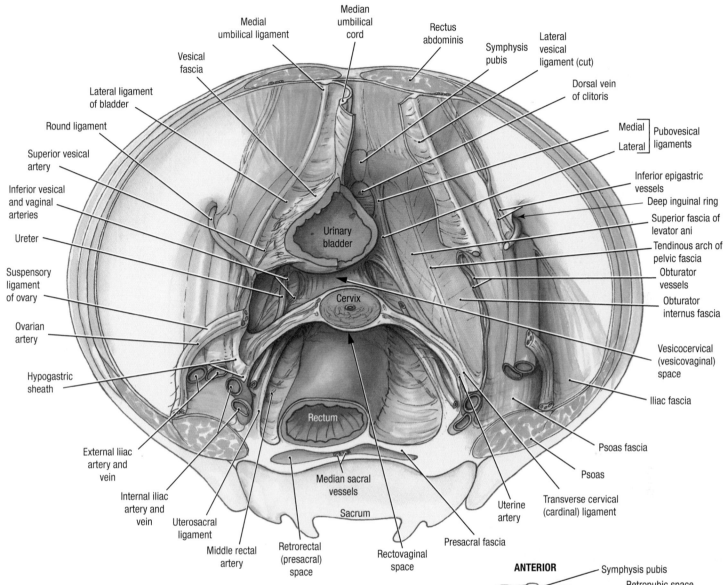

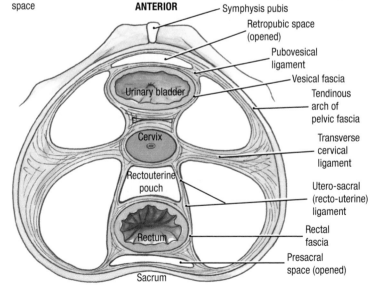

3.34   Pelvic fascia and the supporting mechanism of the cervix and upper vagina

A. Pelvic viscera and endopelvic fascia, superior vew. **B.** Schematic illustration of fascial ligaments and spaces, superior view.

OBSERVE:

1. The parietal pelvic fascia covering the obturator internus and levator ani muscles; the visceral pelvic fascia surrounding the pelvic organs; these membranous fasciae are continuous where the organs penetrate the pelvic floor; forming a tendinous arch of pelvic fascia bilaterally.
2. Anteriorly the tendinous arch formed by the pubovesical ligaments;
3. The subperitoneal endopelvic fascia consisting of a connective tissue matrix around the pelvic organs; this fascia is continuous with both visceral and parietal layers of pelvic fascia; the condensation of this fascia into a thick band the hypogastric sheath containing the vessels to the pelvic viscera from the lateral wall, the ureters and in the male the ductus deferens;
4. The ligamentous extensions of the hypogastric sheath: the lateral ligament of the urinary bladder, the transverse cervical (cardinal) ligament at the base of the broad ligament, and a less prominent lamina posteriorly containing the middle rectal vessels.

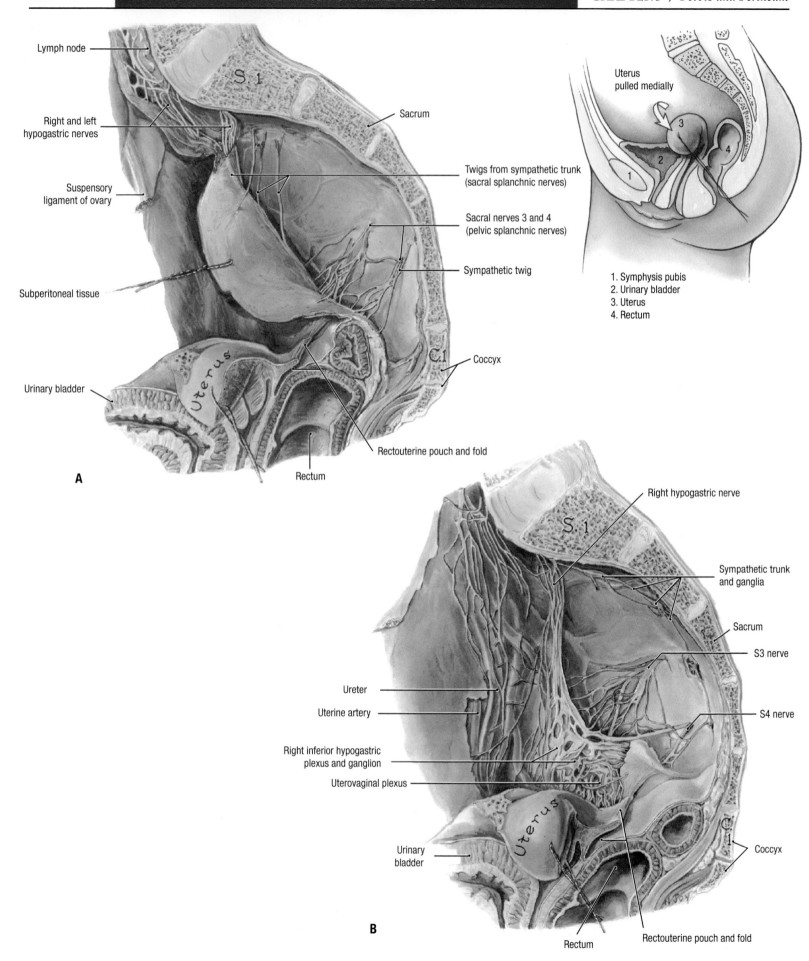

Lymph node

Right and left hypogastric nerves

Suspensory ligament of ovary

Subperitoneal tissue

Urinary bladder

S.1

Sacrum

Twigs from sympathetic trunk (sacral splanchnic nerves)

Sacral nerves 3 and 4 (pelvic splanchnic nerves)

Sympathetic twig

Coccyx

Rectouterine pouch and fold

Rectum

A

Uterus pulled medially

1. Symphysis pubis
2. Urinary bladder
3. Uterus
4. Rectum

Right hypogastric nerve

S.1

Sympathetic trunk and ganglia

Sacrum

S3 nerve

Ureter

Uterine artery

S4 nerve

Right inferior hypogastric plexus and ganglion

Uterovaginal plexus

Urinary bladder

Coccyx

Rectum

Rectouterine pouch and fold

B

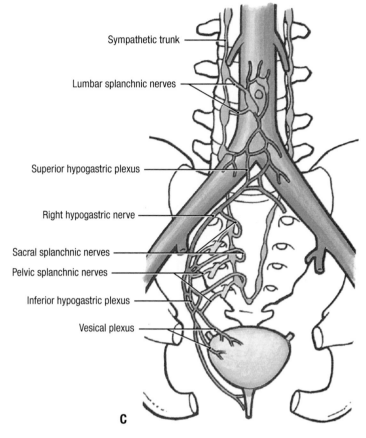

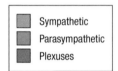

Sympathetic

Parasympathetic

Plexuses

C

3.35   Autonomic nerves of female pelvis

A. Median section, rectum and subperitoneal tissue reflected anteriorly. **B.** Median section, subperitoneal tissue removed. (This is a latter stage in dissection of A.) The right inferior hypogastric plexus continues as the uterovaginal plexus and supplies the uterus, uterine tubes, vagina, urethra, greater vestibular glands, erectile tissue of the clitoris, and bulb of the vestibule. **C.** Innervation of ureters, urinary bladder, and urethra, anterior view. **D.** Innervation of uterus, vagina, uterine tubes, and ovaries.

OBSERVE IN **A:**

1. The rectum and subperitoneal fatty areolar tissue were reflected anteriorly, pulling taut the pelvic splanchnic nerves, sympathetic fibers, and right hypogastric nerve;

2. The parasympathetic pelvic splanchnic nerves arise from the ventral primary rami of S2, S3, and S4; they supply motor fibers to the pelvic organs and sigmoid colon, and vasodilator fibers to the erectile tissue of the clitoris and bulb of the vestibule;

3. The sympathetic sacral splanchnic nerves arise from the sympathetic trunk and join the inferior hypogastric plexuses.

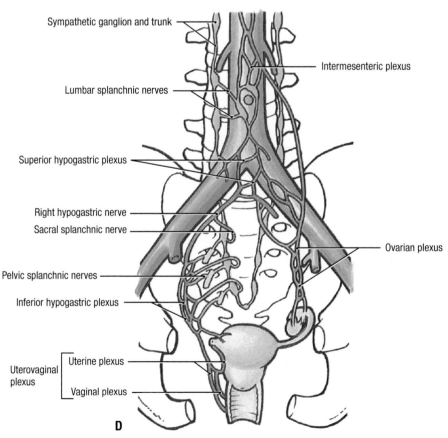

D

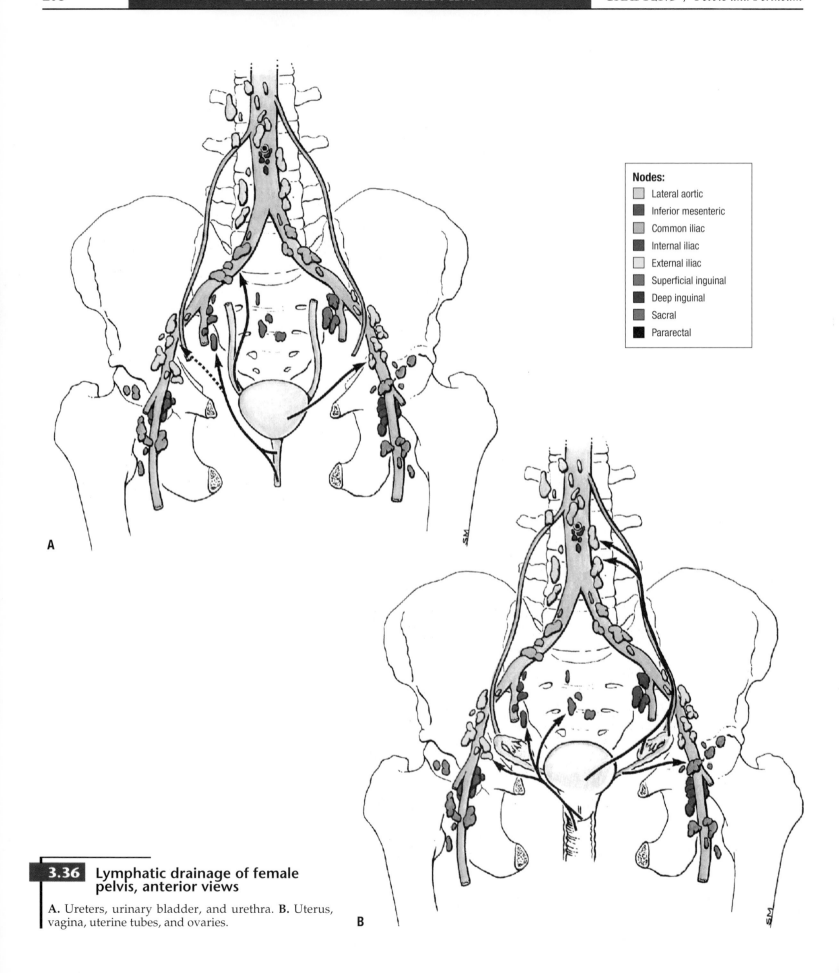

Nodes:
- Lateral aortic
- Inferior mesenteric
- Common iliac
- Internal iliac
- External iliac
- Superficial inguinal
- Deep inguinal
- Sacral
- Pararectal

3.36 Lymphatic drainage of female pelvis, anterior views

A. Ureters, urinary bladder, and urethra. **B.** Uterus, vagina, uterine tubes, and ovaries.

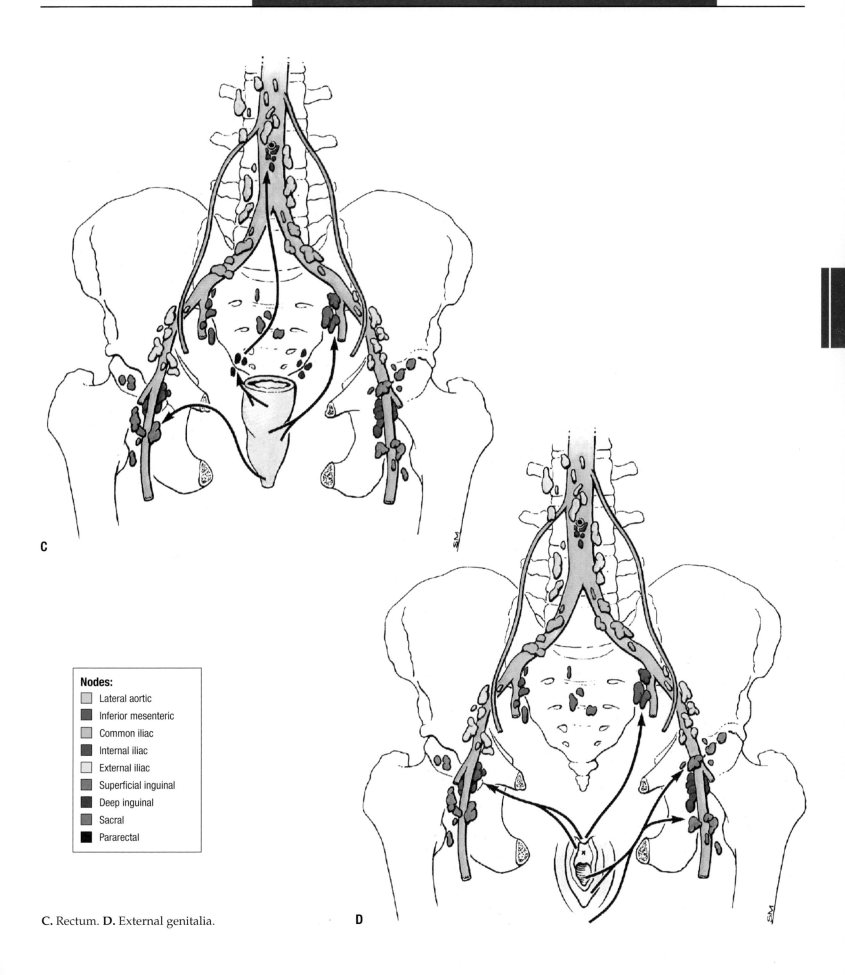

Nodes:

- Lateral aortic
- Inferior mesenteric
- Common iliac
- Internal iliac
- External iliac
- Superficial inguinal
- Deep inguinal
- Sacral
- Pararectal

C. Rectum. **D.** External genitalia.

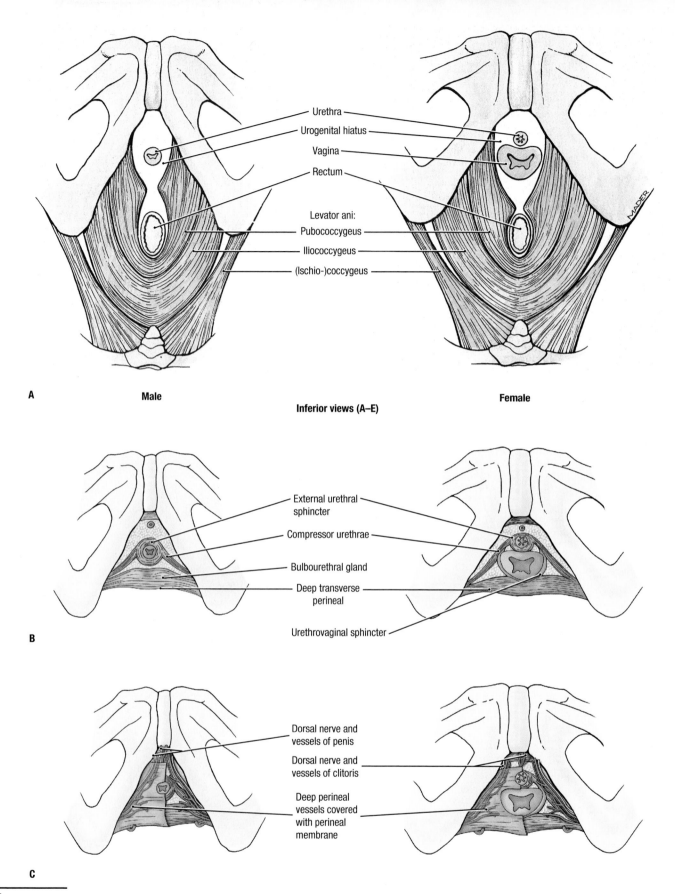

Urethra

Urogenital hiatus

Vagina

Rectum

Levator ani:

Pubococcygeus

Iliococcygeus

(Ischio-)coccygeus

A   Male   Female

Inferior views (A–E)

External urethral
sphincter

Compressor urethrae

Bulbourethral gland

Deep transverse
perineal

Urethrovaginal sphincter

B

Dorsal nerve and
vessels of penis

Dorsal nerve and
vessels of clitoris

Deep perineal
vessels covered
with perineal
membrane

C

3.37 Male and female perineum, inferior views

A. Levator ani. **B.** External urethral sphincter, urethrovaginal sphincter, and compressor urethrae. **C.** Perineal membrane and vessels. **D.** Crura and bulb of penis and clitoris. **E.** Muscles of superficial perineal compartment. **F.** Structures of the perineum in situ. These illustrations show the layers of the perineum built up from deep to superficial. The urethra (and vagina in the female) pierces the perineal membrane an-teriorly, and the rectum lies posteriorly. The perineal membrane is strong, spanning between the ischiopubic rami, and separating the superficial and deep perineal compartments. The perineal vessels are covered by the perineal membrane. In the female, greater vestibular glands lie posterior to the bulb of the vestibule.

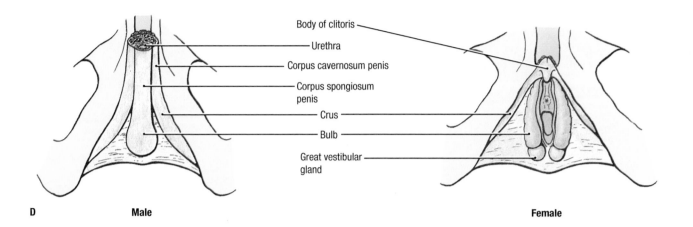

Body of clitoris
Urethra
Corpus cavernosum penis
Corpus spongiosum penis
Crus
Bulb
Great vestibular gland

D   **Male**   **Female**

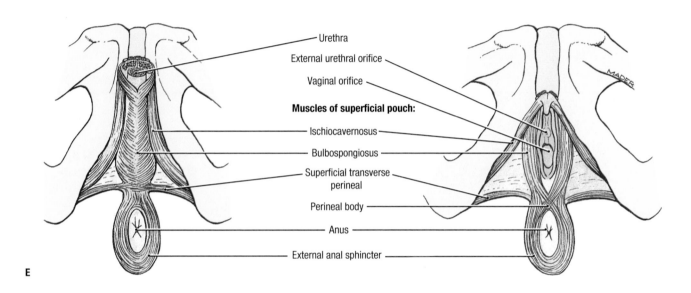

Urethra
External urethral orifice
Vaginal orifice
Muscles of superficial pouch:
Ischiocavernosus
Bulbospongiosus
Superficial transverse perineal
Perineal body
Anus
External anal sphincter

E

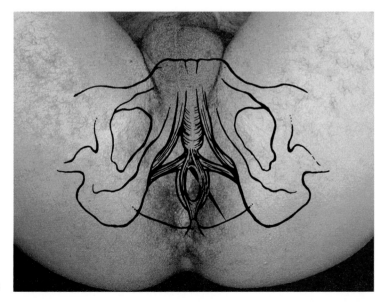

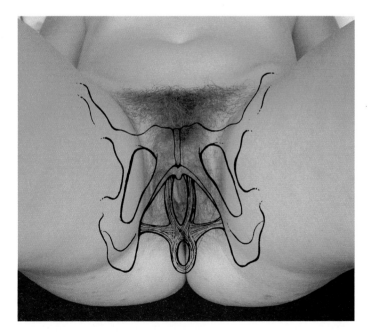

F

Table 3.4. Muscles of Perineum

Muscle	Origin	Insertion	Innervation	Action(s)
External anal sphincter	Skin and fascia surrounding anus and coccyx via anococcygeal ligament	Perineal body	Inferior anal nerve	Closes anal canal; works with bulbospongiosus to support and fix perineal body
Bulbospongiosus	*Male:* median raphe, ventral surface of bulb of penis, and perineal body	*Male:* corpus spongiosum and cavernosa and fascia of bulb of penis		*Male:* compresses bulb of urethra and assists in erection of penis
	Female: perineal body	*Female:* fascia of corpus cavernosa		*Female:* reduces lumen of vagina and assists in erection of clitoris
Ischiocavernosus		Crus of penis or clitoris		Maintains erection of penis or clitoris by compression of crura
Superficial transverse perineal	Internal surface of ischiopubic ramus and ischial tuberosity (compressor urethrae portion only)	Perineal body	Deep branch of perineal nerve, branch of pudendal nerve	Supports perineal body
Deep transverse perineal		Median raphe, perineal body, and external anal sphincter		Fixes perineal body
External urethral sphincter		Surrounds urethra; in males, also ascends anterior aspect of prostate; in females also encloses vagina		*Female:* compresses urethra and vagina *Male:* compresses intermediate (membranous) urethra

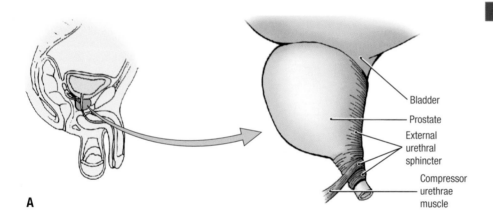

A

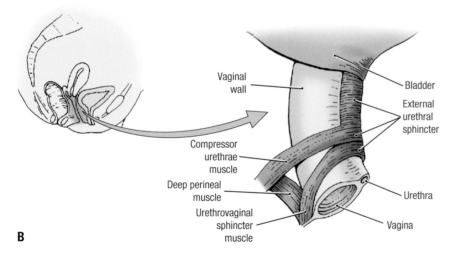

B

Bladder
Prostate
External urethral sphincter
Compressor urethrae muscle

Vaginal wall
Compressor urethrae muscle
Deep perineal muscle
Urethrovaginal sphincter muscle
Bladder
External urethral sphincter
Urethra
Vagina

3.38 **External urethral sphincter, compressor urethrae, and urethrovaginal sphincter, lateral views**

A. Male. The sphincter urethrae is more tubelike. In the male, part of the muscle encircles the intermediate (membranous) part of the urethra, and part extends to the base of the bladder, investing the prostatic urethra anteriorly and anterolaterally. This muscle is called the external urethral sphincter.[1] **B.** Female. The sphincter urethrae is a urogenital sphincter with three parts: 1) a superior part that extends to the base of the bladder, the external urethral sphincter muscle; 2) a part extending inferolaterally to the ischial ramus on each side, the compressor urethrae muscle; and 3) a bandlike part encircling the vagina and urethra, the urethrovaginal sphincter.[2]

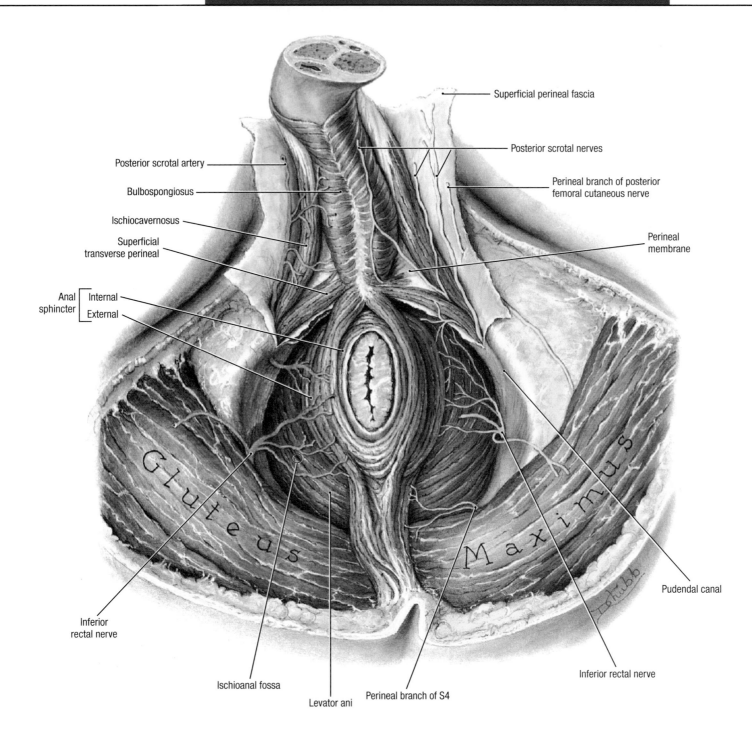

Posterior scrotal artery

Bulbospongiosus

Ischiocavernosus

Superficial
transverse perineal

Anal
sphincter — Internal
— External

Inferior
rectal nerve

Ischioanal fossa

Levator ani

Perineal branch of S4

Superficial perineal fascia

Posterior scrotal nerves

Perineal branch of posterior
femoral cutaneous nerve

Perineal
membrane

Pudendal canal

Inferior rectal nerve

3.39 Male perineum, inferior view

OBSERVE:

1. The anal orifice at the center of the anal triangle is surrounded by the external anal sphincter; there is an ischioanal (ischiorectal) fossa on each side;

2. The superficial fibers of the external anal sphincter anchor the anus anteriorly to the perineal body, or central tendon of the perineum, and posteriorly to the coccyx (in this specimen, to the skin);

3. The ischioanal fossa is bounded medially by the levator ani muscle, laterally by the obturator internus fascia, posteriorly by the gluteus maximus muscle lying superficial to the sacrotuberous ligament, and anteriorly by the perineal membrane;

4. The inferior rectal nerve leaves the pudendal canal and, with the perineal branch of S4, supplies the external anal sphincter; its cutaneous twigs to the anus are removed. The branch hooking around the gluteus maximus muscle replaces the perforating cutaneous nerve;

5. The superficial perineal (Colles') fascia was incised in the midline, freed from its attachment to the base of the perineal membrane, and reflected;

6. The cutaneous nerves and artery are in the superficial perineal compartment;

7. The three paired, superficial perineal muscles are the bulbospongiosus, ischiocavernosus, and superficial transverse perineus;

8. The triangular portion of the perineal membrane is exposed.

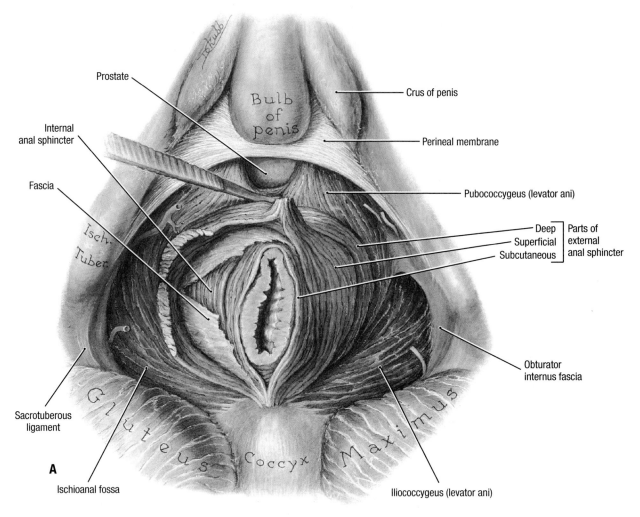

Prostate

Crus of penis

Bulb of penis

Internal anal sphincter

Perineal membrane

Fascia

Pubococcygeus (levator ani)

Deep ⎤ Parts of
Superficial ⎬ external
Subcutaneous ⎦ anal sphincter

Isch. Tuber.

Obturator internus fascia

Sacrotuberous ligament

Gluteus Coccyx Maximus

Ischioanal fossa

Iliococcygeus (levator ani)

A

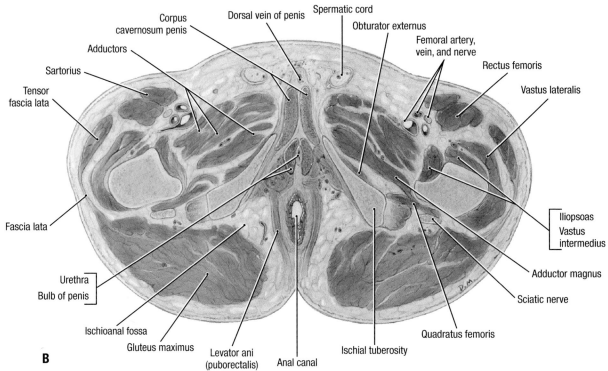

Corpus cavernosum penis

Dorsal vein of penis

Spermatic cord

Obturator externus

Femoral artery, vein, and nerve

Adductors

Rectus femoris

Sartorius

Vastus lateralis

Tensor fascia lata

Iliopsoas
Vastus intermedius

Fascia lata

Adductor magnus

Urethra
Bulb of penis

Sciatic nerve

Ischioanal fossa

Gluteus maximus

Levator ani (puborectalis)

Anal canal

Ischial tuberosity

Quadratus femoris

B

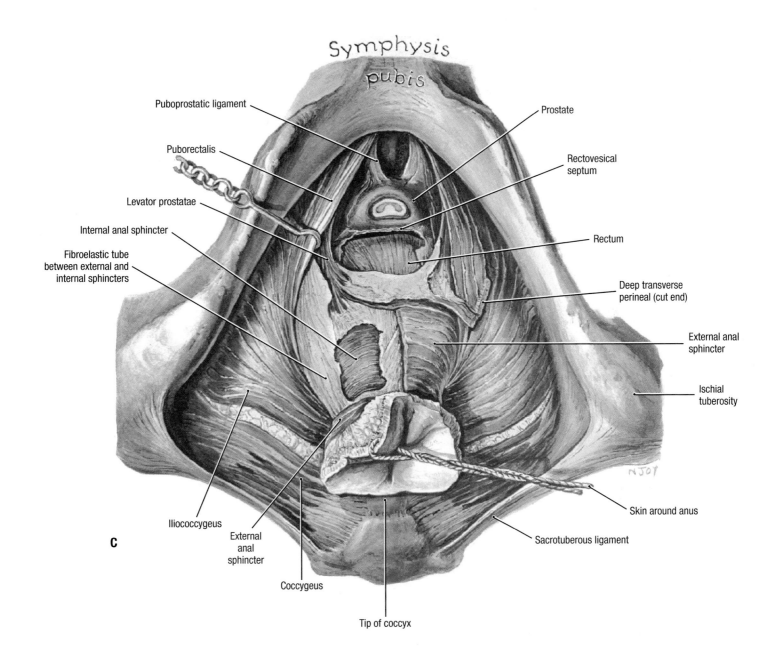

Symphysis pubis

Puboprostatic ligament

Puborectalis

Levator prostatae

Internal anal sphincter

Fibroelastic tube between external and internal sphincters

Iliococcygeus

External anal sphincter

Coccygeus

Tip of coccyx

Prostate

Rectovesical septum

Rectum

Deep transverse perineal (cut end)

External anal sphincter

Ischial tuberosity

Skin around anus

Sacrotuberous ligament

C

3.40　Dissection of male perineum

A. External anal sphincter, inferior view. **B.** Transverse section. **C.** Levator ani and coccygei muscles, and exposure of prostate, inferior view.

OBSERVE:

1. The three parts of the voluntary sphincter: a) subcutaneous, encircling the anal orifice; b) superficial, anchoring the anus in the median plane to the perineal body anteriorly, and to the coccyx posteriorly; and c) deep, forming a wide, encircling band;
2. In **A**, on the left of the figure: The superficial and deep parts of the sphincter are reflected, and the underlying sheet, consisting of areolar tissue, levator ani fibers, and the outer, longitudinal, muscular coat of the gut, is cut to reveal the inner, circular, muscular coat of the gut, which is thickened to form the internal anal sphincter;
3. The anterior free borders of the levator ani muscles meet anterior to the anal canal and are pushed posteriorly to expose the prostate;
4. In **C,** the longitudinal muscle coat of the rectum and its fascia blend with the levator ani muscle and its fasciae to form a fibroelastic tube that descends between the external and internal anal sphincters; from this tube, septa pass through the internal sphincter to the submucous coat, through the external sphincter to the skin, and, as the anal intermuscular septum, inferior to the internal sphincter.

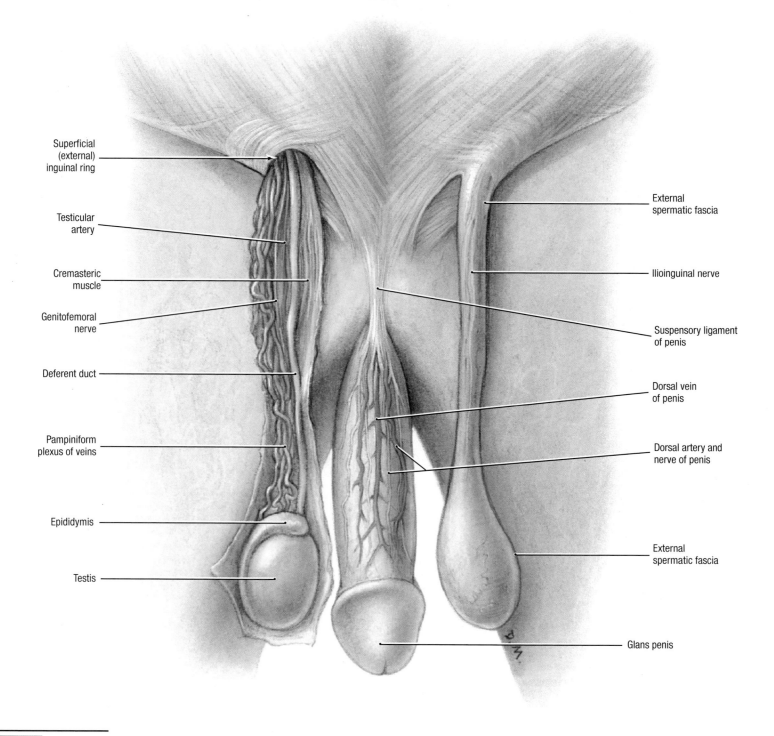

Superficial (external) inguinal ring

Testicular artery

Cremasteric muscle

Genitofemoral nerve

Deferent duct

Pampiniform plexus of veins

Epididymis

Testis

External spermatic fascia

Ilioinguinal nerve

Suspensory ligament of penis

Dorsal vein of penis

Dorsal artery and nerve of penis

External spermatic fascia

Glans penis

3.41   Vessels and nerves of penis and contents of spermatic cord

OBSERVE:

1. The superficial fascia covering the penis is removed to expose the midline deep dorsal vein and the bilateral dorsal arteries and nerves of the penis. The triangular suspensory ligament of the penis attaches to the region of the pubic symphysis and blends with the deep fascia of the penis;

2. On the specimen's left, the spermatic cord passes through the external inguinal ring and picks up a covering of external spermatic fascia from the margins of the external inguinal ring. The ilioinguinal nerve supplies the skin at the base of the penis and the ante-

rior aspect of the scrotum, and the cremasteric vessels supply the coverings of the cord and cremaster muscle;

3. On the specimen's right, the coverings of the spermatic cord and testis are reflected, and the contents of the cord are separated. The spermatic cord contains the deferent duct (with its vessels), the testicular artery (dissected away from the surrounding pampiniform plexus of veins), the genital branch of the genitofemoral nerve, and fibers of the cremaster muscle; lymphatic vessels and autonomic nerve fibers, not shown here, are also present.

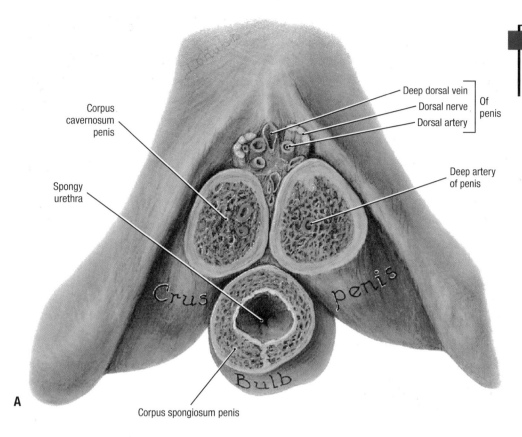

Corpus cavernosum penis

Spongy urethra

Deep dorsal vein ⎤
Dorsal nerve   ⎬ Of penis
Dorsal artery ⎦

Deep artery of penis

Crus   *penis*

Bulb

Corpus spongiosum penis

A

3.42 Root of penis, inferior views

A. Transverse section through crura and bulb of penis. The urethra is dilated within the bulb of the penis. **B.** Transverse section through bulb of penis with crura removed. The bulb is cut shorter than that in **A.** On the right of the figure, the perineal membrane is partially removed, opening the deep perineal pouch.

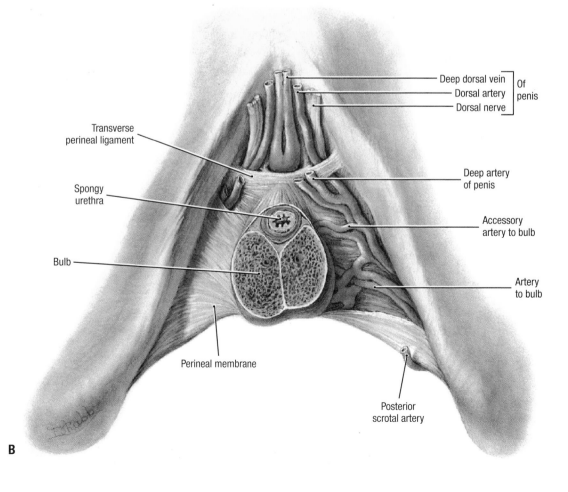

Deep dorsal vein ⎤
Dorsal artery ⎬ Of penis
Dorsal nerve   ⎦

Transverse perineal ligament

Spongy urethra

Deep artery of penis

Accessory artery to bulb

Bulb

Artery to bulb

Perineal membrane

Posterior scrotal artery

B

OBSERVE IN **B**:
1. The fibers of the perineal membrane converge on the bulb and anchor it to the pubic arch;
2. The urethra is bound to the dorsum of the bulb;
3. The septum in the bulb indicates its bilateral origin;
4. The artery to the bulb (here double); the artery to the crus, called the deep artery; and the dorsal artery, which ends in the glans penis. The deep dorsal vein, originally double, ends in the prostatic venous plexus.

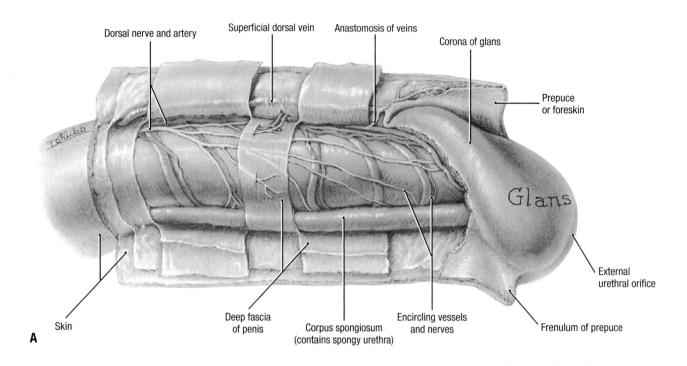

A. Lateral view. Labels: Dorsal nerve and artery, Superficial dorsal vein, Anastomosis of veins, Corona of glans, Prepuce or foreskin, Glans, External urethral orifice, Frenulum of prepuce, Encircling vessels and nerves, Corpus spongiosum (contains spongy urethra), Deep fascia of penis, Skin.

A

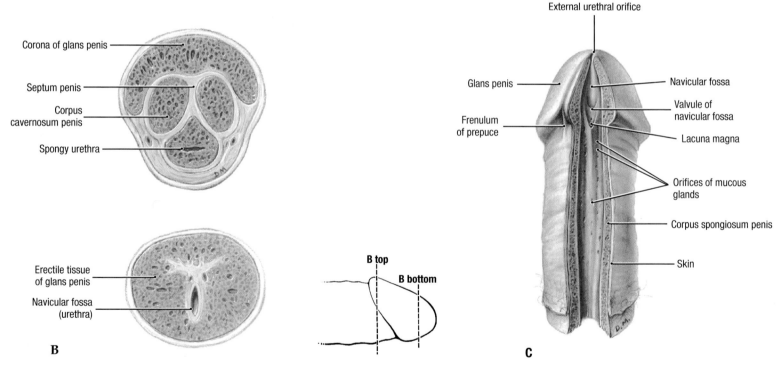

B. Transverse sections. Labels: Corona of glans penis, Septum penis, Corpus cavernosum penis, Spongy urethra, Erectile tissue of glans penis, Navicular fossa (urethra).

B top, **B bottom**

B

C. Spongy urethra. Labels: External urethral orifice, Glans penis, Navicular fossa, Valvule of navicular fossa, Lacuna magna, Frenulum of prepuce, Orifices of mucous glands, Corpus spongiosum penis, Skin.

C

3.43 Penis

A. Lateral view. The three tubular envelopes of the penis and the prepuce are reflected **B.** Transverse sections. One section is taken through the glans penis more proximally (top) and the other more distally (bottom), as indicated by the orientation drawing. **C.** Spongy urethra, interior. A longitudinal incision was made on the urethral surface of the penis and carried through the floor of the urethra, allowing for a view of the dorsal surface of the interior of the urethra.

OBSERVE IN **A:**

1. The skin is carried forward as the prepuce;

2. The loose, laminated, subcutaneous areolar tissue (called the superficial fascia of the penis) is carried forward into the prepuce and contains the superficial dorsal vein; this vein begins in the prepuce, anastomoses with the deep dorsal vein from the glans, and ends in the superficial inguinal veins;

3. The deep fascia of the penis ends at the glans penis;

4. The large, encircling tributaries of the deep dorsal vein, the thread-like companion arteries, and numerous oblique nerves;

5. The vessels and nerves at the neck plunge into the glans penis.

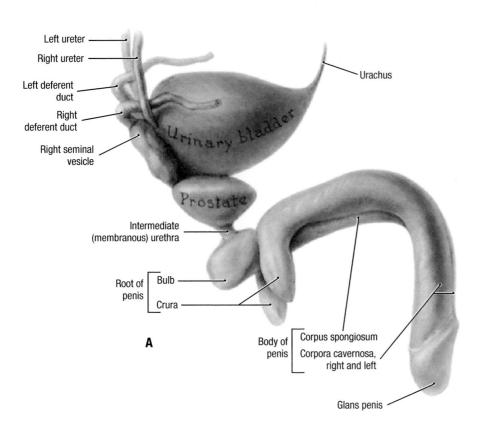

Left ureter

Right ureter

Left deferent duct

Right deferent duct

Right seminal vesicle

Urachus

Urinary bladder

Prostate

Intermediate (membranous) urethra

Root of penis { Bulb / Crura }

Body of penis { Corpus spongiosum / Corpora cavernosa, right and left }

Glans penis

A

3.44 Male urogenital system

A. Inferior components of genital and urinary tracts, lateral view. **B.** Dissection of corpora cavernosa and corpus spongiosum, lateral view. The corpus spongiosum is separated from the corpora cavernosa. The natural flexures are preserved.

OBSERVE:
1. The corpora cavernosa is bent where the penis is suspended by the suspensory ligament of the penis to the pubic symphysis;
2. The corpus spongiosum extends posteriorly from the bulb of the penis and terminates anteriorly at the glans; the glans fits like a "cap" on the ends of the corpora cavernosa.

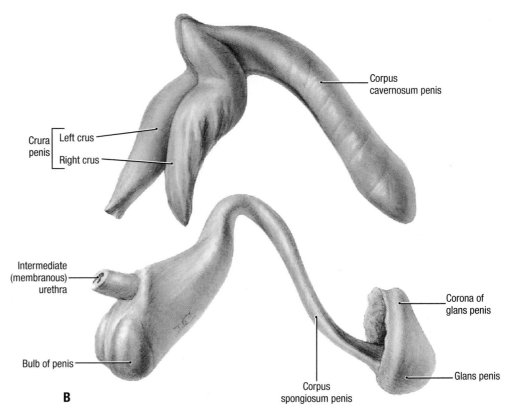

Crura penis { Left crus / Right crus }

Corpus cavernosum penis

Intermediate (membranous) urethra

Bulb of penis

Corpus spongiosum penis

Corona of glans penis

Glans penis

B

3.45 Female perineum—I, inferior view

OBSERVE ON THE SPECIMEN'S RIGHT:
1. A long digital, or finger-like, process of fat lies deep to the subcutaneous fatty tissue and descends far into the labium majus;
2. The round ligament of the uterus ends as a branching band of fascia that spreads out superficial to the fatty digital process; the external pudendal vessels cross the process;

OBSERVE ON THE SPECIMEN'S LEFT:
3. Most of the digital process of fat is removed;
4. The posterior labial vessels and nerves (S2, S3) are joined by the perineal branch of the posterior femoral cutaneous nerve (S1, S2, S3) and run anteriorly almost to the mons pubis; the vessels there anastomose with the external pudendal vessels and the nerves meeting the ilioinguinal nerve (L1).

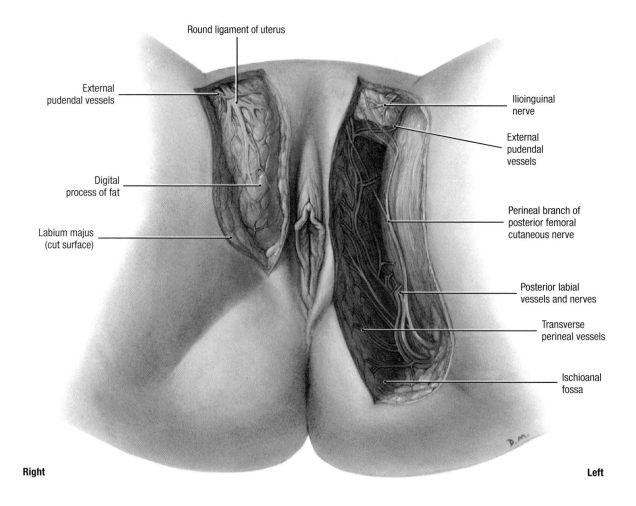

Round ligament of uterus

External pudendal vessels

Digital process of fat

Labium majus (cut surface)

Ilioinguinal nerve

External pudendal vessels

Perineal branch of posterior femoral cutaneous nerve

Posterior labial vessels and nerves

Transverse perineal vessels

Ischioanal fossa

Right   **Left**

3.46 Female perineum—II, inferior view

OBSERVE:
1. The thickness of the superficial fatty tissue at the mons pubis and the encapsulated digital process of fat deep to this; the suspensory ligament of the clitoris descends from the linea alba and symphysis pubis;
2. The prepuce of the clitoris, thrown like a "hood" over the clitoris, and the anterior ends of the labia minora unite to form the frenulum of the clitoris;
3. There are three muscles on each side: bulbospongiosus, ischiocavernosus, and superficial transverse perineus; when slightly separated, they reveal the perineal membrane. The bulbospongiosus muscle overlies the bulb of the vestibule. In the male, the muscles of the two sides are united by a median raphe; in the female, the orifice of the vagina separates the two;
4. The pinpoint orifices of the right and left paraurethral ducts are below the urethral orifice;
5. The anterior recess of the ischioanal fossa lies deep to the urogenital diaphragm.

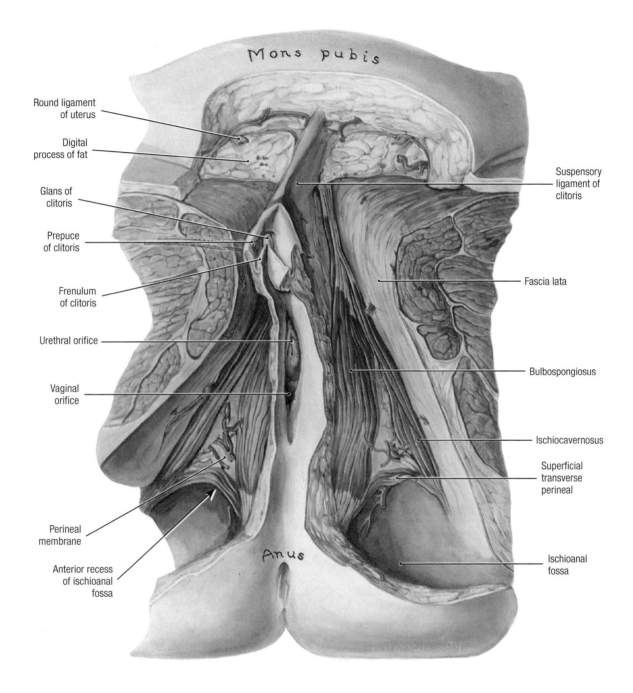

Mons pubis

Round ligament of uterus

Digital process of fat

Glans of clitoris

Prepuce of clitoris

Frenulum of clitoris

Urethral orifice

Vaginal orifice

Perineal membrane

Anterior recess of ischioanal fossa

Suspensory ligament of clitoris

Fascia lata

Bulbospongiosus

Ischiocavernosus

Superficial transverse perineal

Ischioanal fossa

Anus

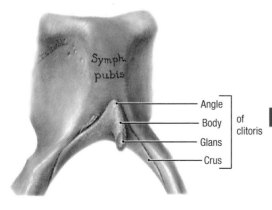

Symph. pubis

Angle

Body   of clitoris

Glans

Crus

3.47   Clitoris, inferior view

The body of the clitoris comprises two corpora cavernosa that are bent, suspended by a suspensory ligament, and capped by a glans. The crura are covered by the paired ischiocavernosus muscles. The bulbs of the vestibule and the commissure of the bulbs are represented in the male by the bulb and body of the corpus spongiosum. However, these are not regarded as part of the clitoris and are not traversed by the urethra.

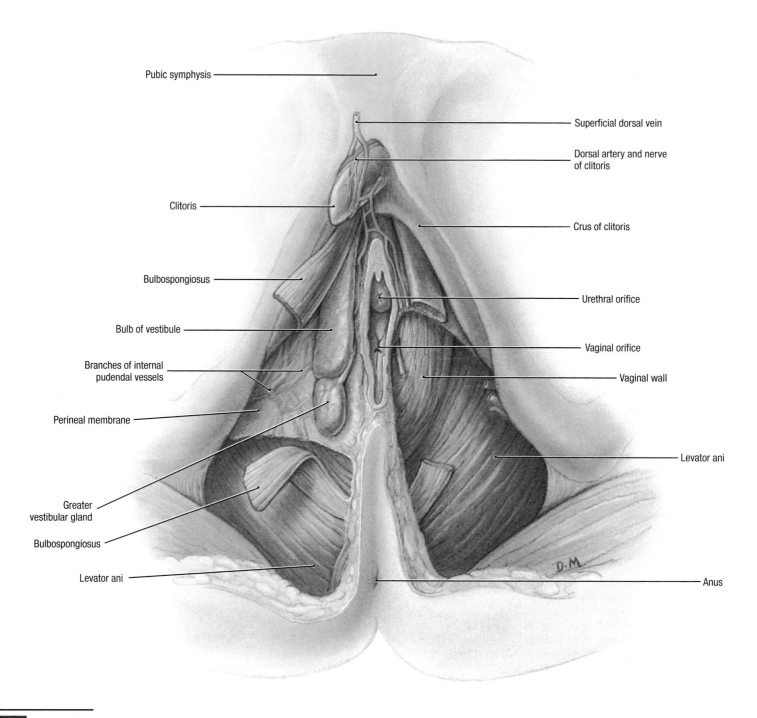

Pubic symphysis

Superficial dorsal vein

Dorsal artery and nerve of clitoris

Clitoris

Crus of clitoris

Bulbospongiosus

Urethral orifice

Bulb of vestibule

Vaginal orifice

Branches of internal pudendal vessels

Vaginal wall

Perineal membrane

Levator ani

Greater vestibular gland

Bulbospongiosus

Levator ani

Anus

3.48   **Female perineum—III, inferior view**

The bulbospongiosus muscle is divided and reflected on the right side, and largely excised on the left side. The bulb of the vestibule on the left has been partially removed.

OBSERVE:
1. The glans clitoris is pulled over to the specimen's right side, and the dorsal vessels and nerve of the clitoris run to it;
2. The bulb of the vestibule is split by the vagina so that it appears as two masses of elongated erectile tissue that lie along the sides of the vaginal orifice;

3. Veins connect the bulbs of the vestibule to the glans of the clitoris;
4. On the specimen's right, the greater vestibular gland is situated at the posterior end of the bulb and is covered with bulbospongiosus muscle; it has a long duct (approximately 1.9 mm) that opens into the vestibule;
5. On the specimen's left side, the perineal membrane is cut away, thereby revealing the vaginal wall.

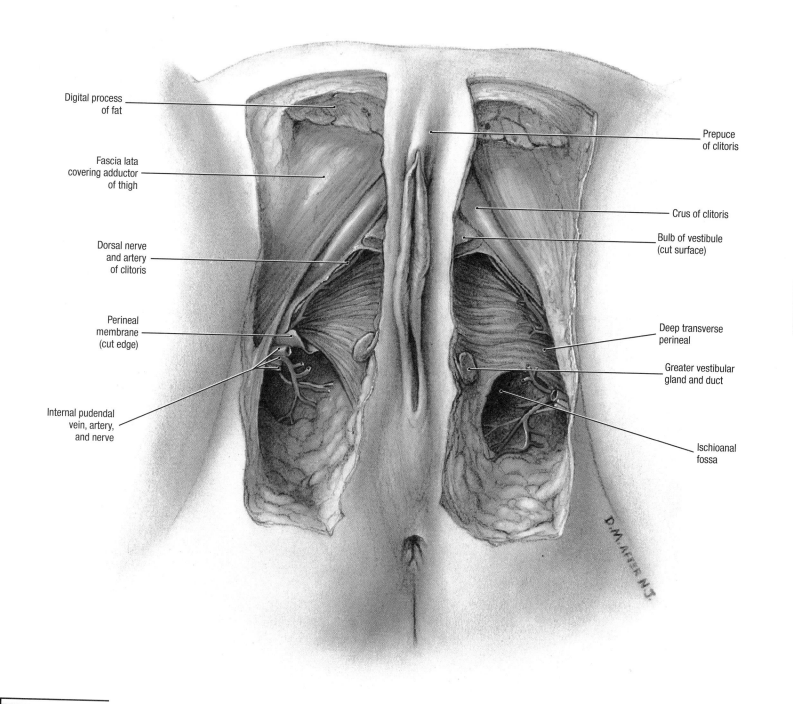

Digital process
of fat

Fascia lata
covering adductor
of thigh

Dorsal nerve
and artery
of clitoris

Perineal
membrane
(cut edge)

Internal pudendal
vein, artery,
and nerve

Prepuce
of clitoris

Crus of clitoris

Bulb of vestibule
(cut surface)

Deep transverse
perineal

Greater vestibular
gland and duct

Ischioanal
fossa

3.49 Female perineum—IV, inferior view

The bulbs of the vestibule have been removed, except at their pubic ends, but the greater vestibular glands and ducts remain; the perineal membrane is removed, except for a marginal fringe;

OBSERVE:

1. The deep transverse perineal is shown on both sides as thin striated muscle;

2. The dorsal nerve and artery to the clitoris run anteriorly and give twigs to the bulb and crus;

3. The greater vestibular glands are located in the superficial perineal pouch.

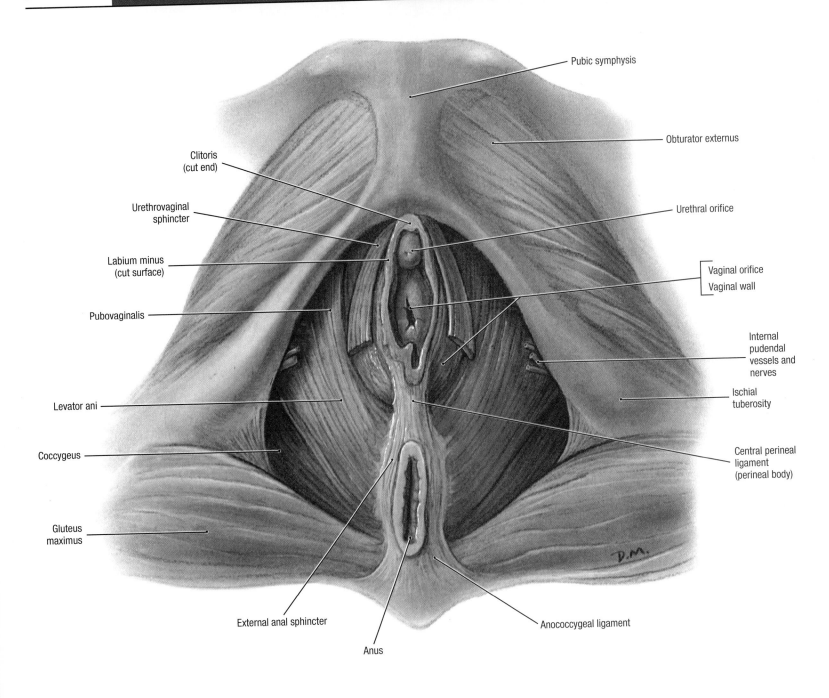

Pubic symphysis

Obturator externus

Clitoris
(cut end)

Urethral orifice

Urethrovaginal
sphincter

Labium minus
(cut surface)

Vaginal orifice
Vaginal wall

Pubovaginalis

Internal
pudendal
vessels and
nerves

Levator ani

Ischial
tuberosity

Coccygeus

Central perineal
ligament
(perineal body)

Gluteus
maximus

D.M.

External anal sphincter

Anococcygeal ligament

Anus

3.50   Female perineum—V, inferior view

The perineal membrane and deep transverse perineus have been removed.

OBSERVE:
1. The anterior parts of the levator ani (pubovaginales) muscle meet posterior to the vaginal orifice;

2. The sphincter urethrae rests on the urethra and straddles the vagina;
3. The labia minora, cut short, bounds the vestibule of the vagina;

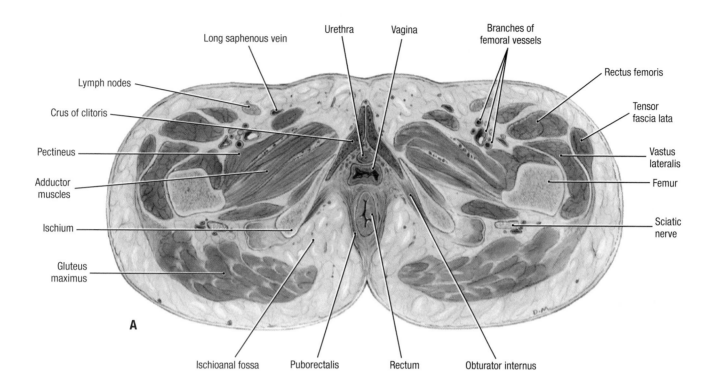

A

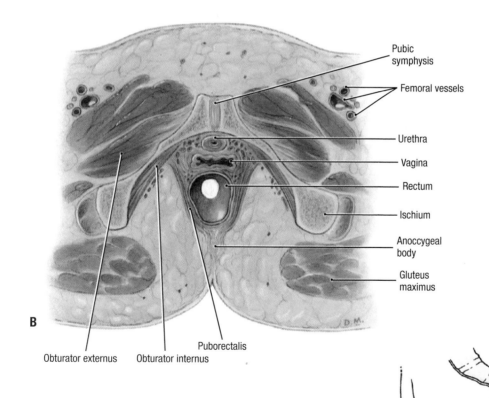

B

3.51 Transverse sections of female perineum

A. Section through vagina, urethra, and crura of clitoris. **B.** Section through vagina and urethra at base of urinary bladder.

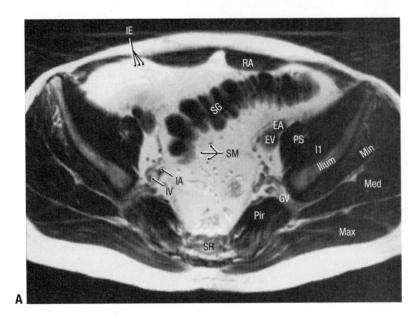

A

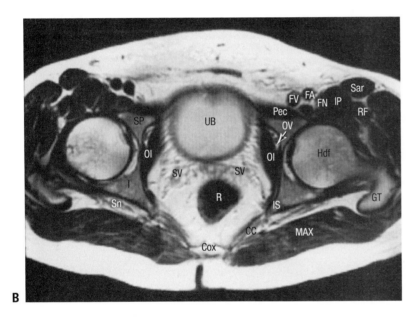

B

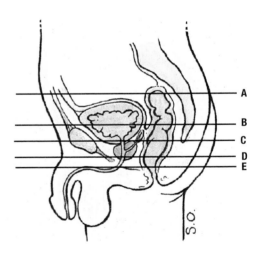

3.52   Transverse (axial) MRIs of the male pelvis and perineum

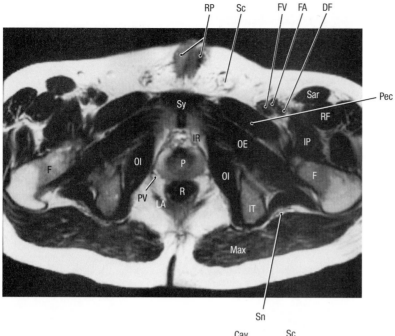

C

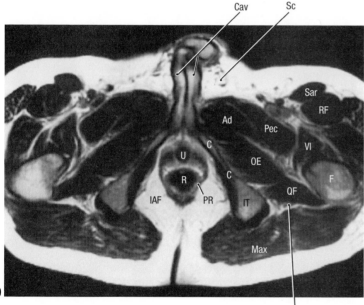

D

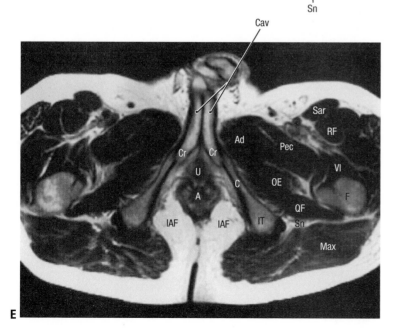

E

A	Anus
Ad	Adductor muscles
C	Conjoint ramus
Cav	Corpus cavernosum penis
CC	Coccygeus
Cox	Coccyx
Cr	Crus of penis
DF	Deep femoral artery
EA	External iliac artery
EV	External iliac vein
F	Femur
FA	Femoral artery
FN	Femoral nerve
FV	Femoral vein
GT	Greater trochangter
GV	Superior gluteal vein
Hd F	Head of femur
I	Body of ischium
IA	Internal iliac artery
IAF	Ischioanal fossa
IE	Inferior epigastric vessels
IL	Iliacus
IR	Inferior ramus of pubis
IP	Iliopsoas
IS	Ischial spine
IT	Ischial tuberosity
IV	Internal iliac vein
LA	Levator ani
Max	Gluteus maximus
Med	Gluteus medius
Min	Gluteus minimus
OE	Obturator externus
OI	Obturator internus
OV	Obturator vessels and nerve
P	Prostate
Pec	Pectineus
Pir	Piriformis
PR	Puborectalis
Ps	Psoas
PV	Pelvic vessels and nerves
QF	Rectus femoris
R	Rectum
RA	Rectus abdominis
RF	Rectus femoris
RP	Root of penis
Sar	Sartorius
Sc	Spermatic cord
SR	Sacrum
SG	Sigmoid colon
SM	Sigmoidal vessels inmesentry of sigmoid colon
Sn	Sciatic nerve
SP	Superior ramus of pubis
SV	Seminal vesicle
Sy	Symphysis pubis
U	Urethra
UB	Urinary bladder
VI	Vastus intermedius

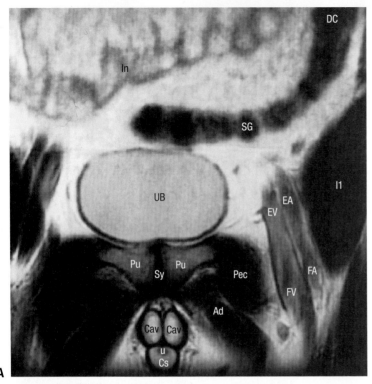

A

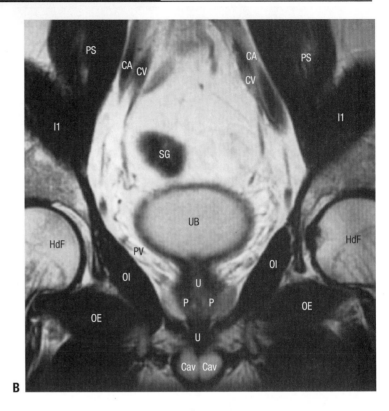

B

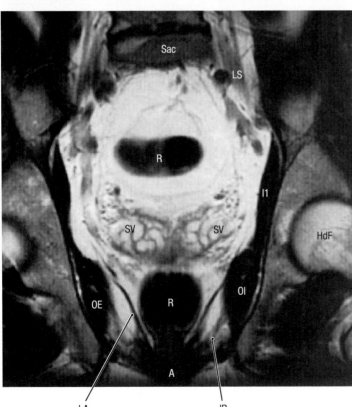

C

A	Anus	LA	Levator ani
Ad	Adductors	LS	Lumbosacral trunk
CA	Common iliac artery	OE	Obturator externus
Cav	Corpus cavernosum penis	OI	Obturator internus
		P	Prostate
Cs	Corpus spongiosum penis	Pec	Pectineus
		PS	Psoas
CV	Common iliac vein	Pu	Pubic bone
DC	Descending colon	PV	Pelvic vessels and nerves
EA	External iliac artery		
EV	External iliac vein	R	Rectum
FA	Femoral artery	Sac	Sacrum
FV	Femoral vein	SG	Sigmoid colon
Hd F	Head of femur	SV	Seminal vesicle
Il	Iliacus	Sy	Symphysis pubis
In	Intestine	U	Urethra
IR	Inferior rectal nerve and vessels	UB	Urinary bladder

3.53 Coronal MRIs (magnetic resonance images) of the male pelvis and perineum

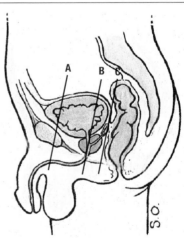

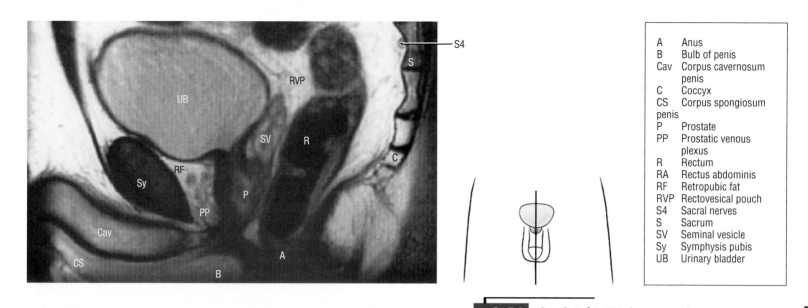

A	Anus
B	Bulb of penis
Cav	Corpus cavernosum penis
C	Coccyx
CS	Corpus spongiosum penis
P	Prostate
PP	Prostatic venous plexus
R	Rectum
RA	Rectus abdominis
RF	Retropubic fat
RVP	Rectovesical pouch
S4	Sacral nerves
S	Sacrum
SV	Seminal vesicle
Sy	Symphysis pubis
UB	Urinary bladder

3.54 Sagittal MRI (magnetic resonance image) of the male pelvis

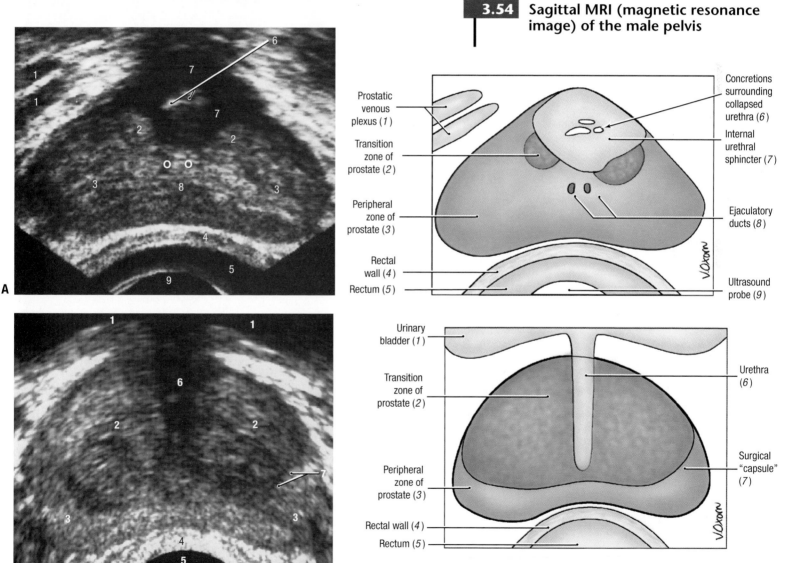

Prostatic venous plexus (1)

Transition zone of prostate (2)

Peripheral zone of prostate (3)

Rectal wall (4)

Rectum (5)

Concretions surrounding collapsed urethra (6)

Internal urethral sphincter (7)

Ejaculatory ducts (8)

Ultrasound probe (9)

Urinary bladder (1)

Transition zone of prostate (2)

Peripheral zone of prostate (3)

Rectal wall (4)

Rectum (5)

Urethra (6)

Surgical "capsule" (7)

3.55 Axial (transverse) transrectal ultrasound scans through prostate

A. Normal prostate of young male. **B.** Benign prostatic hyperplasia. In **B,** note the enlarged transition zone. *The transition zone of the prostate normally starts becoming hyperplastic after age 30.* The red line indicates the site of scans **A** and **B.** The numbers in parentheses correspond to labels on the ultrasound scan.

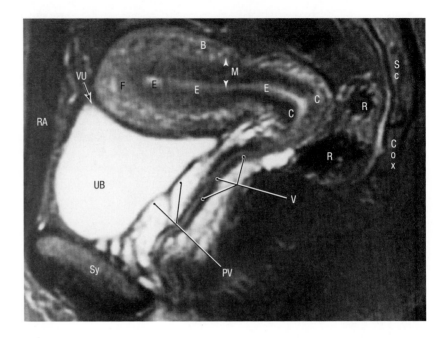

B	Body of uterus
C	Cervix of uterus
Cox	Coccyx
E	Endometrium
F	Fundus of uterus
M	Myometrium
PV	Perivaginal veins
R	Rectum
RA	Rectus abdominis
Sc	Sacrum
Sy	Symphysis pubis
UB	Urinary bladder
V	Vagina
VU	Vesicouterine pouch

3.56 Sagittal MRI (magnetic resonance image) of the female pelvis

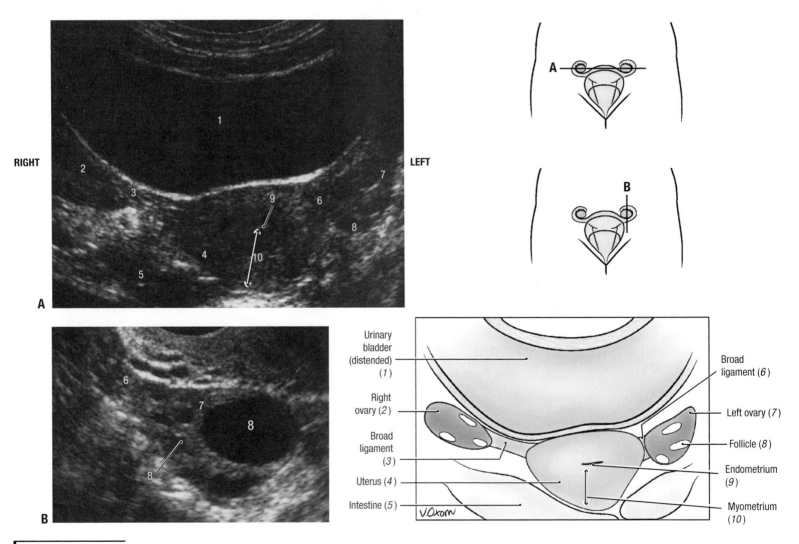

Urinary bladder (distended) (1)

Right ovary (2)

Broad ligament (3)

Uterus (4)

Intestine (5)

Broad ligament (6)

Left ovary (7)

Follicle (8)

Endometrium (9)

Myometrium (10)

V. Oxorn

3.57 Ultrasound scans of female pelvis

A. Transabdominal axial (transverse) scan through uterus and ovaries. **B.** Transvaginal sagittal scan of left ovary. The red line on each orientation drawing indicates the site of the scan. The numbers in parentheses correspond to labels on the ultrasound scans. In **B,** note the F-dominant follicle.

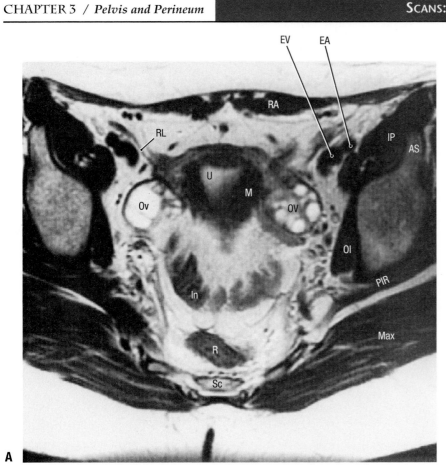

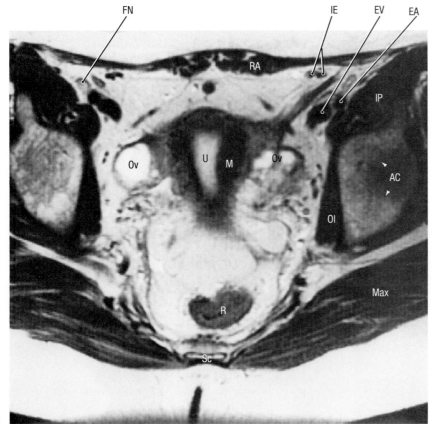

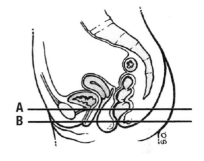

3.58 Transverse (axial) MRIs of the female pelvis and perineum

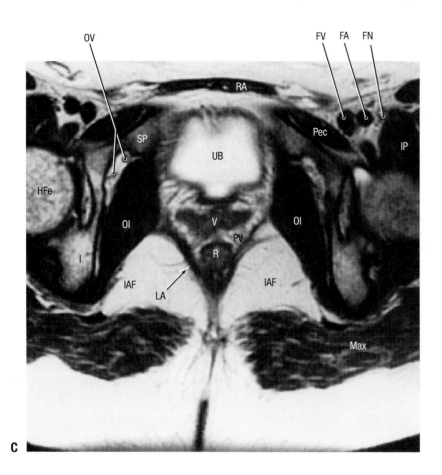

C

A	Anus
Ac	Acetabulum
Ad	Adductor muscles
AS	Anterior superior iliac spine
C	Conjoint ramus
EA	External iliac artery
EV	External iliac vein
FA	Femoral artery
FN	Femoral nerve
FV	Femoral vein
H Fe	Head of femur
I	Ilium
IAF	Ischioanal fossa
IE	Inferior epigastric vessels
In	Intestine
IP	Iliopsoas
IT	Ischial tuberosity
LA	Levator ani
LM	Labia majora
M	Myometrium
Max	Gluteus maximus

OE	Obturator externus
OI	Obturator internus
Ov	Ovary
OV	Obturator vessels
Pec	Pectineus
PIR	Piriformis
Pm	Perineal membrane
Pu	Pubic bone
PV	Perivaginal veins
QF	Quadratus femoris
R	Rectum
RA	Rectus abdominis
RL	Round ligament
Sc	Sacrum
SP	Superior ramus of pubis
Sy	Symphysis pubis
U	Uterus
UB	Urinary bladder
Ur	Urethra
V	Vagina
Ve	Vestibule

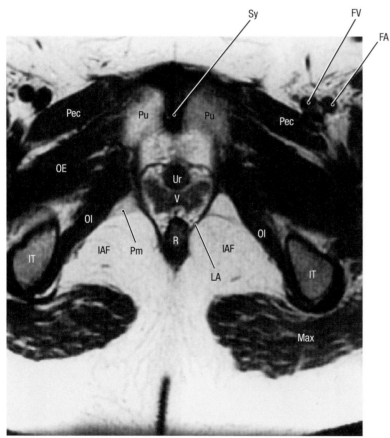

D

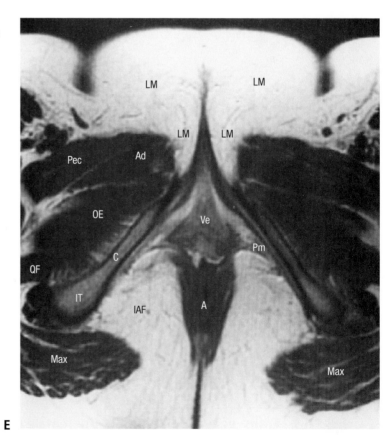

E

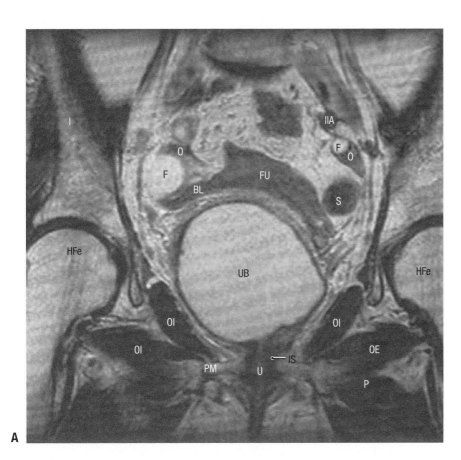

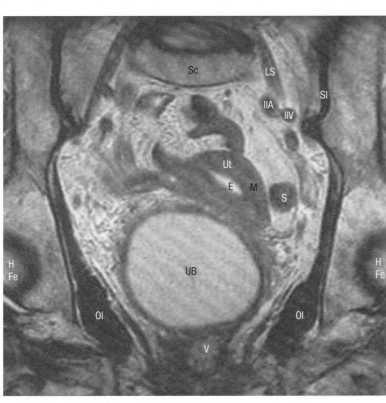

BL	Broad ligament
E	Endometrium
F	Follicle
FU	Fundus of uterus
Hfe	Head of femur
I	Ilium
IIA	Internal iliac artery
IIV	Internal iliac vein
IS	Internal urethral sphincter
LS	Lumbosacral trunk
M	Myometrium
O	Ovary
OE	Obturator externus
OI	Obturator internus
P	Pectineus
PM	Perineal membrane
S	Sigmoid colon
Sc	Sacrum
Ut	Uterus
U	Urethra
UB	Urinary bladder
V	Vagina

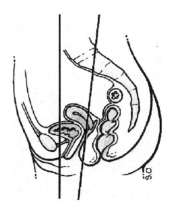

3.59 Coronal MRIs of female pelvis

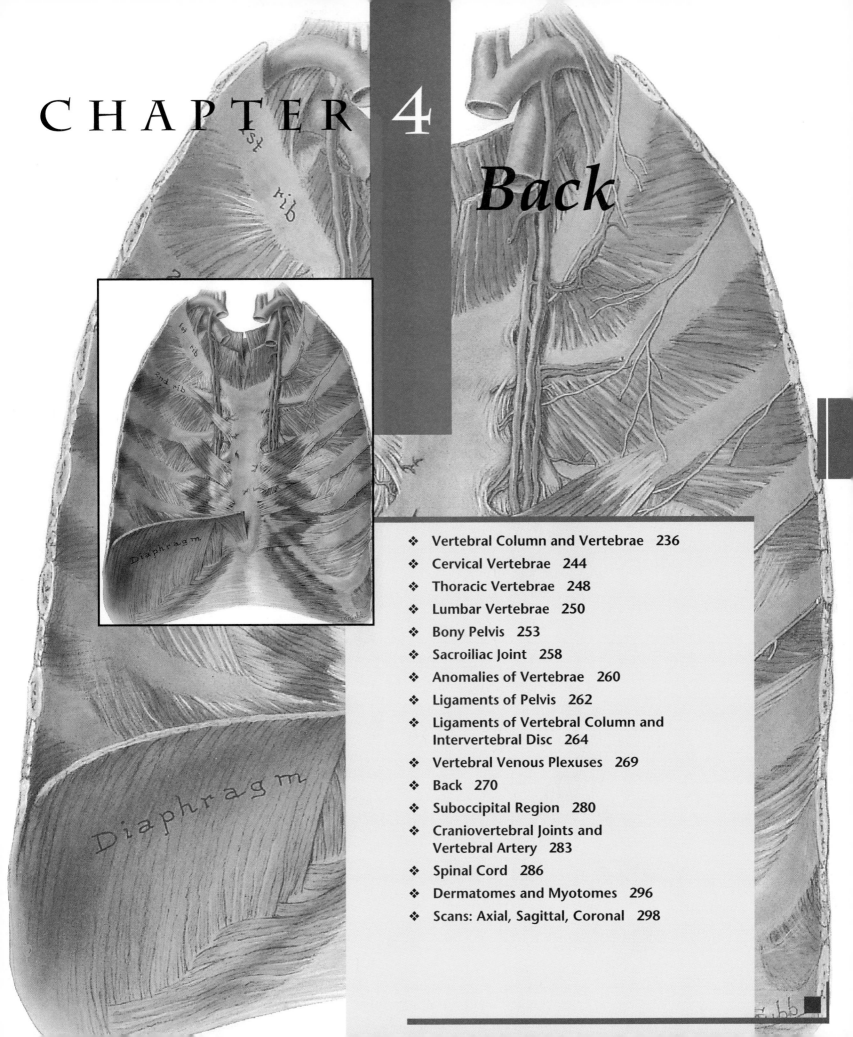

CHAPTER 4

Back

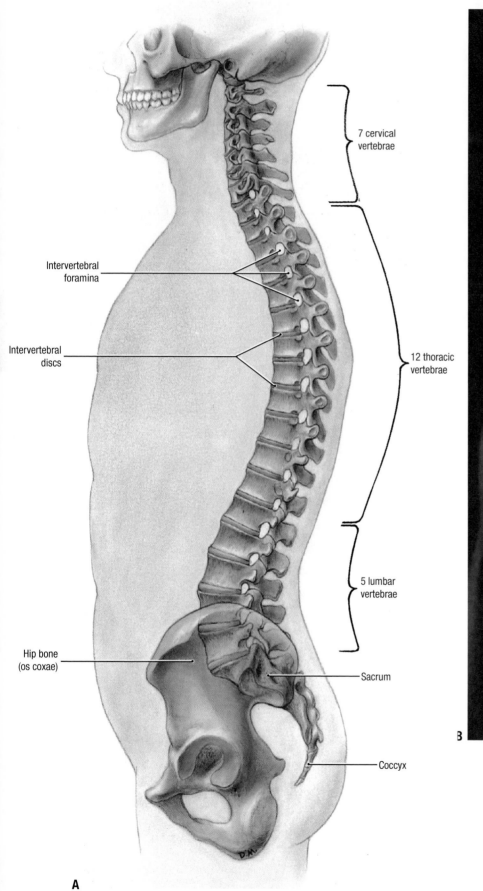

7 cervical vertebrae

Intervertebral foramina

Intervertebral discs

12 thoracic vertebrae

5 lumbar vertebrae

Hip bone (os coxae)

Sacrum

Coccyx

A

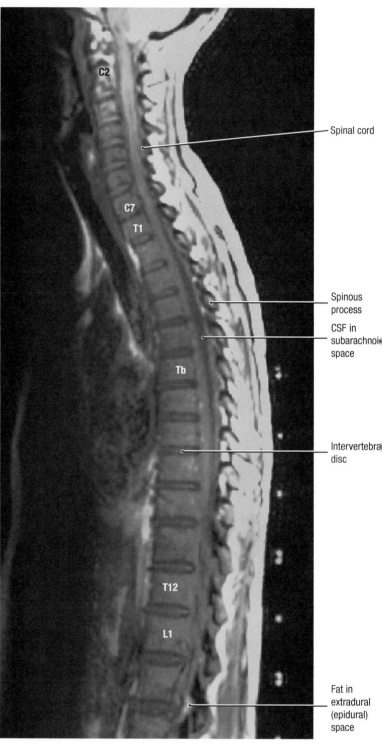

C2

C7

T1

Tb

T12

L1

Spinal cord

Spinous process

CSF in subarachnoid space

Intervertebral disc

Fat in extradural (epidural) space

B

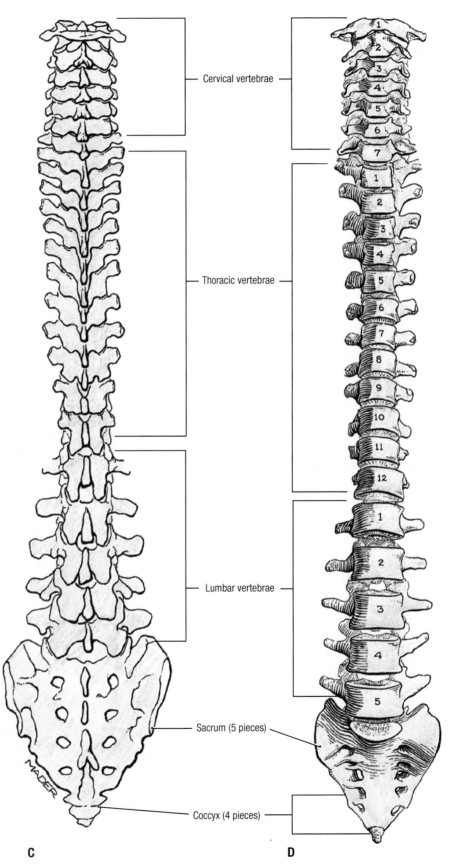

Cervical vertebrae

Thoracic vertebrae

Lumbar vertebrae

Sacrum (5 pieces)

Coccyx (4 pieces)

C **D**

4.1 Vertebral column

A. Lateral view. **B.** Sagittal MRI, lateral view. **C.** Posterior view. **D.** Anterior view.

OBSERVE:

1. The vertebral column comprises 24 separate (presacral) vertebrae and two composite vertebrae, the sacrum and coccyx; of the 24 separate vertebrae, 12 support ribs (thoracic), 7 are in the neck (cervical), and 5 are in the lumbar region (lumbar);
2. Vertebrae forming the posterior walls of the bony cavities (the thoracic vertebrae posterior to the thoracic cavity, and the sacrum and coccyx posterior to the pelvic cavity) are concave anteriorly; elsewhere (in the cervical and lumbar regions), by way of compensation, they are convex anteriorly (**A** and **B**);
3. The transverse processes of the atlas (C1) are spread widely; those of C7 spread almost as far, and those of C2 to C6 spread less. The spread diminishes progressively from T1 to T12; in the lumbar region, it is greatest at L3 (**C** and **D**).
4. In **A,** the intervertebral foramina are where the spinal nerves exit the vertebral (spinal) canal; there are 8 cervical, 12 thoracic, 5 lumbar, 5 sacral, and 1 to 2 coccygeal nerves (see Figure 4.52).
5. In **B,** note the size and shape of the vertebral bodies, the direction of the spinous processes, and the spinal cord in the vertebral canal.

Curvatures: **Vertebral column:**

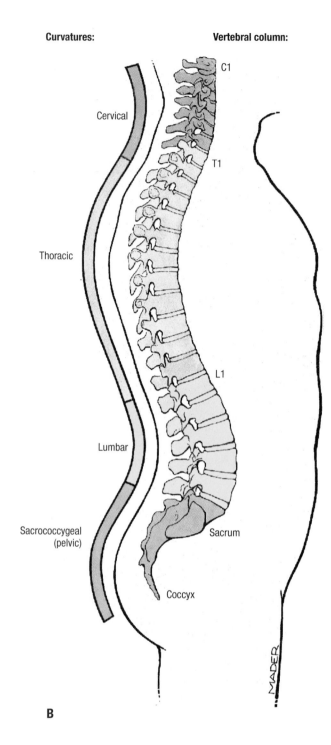

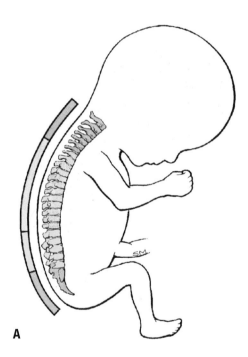

A

4.2   Curvatures of vertebral column, lateral views

A. Fetus. **B.** Adult. Cervical vertebrae are red, thoracic vertebrae are brown, and lumbar vertebrae are yellow; the sacrum and coccyx are orange.

OBSERVE:

1. In **A,** note the C-shaped curvature of the fetal spine; the curvature is concave anteriorly;
2. The thoracic and sacrococcygeal curves are primary curves; the cervical and lumbar curves are secondary curves, which develop after birth; the cervical curve develops when the child begins to hold the

head up, and the lumbar curve develops when the child begins to walk.

3. In **B,** the four curvatures of the adult vertebral column include (a) the cervical curve, which is convex anteriorly and lies between vertebrae C1 and T2; (b) the thoracic curve, which is concave anteriorly, between vertebrae T2 and T12; (c) the lumbar curve, convex anteriorly and lying between T12 and the lumbosacral joint; and (d) the sacrococcygeal (pelvic) curve, concave anteriorly and spanning from the lumbosacral joint to the tip of the coccyx;

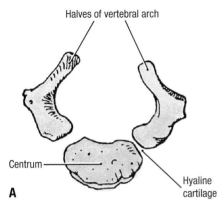

Halves of vertebral arch

Centrum

Hyaline cartilage

A

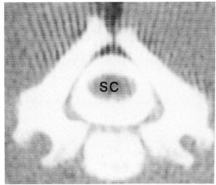

SC

B

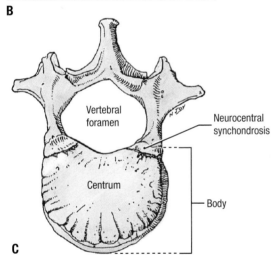

Vertebral foramen

Neurocentral synchondrosis

Centrum

Body

C

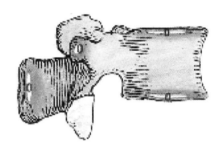

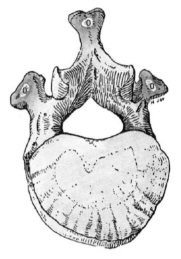

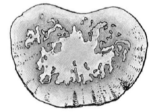

**Epiphyseal plate removed
from the vertebra above**

D

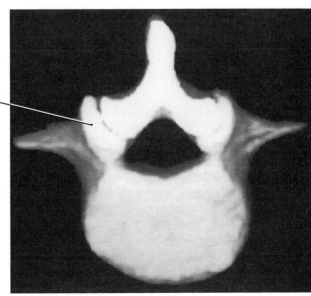

Superior articular process of vertebra below

E

| 4.3 | **Development of vertebrae** |

A. Vertebra at birth, superior view. At birth, a vertebra consists of three bony parts (two halves of the bony arch and the centrum) united by hyaline cartilage; **B.** Transverse CT scan. Note the three bony parts of a vertebra at birth and the contrast material around the spinal cord (*SC*), filling the dural sac; **C.** Fused vertebra, superior view. At age 2, the halves of each vertebral (neural) arch begin to fuse together from the lumbar to the cervical region; At approximately age 7, the arches begin to fuse to the centrum in sequence from the cervical to lumbar regions; **D.** Centers of ossification (top, lateral view; middle and bottom, inferior views). During puberty, secondary centers of ossification (*O*) appear at the tips of the spinous and transverse processes. Epiphyseal plates for the body consist of a plate of hyaline cartilage and a circumferential bony ring. **E.** Three-dimensional, computer-generated image of vertebra, inferior view. The secondary centers of ossification have fused in this 18 year old.

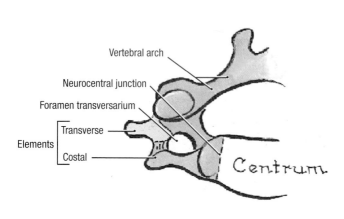

Cervical vertebra

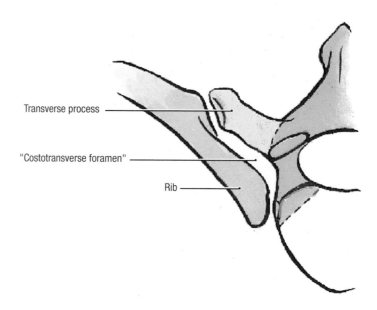

Thoracic vertebra

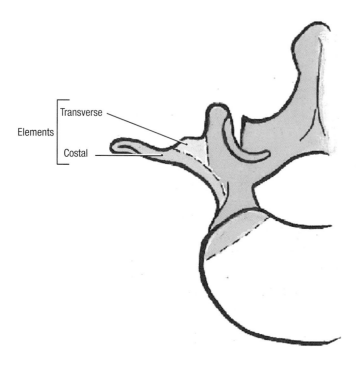

Lumbar vertebra

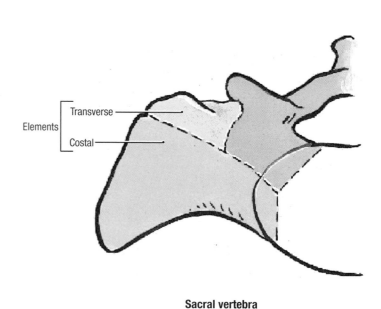

Sacral vertebra

4.4   Homologous parts of vertebrae, superior view

OBSERVE:

1. The centrum (uncolored), the vertebral arch (dark pink) and its process (pink), and the rib, or costal, element (yellow);
2. A rib, or costa, is a free element in the thoracic region; in the cervical and lumbar regions, it is represented by the anterior part of a transverse process, and in the sacrum, by the anterior part of the lateral mass;
3. The heads of the ribs (thoracic region) articulate with the sides of the vertebral bodies posterior to the neurocentral junctions, i.e., not with the centra, but with the neural arches.

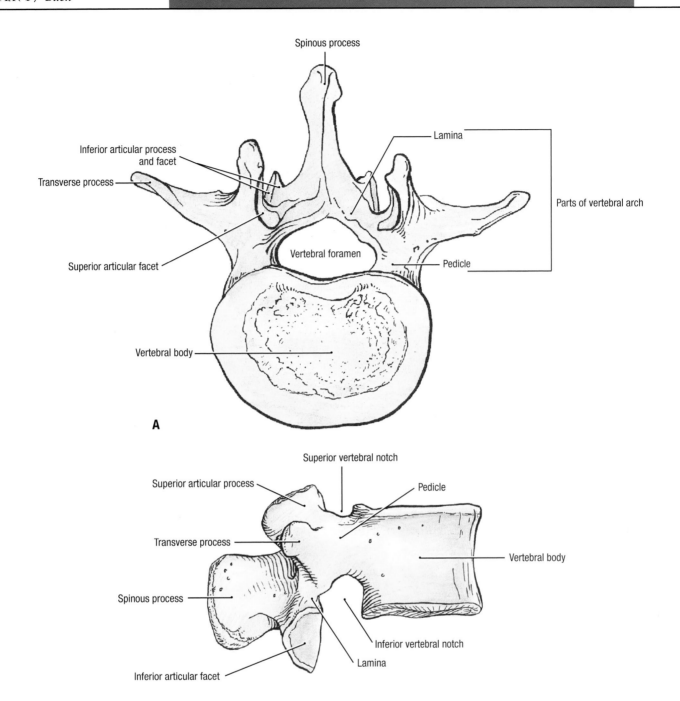

A. Superior view. **B.** Lateral view.

4.5 Typical vertebra

A. Superior view. **B.** Lateral view. A typical vertebra (2nd lumbar vertebra) comprises the following parts:

1. A vertebral body, situated anteriorly; its function is to support weight. Like other long bones, it is narrow about its middle and expanded at both ends; these ends are articular and have epiphyses during growth;

2. A vertebral arch, posterior to the body; with the body, this arch encloses the vertebral foramen. Collectively, the vertebral foramina constitute the vertebral canal, which houses the spinal cord. The function of a vertebral arch is to protect the cord; the vertebral arch consists of two stout, rounded pedicles, one on each side, that spring from the body and are united posteriorly by two flat plates, or laminae;

3. Three processes, two transverse and one spinous; they afford attachment to muscles and are the levers that help move the vertebrae;

4. Four articular processes, two superior and two inferior; each articular process has an articular facet. The articular processes project superiorly and inferiorly, respectively, from the vertebral arch and come into apposition with the articular facet of the corresponding processes of the vertebrae above and below; the direction of the articular facets determines the nature of the movement between adjacent vertebrae and prevents the vertebrae from slipping anteriorly.

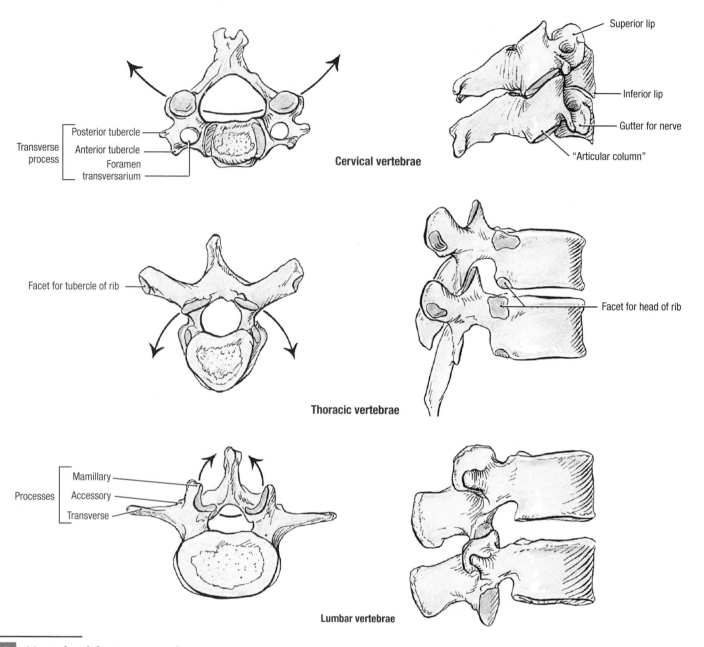

Cervical vertebrae

Transverse process
— Posterior tubercle
— Anterior tubercle
— Foramen transversarium

Superior lip
Inferior lip
Gutter for nerve
"Articular column"

Thoracic vertebrae

Facet for tubercle of rib

Facet for head of rib

Lumbar vertebrae

Processes
— Mamillary
— Accessory
— Transverse

4.6 Vertebral features and movements, superior (left) and lateral (right) views

OBSERVE:

1. The most distinctive feature of the cervical vertebrae is the presence of foramina transversaria, whereas all thoracic vertebrae have facets for articulation with the heads of ribs; the absence of these two features is distinctive of the large lumbar vertebrae;

2. The bodies of cervical and lumbar vertebrae are greater in the transverse diameter than in the anteroposterior, and the vertebral foramina are triangular; in thoracic vertebrae, the two diameters are approximately equal, and the foramina are circular. The superior surface of the body of a cervical vertebra ends at each side in an upturned, superior lip; hence, it is concave from side to side, and the inferior surface ends anteriorly in a downturned, inferior lip. The superior and inferior surfaces of thoracic and lumbar bodies are flat;

3. A transverse process in the cervical region points laterally, inferiorly, and anteriorly, ending in two tubercles with a gutter between them. In the thoracic region, it points laterally, posteriorly, and su-

periorly, has a facet for the tubercle of a rib, and is stout. In the lumbar region, it points laterally, and is long and slender;

4. Spinous processes are bifid in cervical, spine-like in thoracic, and oblong in lumbar vertebrae;

5. Articular processes in the cervical region collectively form a cylinder. In the thoracic and lumbar regions, the superior articular facets lie posterior to the pedicles and the inferior facets are anterior to the laminae; superior articular facets in the cervical region face mainly superiorly, in the thoracic region, mainly posteriorly, and in the lumbar region, mainly medially. The change in direction is gradual from cervical to thoracic, but abrupt from thoracic to lumbar;

6. Movements (indicated by arrows): In all three regions, the articular processes permit flexion, extension, and side-to-side movement; cervical vertebrae allow one to look sideways up, and thoracic vertebrae allow rotation, whereas lumbar vertebrae permit limited rotation.

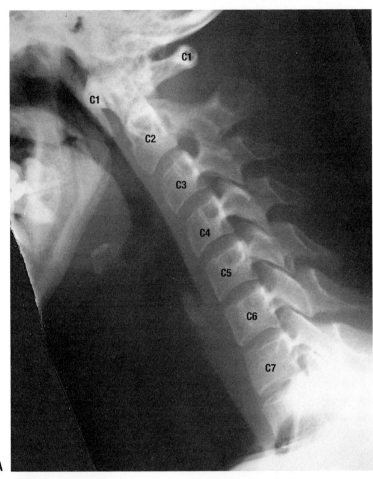

A

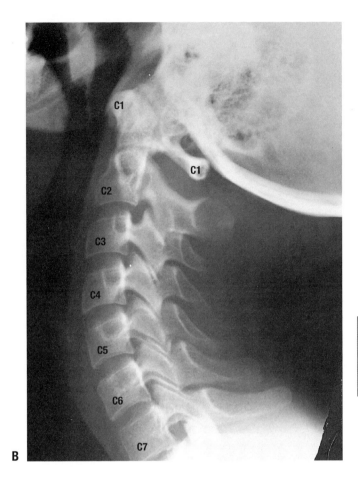

B

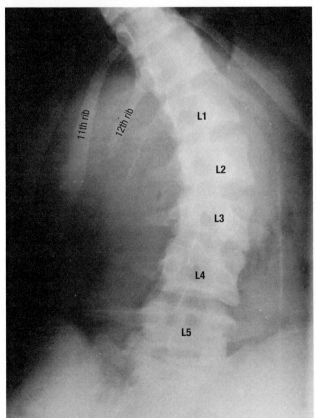

C

4.7　**Movements of vertebral column**

A. Lateral radiograph of the flexed cervical spine. **B.** Lateral radiograph of the extended cervical spine. **C.** Anteroposterior radiograph of the lumbar spine during lateral bending.

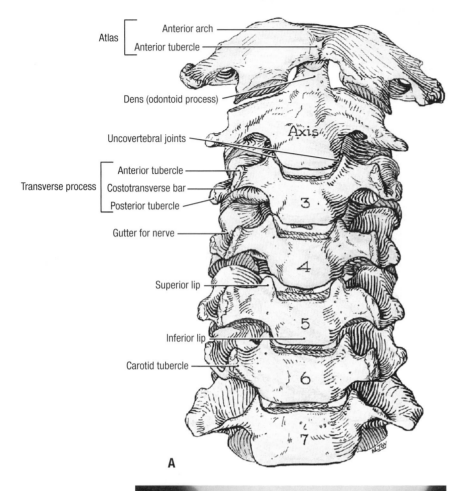

Atlas {
Anterior arch
Anterior tubercle

Dens (odontoid process)

Axis

Uncovertebral joints

Transverse process {
Anterior tubercle
Costotransverse bar
Posterior tubercle

3

Gutter for nerve

4

Superior lip

5

Inferior lip

Carotid tubercle

6

7

A

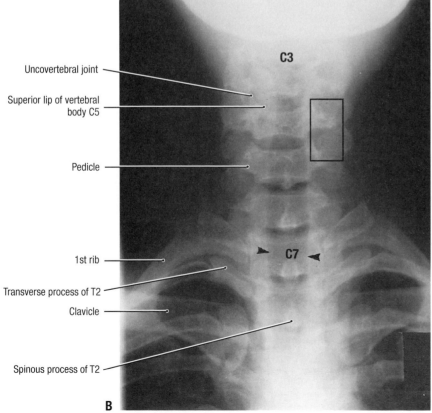

Uncovertebral joint

Superior lip of vertebral body C5

C3

Pedicle

C7

1st rib

Transverse process of T2

Clavicle

Spinous process of T2

B

4.8   Cervical spine

A. Articulated cervical vertebrae, anterior view. **B.** Radiograph, anteroposterior view. **C.** Articulated cervical vertebrae, lateral view. **D.** Radiograph, lateral view.

OBSERVE IN **A** AND **B:**
1. The superior surfaces of vertebral bodies C3 to C7 have lateral, upturned lips that articulate with the vertebrae above (joints of Luschka).
2. In **B,** the margins of the (black) column of air in the trachea (*arrowheads*);
3. In **B,** the laterally located column of articular processes and the overlapping transverse processes (boxed area).

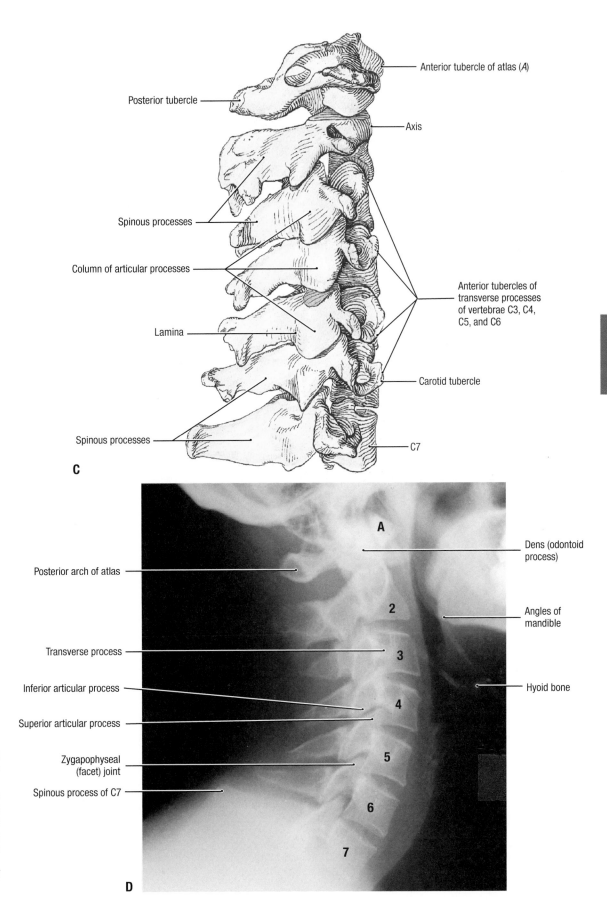

Anterior tubercle of atlas (*A*)

Posterior tubercle

Axis

Spinous processes

Column of articular processes

Anterior tubercles of transverse processes of vertebrae C3, C4, C5, and C6

Lamina

Carotid tubercle

Spinous processes

C7

C

Dens (odontoid process)

Posterior arch of atlas

A

2

Angles of mandible

Transverse process

3

Inferior articular process

4

Hyoid bone

Superior articular process

5

Zygapophyseal (facet) joint

Spinous process of C7

6

7

D

OBSERVE IN **C** AND **D**:

4. The bodies of the 2nd to 7th cervical vertebrae are numbered;

5. Anterior arch of the atlas (*A*) is in a plane anterior to the curved line joining the anterior borders of the vertebral bodies;

6. The spinous process of C7, the vertebra prominens;

7. The bifid spinous processes of cervical vertebrae.

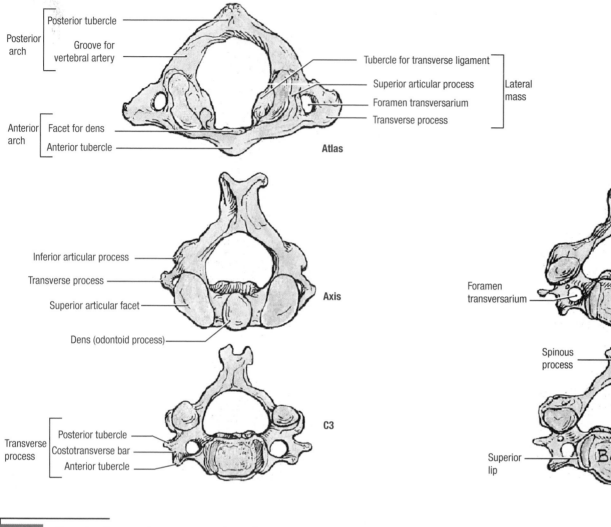

Atlas

Posterior arch
- Posterior tubercle
- Groove for vertebral artery

Tubercle for transverse ligament
Superior articular process
Foramen transversarium
Transverse process — Lateral mass

Anterior arch
- Facet for dens
- Anterior tubercle

Axis

Inferior articular process
Transverse process
Superior articular facet
Dens (odontoid process)

C3

Transverse process
- Posterior tubercle
- Costotransverse bar
- Anterior tubercle

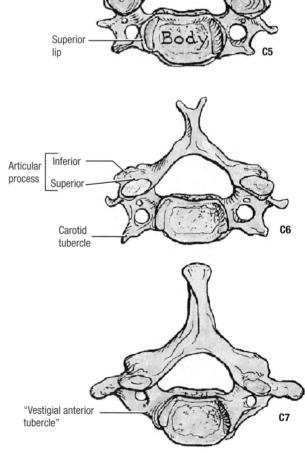

C4

Foramen transversarium

C5

Spinous process
Superior lip
Body

C6

Articular process
- Inferior
- Superior

Carotid tubercle

C7

"Vestigial anterior tubercle"

4.9   Cervical vertebrae, superior view

OBSERVE:
1. C3 through C6 are "typical" cervical vertebrae, and C1, C2, and C7 are "atypical";
2. The vertebral bodies of typical cervical vertebrae, transversely elongated, are of equal depth anteriorly and posteriorly; their superior surfaces with lateral lips, resembling seats with upturned side arms, bear facets that articulate with the vertebrae above at the uncovertebral joints. *Arthritic expansion of these joints encroach on the vertebral canal (spinal cord) and the foramen transversarium (vertebral artery)*;
3. The body of the atlas is missing: it is joined to the axis at the dens; the anterior arch on the atlas lies anterior to the dens and articulates with it;
4. The vertebral foramina are large and triangular;
5. The superior and inferior vertebral notches are nearly equal in depth;
6. The spinous processes are short and bifid, except that of the atlas, which is reduced to a tubercle, and that of C7 (vertebra prominens), which is long and nonbifid. The spinous process of the axis is massive;
7. The transverse processes are short, perforated, and end laterally in anterior and posterior tubercles with a gutter between them; those of the atlas and C7 are long and have one (posterior) tubercle, as does the axis, but it is short;

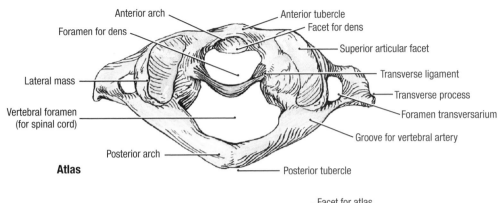

Anterior arch · Anterior tubercle · Foramen for dens · Facet for dens · Superior articular facet · Lateral mass · Transverse ligament · Transverse process · Vertebral foramen (for spinal cord) · Foramen transversarium · Groove for vertebral artery · Posterior arch · Posterior tubercle

Atlas

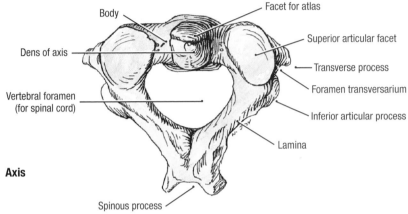

Body · Facet for atlas · Dens of axis · Superior articular facet · Transverse process · Foramen transversarium · Vertebral foramen (for spinal cord) · Inferior articular process · Lamina · Spinous process

Axis

4.10   Atlas and axis, superior views

OBSERVE:

1. The large vertebral foramen of the atlas is divided into two foramina by the transverse ligament; in the larger, posterior foramen, the spinal cord lies loosely, whereas in the smaller, anterior foramen, the dens of the axis fits tightly;

2. The dens of the axis articulates anteriorly with the anterior arch of the atlas and posteriorly with the transverse ligament, which forms an arc of a circle.

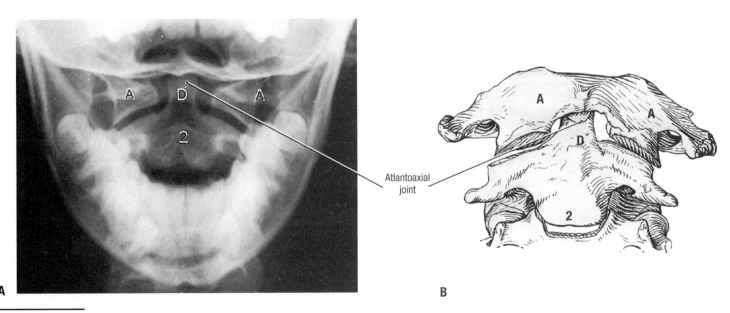

A

B

Atlantoaxial joint

4.11   Atlantoaxial joint

A. Anteroposterior radiograph, taken through the open mouth.
B. Articulated atlas and axis, anterior view.

OBSERVE:

1. The atlantoaxial joint consists of two lateral and one medial articulation;

2. The body of the axis (*2*), with the dens, or odontoid process (*D*), projecting superiorly between the lateral masses of the atlas (*A*) to articulate with the anterior arch of the atlas (medial articulation);

3. The synovial joint between the lateral masses of C1 and the superior articular facets of C2, forming the lateral articulations.

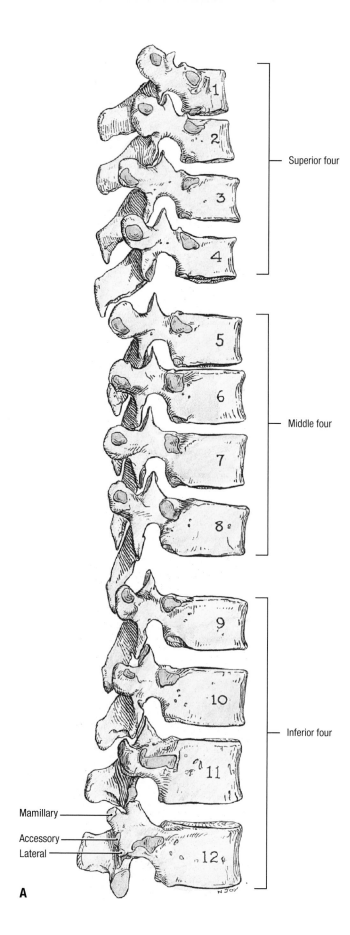

Superior four

Middle four

Inferior four

Mamillary
Accessory
Lateral

A

4.12 Thoracic vertebrae

A. Lateral view. **B.** Superior view.

OBSERVE:
1. The middle four vertebrae are typically thoracic; the superior four have some cervical features, and the inferior four have some lumbar features. The cervical features of T1 include the superior vertebral notches and the upturned, lateral lips on the body. The lumbar features of T12 include the lateral direction of the inferior articular processes and the mamillary, accessory, and lateral processes;
2. The body is deeper posteriorly than anteriorly, with flat superior and inferior surfaces; the surface area (weight-bearing surface) increases from T1 to T12. Note the triangular shape of the middle four, which have almost equal transverse and anteroposterior diameters; the transverse diameter increases toward the cervical and lumbar ends of the series;
3. There are two articular facets on each vertebral body, except T10, T11, and T12, which have one facet on the pedicle;
4. The vertebral foramina are circular and become triangular toward the cervical and lumbar ends;
5. The spinous processes of the middle four are long, overlapping, and nearly vertical; those of the 1st, 2nd, 11th, and 12th are nearly horizontal, and those of the 3rd, 4th, 9th, and 10th are oblique;
6. The length of the transverse processes diminishes progressively from T1 to T12; T1 to T10 have rib facets on their transverse processes that are concave and placed anteriorly on T1 to T7, and flat and superiorly placed on T8 to T10.

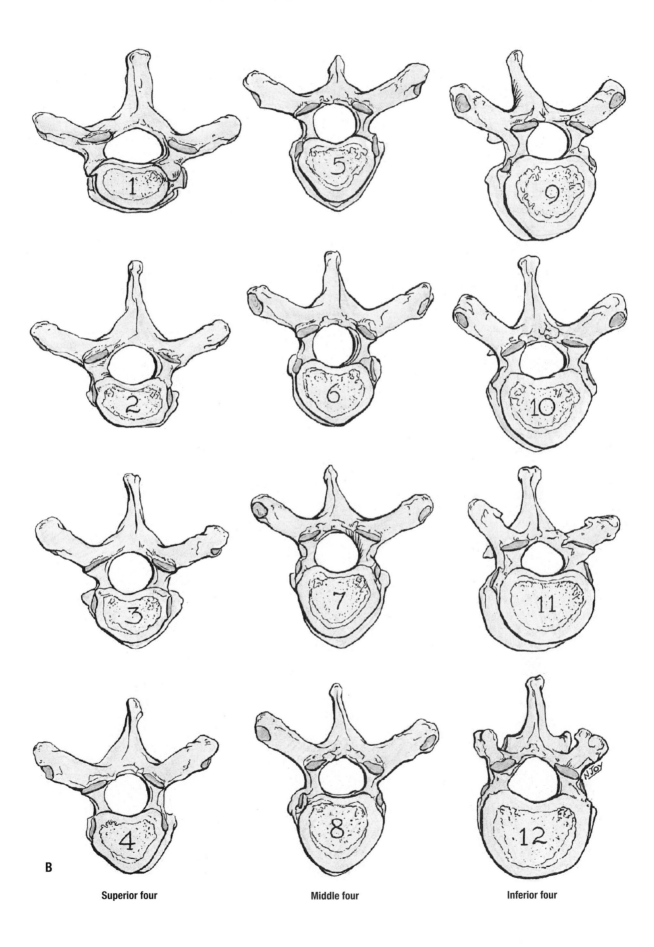

B

Superior four   Middle four   Inferior four

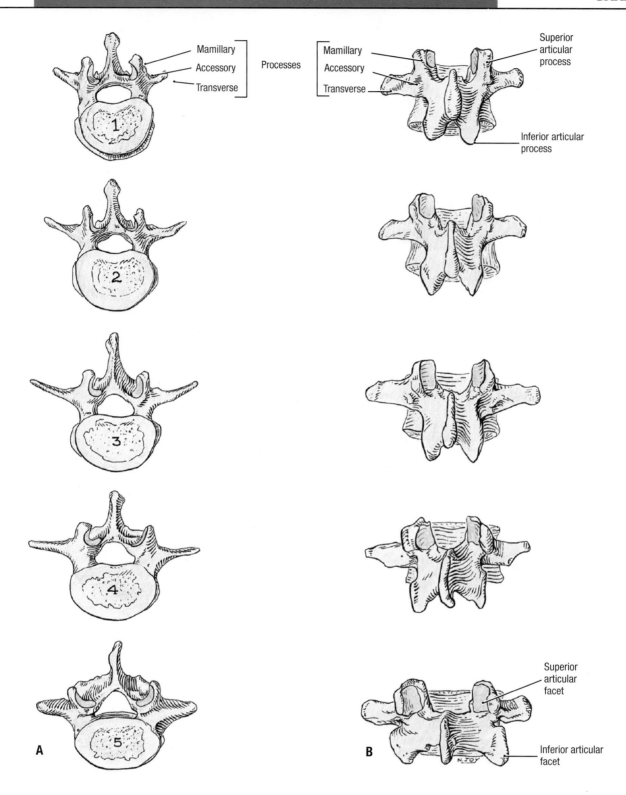

4.13   Lumbar vertebrae

A. Superior view. **B.** Posterior view. **C.** Lateral view. **D.** Radiograph, lateral view.

OBSERVE:
1. The kidney-shaped bodies are greater in transverse than in antero-posterior diameter; the bodies of L1 and L2 are deeper posteriorly, L4 and L5 are deeper anteriorly, and L3 is transitional;

2. The vertebral foramina are small and triangular, with "pinched" lateral angles in L5;
3. The slight, superior vertebral notches;
4. The large, oblong, horizontal spinous processes;
5. The long, slender, horizontal transverse processes. That of L3 projects farthest; that of L5 spreads anteriorly onto the body, is conical, and its apex has a superior tilt. Note the mamillary process (for the

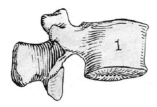

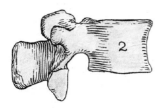

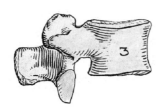

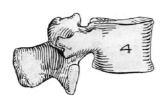

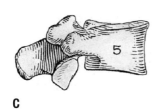

F	Zygopophyseal (facet joint)
DS	Intervertebral disc space
IA	Inferior anticular process
IV	Intervertebral foramen
P	Pedicle
PR	Sacral promentory
SA	Superior anticular process
SP	Spinous process
T12-L5 Vertebral bodies	

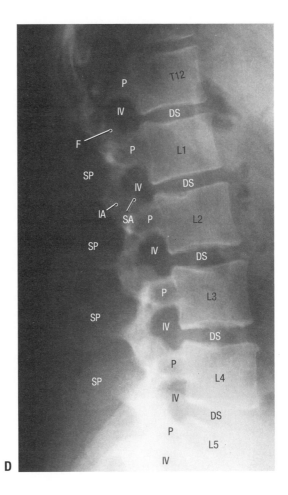

C

origin of the multifidus muscle) on the superior articular process and the accessory process (for insertion of the longissimus muscle) on the transverse process;

6. The superior articular processes face each other and grasp the inferior processes of the vertebra above;

7. The inferior articular processes are close together in L1, but far apart in L5 and face more anteriorly;

8. In D, the angulation at the lumbosacral junction produces the sacral promontory;

9. Intervertebral foramen is bounded superiorly and inferiorly by the pedicles, anteriorly by vertebral bodies and intervertebral disc, and posteriorly by the articular process.

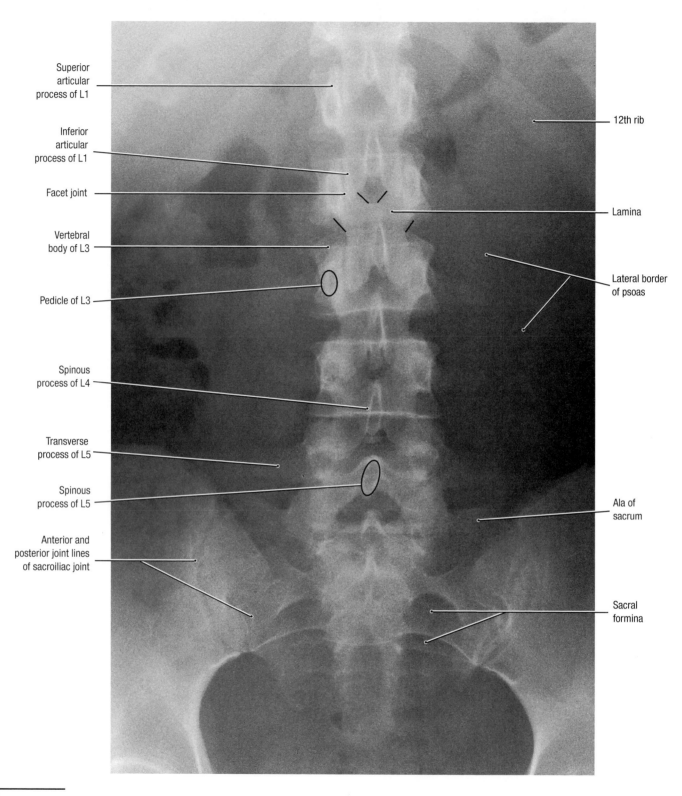

Superior articular process of L1

12th rib

Inferior articular process of L1

Facet joint

Lamina

Vertebral body of L3

Pedicle of L3

Lateral border of psoas

Spinous process of L4

Transverse process of L5

Spinous process of L5

Ala of sacrum

Anterior and posterior joint lines of sacroiliac joint

Sacral formina

4.14   Radiograph of inferior thoracic and lumbosacral spine, anteroposterior view

OBSERVE:
1. The articulation of the 12th rib with T12;
2. The bodies and processes of the five lumbar vertebrae; the spinous and transverse processes of L5 are labeled;
3. The sinuous sacroiliac joint;
4. The lateral margin of the right and left psoas major muscles.

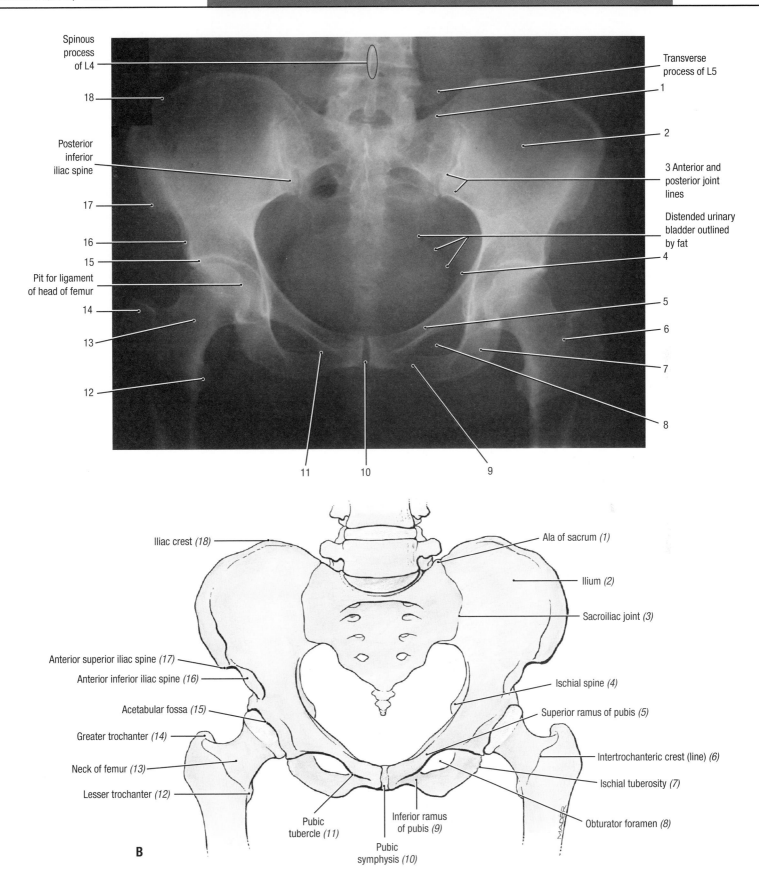

Spinous process of L4

Transverse process of L5

18

1

2

Posterior inferior iliac spine

3 Anterior and posterior joint lines

Distended urinary bladder outlined by fat

17

16

15

4

Pit for ligament of head of femur

14

5

13

6

12

7

8

11   10   9

Iliac crest *(18)*

Ala of sacrum *(1)*

Ilium *(2)*

Sacroiliac joint *(3)*

Anterior superior iliac spine *(17)*

Anterior inferior iliac spine *(16)*

Ischial spine *(4)*

Acetabular fossa *(15)*

Superior ramus of pubis *(5)*

Greater trochanter *(14)*

Intertrochanteric crest (line) *(6)*

Neck of femur *(13)*

Ischial tuberosity *(7)*

Lesser trochanter *(12)*

Obturator foramen *(8)*

Pubic tubercle *(11)*

Inferior ramus of pubis *(9)*

Pubic symphysis *(10)*

B

4.15 **Pelvis, anterior views**

A. Radiograph of pelvis. **B.** Bony pelvis with articulated femora.

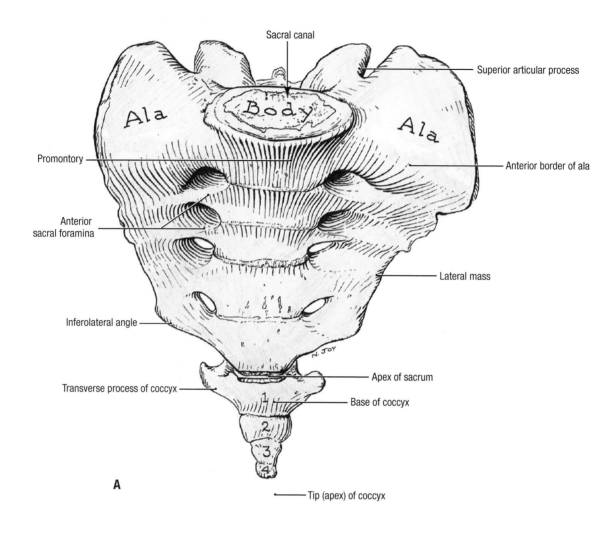

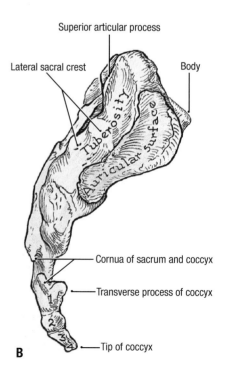

4.16 Sacrum and coccyx

A. Anterior view. **B.** Lateral view. **C.** Posterior view. **D.** Sacrum in youth, anterior view.

OBSERVE IN **A:**

1. The five sacral bodies are demarcated by four transverse lines that end laterally in four pairs of anterior sacral foramina;
2. The foramina of the two sides are approximately equidistant throughout; their margins are rounded laterally, but sharp elsewhere, indicating the courses of the emerging nerves;
3. The coccyx has four pieces; the first has a pair of transverse processes and a pair of cornua; the other three pieces are nodular.

OBSERVE IN **B:**

4. Anterosuperiorly, the auricular, ear-shaped surface articulates with the ilium of the hip bone (os coxae);
5. Posterosuperiorly, note the sacral tuberosity for the attachment of the dorsal sacroiliac and interosseous sacroiliac ligaments;
6. Inferiorly, the apex of the sacrum articulates with the coccyx, which is concave anteriorly.

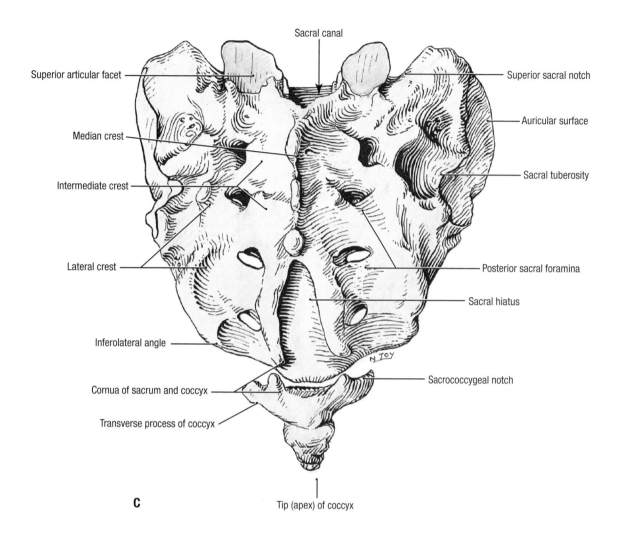

Sacral canal

Superior articular facet

Median crest

Intermediate crest

Lateral crest

Inferolateral angle

Cornua of sacrum and coccyx

Transverse process of coccyx

Superior sacral notch

Auricular surface

Sacral tuberosity

Posterior sacral foramina

Sacral hiatus

Sacrococcygeal notch

C

Tip (apex) of coccyx

OBSERVE IN **C:**

7. The absence of the 4th and 5th sacral spines and laminae;
8. The superior articular processes, intermediate crest, and sacral and coccygeal cornua are serially homologous; likewise are the superior sacral notch, four dorsal sacral foramina, and sacrococcygeal notch;
9. A straight probe could be passed through a lower posterior sacral foramen, across the sacral canal, and through an anterior sacral foramen.

OBSERVE IN **D:**

10. The costal elements begin to fuse with each other at about the time of puberty. The bodies begin to fuse from inferior to superior at approximately the 17th to 18th year, with fusion completed by the 23rd year. A gap may persist between the 2nd and 3rd bodies until the 24th year, and between the 1st and 2nd bodies until the 33rd year.

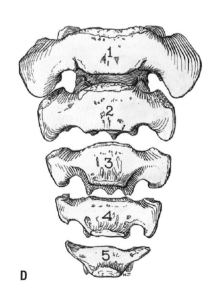

D

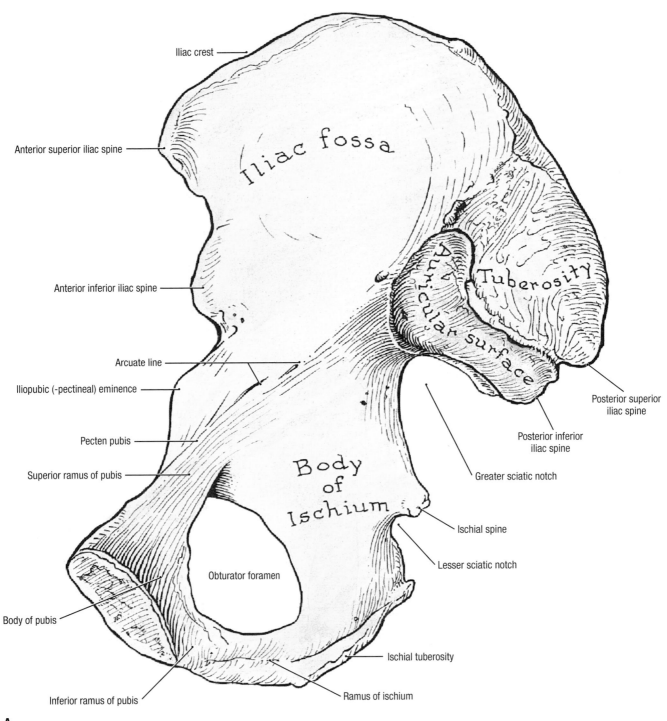

Iliac crest

Iliac fossa

Anterior superior iliac spine

Anterior inferior iliac spine

Tuberosity

Auricular surface

Arcuate line

Iliopubic (-pectineal) eminence

Posterior superior
iliac spine

Pecten pubis

Posterior inferior
iliac spine

Superior ramus of pubis

Greater sciatic notch

Body
of
Ischium

Ischial spine

Lesser sciatic notch

Obturator foramen

Body of pubis

Ischial tuberosity

Inferior ramus of pubis

Ramus of ischium

A

4.17 Hip bone (os coxae)

A. Medial view. **B.** Lateral view.

OBSERVE:

1. Each hip bone consists of three bones: ilium, ischium, and pubis;
2. The ilium is the superior, larger part of the hip bone, forming the superior part of the acetabulum; the deep socket on the lateral aspect of the hip bone articulates with the head of the femur;

3. The ischium forms the posteroinferior part of the acetabulum and hip bone.
4. The pubis forms the anterior part of the acetabulum and anteromedial part of the hip bone;
5. In anatomic position, the anterior superior iliac spine and pubic tu-

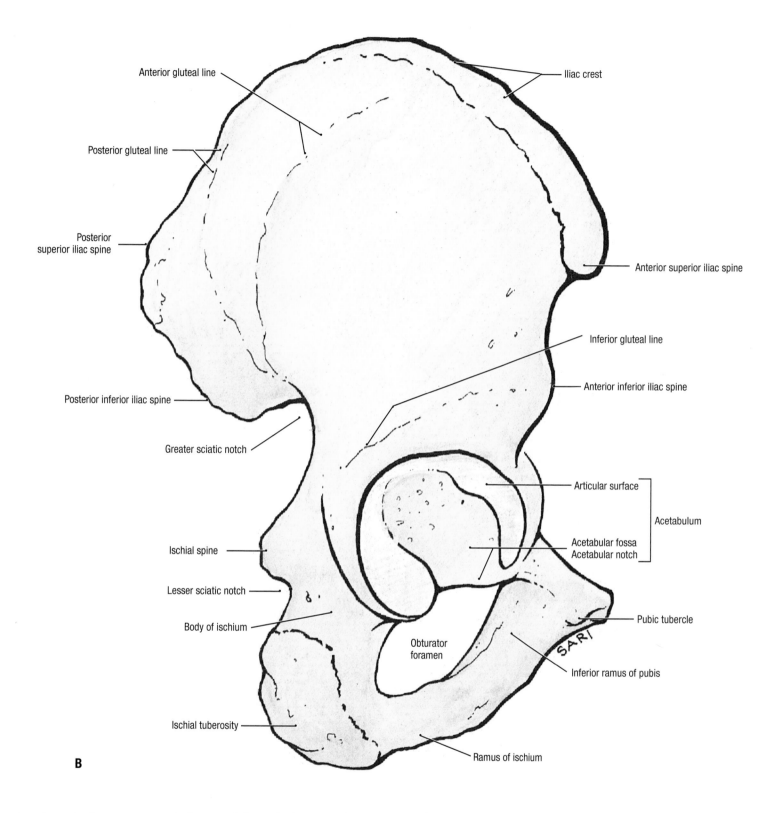

Anterior gluteal line

Posterior gluteal line

Posterior superior iliac spine

Posterior inferior iliac spine

Greater sciatic notch

Ischial spine

Lesser sciatic notch

Body of ischium

Ischial tuberosity

Iliac crest

Anterior superior iliac spine

Inferior gluteal line

Anterior inferior iliac spine

Articular surface

Acetabulum

Acetabular fossa
Acetabular notch

Pubic tubercle

Obturator foramen

Inferior ramus of pubis

Ramus of ischium

SARI

B

bercle are in the same coronal plane, and the ischial spine and superior end of the pubic symphysis are in the same horizontal plane;

6. The internal aspect of the body of the pubis faces superiorly, and the acetabulum faces inferolaterally;
7. The obturator foramen lies inferomedial to the acetabulum.

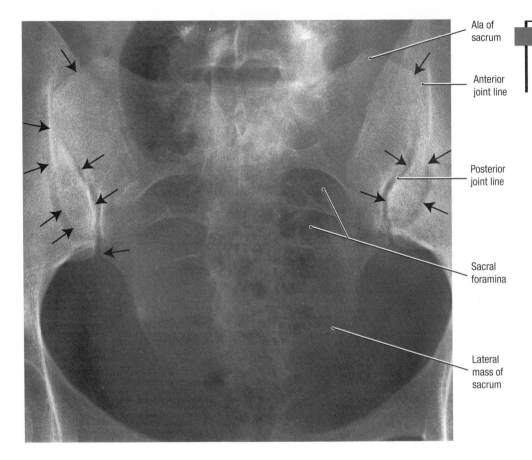

Ala of sacrum

Anterior joint line

Posterior joint line

Sacral foramina

Lateral mass of sacrum

4.18 Imaging of the sacroiliac joint

A. Radiograph, anteroposterior view. **B.** CT (computed tomographic) scan, axial (transverse) plane. The sacroiliac joint is indicated by arrows. Note that the articular surfaces of the ilium and sacrum have irregular shapes which result in partial interlocking of the bones. The sacroiliac joint is oblique with the anterior aspect of the joint situated lateral to the posterior aspect of the joint.

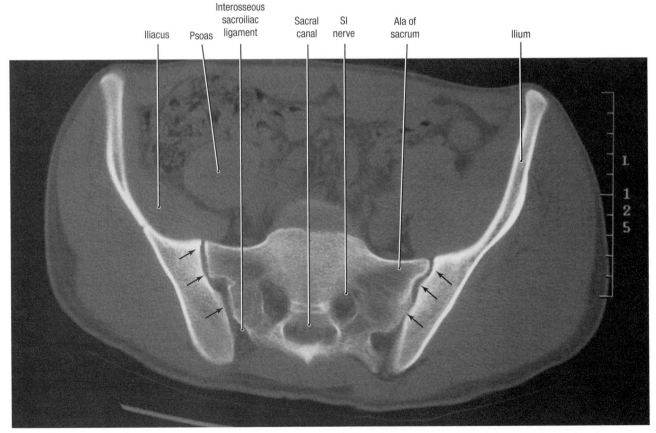

Iliacus Psoas Interosseous sacroiliac ligament Sacral canal SI nerve Ala of sacrum Ilium

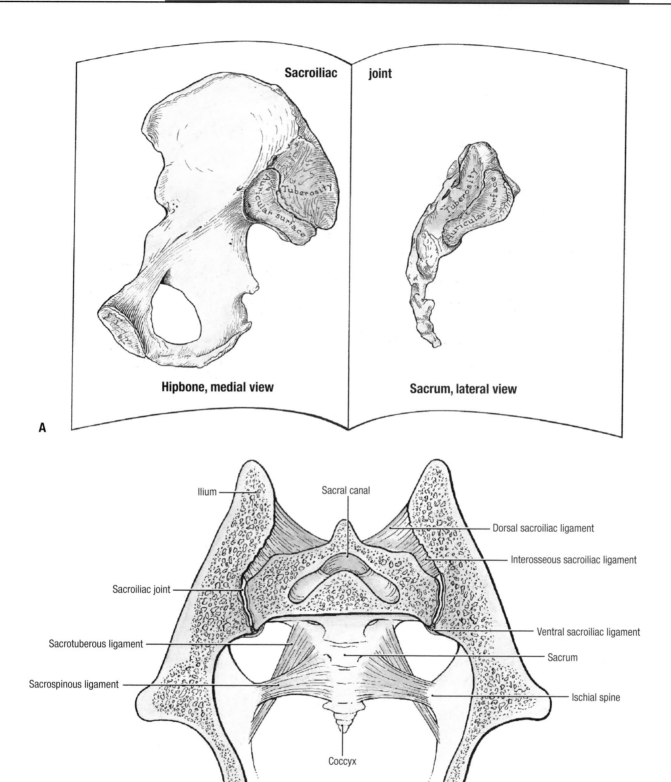

Sacroiliac   joint

Hipbone, medial view   Sacrum, lateral view

A

Ilium

Sacral canal

Dorsal sacroiliac ligament

Interosseous sacroiliac ligament

Sacroiliac joint

Ventral sacroiliac ligament

Sacrotuberous ligament

Sacrum

Sacrospinous ligament

Ischial spine

Coccyx

B

4.19 **Ligaments and articular surfaces of sacroiliac joint**

A. Articular surfaces, medial and lateral views. **B.** Coronal section. Note the transversely oriented sacroiliac joints and the strong interosseous sacroiliac ligament that lies anterior to the dorsal sacroiliac ligament and consists of short fibers connecting the sacral tuberosity to the ilium.

OBSERVE IN **A**:
1. The auricular surface (articular area, in blue) of the sacrum and hip bone;
2. The roughened areas superior and posterior to the auricular areas (orange) for the attachment of the interosseous sacroiliac ligament.

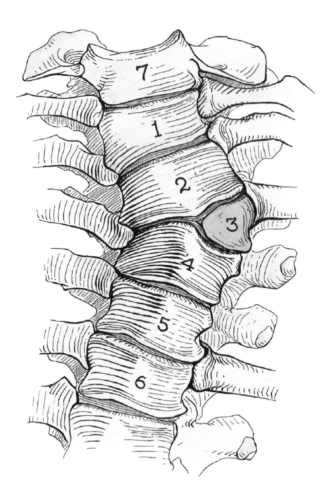

A

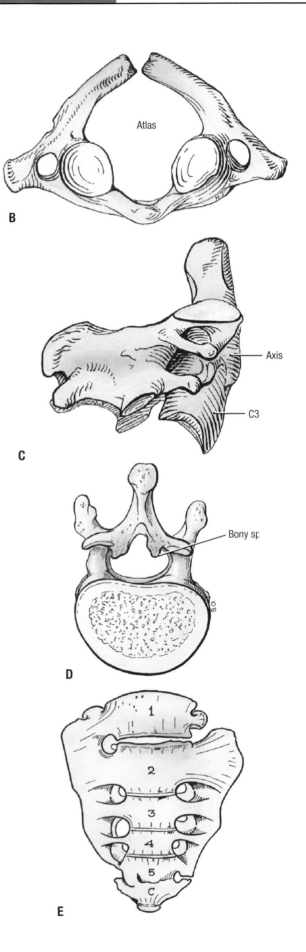

B

C

D

E

4.20   Anomalies of the vertebrae

A. Hemivertebra, anterior view. The entire right half of T3 and the corresponding rib are absent. The left lamina and the spine are fused with those of T4, and the left intervertebral foramen is reduced in size. *Observe the associated scoliosis (lateral curvature of the spine).* **B.** Unfused posterior arch of the atlas, inferior view. The centrum has fused to the right and left halves of the vertebral arch, but the arch has not fused in the midline posteriorly. **C.** Synostosis (fusion) of vertebrae C2 (axis) and C3, lateral view. **D.** Ossifying ligamenta flava, superior view. *Sharp, bony spurs commonly grow from the laminae inferiorly into the ligamenta flava, thereby reducing the lengths of these elastic bands. Hence, when the vertebral column is flexed, they are likely to be torn. Restricted to the thoracic and lumbar regions, and most common and largest on T11, they diminish in size and frequency cranially to T1 and caudally to L5.* **E.** Transitional lumbosacral vertebra, anterior view. Here, the 1st sacral vertebra is partly free (lumbarized). Not uncommonly, the 5th lumbar vertebra is partly fused to the sacrum (sacralized).

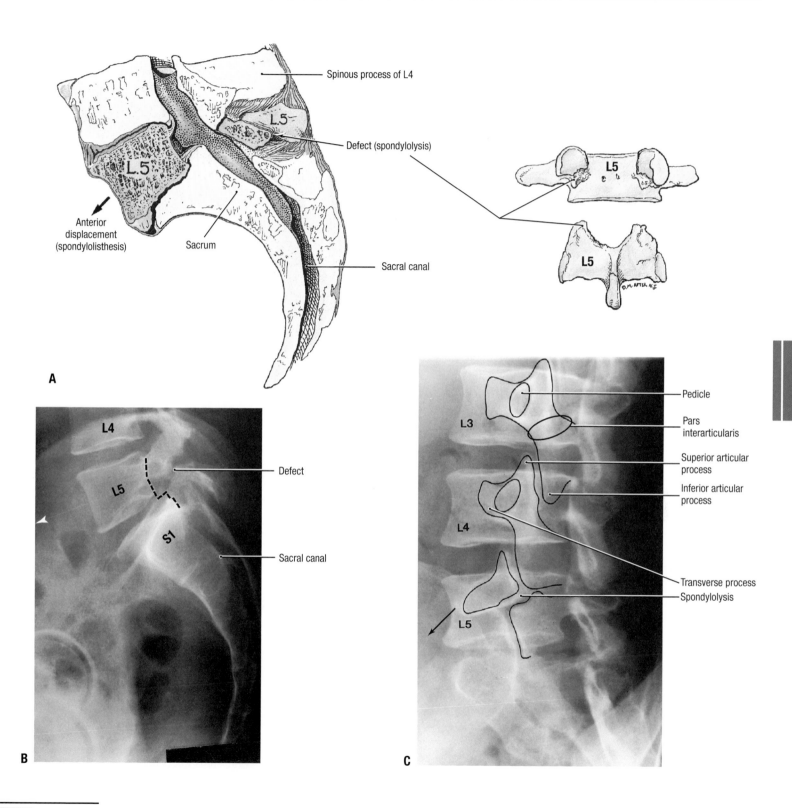

A. Sagittal section (left) and posterior view (right).

Spinous process of L4

Defect (spondylolysis)

Anterior displacement (spondylolisthesis)

Sacrum

Sacral canal

L5

D.M. AFTER N.J.

B.

L4

L5

Defect

S1

Sacral canal

C.

L3

L4

L5

Pedicle

Pars interarticularis

Superior articular process

Inferior articular process

Transverse process

Spondylolysis

4.21   Spondylolysis and Spondylolisthesis

A. Sagittal section (left) and posterior view (*right*). *L5 vertebra has an oblique defect, spondylolysis, through the pars interarticularis. The defect may be traumatic or congenital in origin. The pars interarticularis is the region of the lamina of a lumbar vertebra that is located between the superior and inferior articular processes. Also, the vertebral body of L5 has slipped anteriorly (spondylolisthesis).* **B.** Lateral radiograph. The *dotted line* follow-

ing the posterior vertebral margins of L5 and the sacrum shows the anterior displacement of L5 (*arrow*). **C.** Oblique radiograph. Note the superimposed outline of a dog: the head is the transverse process, the eye is the pedicle, and the ear is the superior articular process. *The lucent cleft across the "neck" of the dog is the spondylolysis, the anterior displacement (arrow) is the spondylolisthesis.*

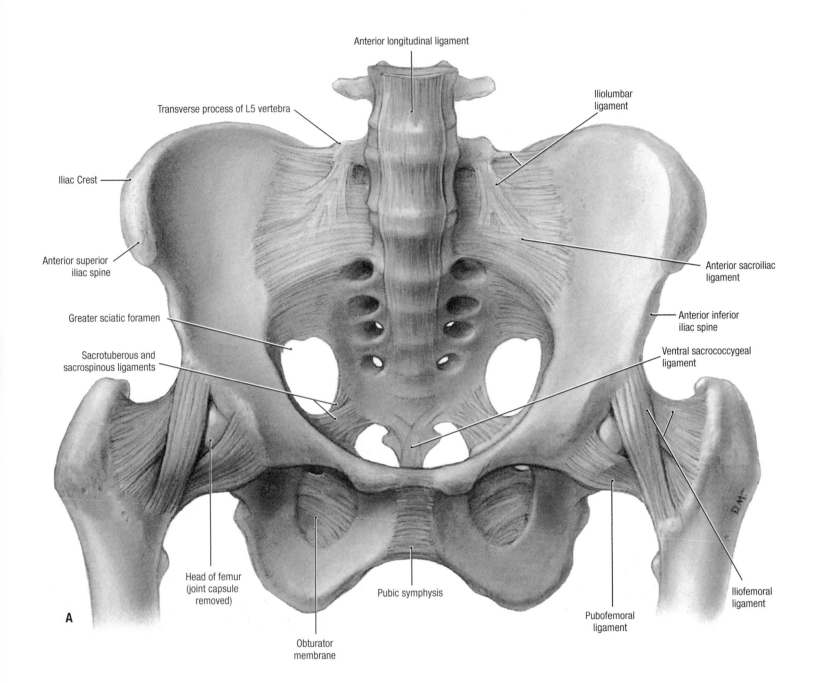

Anterior longitudinal ligament

Transverse process of L5 vertebra

Iliolumbar ligament

Iliac Crest

Anterior superior iliac spine

Anterior sacroiliac ligament

Greater sciatic foramen

Anterior inferior iliac spine

Sacrotuberous and sacrospinous ligaments

Ventral sacrococcygeal ligament

Head of femur (joint capsule removed)

Pubic symphysis

Iliofemoral ligament

Pubofemoral ligament

A

Obturator membrane

4.22 Lumbar and pelvic ligaments

A. Anterior view. **B.** Posterior view.

OBSERVE:
1. The iliolumbar ligaments unite the ilia and transverse processes of L5; the lumbosacral portion of the ligaments descends to the alae of the sacrum and blends with the anterior sacroiliac ligaments;
2. The sacrococcygeal ligaments correspond to the anterior and posterior longitudinal ligaments of the other intervertebral joints;

3. Note the posterior sacroiliac ligaments between the sacrum and tuberosity of the ilium; short fibers pass between the first and second transverse tubercles of the sacrum and the iliac tuberosity, and long fibers pass between the posterior superior iliac spine and third and fourth transverse tubercles of the sacrum;
4. The anterior sacroiliac ligaments unite the anterior aspect of the joint;
5. The sacrotuberous ligaments attach the sacrum, ilium, and coccyx

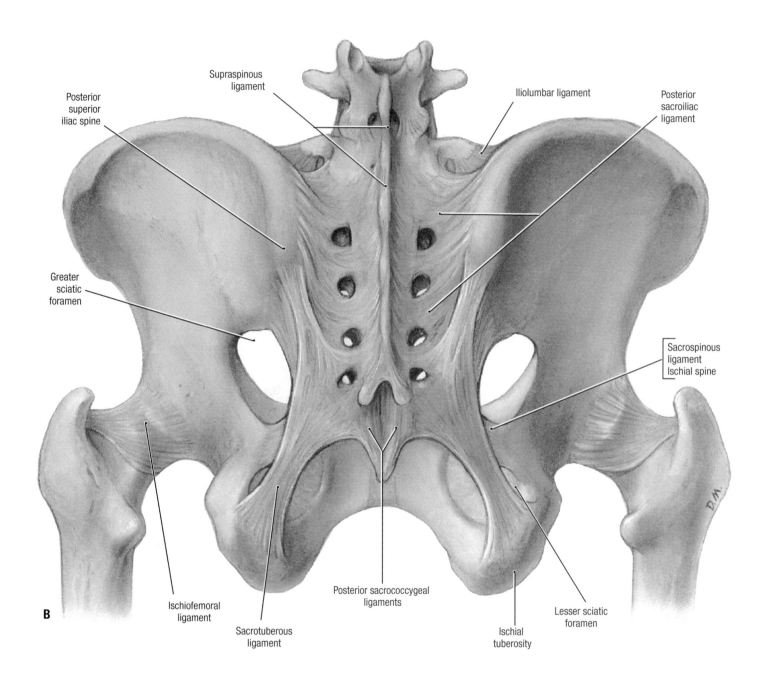

Supraspinous ligament

Posterior superior iliac spine

Iliolumbar ligament

Posterior sacroiliac ligament

Greater sciatic foramen

Sacrospinous ligament
Ischial spine

B

Ischiofemoral ligament

Sacrotuberous ligament

Posterior sacrococcygeal ligaments

Ischial tuberosity

Lesser sciatic foramen

to the ischial tuberosity; the sacrospinous ligaments unite the sacrum and coccyx to the ischial spine. The sacrotuberous and sacrospinous ligaments convert the sciatic notches of the hip bones into greater and lesser sciatic foramina.

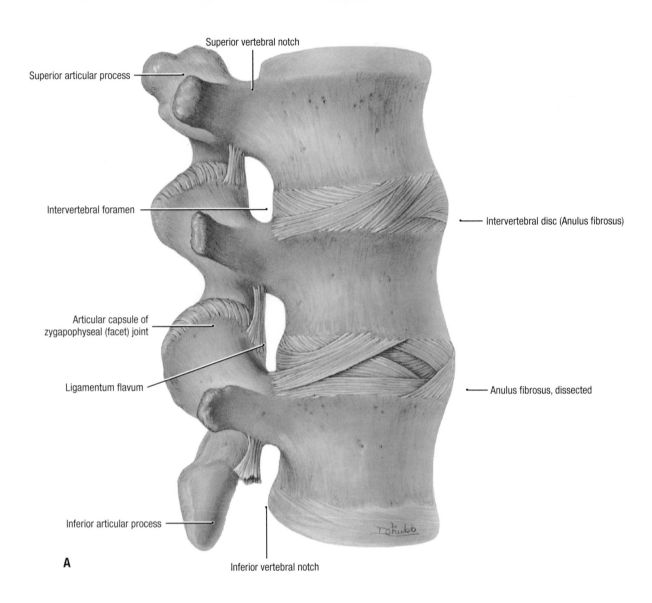

Superior vertebral notch

Superior articular process

Intervertebral foramen

Intervertebral disc (Anulus fibrosus)

Articular capsule of
zygapophyseal (facet) joint

Ligamentum flavum

Anulus fibrosus, dissected

Inferior articular process

A

Inferior vertebral notch

4.23 Intervertebral disc

A. Lateral view. Sections have been removed from the superficial layers of the inferior disc to show the direction of the fibers. **B.** Schematic of intervertebral disc, anterior view.

OBSERVE:
1. The anulus fibrosus is arranged in layers of parallel fibers that crisscross those of the next layer;
2. An intervertebral foramen, resulting from the apposition of a superior and inferior vertebral notch, is bounded superiorly and inferiorly by pedicles, anteriorly by an intervertebral disc and parts of the two bodies united by that disc, and posteriorly by a capsular ligament and parts of the two articular processes united by that capsular ligament. The anterior part of the capsule is strengthened by the lateral border of the ligamentum flavum;
3. In B, note that the center of the disc is filled with fibrogelatinous pulp, the nucleus pulposus, which acts as a shock absorber. *As a result of aging, the nucleus pulposus becomes increasingly fibrocartilaginous and contains less water.*

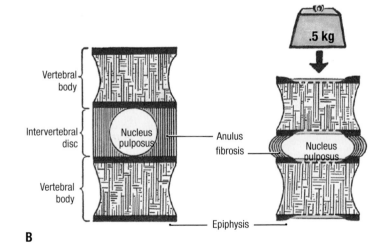

.5 kg

Vertebral
body

Intervertebral
disc

Nucleus
pulposus

Anulus
fibrosis

Vertebral
body

Nucleus
pulposus

Epiphysis

B

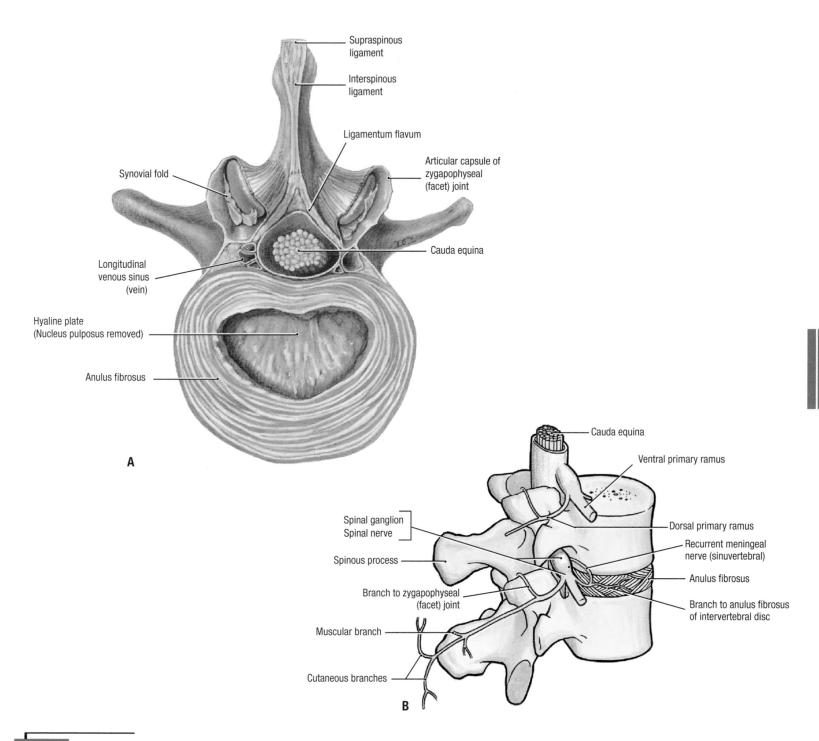

4.24   Intervertebral disc and ligaments

A. Transverse section, superior view. The nucleus pulposus has been removed, and the cartilaginous epiphyseal plate exposed. **B.** Innervation of vertebral joint and intervertebral disc, posterolateral view.

OBSERVE IN **A:**
1. The rings of the anulus fibrosus are fewer posteriorly;
2. The continuity of the following ligaments: flavum, interspinous, and supraspinous, and the articular capsule of the zygapophyseal (facet) joint;
3. The synovial fold contains a pad of fat;
4. The longitudinal vertebral venous sinuses (veins) extend extradurally throughout the length of the vertebral canal (Figure 4.27).

5. The cauda equina of the spinal cord lies free within the subarachnoid space.

OBSERVE IN **B:**
6. The sensory innervation of the zygapophyseal (facet) joint is from a medial branch of the dorsal primary ramus;
7. The outer third of the anulus fibrosus has sensory and vasomotor innervation; the posterolateral aspect of the anulus is innervated by branches from the ventral primary ramus, and the posterior aspect by the recurrent meningeal nerves.

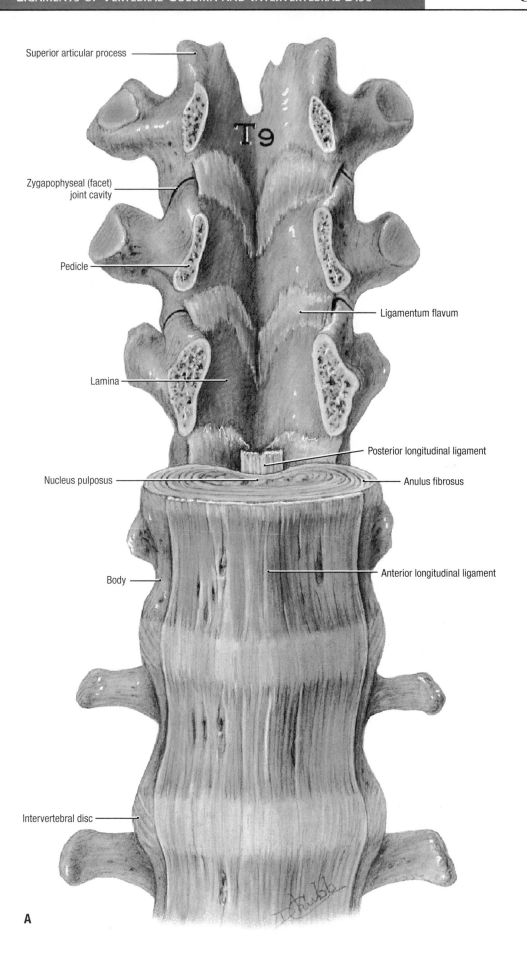

Superior articular process

Zygapophyseal (facet) joint cavity

Pedicle

Ligamentum flavum

Lamina

Posterior longitudinal ligament

Nucleus pulposus

Anulus fibrosus

Body

Anterior longitudinal ligament

Intervertebral disc

T9

A

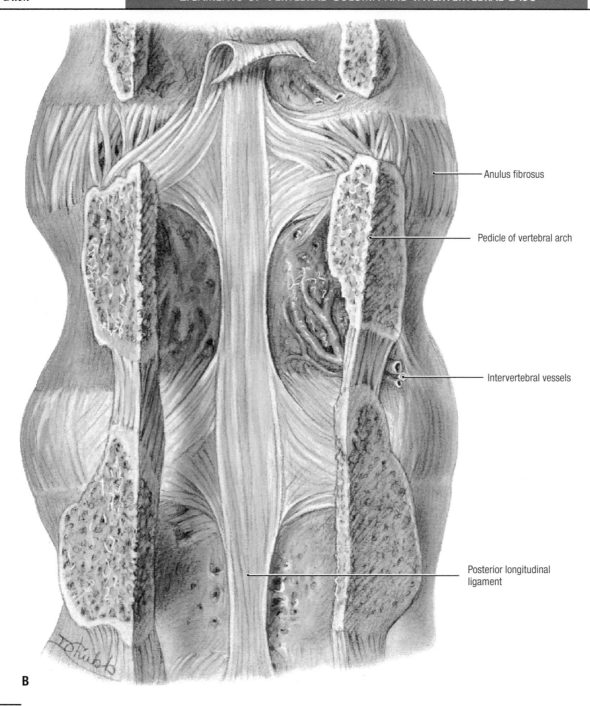

Anulus fibrosus

Pedicle of vertebral arch

Intervertebral vessels

Posterior longitudinal
ligament

B

4.25   Anterior and posterior longitudinal ligaments

A. Anterior longitudinal ligament and ligamenta flava, anterior view. The pedicles of T9 to T11 were sawed through, and their bodies are shown in **B. B.** Posterior longitudinal ligament, posterior view.

OBSERVE IN **A:**
1. The anterior and posterior longitudinal ligaments are ligaments of the bodies; the ligamenta flava are ligaments of the vertebral arches;
2. The anterior longitudinal ligament consists of broad, strong, fibrous bands that are attached to the intervertebral discs and vertebral bodies anteriorly; they have foramina for arteries and veins passing to and from the vertebral bodies;
3. The ligamenta flava, composed of elastic fibers, extend between adjacent laminae; those of opposite sides meet and blend in the median plane. They extend laterally to the articular processes, where they blend with the capsule of the zygapophyseal joint. Cranially,

they are in series with the posterior atlantoaxial and posterior atlanto-occipital membranes.

OBSERVE IN **B:**
4. The posterior longitudinal ligament, a taut, but somewhat flimsy, band passing from disc to disc, spans the posterior surfaces of the vertebral bodies and renders smooth the anterior wall of the vertebral canal;
5. The diamond shape of the ligament posterior to each disc, where it gives and receives fibers;
6. The ligament extends to the sacrum inferiorly and becomes the strong tectorial membrane cranially;
7. The intervertebral veins drain blood from the venous plexuses of the spinal canal; they drain into the vertebral, intercostal, lumbar, or lateral sacral veins (See Fig. 4.27).

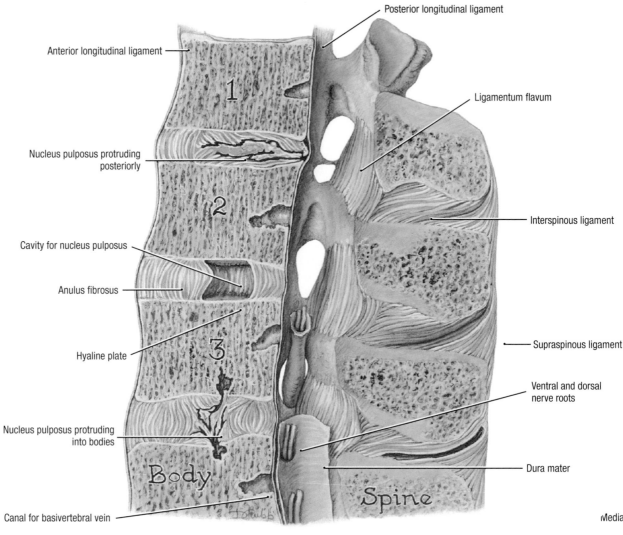

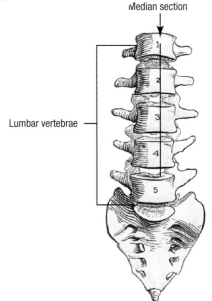

4.26 Lumbar region of vertebral column, median section

OBSERVE:

1. The nucleus pulposus of the normal disc between L2 and L3 has been removed from the enclosing anulus fibrosus;
2. The ligamentum flavum extends from the superior border and adjacent part of the posterior aspect of one lamina to the inferior border and adjacent part of the anterior aspect of the lamina above, and extends laterally to the intervertebral foramen;
3. The interspinous ligament unites obliquely the superior and inferior borders of two adjacent spines; elastic fibers are sparse;
4. The supraspinous ligament extends as far inferiorly as L4 or L5;
5. The bursa between L3 and L4 spines is presumably the result of habitual hyperextension, which brings the lumbar spines into contact;
6. *Two degenerative changes: (a) The pulp of the disc between L1 and L2 has herniated posteriorly through the anulus; spinal nerves are vulnerable to the pressure of an extruded nucleus pulposus through a torn anulus fibrosus (the most common site of a disc lesion is between L5 and S1), and (b) the pulp of the disc between L3 and L4 has herniated through the cartilaginous epiphyseal plates into the bodies of the vertebrae superiorly and inferiorly.*

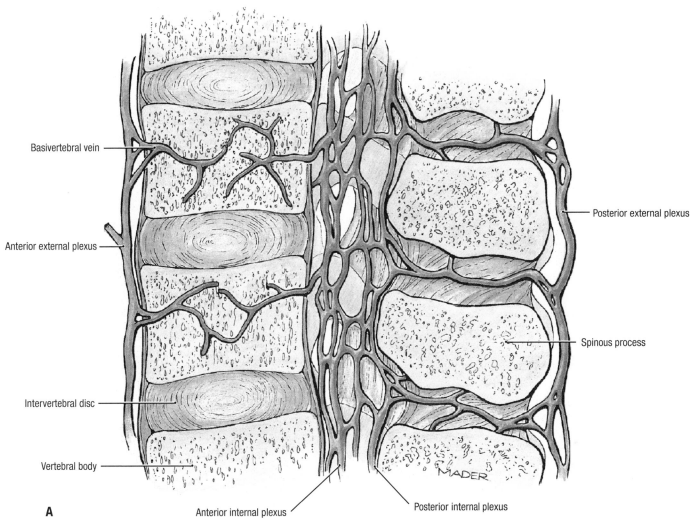

Basivertebral vein

Anterior external plexus

Intervertebral disc

Vertebral body

Posterior external plexus

Spinous process

Posterior internal plexus

A

Anterior internal plexus

4.27   **Vertebral venous plexuses**

A. Median section of lumbar spine. **B.** Superior view of lumbar vertebra with the vertebral body sectioned transversely.

OBSERVE:

1. There are internal and external plexuses, communicating with each other and with both segmental systemic veins and the portal system. *Infection and tumors can spread from the systemic and portal areas (e.g., prostate, breast) to the vertebral venous system and lodge in the vertebrae, spinal cord, brain, or skull;*

2. The internal plexus: The vertebral canal contains a plexus of thin-walled, valveless veins that surround the dura mater of the spinal cord and the posterior longitudinal ligament like a basket. Anterior and posterior longitudinal channels (venous sinuses) can be discerned in this plexus. Cranially, the internal plexus communicates through the foramen magnum with the occipital and basilar sinuses; at each spinal segment, the plexus receives veins from the spinal cord and a basivertebral vein from the vertebral body. The plexus is drained by intervertebral veins that pass through the intervertebral and sacral foramina to the vertebral, intercostal, lumbar, and lateral sacral veins;

3. The external plexus: Through the body of each vertebra come veins that form a small anterior external vertebral plexus, and through the ligamenta flava pass veins that form a well-marked posterior external vertebral plexus. In the cervical region, these plexuses communicate freely with the occipital and deep cervical veins,

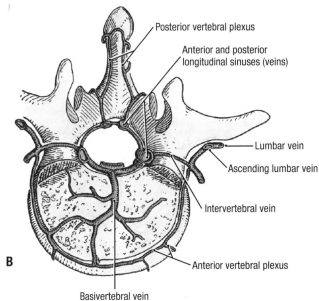

Posterior vertebral plexus

Anterior and posterior longitudinal sinuses (veins)

Lumbar vein

Ascending lumbar vein

Intervertebral vein

B

Anterior vertebral plexus

Basivertebral vein

which receive blood from the sigmoid sinus and mastoid and condyloid emissary veins. In the thoracic, lumbar, and pelvic regions, the azygos (or hemiazygos), ascending lumbar, and lateral sacral veins, respectively, further link segment to segment.

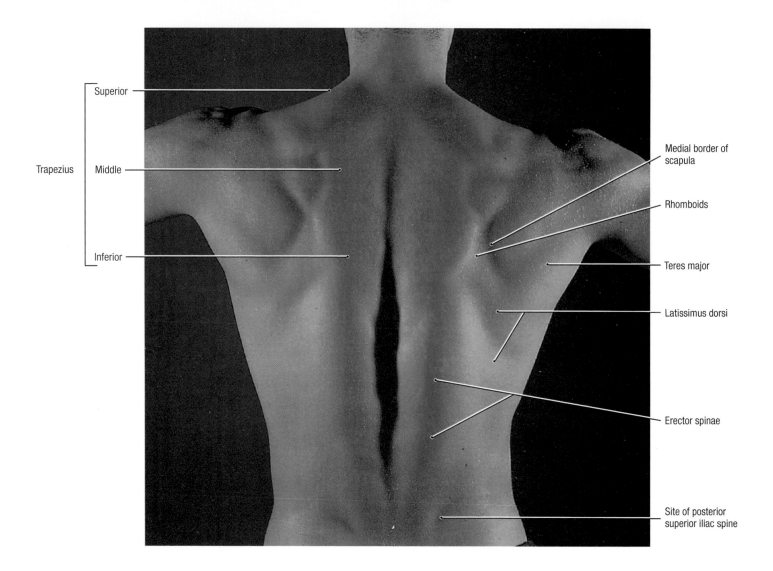

4.28   **Surface anatomy of back, posterior view**

OBSERVE:

1. The upper limbs are elevated, so the scapulae have moved laterally on the thoracic wall, enabling visualization of the rhomboid muscles;
2. The superior, middle, and inferior parts of the trapezius muscle;
3. The latissimus dorsi and teres major muscles form the posterior axillary fold;
4. The deep, midline furrow separates the lateral bulges of the erector spinae group of muscles;
5. The dimples (depressions) indicate the site of the posterior superior iliac spines, which usually lie at the level of the sacroiliac joint.

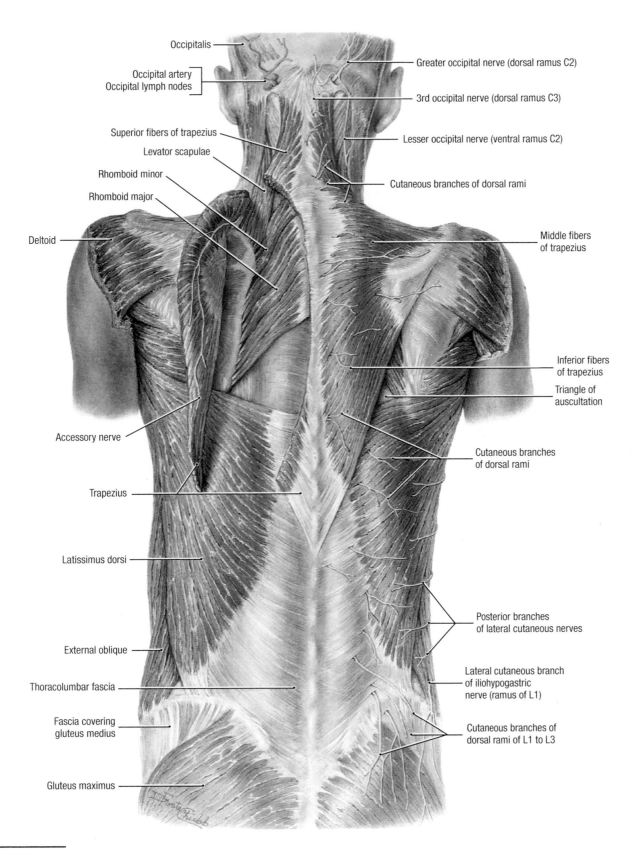

Occipitalis

Occipital artery
Occipital lymph nodes

Superior fibers of trapezius

Levator scapulae

Rhomboid minor

Rhomboid major

Deltoid

Accessory nerve

Trapezius

Latissimus dorsi

External oblique

Thoracolumbar fascia

Fascia covering
gluteus medius

Gluteus maximus

Greater occipital nerve (dorsal ramus C2)

3rd occipital nerve (dorsal ramus C3)

Lesser occipital nerve (ventral ramus C2)

Cutaneous branches of dorsal rami

Middle fibers
of trapezius

Inferior fibers
of trapezius

Triangle of
auscultation

Cutaneous branches
of dorsal rami

Posterior branches
of lateral cutaneous nerves

Lateral cutaneous branch
of iliohypogastric
nerve (ramus of L1)

Cutaneous branches of
dorsal rami of L1 to L3

4.29   **Superficial muscles of back, posterior view**

On the left, the trapezius muscle is reflected. Observe two layers: a) the trapezius and latissimus dorsi muscles, and b) the levator scapulae and rhomboids minor and major; these muscles help attach the upper limb to the trunk.

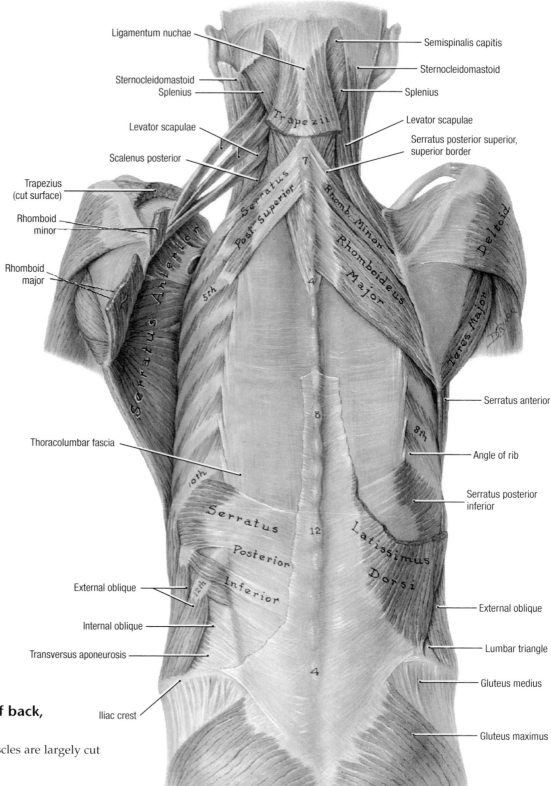

Ligamentum nuchae

Sternocleidomastoid
Splenius

Levator scapulae

Scalenus posterior

Trapezius
(cut surface)

Rhomboid
minor

Rhomboid
major

Thoracolumbar fascia

External oblique

Internal oblique

Transversus aponeurosis

Iliac crest

Semispinalis capitis

Sternocleidomastoid

Splenius

Levator scapulae

Serratus posterior superior,
superior border

Serratus anterior

Angle of rib

Serratus posterior
inferior

External oblique

Lumbar triangle

Gluteus medius

Gluteus maximus

4.30 **Intermediate muscles of back,
posterior view**

The trapezius and latissimus dorsi muscles are largely cut
away on both sides.

OBSERVE:

1. On the right are the levator scapulae and rhomboid muscles, and
   the serratus posterior superior, extending superior to the rhomboid
   minor muscles;
2. On the left, the rhomboid muscles have been severed, allowing the
   vertebral border of the scapula to be raised from the thoracic wall.
   Also note the digitations of levator scapulae muscles;
3. The serratus posterior superior and inferior form the intermediate
   layer of muscles, passing from the vertebral spines to the ribs; the

two muscles slope in opposite directions and are muscles of respiration;
4. The thoracolumbar fascia extends laterally to the angles of the ribs,
   becomes thin superiorly, passes deep to the serratus posterior superior muscle, and is reinforced inferiorly by the latissimus dorsi
   and serratus posterior inferior muscles.

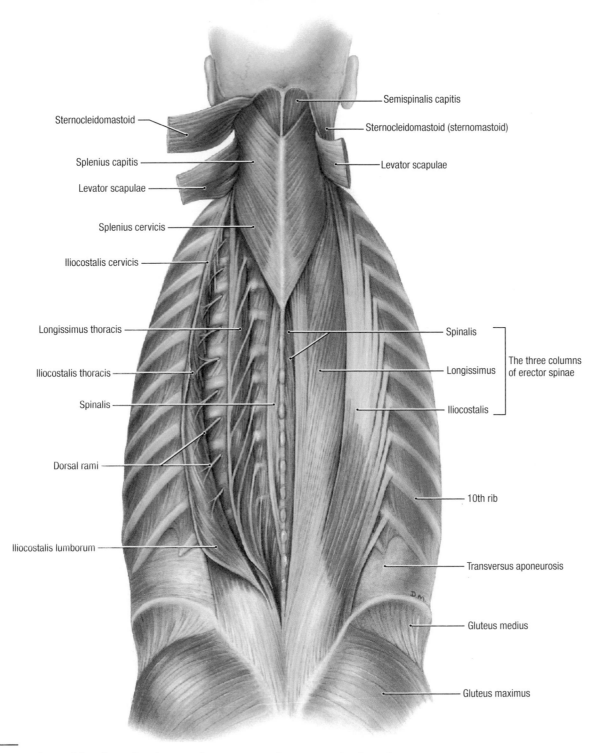

Semispinalis capitis

Sternocleidomastoid

Sternocleidomastoid (sternomastoid)

Splenius capitis

Levator scapulae

Levator scapulae

Splenius cervicis

Iliocostalis cervicis

Longissimus thoracis

Spinalis

The three columns of erector spinae

Iliocostalis thoracis

Longissimus

Spinalis

Iliocostalis

Dorsal rami

10th rib

Iliocostalis lumborum

Transversus aponeurosis

Gluteus medius

Gluteus maximus

4.31   **Deep muscles of back: splenius and erector spinae, posterior view**

OBSERVE:

1. The splenius capitis muscle attaches to the mastoid process deep to the sternocleidomastoid muscle, and the splenius cervicis muscle attaches to the 1st, 2nd, and 3rd cervical transverse processes deep to the levator scapulae muscle;

2. On the right of the body, note the erector spinae muscles in situ, lying between the spinous processes medially and the angles of the ribs laterally, and splitting into three longitudinal columns: iliocostalis laterally, longissimus in the middle, and spinalis medially;

3. On the left of the body, the spinalis muscle, the thinnest and most

medial of the erector spinae muscles, runs from inferior to more superior spinous processes, variably extending as high as the cervical region. The longissimus muscle, the intermediate column, is pulled laterally to show the insertion into the transverse processes and ribs; not shown here are its extensions to the neck and head, longissimus cervicis and capitis. The iliocostalis muscle, the most lateral, consists of three parts: iliocostalis lumborum, iliocostalis thoracis, and iliocostalis cervicis, inserting on the posterior tubercles of inferior cervical vertebrae.

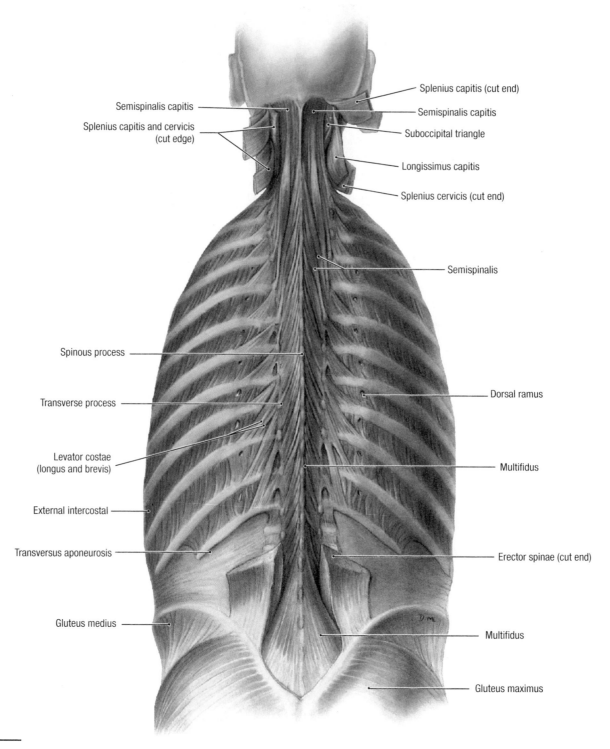

Semispinalis capitis

Splenius capitis and cervicis
(cut edge)

Splenius capitis (cut end)

Semispinalis capitis

Suboccipital triangle

Longissimus capitis

Splenius cervicis (cut end)

Semispinalis

Spinous process

Transverse process

Dorsal ramus

Levator costae
(longus and brevis)

Multifidus

External intercostal

Transversus aponeurosis

Erector spinae (cut end)

Gluteus medius

Multifidus

Gluteus maximus

4.32   Deep muscles of back: semispinalis and multifidus, posterior view

OBSERVE:

1. The semispinalis, multifidus, and rotatores muscles, constitute the transversospinalis group of deep muscles. In general, their bundles pass obliquely in a superomedial direction, from transverse processes to spinous processes in successively deeper layers. The bundles of semispinalis span approximately five interspaces, those of multifidus approximately three, and those of rotatores, one or two.

2. The semispinalis (thoracis, cervicis, and capitis) muscles extend from the lower thoracic region to the skull; the semispinalis capitis, a powerful extensor muscle, originates from the lower cervical and upper thoracic vertebrae and inserts into the occipital bone between the superior and inferior nuchal lines;

3. The multifidus muscle extends from the sacrum to the spine of the axis, emerges from the lumbosacral region from the aponeurosis of the erector spinae, the sacrum, and mamillary processes of the lumbar vertebrae, and inserts into spinous processes approximately three segments higher.

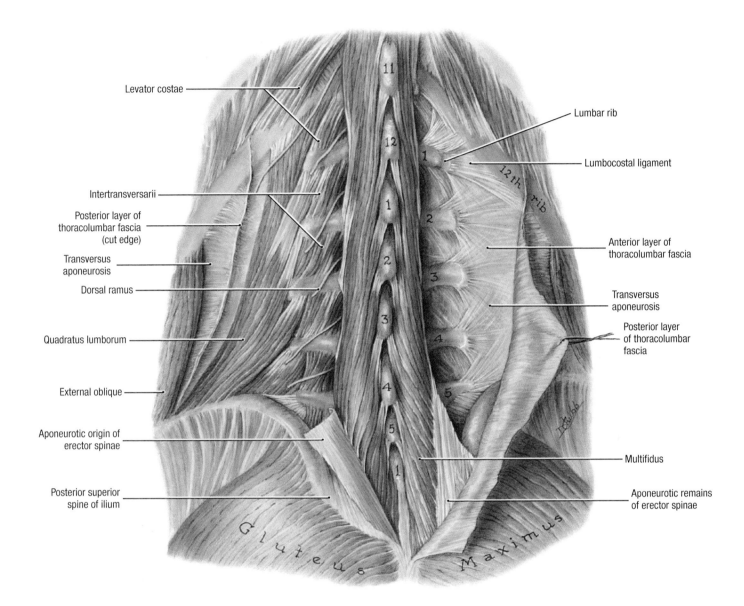

Levator costae

Intertransversarii

Posterior layer of
thoracolumbar fascia
(cut edge)

Transversus
aponeurosis

Dorsal ramus

Quadratus lumborum

External oblique

Aponeurotic origin of
erector spinae

Posterior superior
spine of ilium

Lumbar rib

Lumbocostal ligament

Anterior layer of
thoracolumbar fascia

Transversus
aponeurosis

Posterior layer
of thoracolumbar
fascia

Multifidus

Aponeurotic remains
of erector spinae

4.33 **Back: multifidus, quadratus lumborum, and
lumbar fascia, posterior view**

OBSERVE:
1. On the right: After removal of erector spinae, the anterior layer of
thoracolumbar fascia is attached in a fan-shaped manner to the tips
of transverse processes; also note a short lumbar rib (see Fig. 4.35);

2. On the left: After removal of the posterior layer of thoracolumbar
fascia, the lateral border of the quadratus lumborum muscle is
oblique, and the medial border is in continuity with the intertransversarii.

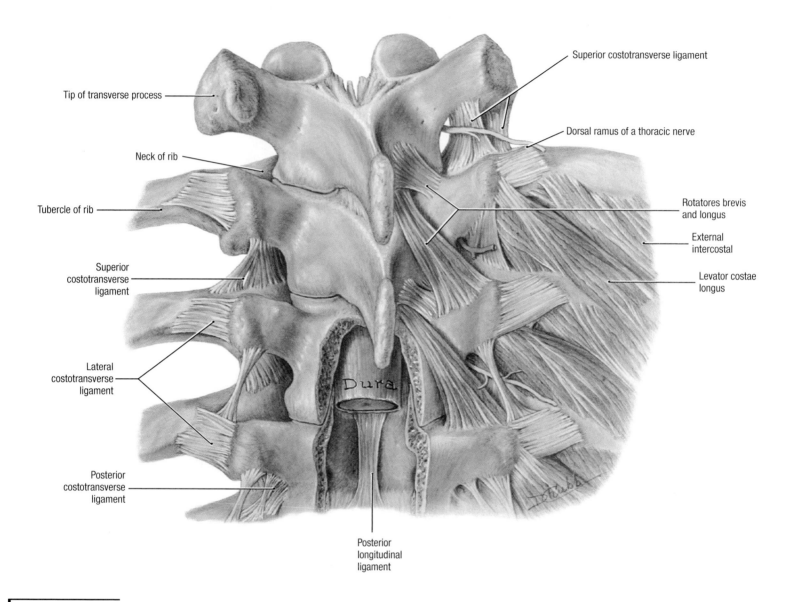

Tip of transverse process

Neck of rib

Tubercle of rib

Superior costotransverse ligament

Lateral costotransverse ligament

Posterior costotransverse ligament

Dura

Posterior longitudinal ligament

Superior costotransverse ligament

Dorsal ramus of a thoracic nerve

Rotatores brevis and longus

External intercostal

Levator costae longus

4.34   Rotatores and costotransverse ligaments, posterior view

OBSERVE:
1. Of the three layers of transversospinalis, or oblique, muscles of the back (semispinalis, multifidus, rotatores), the rotatores are the deepest and shortest; they pass from the root of one transverse process superomedially to the junction of the transverse process and lamina of the vertebra above. Some (rotatores longi) span two vertebrae;

2. The levatores costarum pass from the tip of one transverse process inferiorly to the rib below; some (levatores longi) span two ribs;
3. The superior costotransverse ligament splits laterally into two sheets, between which lie the levator costae and external intercostal; the dorsal ramus of a thoracic nerve passes posterior to this ligament;
4. The lateral costotransverse ligament is strong and joins the tubercle of the rib to the tip of the transverse process.

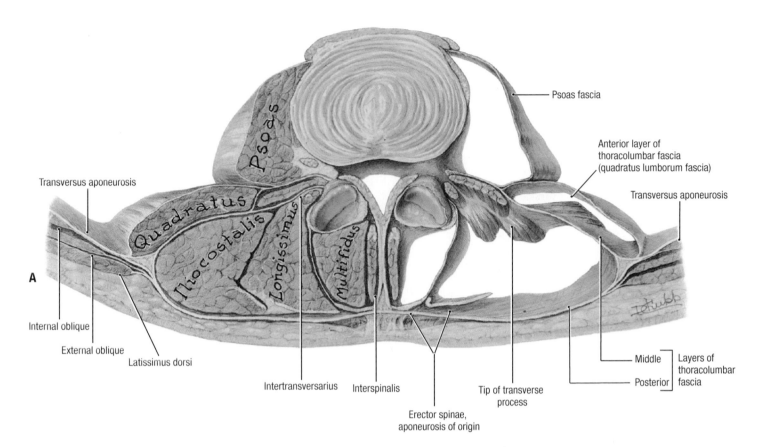

A. At level of lumbar spine. On the left, the muscles are seen within their sheaths or compartments; on the right, the sheaths are empty.

Labels: Transversus aponeurosis, Internal oblique, External oblique, Latissimus dorsi, Intertransversarius, Interspinalis, Erector spinae, aponeurosis of origin, Tip of transverse process, Middle, Posterior, Layers of thoracolumbar fascia, Transversus aponeurosis, Anterior layer of thoracolumbar fascia (quadratus lumborum fascia), Psoas fascia, Quadratus, Psoas, Iliocostalis, Longissimus, Multifidus

4.35　Transverse section of back muscles

A. At level of lumbar spine. On the left, the muscles are seen within their sheaths or compartments; on the right, the sheaths are empty. **B.** At level of thoracic spine. This transverse section shows erector spinae muscles in three columns, and the transversospinalis muscle in three layers.

OBSERVE:

1. The aponeurosis of the transversus abdominis muscle splits into two strong sheets, the anterior and posterior layers of the thoracolumbar fascia, which enclose the deep muscles of the back;
2. The posterior layer of the thoracolumbar fascia is reinforced by the latissimus dorsi muscle and, at a higher level, the serratus posterior inferior muscle;
3. Fascial layers cover the quadratus lumborum and psoas muscles;
4. The ends of intertransversarius, longissimus, and quadratus lumborum muscles attach to a transverse process.

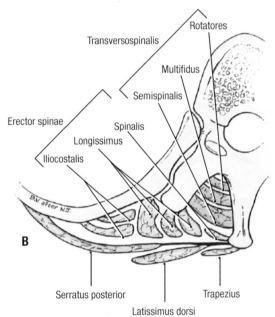

Labels: Transversospinalis, Rotatores, Multifidus, Semispinalis, Erector spinae, Spinalis, Longissimus, Iliocostalis, Serratus posterior, Latissimus dorsi, Trapezius

Table 4.1. Intrinsic Back Muscles[a]

Muscles	Origin	Insertion	Nerve Supply[b]	Main Actions
Superficial layer				
Splenius	Arises from ligamentum nuchae and spinous processes of C7–T3 or T4 vertebrae	*Spenius capitis:* fibers run superolaterally to mastoid process of temporal bone and lateral third of superior nuchal line of occipital bone *Splenius cervicis:* posterior tubercles of transverse processes of C1–C3 or C4 vertebrae		*Acting alone,* they laterally bend to side of active muscles; *acting together,* they extend head and neck
Intermediate layer				
Erector spine	Arises by a broad tendon from posterior part of iliac crest, posterior surface of sacrum, sacral and inferior lumbar spinous processes, and supraspinous ligament	*Iliocostalis:* lumborum, thoracis, and cervicis; fibers run superiorly to angles of lower ribs and cervical transverse processes *Longissimus:* thoracis, cervicis, and capitis; fibers run superiorly to ribs between tubercles and angles, to transverse processes in thoracic and cervical regions, and to mastoid process of temporal bone *Spinalis:* thoracis, cervicis, and capitis; fibers run superiorly to spinous processes in the upper thoracic region and to skull	Dorsal rami of spinal nerves	*Acting bilaterally,* they extend vertebral column and head; as back is flexed they control movement by gradually lengthening their fibers; *acting unilaterally,* they laterally bend vertebral column
Deep layer				
Transversospinal	Semispinalis arises from thoracic and cervical transverse processes	*Semispinalis:* thoracis, cervicis, and capitis; fibers run superomedially and attach to occipital bone and spinous processes in thoracic and cervical regions, spanning four to six segments		Extend head and thoracic and cervical regions of vertebral column and rotate them contralaterally
	Multifidus arises from sacrum and ilium, transverse processes of T1–T3, and articular processes of C4–C7	Fibers pass superomedially to spinous processes, spanning two to four segments		Stabilizes vertebrae during local movements of vertebral column
	Rotatores arise from transverse processes of vertebrae; best developed in thoracic region	Pass superomedially and attach to junction of lamina and transverse process of vertebra of origin or into spinous process above their origin, spanning one to two segments		Stabilize vertebrae and assist with local extension and rotary movements of vertebral columns
Minor deep layer				
Interspinales	Superior surfaces of spinous processes of cervical and lumbar vertebrae	Inferior surfaces of spinous processes of vertebrae superior to vetebrae of origin	Dorsal rami of spinal nerves	Aid in extension and rotation of vertebral column
Intertransversarii	Transverse processes of cervical and lumbar vertebrae	Transverse processes of adjacent vertebrae	Dorsal and ventral rami of spinal nerves	Aid in lateral bending of vertebral column; acting bilaterally, they stabilize vertebral column
Levatores costarum	Tips of transverse processes of C7 and T1–T11 vertebrae	Pass inferolaterally and insert on rib between its tubercle and angle	Dorsal rami of C8–T11 spinal nerves[c]	Elevate ribs, assisting inspiration Assist with lateral bending of vertebral column

[a] See figures on opposite page.
[b] Most back muscles are innervated by dorsal rami of spinal nerves, but a few are innervated by ventral rami. Anterior intertransversarii of cervical region are supplied by ventral rami.
[c] Levatores costarum were once said to be innervated by ventral rami, but investigators now agree that they are innervated by dorsal rami.

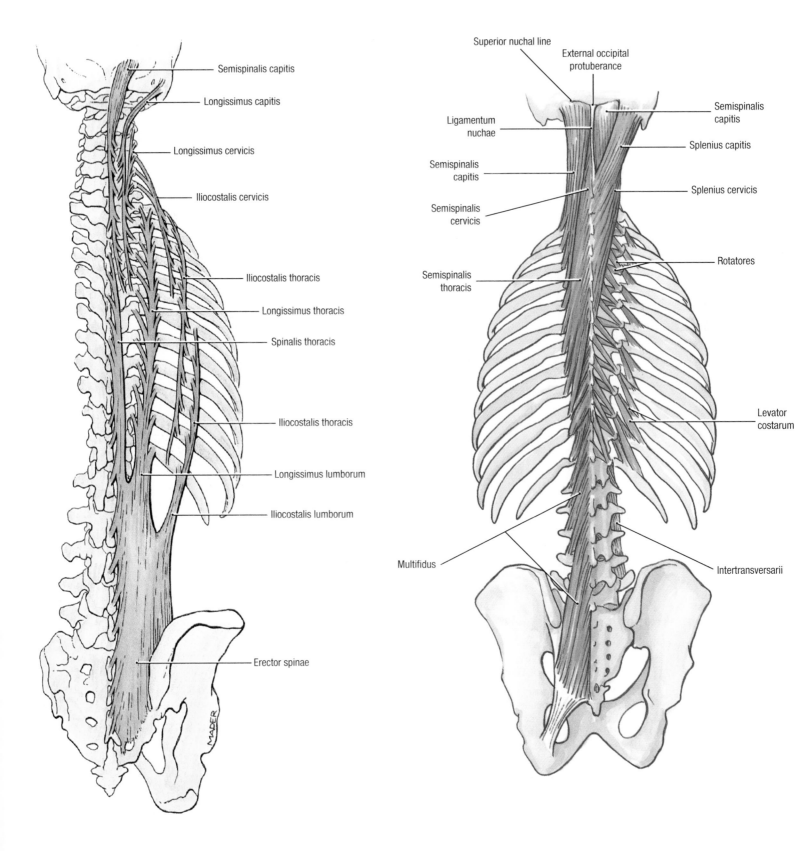

Semispinalis capitis

Longissimus capitis

Longissimus cervicis

Iliocostalis cervicis

Iliocostalis thoracis

Longissimus thoracis

Spinalis thoracis

Iliocostalis thoracis

Longissimus lumborum

Iliocostalis lumborum

Erector spinae

Superior nuchal line

External occipital protuberance

Ligamentum nuchae

Semispinalis capitis

Semispinalis cervicis

Semispinalis thoracis

Multifidus

Semispinalis capitis

Splenius capitis

Splenius cervicis

Rotatores

Levator costarum

Intertransversarii

MADER

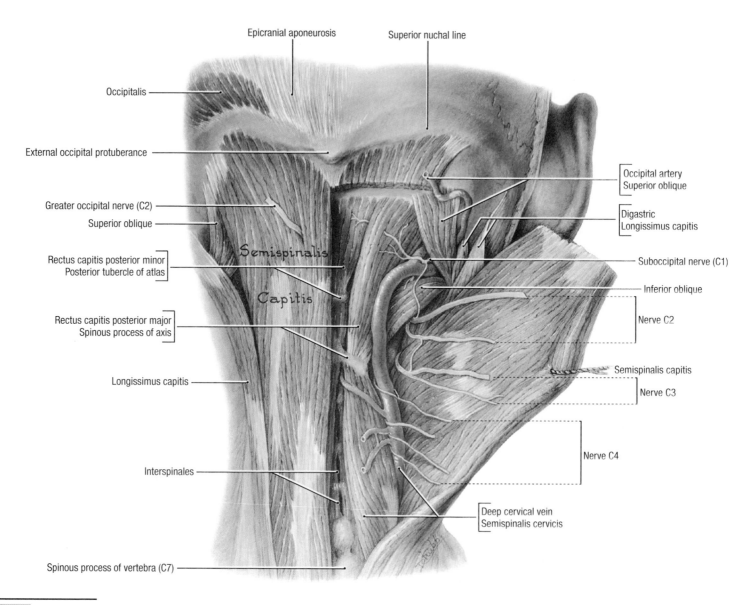

Epicranial aponeurosis

Superior nuchal line

Occipitalis

External occipital protuberance

Greater occipital nerve (C2)

Superior oblique

Rectus capitis posterior minor
Posterior tubercle of atlas

Rectus capitis posterior major
Spinous process of axis

Longissimus capitis

Interspinales

Spinous process of vertebra (C7)

Semispinalis

Capitis

Occipital artery
Superior oblique

Digastric
Longissimus capitis

Suboccipital nerve (C1)

Inferior oblique

Nerve C2

Semispinalis capitis

Nerve C3

Nerve C4

Deep cervical vein
Semispinalis cervicis

4.36 Suboccipital region-I, posterior view

The trapezius, sternocleidomastoid, and splenius muscles are removed.

OBSERVE:

1. The semispinalis capitis, the great extensor muscle of the head and neck, forms the posterior wall of the suboccipital region. It is pierced by the greater occipital nerve (C2, dorsal ramus) and has free medial and lateral borders at this high level. The right semispinalis muscle is divided and turned laterally;

2. The greater occipital nerve, when followed caudally, leads to the inferior border of the inferior oblique muscle, around which it turns. Following the inferior border of the inferior oblique muscle medi-ally from the nerve leads to the spinous process of the axis; followed laterally, this leads to the transverse process of the atlas;

3. Five muscles (all paired) are attached to the spinous process of the axis: inferior oblique, rectus capitis posterior major, semispinalis cervicis, multifidus, and interspinalis; the latter two are largely concealed by the semispinalis cervicis;

4. The occipital veins along with the suboccipital nerve (C1, dorsal ramus), emerge through the suboccipital triangle to join the deep cervical vein;

5. The suboccipital triangle is bounded by three muscles: inferior oblique, superior oblique, and rectus capitis posterior major.

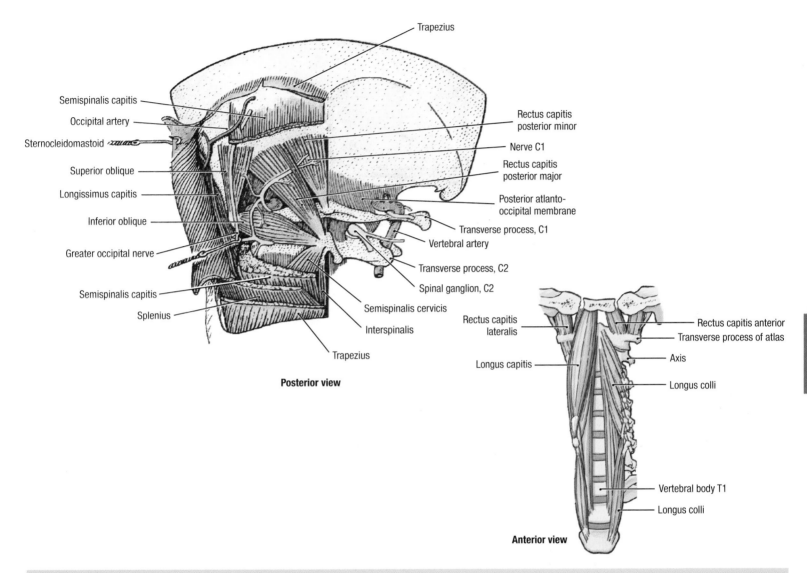

Posterior view

Anterior view

Table 4.2. Muscles of the Atlanto-Occipital and Atlantoaxial Joints

Movements of Atlanto-occipital Joints:

Flexion	Extension	Lateral Bending
Longus capitis	Rectus capitis posterior major and minor	Sternocleidomastoid
Rectus capitis anterior	Superior oblique	Superior and inferior oblique
Anterior fibers of	Semispinalis capitis	Rectus capitis lateralis
sternocleidomastoid	Splenius capitis	Longissimus capitis
	Longissimus capitis	Splenius capitis
	Trapezius	

Rotation at Atlantoaxial Joints[a]:

Ipsilateral[b]	Contralateral
Inferior oblique	Sternocleidomastoid
Rectus capitis posterior, major and minor	Semispinalis capitis
Longissimus capitis	
Splenius capitis	

[a]Rotation is the specialized movement at these joints. Movement of one joint involves the other.
[b]Same side to which head is rotated.

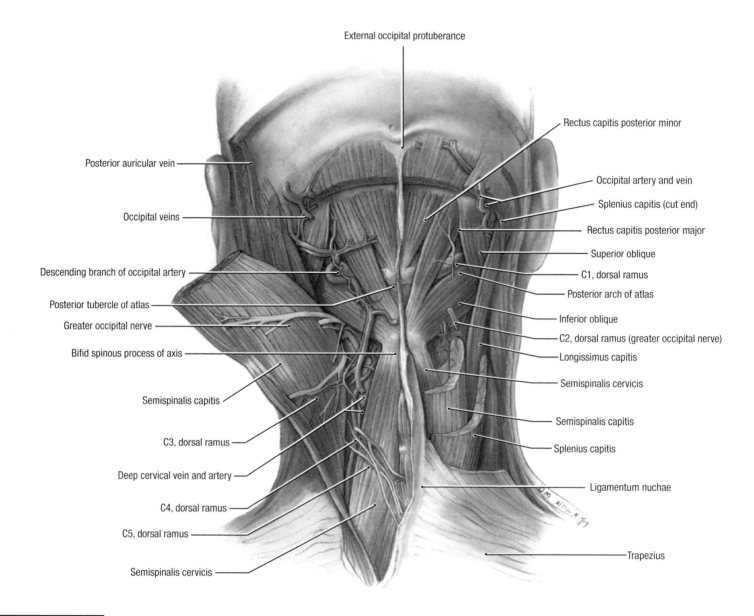

External occipital protuberance

Posterior auricular vein

Occipital veins

Descending branch of occipital artery

Posterior tubercle of atlas

Greater occipital nerve

Bifid spinous process of axis

Semispinalis capitis

C3, dorsal ramus

Deep cervical vein and artery

C4, dorsal ramus

C5, dorsal ramus

Semispinalis cervicis

Rectus capitis posterior minor

Occipital artery and vein

Splenius capitis (cut end)

Rectus capitis posterior major

Superior oblique

C1, dorsal ramus

Posterior arch of atlas

Inferior oblique

C2, dorsal ramus (greater occipital nerve)

Longissimus capitis

Semispinalis cervicis

Semispinalis capitis

Splenius capitis

Ligamentum nuchae

Trapezius

4.37   Suboccipital region-II, posterior view

The semispinalis capitis is reflected on the left and removed on the right side of the body.

OBSERVE:

1. The suboccipital region contains four pairs of structures: two straight muscles, the rectus capitis posterior major and minor; two oblique muscles, the superior oblique and inferior oblique; two nerves (dorsal primary rami), C1 suboccipital (motor) and C2 greater occipital (sensory); and two arteries, the occipital and vertebral;

2. The ligamentum nuchae, which represents the cervical part of the supraspinous ligament, is a median, thin, fibrous partition attached to the spinous processes of cervical vertebrae and the external occipital crest; its posterior border gives origin to the trapezius muscle and extends superiorly to the external occipital protuberance (inion);

3. The rectus capitis posterior minor muscle arises from the posterior tubercle of the atlas and thus lies on a deeper plane than the rectus capitis posterior major muscle, which arises from a spinous process;

4. The suboccipital nerve (C1, dorsal ramus) supplies the three muscles bounding the suboccipital triangle and also the rectus capitis minor muscle, and communicates with the greater occipital nerve;

5. The descending branch of the occipital artery anastomoses with the deep cervical artery, a branch of the subclavian;

6. The longissimus capitis muscle is the only section of erector spinae to reach the skull;

7. The posterior arch of the atlas forms the floor of the sub-occipital triangle.

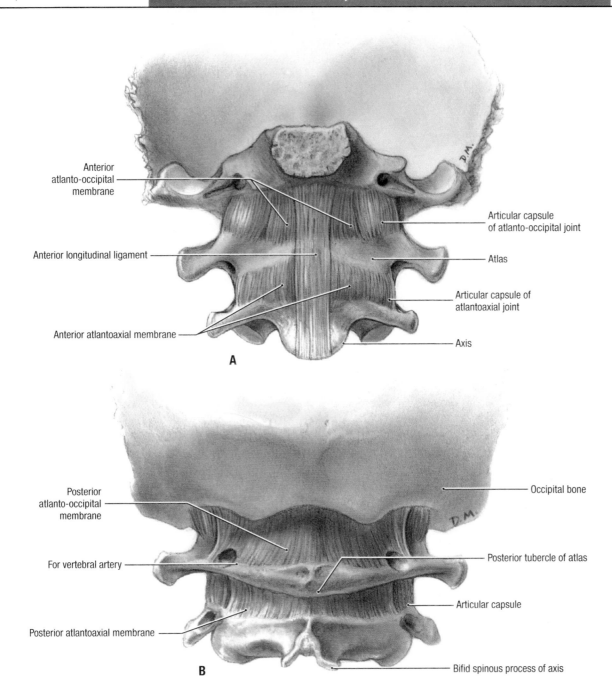

Anterior atlanto-occipital membrane

Anterior longitudinal ligament

Anterior atlantoaxial membrane

Articular capsule of atlanto-occipital joint

Atlas

Articular capsule of atlantoaxial joint

Axis

A

Posterior atlanto-occipital membrane

For vertebral artery

Posterior atlantoaxial membrane

Occipital bone

Posterior tubercle of atlas

Articular capsule

Bifid spinous process of axis

B

4.38 Ligaments of atlanto-occipital and atlantoaxial joints, and vertebral artery

A. Anterior view. **B.** Posterior view. **C.** Posterior view, vertebral artery.

OBSERVE:

1. In **A,** the anterior longitudinal ligament blends in the midline with the anterior atlanto-occipital and anterior atlantoaxial membranes, and laterally with the facet joints;

2. In **B,** the posterior atlanto-occipital membrane lies between the foramen magnum and superior surface of the posterior arch of the atlas, and the posterior atlantoaxial membrane lies between the inferior surface of the posterior arch of the atlas and the laminae of the axis; it is continuous with the ligamentum flava;

3. In **C,** the vertebral arteries enter the skull through the foramen magnum and join to form the basilar artery.

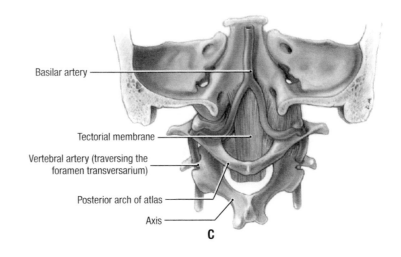

Basilar artery

Tectorial membrane

Vertebral artery (traversing the foramen transversarium)

Posterior arch of atlas

Axis

C

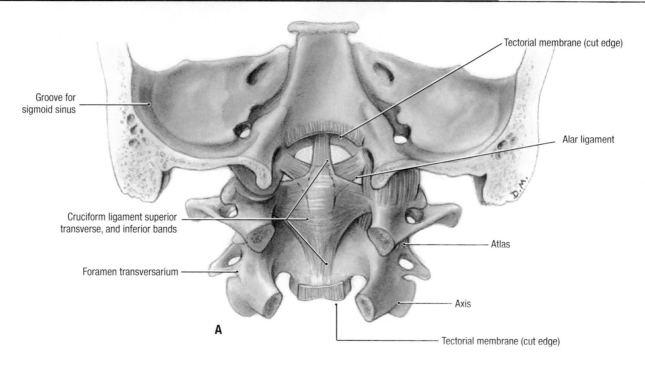

Tectorial membrane (cut edge)

Groove for sigmoid sinus

Alar ligament

Cruciform ligament superior transverse, and inferior bands

Foramen transversarium

Atlas

Axis

Tectorial membrane (cut edge)

A

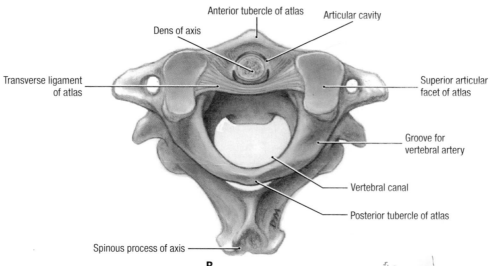

Anterior tubercle of atlas

Dens of axis

Articular cavity

Transverse ligament of atlas

Superior articular facet of atlas

Groove for vertebral artery

Vertebral canal

Posterior tubercle of atlas

Spinous process of axis

B

4.39   Atlanto-occipital and atlantoaxial joints

A. Posterior view. **B.** Superior view. **C.** Median section through the dens, lateral view.

OBSERVE:

1. In **A,** note the alar ligaments and cruciform ligament, consisting of superior, transverse, and inferior bands;
2. In **B,** the large vertebral foramen of the atlas is divided into two foramina by the transverse ligament; in the larger, posterior foramen, the spinal cord lies loosely, and in the smaller, anterior foramen, the dens of the axis fits tightly.
3. In **C,** the layers of tissue, from posterior to anterior, are: dura mater, posterior longitudinal ligament continued superiorly as the tectorial membrane, transverse ligament of the atlas, inferior and superior bands of the cruciform ligament, and the apical ligament of dens, stretching from the apex of the dens to the occipital bone.

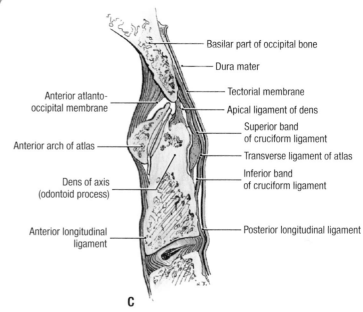

Basilar part of occipital bone

Dura mater

Tectorial membrane

Apical ligament of dens

Superior band of cruciform ligament

Transverse ligament of atlas

Inferior band of cruciform ligament

Posterior longitudinal ligament

Anterior atlanto-occipital membrane

Anterior arch of atlas

Dens of axis (odontoid process)

Anterior longitudinal ligament

C

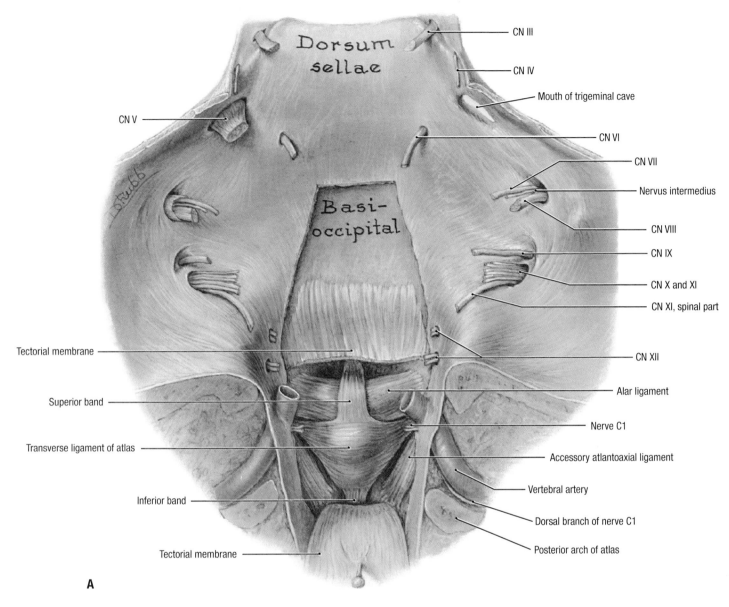

A

CN III
CN IV
Mouth of trigeminal cave
CN V
CN VI
CN VII
Nervus intermedius
CN VIII
CN IX
CN X and XI
CN XI, spinal part
Tectorial membrane
CN XII
Superior band
Alar ligament
Transverse ligament of atlas
Nerve C1
Accessory atlantoaxial ligament
Vertebral artery
Inferior band
Dorsal branch of nerve C1
Posterior arch of atlas
Tectorial membrane

Dorsum sellae

Basi-occipital

4.40 Craniovertebral joints and vertebral artery

A. Posterior view. **B.** Lateral view.

OBSERVE:
1. The bow-shaped transverse ligament of the atlas, with the addition of a superior and inferior longitudinal band, becomes a cruciform ligament that stretches from the axis to the occipital bone;
2. The alar ligament passes from the sides of the apex of the dens posterolaterally, and superior to the transverse ligament to the medial sides of the occipital condyles;
3. The sites where the last 10 pairs of cranial nerves and the first pair of cervical nerves pass through the dura, noting: (a) they are in numerical sequence craniocaudally, and (b) nerves III, IV, and VI, which supply the muscles of the eye, and XII, which supplies the muscles of the tongue, are nearly in vertical line with each other and with the ventral or motor root of C1;
4. In **B,** the vertebral artery arises from the subclavian artery and passes through the foramina transversaria of the superior six cervical vertebrae.

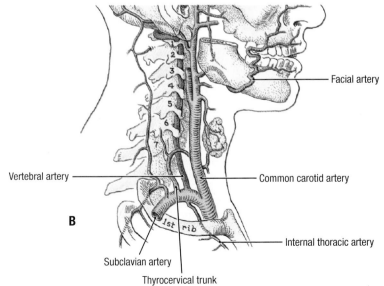

B

Facial artery
Vertebral artery
Common carotid artery
Internal thoracic artery
Subclavian artery
Thyrocervical trunk
1st rib

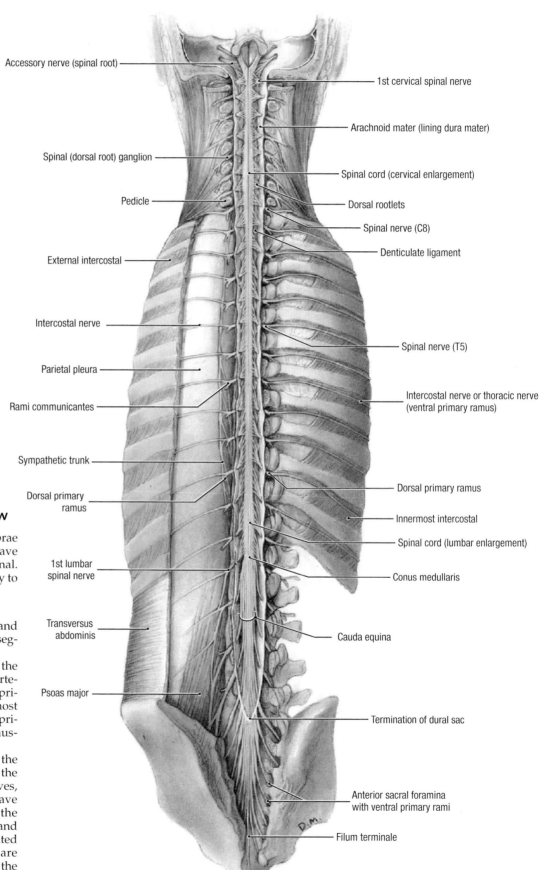

Accessory nerve (spinal root)

1st cervical spinal nerve

Arachnoid mater (lining dura mater)

Spinal (dorsal root) ganglion

Spinal cord (cervical enlargement)

Pedicle

Dorsal rootlets

Spinal nerve (C8)

Denticulate ligament

External intercostal

Intercostal nerve

Spinal nerve (T5)

Parietal pleura

Rami communicantes

Intercostal nerve or thoracic nerve (ventral primary ramus)

Sympathetic trunk

Dorsal primary ramus

Dorsal primary ramus

Innermost intercostal

Spinal cord (lumbar enlargement)

1st lumbar spinal nerve

Conus medullaris

Transversus abdominis

Cauda equina

Psoas major

Termination of dural sac

Anterior sacral foramina with ventral primary rami

Filum terminale

Left　　**Right**

4.41

Spinal cord in situ, posterior view

The vertebral (neural) arches of the vertebrae and the posterior aspect of the sacrum have been removed to expose the vertebral canal. The dural sac has been cut open posteriorly to reveal the spinal cord and nerve roots.

OBSERVE:

1. The spinal cord terminates between L1 and L2, and the dural sac at the 2nd sacral segment;
2. On the right: (a) the ribs articulate with the transverse processes of the thoracic vertebrae, (b) the intercostal nerves (ventral primary rami) pass posterior to the innermost intercostal muscles, and (c) the dorsal primary rami innervate the deep back muscles;
3. On the left: (a) note the formation of the brachial and lumbosacral plexuses by the ventral primary rami of the spinal nerves, (b) the ribs and intercostal muscles have been removed posteriorly to expose the parietal pleura and sympathetic trunk, and (c) the spinal (dorsal root) ganglia, located at the intervertebral foramina, are bounded superiorly and inferiorly by the pedicles.

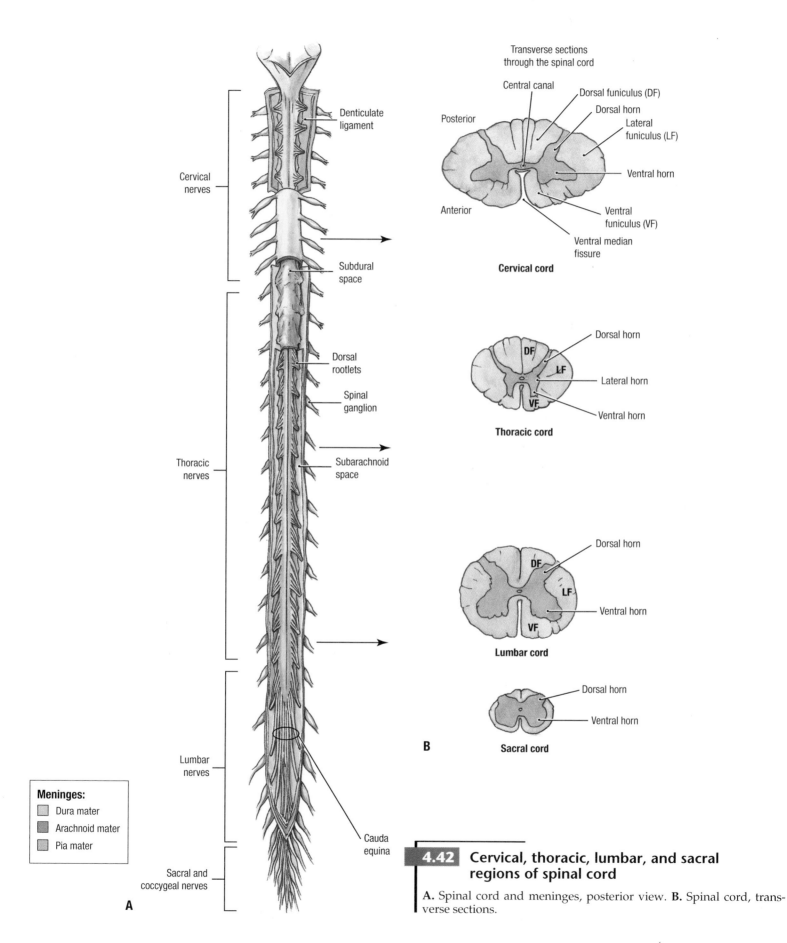

Transverse sections
through the spinal cord

Central canal

Dorsal funiculus (DF)

Dorsal horn

Lateral
funiculus (LF)

Posterior

Ventral horn

Anterior

Ventral
funiculus (VF)

Ventral median
fissure

Cervical cord

Denticulate
ligament

Cervical
nerves

Subdural
space

Dorsal horn

DF

LF

Lateral horn

VF

Ventral horn

Thoracic cord

Dorsal
rootlets

Spinal
ganglion

Thoracic
nerves

Subarachnoid
space

Dorsal horn

DF

LF

Ventral horn

VF

Lumbar cord

Dorsal horn

Ventral horn

B

Sacral cord

Meninges:

Dura mater

Arachnoid mater

Pia mater

Lumbar
nerves

Cauda
equina

Sacral and
coccygeal nerves

A

4.42 **Cervical, thoracic, lumbar, and sacral
regions of spinal cord**

A. Spinal cord and meninges, posterior view. **B.** Spinal cord, transverse sections.

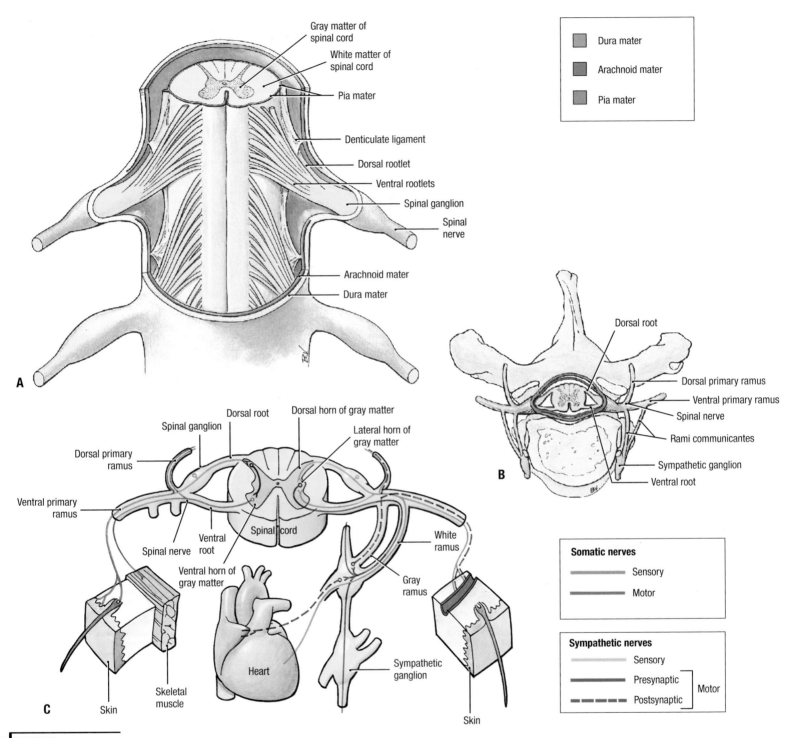

Gray matter of spinal cord
White matter of spinal cord
Pia mater
Denticulate ligament
Dorsal rootlet
Ventral rootlets
Spinal ganglion
Spinal nerve
Arachnoid mater
Dura mater

A

Dura mater
Arachnoid mater
Pia mater

Dorsal root
Dorsal primary ramus
Ventral primary ramus
Spinal nerve
Rami communicantes
Sympathetic ganglion
Ventral root

B

Spinal ganglion
Dorsal root
Dorsal horn of gray matter
Lateral horn of gray matter
Dorsal primary ramus
Ventral primary ramus
Spinal nerve
Ventral root
Ventral horn of gray matter
Spinal cord
White ramus
Gray ramus
Heart
Sympathetic ganglion
Skeletal muscle
Skin
Skin

C

Somatic nerves
Sensory
Motor

Sympathetic nerves
Sensory
Presynaptic ⎤
Postsynaptic ⎦ Motor

4.43   Formation of spinal nerves

A. Anterior view. **B.** Superior view. **C.** Components of a typical spinal nerve.

OBSERVE:
1. The dural sac consists of the dura mater and arachnoid mater. The pia mater covers the spinal cord and projects laterally as the denticulate ligaments, which separate the rows of dorsal and ventral rootlets;
2. Cerebrospinal fluid circulates between the pia and arachnoid in the subarachnoid space;
3. On each side, two rows of rootlets attach to the cord; the dorsal fil-aments carry sensory information to the CNS, and the ventral filaments convey motor information from the CNS to the periphery;
4. Several rootlets combine to form dorsal and ventral roots at each segment;
5. The swollen area on the dorsal root, the spinal (dorsal root) ganglion, contains cell bodies of sensory neurons;
6. Dorsal and ventral roots unite to form a spinal nerve;
7. The dura and arachnoid continue as a sheath around nerves leaving the spinal cord.

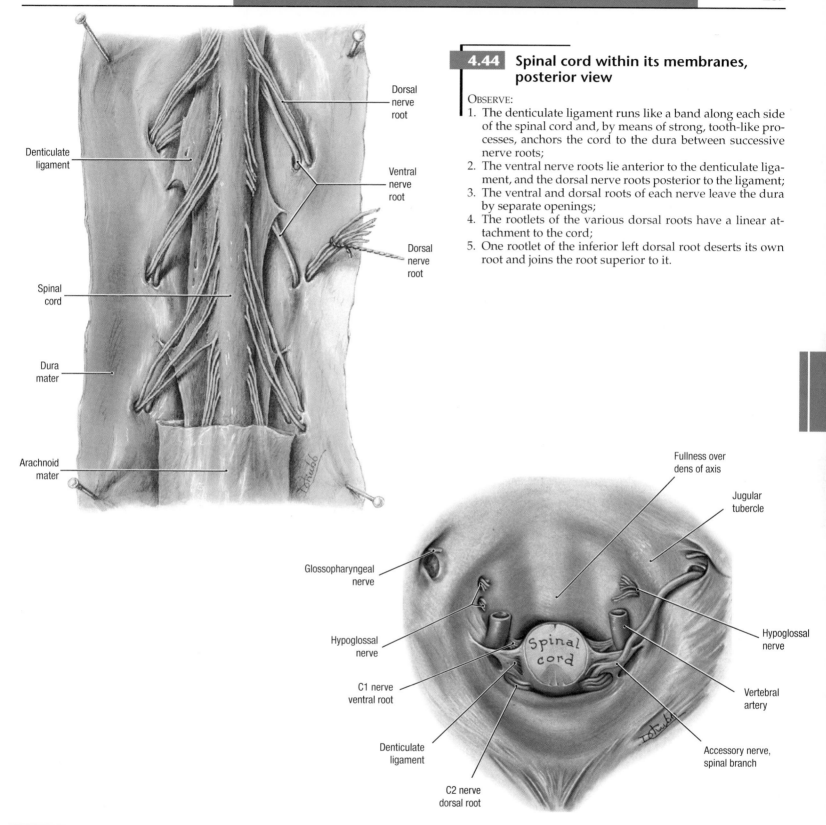

Dorsal nerve root

Denticulate ligament

Ventral nerve root

Dorsal nerve root

Spinal cord

Dura mater

Arachnoid mater

4.44 Spinal cord within its membranes, posterior view

OBSERVE:
1. The denticulate ligament runs like a band along each side of the spinal cord and, by means of strong, tooth-like processes, anchors the cord to the dura between successive nerve roots;
2. The ventral nerve roots lie anterior to the denticulate ligament, and the dorsal nerve roots posterior to the ligament;
3. The ventral and dorsal roots of each nerve leave the dura by separate openings;
4. The rootlets of the various dorsal roots have a linear attachment to the cord;
5. One rootlet of the inferior left dorsal root deserts its own root and joins the root superior to it.

Fullness over dens of axis

Jugular tubercle

Glossopharyngeal nerve

Hypoglossal nerve

Hypoglossal nerve

C1 nerve ventral root

Vertebral artery

Denticulate ligament

Accessory nerve, spinal branch

C2 nerve dorsal root

4.45 Structures of vertebral canal seen through foramen magnum, superior view

OBSERVE:
1. Anteriorly, the fullness over the dens of the axis is created by the transverse ligament of the atlas, which curves tightly posterior to the dens;
2. The spinal cord (or medulla), vertebral arteries, spinal roots of the accessory nerves (CNXI), and most superior tooth of the denticulate ligament pass through the foramen magnum within the meninges;
3. The hypoglossal nerve (CNXII) leaves the dura mater through two openings that are close together on the right side and separated on the left;
4. In this specimen, the first cervical nerve has no posterior root.

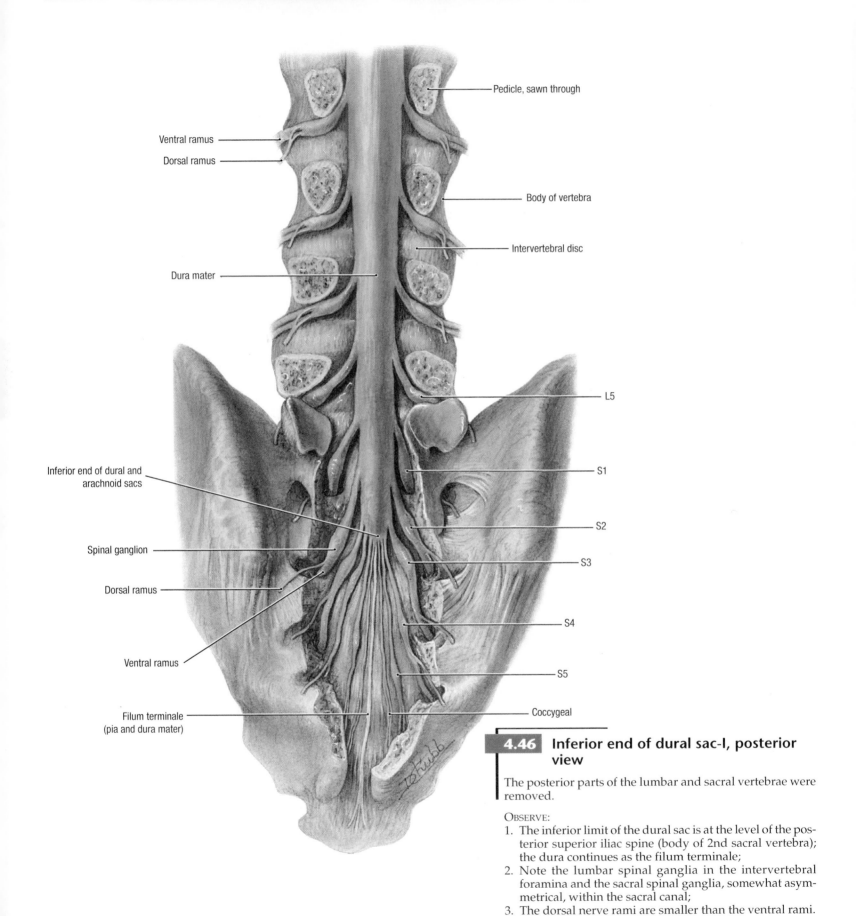

Pedicle, sawn through

Ventral ramus

Dorsal ramus

Body of vertebra

Intervertebral disc

Dura mater

L5

Inferior end of dural and
arachnoid sacs

S1

S2

Spinal ganglion

S3

Dorsal ramus

S4

Ventral ramus

S5

Filum terminale
(pia and dura mater)

Coccygeal

4.46   Inferior end of dural sac-I, posterior
view

The posterior parts of the lumbar and sacral vertebrae were
removed.

OBSERVE:
1. The inferior limit of the dural sac is at the level of the posterior superior iliac spine (body of 2nd sacral vertebra);
   the dura continues as the filum terminale;
2. Note the lumbar spinal ganglia in the intervertebral
   foramina and the sacral spinal ganglia, somewhat asymmetrical, within the sacral canal;
3. The dorsal nerve rami are smaller than the ventral rami.

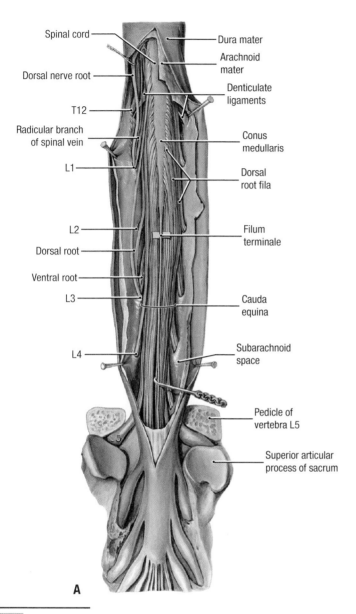

A

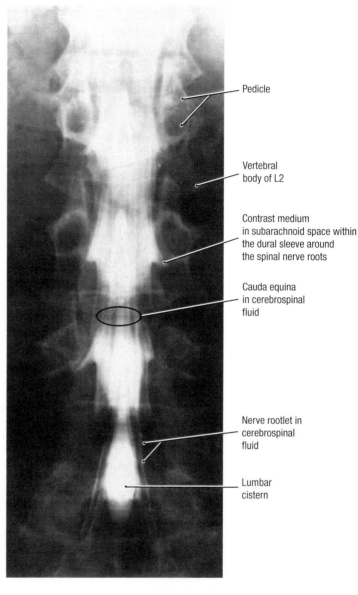

B

4.47 Inferior end of dural sac-II, posterior view

A. Inferior end of dural sac, opened, posterior view. **B.** Myelogram of the lumbar region of the vertebral column. Contrast medium was injected into the subarachnoid place. **C.** Termination of spinal cord, in situ, sagittal section.

OBSERVE IN **A**:
1. The inferior margin of the denticulate ligament is variable in level and asymmetrical;
2. A radicular branch of a spinal vein accompanies the dorsal root of nerve L1;
3. The conus medullaris, or conical lower end of the spinal cord, continues as a glistening thread, the filum terminale, which descends with the posterior and anterior nerve roots; these constitute the cauda equina;
4. The subarachnoid space is enclosed by arachnoid mater; the subdural space is the potential space between the dura mater and arachnoid mater.

OBSERVE IN **C**:
5. In the adult, the spinal cord usually ends at the level of the disc between L1 and L2;
6. The subarachnoid space usually ends at the level of the disc between S1 and S2, but it can be more inferior;
7. Variations: 95% of cords end within the limits of the bodies of L1 and L2, whereas 3% end posterior to the inferior half of T12, and 2% posterior to L3.

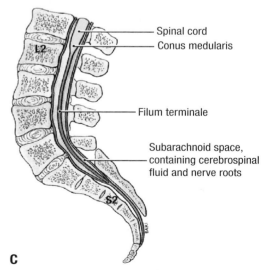

C

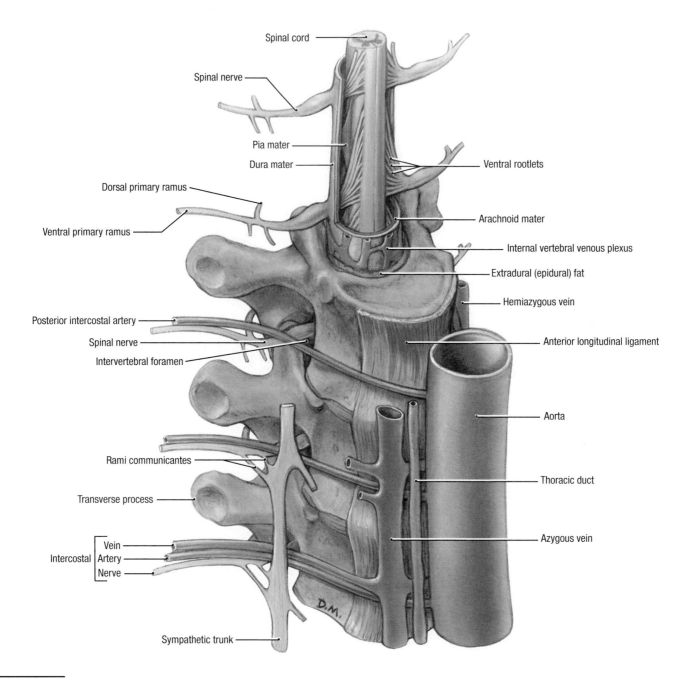

Spinal cord

Spinal nerve

Pia mater

Dura mater — Ventral rootlets

Dorsal primary ramus

Ventral primary ramus — Arachnoid mater

Internal vertebral venous plexus

Extradural (epidural) fat

Hemiazygous vein

Posterior intercostal artery

Spinal nerve — Anterior longitudinal ligament

Intervertebral foramen

Aorta

Rami communicantes

Thoracic duct

Transverse process

Vein
Intercostal Artery — Azygous vein
Nerve

Sympathetic trunk

4.48   Spinal cord and prevertebral structures, anterolateral view

The vertebrae have been removed superiorly to expose the spinal cord and meninges.

OBSERVE:
1. The aorta descends to the left of the midline, with the thoracic duct and azygos vein to its right;
2. The azygos vein is on the right side of the vertebral bodies, and the hemiazygos vein is on the left;
3. The thoracic sympathetic trunk and ganglia; the rami communicantes connect the sympathetic ganglia with the spinal nerve;

4. The dural sac of the spinal cord consists of dura mater and archnoid mater; a sleeve of dura mater surrounds the spinal nerves and blends with the sheath of the spinal nerve;
5. The spinal cord is covered with pia mater and anchored laterally by the denticulate ligaments;
6. The dura mater is separated from the walls of the vertebral canal by extradural (epidural) fat, the internal vertebral venous plexus, and areolar tissue.

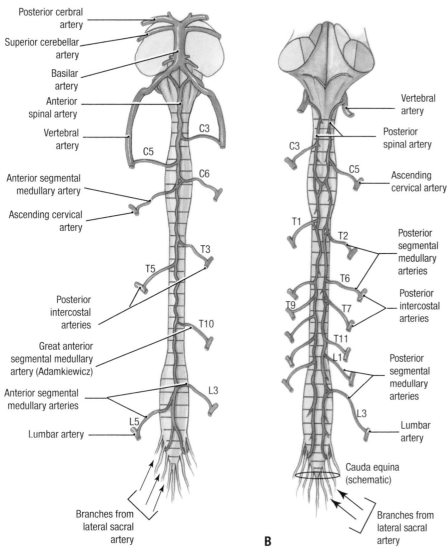

A

B

4.49 Blood vessels of spinal cord

A. Arterial supply, anterior view. **B.** Arterial supply, posterior view. **C.** Arterial supply and venous drainage, transverse section.

OBSERVE:
1. The pattern of arterial supply from three longitudinal vessels: one anterior and two posterior spinal arteries;
2. The anterior and posterior spinal arteries are reinforced at irregular intervals by anterior and posterior segmental medullary arteries, at levels where these arteries do not occur, radicular arteries supply the dorsal and ventral roots, but they do not reinforce the spinal arteries;
3. The great anterior segmental medullary artery ("Adamkiewicz artery") occurs on the left side in 65% of people. It reinforces the circulation to 2/3 of the spinal cord;
4. Distribution of the veins is similar to that of the arteries. The spinal veins are arranged longitudinally; they communicate with each other and are drained by up to 12 anterior and posterior medullary and radicular veins. The veins join the internal vertebral venous plexus, which lies in the extradural space.

POSTERIOR

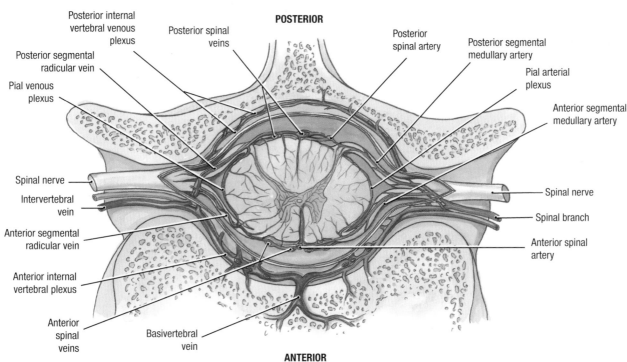

C

ANTERIOR

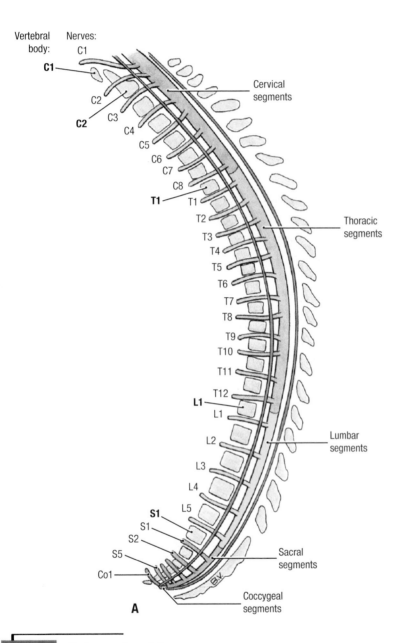

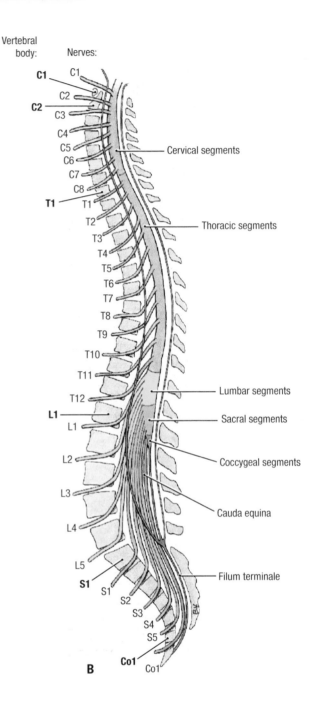

4.50   Subarachnoid space

A. Spinal cord at 12 weeks gestation, sagittal section. **B.** Spinal cord of an adult, sagittal section. Early in development, the spinal cord and vertebral (spinal) canal are nearly equal in length. The canal grows longer, so spinal nerves have an increasingly longer course to reach the intervertebral foramen at the correct level for their exit. Descending the cord, the spinal nerves become increasingly oblique in their courses. The spinal cord proper terminates at L2, and the remaining spinal nerves, seeking their intervertebral foramen of exit, form the cauda equina. At S2, the subarachnoid space ceases. *Thus, spinal taps to obtain a sample of cerebrospinal fluid, are usually conducted between vertebral levels L3 and S2.*

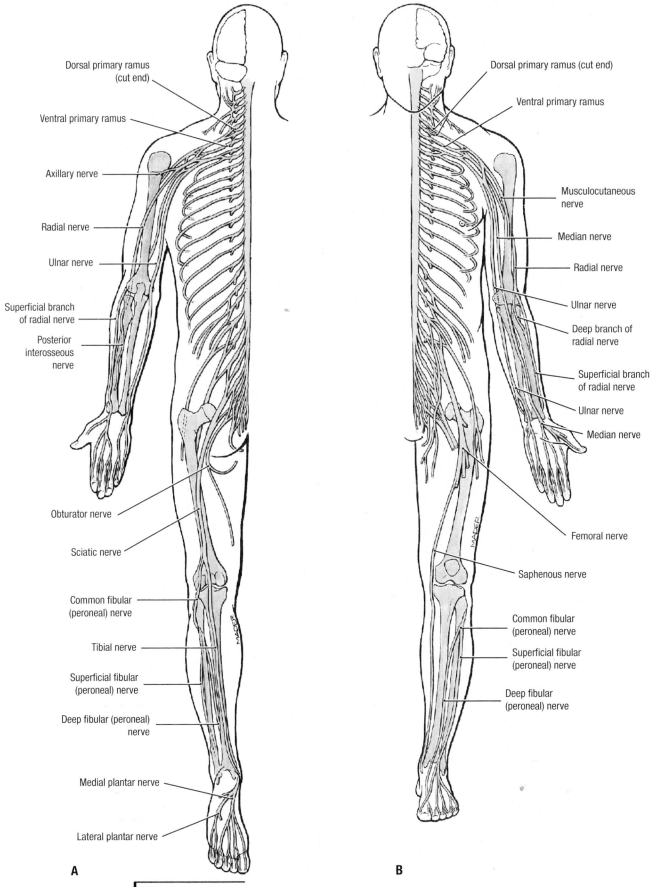

Dorsal primary ramus
(cut end)

Ventral primary ramus

Axillary nerve

Radial nerve

Ulnar nerve

Superficial branch
of radial nerve

Posterior
interosseous
nerve

Obturator nerve

Sciatic nerve

Common fibular
(peroneal) nerve

Tibial nerve

Superficial fibular
(peroneal) nerve

Deep fibular (peroneal)
nerve

Medial plantar nerve

Lateral plantar nerve

Dorsal primary ramus (cut end)

Ventral primary ramus

Musculocutaneous
nerve

Median nerve

Radial nerve

Ulnar nerve

Deep branch of
radial nerve

Superficial branch
of radial nerve

Ulnar nerve

Median nerve

Femoral nerve

Saphenous nerve

Common fibular
(peroneal) nerve

Superficial fibular
(peroneal) nerve

Deep fibular
(peroneal) nerve

A   B

4.51 **Overview of somatic nervous system.**

A. Posterior view. **B.** Anterior view.

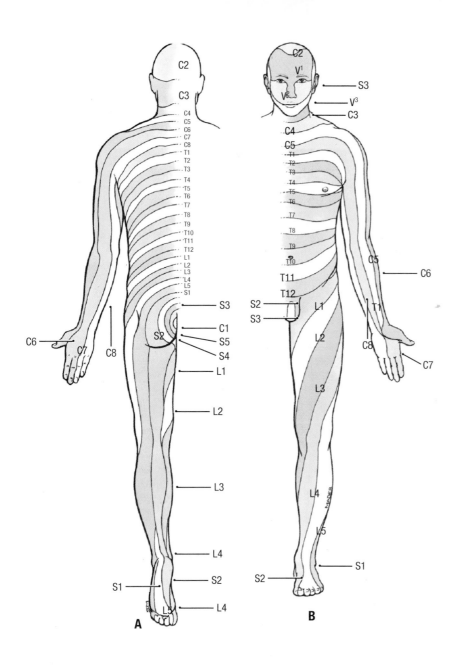

A

B

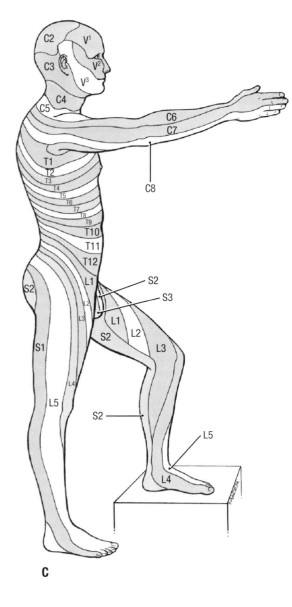

C

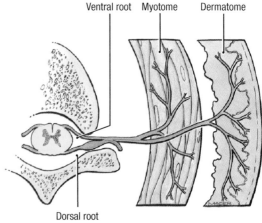

Ventral root   Myotome   Dermatome

Dorsal root

4.52 Dermatomes

A. Posterior view. **B.** Anterior view. **C.** Lateral view. A dermatome is an area of skin supplied by the dorsal (sensory) root of a spinal nerve. In the head and trunk, each segment is horizontally disposed, except C1, which has no sensory component. The dermatomes of the limbs from the 5th cervical to the 1st thoracic, and from the 3rd lumbar to the 2nd sacral vertebrae, extend as a series of bands from the midline of the trunk posteriorly into the limbs. Note that there is considerable overlapping of adjacent dermatomes, i.e., each segmental nerve overlaps the territories of its neighbors. *As a result, no anesthesia occurs unless two or more consecutive dorsal roots have lost their functions.*

4.53 Segmental innervation: dermatome and myotome, schematic transverse section

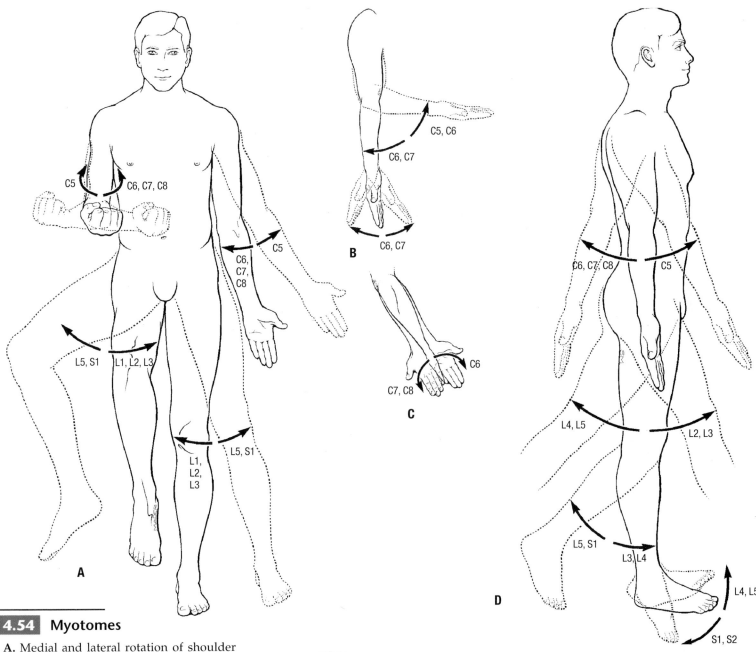

4.54 Myotomes

A. Medial and lateral rotation of shoulder and hip, abduction and adduction of shoulder and hip, anterior view. **B.** Flexion and extension of elbow and wrist, lateral view. **C.** Pronation and supination of forearm, anterior view. **D.** Flexion and extension of shoulder, hip, and knee, dorsiflexion and plantar flexion of ankle, lateral view. A myotome is the segmental innervation of skeletal muscle by the ventral (motor) root(s) of the spinal nerve(s) (Figure 4.55). When adjacent myotomes fuse during embryonic development, the resultant muscle can be innervated by one or both of its segmental spinal nerves. In this diagram, the myotomes have been generalized to apply to movements of the joints of the upper and lower extremities.

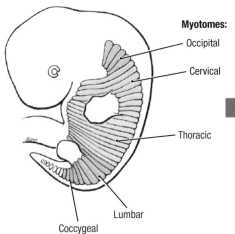

Myotomes:
- Occipital
- Cervical
- Thoracic
- Lumbar
- Coccygeal

4.55 Myotome region of somites

Initially, the muscles of the trunk and limbs are segmental, but during development, various segments fuse, and the distinctive segmental pattern is lost (except for the intercostal muscles of the thorax).

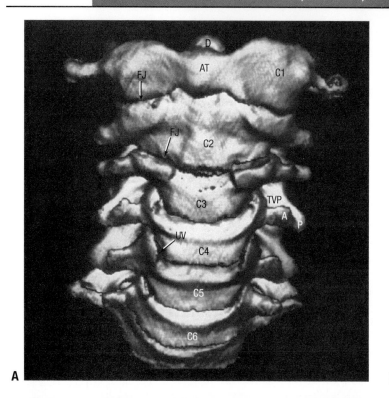

A

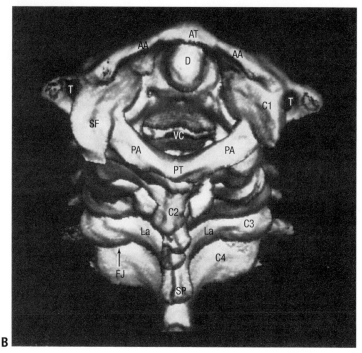

B

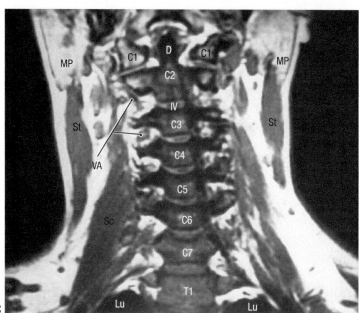

C

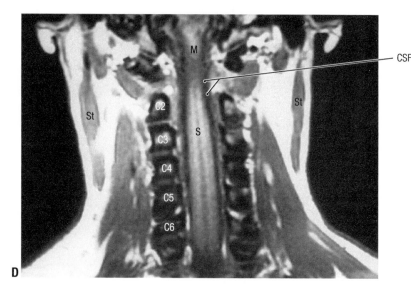

D

4.56 Imaging of spine

A and **B.** Three-dimensional computer-generated images of cervical spine, anterior (**A**) and poster (**B**) views. **C** and **D.** T1 coronal MRIs of cervical spine, posterior view.

AA	Anterior arch of C1	M	Medulla oblongata	T	Foramen transversarium
AT	Anterior tubercle of C1	MP	Mastoid process	TVP	Transverse process
C1–T1	vertebrae	PA	Posterior arch of C1	UV	Uncovertebral joint
CSF	Cerebrospinal fluid in subarachnoid space	PT	Posterior tubercle of C1	VA	Vertebral artery
D	Dens (odontoid) process of C2	S	Spinal cord	VC	Vertebral canal
FJ	Zygapophyseal (facet) joint	Sc	Scalene muscles		
IV	Intervertebral disc	SF	Superior articular facet of C1		
La	Lamina	Sp	Spinous process		
Lu	Lungs	St	Sternomastoid		

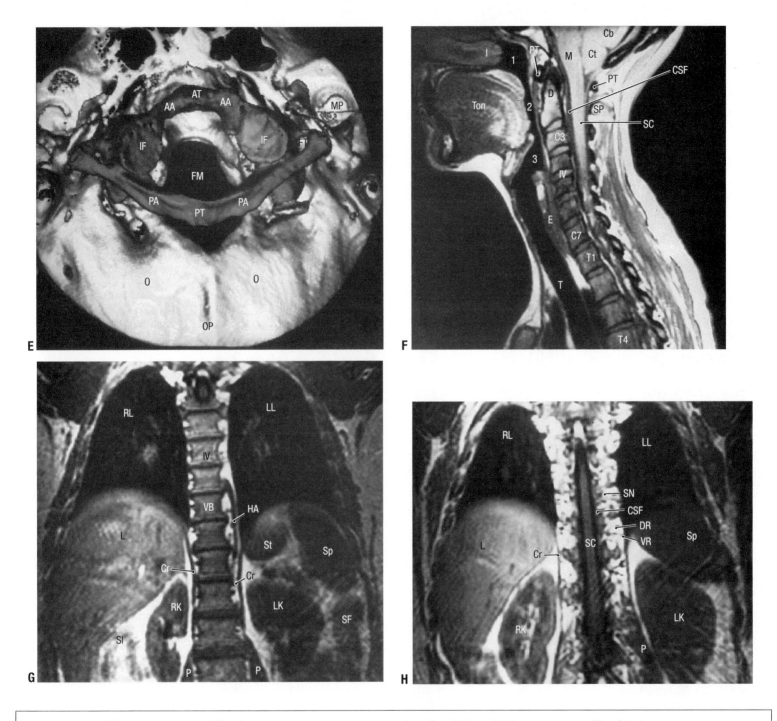

AA	Anterior arch of C1	FM	Foramen magnum	O	Occipital bone of skull	SN	Spinal nerve
AT	Anterior tubercle of C1	FT	Foramen transversarium	OP	External occipital protuberance	SP	Spinous process
C3-T4	Vertebral bodies	HA	Hemiazygos vein	P	Psoas muscle	Sp	Spleen
Cb	Cerebellum	I	Inferior concha	PA	Posterior arch of C1	St	Stomach
Cr	Crus of diaphragm	IF	Inferior articular facet of C1	PT	Posterior tubercle of C1	T	Trachea
CSF	Cerebrospinal fluid in subarachnoid	IV	Intervertebral disc	RK	Right Kidney	Ton	Tongue
	space	L	Liver	RL	Right lung	VB	Vertebral body
Dt	Tonsil of cerebellum	LK	Left kidney	SC	Spinal cord	VR	Ventral primary ramus
D	Dens (odontoid) process of C2	LL	Left lung	SF	Slenic flexure	1	Nasopharynx
DR	Dorsal primary ramus	M	Medulla oblongata	SG	Suprarenal gland	2	Oropharynx
E	Esophagus	MP	Mastoid process	SI	Small intestine	3	Laryngopharynx

E. Three-dimensional computer-generated image of base of skull and atlas (C1), posteroinferior view. **F.** T1 sagittal MRI of cervical and upper thoracic spine, lateral view. **G** and **H.** T1 coronal MRIs of thoracic spine and spinal cord.

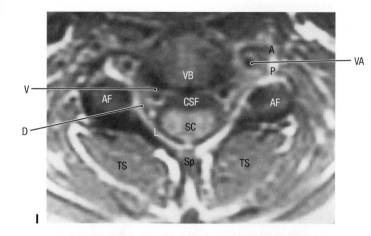

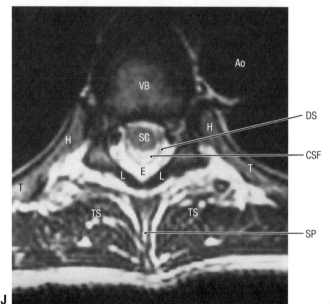

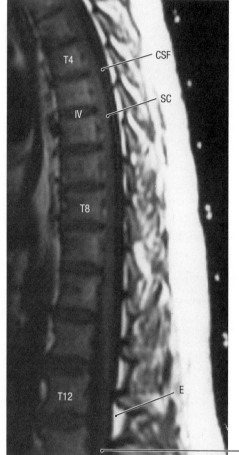

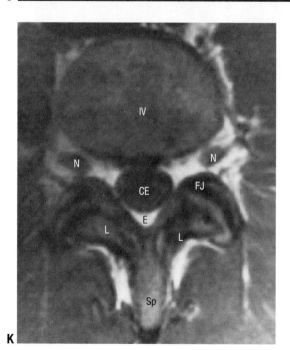

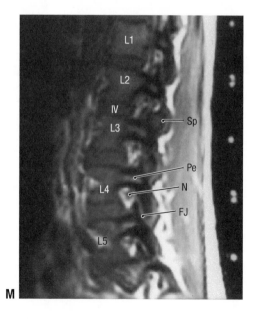

I. T1 axial (transverse) MRI of cervical spine. **J.** T2 axial (transverse) MRI of thoracic spine. **K.** T1 axial (transverse) MRI of lumbar spine. **L.** T1 sagittal MRI of thoracic and upper lumbar spine. **M.** T1 sagittal MRI of lumbar spine.

A	Anterior tubercle
AF	Articular facet
Ao	Aorta
CE	Cauda equina in cerebrospinal fluid
CM	Condus medullaris
CSF	Cerebrospinal fluid in subarachnoid space
D	Dorsal rootlet
DS	Dural sac
E	Epidural (extradural) fat
FJ	Zygapophyseal (facet) joint
H	Head of rib
IV	Intervertebral disc
L	Lamina
N	Spinal nerve in intervertebral foramen
P	Posterior tubercle
Pe	Pedicle
SC	Spinal cord
Sp	Spinous process
T	Tubercle of rib
T4-L5	Vertebral bodies
TS	Transversospinalis muscles
V	Ventral rootlet
VA	Vertebral artery in foramen transversarium
VB	Vertebral body

C H A P T E R   **5**

Lower
Limb

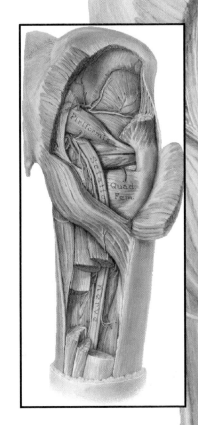

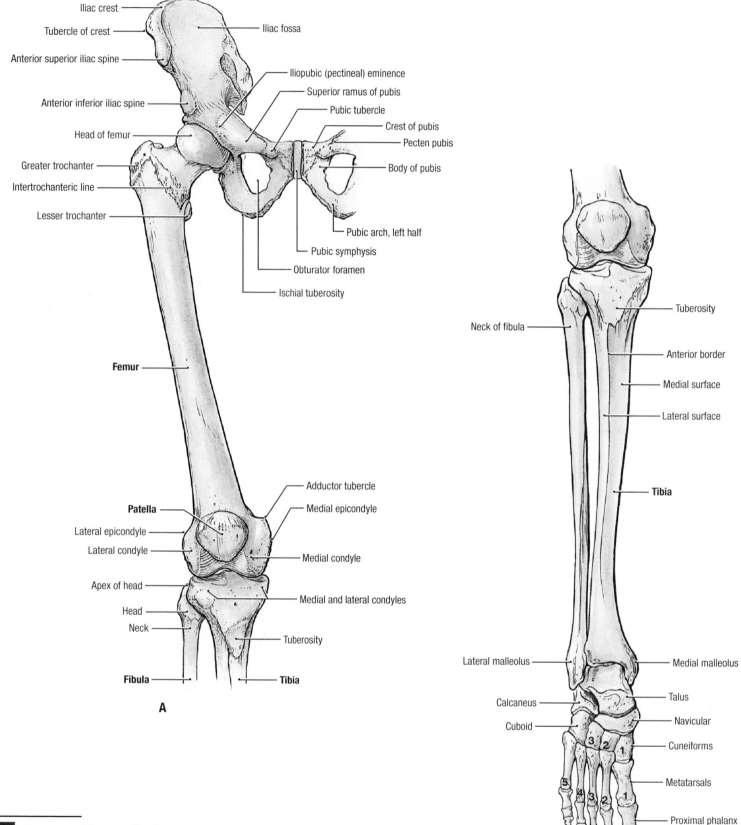

Iliac crest

Tubercle of crest

Anterior superior iliac spine

Anterior inferior iliac spine

Head of femur

Greater trochanter

Intertrochanteric line

Lesser trochanter

Iliac fossa

Iliopubic (pectineal) eminence

Superior ramus of pubis

Pubic tubercle

Crest of pubis

Pecten pubis

Body of pubis

Pubic arch, left half

Pubic symphysis

Obturator foramen

Ischial tuberosity

Femur

Adductor tubercle

Medial epicondyle

Patella

Lateral epicondyle

Lateral condyle

Medial condyle

Apex of head

Head

Neck

Medial and lateral condyles

Tuberosity

Fibula

Tibia

A

Neck of fibula

Tuberosity

Anterior border

Medial surface

Lateral surface

Tibia

Lateral malleolus

Medial malleolus

Calcaneus

Talus

Cuboid

Navicular

Cuneiforms

Metatarsals

Proximal phalanx

Distal phalanx

5.1   **Bones of lower limb**

A. Anterior view.

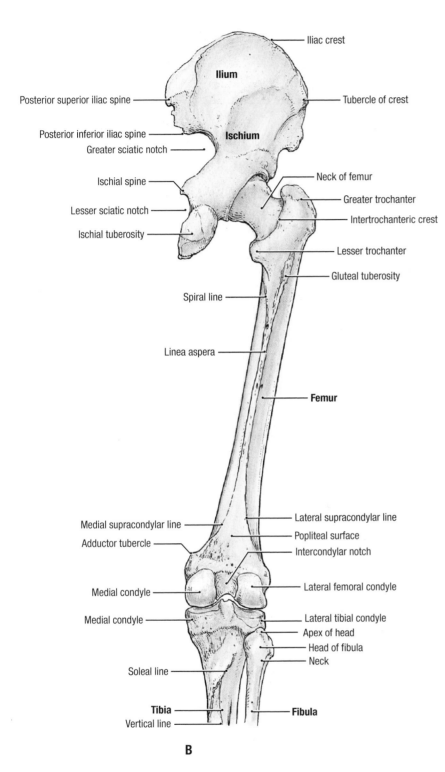

Iliac crest

Ilium

Posterior superior iliac spine

Tubercle of crest

Posterior inferior iliac spine

Ischium

Greater sciatic notch

Neck of femur

Ischial spine

Greater trochanter

Lesser sciatic notch

Intertrochanteric crest

Ischial tuberosity

Lesser trochanter

Gluteal tuberosity

Spiral line

Linea aspera

Femur

Medial supracondylar line

Lateral supracondylar line

Adductor tubercle

Popliteal surface

Intercondylar notch

Medial condyle

Lateral femoral condyle

Medial condyle

Lateral tibial condyle

Apex of head

Head of fibula

Soleal line

Neck

Tibia

Fibula

Vertical line

B

B. Posterior view.

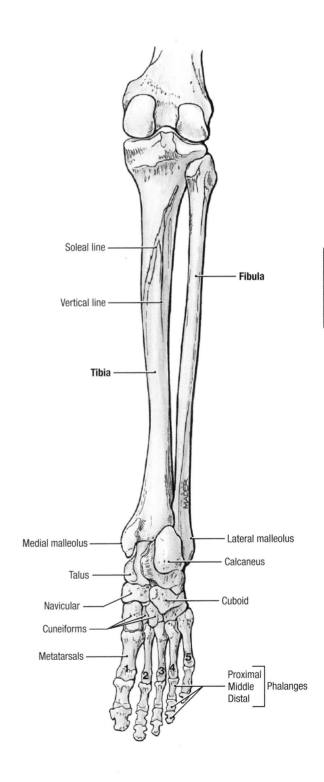

Soleal line

Fibula

Vertical line

Tibia

Medial malleolus

Lateral malleolus

Calcaneus

Talus

Navicular

Cuboid

Cuneiforms

Metatarsals

Proximal
Middle   Phalanges
Distal

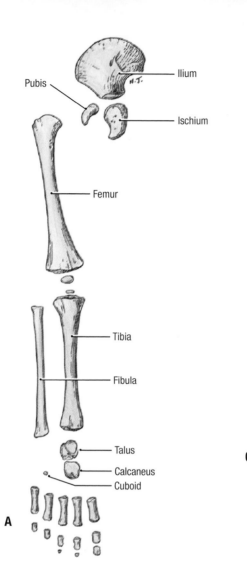

Pubis

Ilium

Ischium

Femur

Tibia

Fibula

Talus

Calcaneus

Cuboid

A

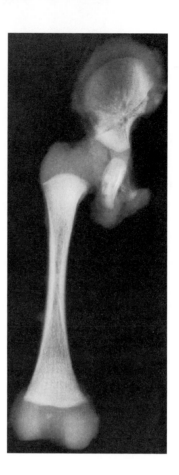

C

5.2   Lower limb development

A. Anterior view. Bones of lower limb at birth. The hip bone can be divided into three primary parts: ilium, ischium, and pubis. The diaphyses (shaft) of the long bones are well ossified. Some epiphyses (growth plates) and tarsal bones have begun to ossify, including the distal epiphysis of the femur, proximal epiphysis of the tibia, calcaneus, talus, and cuboid. **B.** Epiphyses at proximal end of femur, posterior view. The epiphysis of the head begins to ossify during the 1st year, that of the greater trochanter before the 5th year, and that of the lesser trochanter before the 14th year. These usually fuse completely with the body (shaft) before the end of the 18th year, and always by the 20th. **C** and **D.** Anteroposterior radiographs of postmortem specimens of newborns show the bony (white) and cartilaginous (gray) components of the femur and hip bone (os coxae).

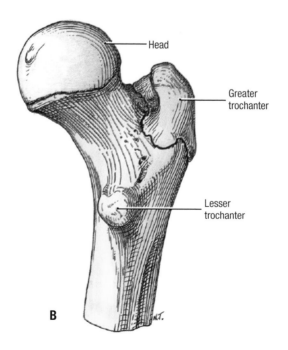

Head

Greater trochanter

Lesser trochanter

B

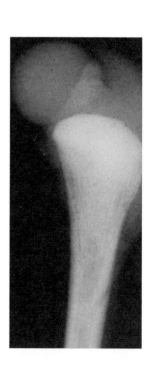

D

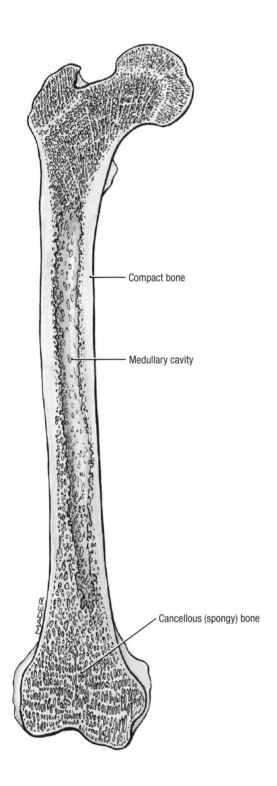

A

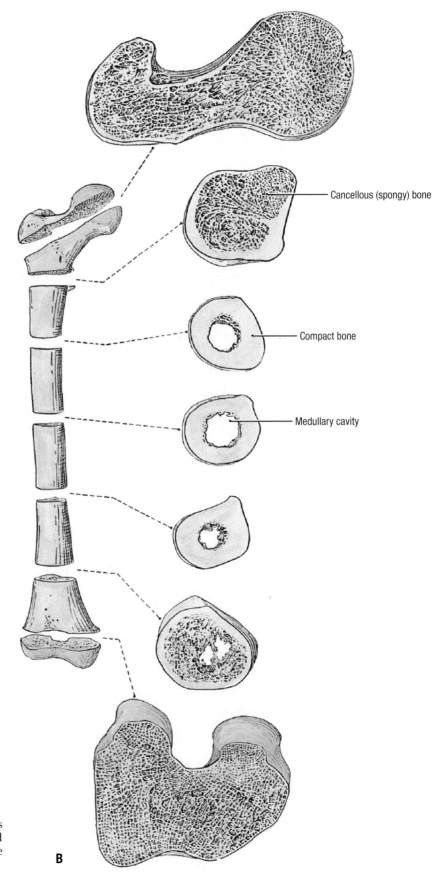

B

5.3 Coronal and transverse sections through femur

A. Coronal section. **B.** Transverse sections. These sections demonstrate the differences in thickness between compact and cancellous (spongy) bone throughout the bone, as well as the width and extent of the medullary cavity (canal).

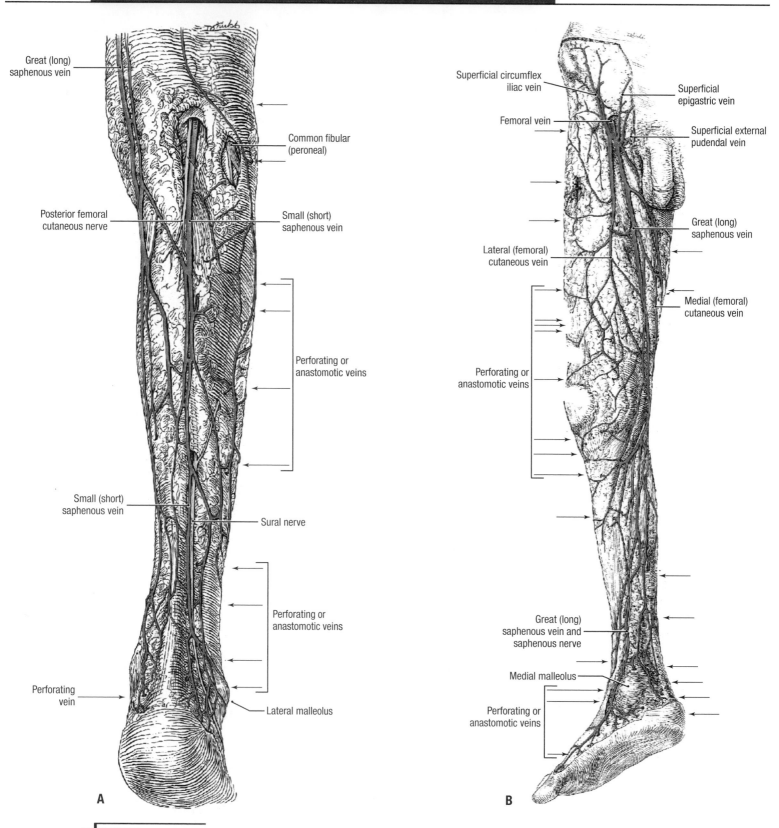

Great (long) saphenous vein

Common fibular (peroneal)

Posterior femoral cutaneous nerve

Small (short) saphenous vein

Perforating or anastomotic veins

Small (short) saphenous vein

Sural nerve

Perforating or anastomotic veins

Perforating vein

Lateral malleolus

Superficial circumflex iliac vein

Superficial epigastric vein

Femoral vein

Superficial external pudendal vein

Great (long) saphenous vein

Lateral (femoral) cutaneous vein

Medial (femoral) cutaneous vein

Perforating or anastomotic veins

Great (long) saphenous vein and saphenous nerve

Medial malleolus

Perforating or anastomotic veins

A   **B**

5.4 Superficial lymphatic drainage of lower limb

A. Anteromedial view. **B.** Posterolateral view. The superficial lymphatic vessels accompany the saphenous veins and their tributaries in the superficial fascia. The lymphatic vessels along the great saphenous vein drain into the superficial inguinal lymph nodes; those along the small saphenous vein drain into the popliteal lymph nodes. Lymph from the superficial inguinal nodes drains to the external iliac and deep inguinal nodes. Lymph from the popliteal nodes ascends through deep lymphatic vessels accompanying the deep blood vessels to the deep inguinal nodes.

5.5 | Superficial veins of lower limb

A. Posterior view. **B.** Anteromedial view. **C.** Lateral view. **D.** Medial view. Note that the superficial veins of the lower limb lie in the subcutaneous fat. *When these veins become enlarged and tortuous, their valves become incompetent and they are termed "varicose veins."* The arrows indicate where anastomotic veins perforate the deep fascia and bring the superficial and deep veins into communication with each other.

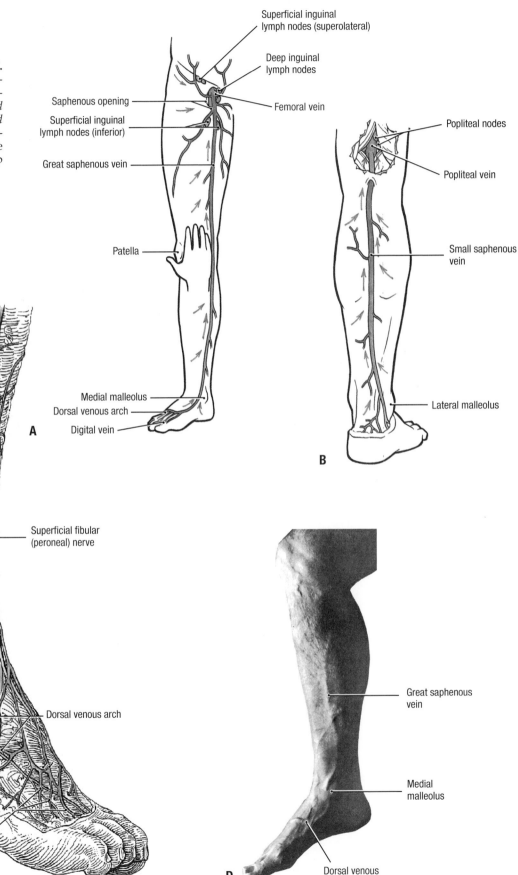

A.

- Superficial inguinal lymph nodes (superolateral)
- Deep inguinal lymph nodes
- Saphenous opening
- Superficial inguinal lymph nodes (inferior)
- Femoral vein
- Great saphenous vein
- Patella
- Medial malleolus
- Dorsal venous arch
- Digital vein

B.

- Popliteal nodes
- Popliteal vein
- Small saphenous vein
- Lateral malleolus

C.

- Small (short) saphenous vein
- Sural nerve
- Superficial fibular (peroneal) nerve
- Dorsal venous arch
- Lateral malleolus
- Common dorsal digital veins

D.

- Great saphenous vein
- Medial malleolus
- Dorsal venous arch of foot

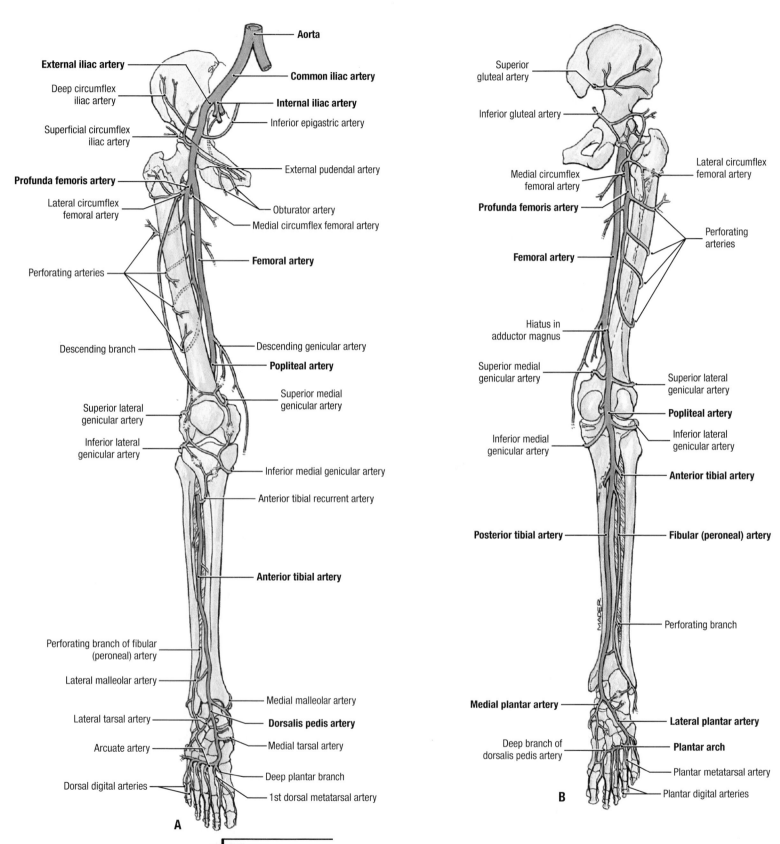

Aorta

External iliac artery

Deep circumflex
iliac artery

Common iliac artery

Superficial circumflex
iliac artery

Internal iliac artery

Inferior epigastric artery

Profunda femoris artery

Lateral circumflex
femoral artery

External pudendal artery

Perforating arteries

Obturator artery

Medial circumflex femoral artery

Femoral artery

Descending branch

Descending genicular artery

Popliteal artery

Superior medial
genicular artery

Superior lateral
genicular artery

Inferior lateral
genicular artery

Inferior medial genicular artery

Anterior tibial recurrent artery

Anterior tibial artery

Perforating branch of fibular
(peroneal) artery

Lateral malleolar artery

Medial malleolar artery

Lateral tarsal artery

Dorsalis pedis artery

Arcuate artery

Medial tarsal artery

Dorsal digital arteries

Deep plantar branch

1st dorsal metatarsal artery

A

Superior
gluteal artery

Inferior gluteal artery

Lateral circumflex
femoral artery

Medial circumflex
femoral artery

Profunda femoris artery

Perforating
arteries

Femoral artery

Hiatus in
adductor magnus

Superior medial
genicular artery

Superior lateral
genicular artery

Popliteal artery

Inferior medial
genicular artery

Inferior lateral
genicular artery

Anterior tibial artery

Posterior tibial artery

Fibular (peroneal) artery

Perforating branch

Medial plantar artery

Lateral plantar artery

Deep branch of
dorsalis pedis artery

Plantar arch

Plantar metatarsal artery

Plantar digital arteries

B

5.6   Overview of arteries of lower limb

A. Anterior view. **B.** Posterior view.

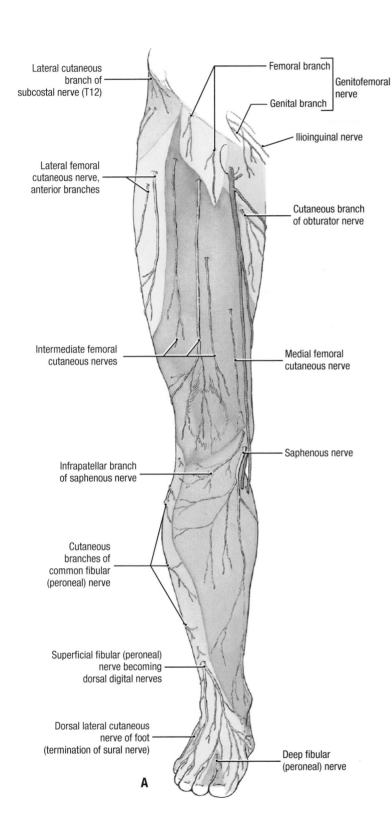

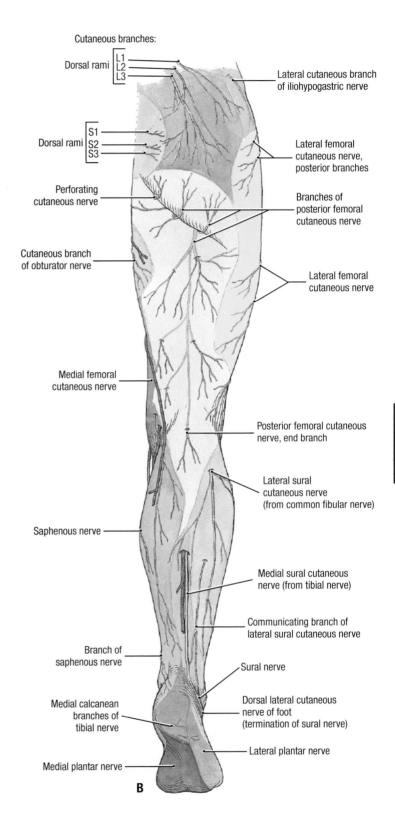

Labels for A (Anterior view):

Lateral cutaneous branch of subcostal nerve (T12)

Femoral branch
Genital branch
Genitofemoral nerve

Ilioinguinal nerve

Lateral femoral cutaneous nerve, anterior branches

Cutaneous branch of obturator nerve

Intermediate femoral cutaneous nerves

Medial femoral cutaneous nerve

Saphenous nerve

Infrapatellar branch of saphenous nerve

Cutaneous branches of common fibular (peroneal) nerve

Superficial fibular (peroneal) nerve becoming dorsal digital nerves

Dorsal lateral cutaneous nerve of foot (termination of sural nerve)

Deep fibular (peroneal) nerve

A

Labels for B (Posterior view):

Cutaneous branches:
Dorsal rami { L1 L2 L3 }

Lateral cutaneous branch of iliohypogastric nerve

Dorsal rami { S1 S2 S3 }

Lateral femoral cutaneous nerve, posterior branches

Perforating cutaneous nerve

Branches of posterior femoral cutaneous nerve

Cutaneous branch of obturator nerve

Lateral femoral cutaneous nerve

Medial femoral cutaneous nerve

Posterior femoral cutaneous nerve, end branch

Lateral sural cutaneous nerve (from common fibular nerve)

Saphenous nerve

Medial sural cutaneous nerve (from tibial nerve)

Communicating branch of lateral sural cutaneous nerve

Branch of saphenous nerve

Sural nerve

Medial calcanean branches of tibial nerve

Dorsal lateral cutaneous nerve of foot (termination of sural nerve)

Lateral plantar nerve

Medial plantar nerve

B

5.7 Cutaneous nerves of lower limb

A. Anterior view. **B.** Posterior view. In **B,** the medial sural cutaneous nerve (*sural* is Latin for the calf) is joined just proximal to the ankle by a communicating branch of the lateral sural cutaneous nerve to form the sural nerve. The level of the junction is variable, and is low in this specimen.

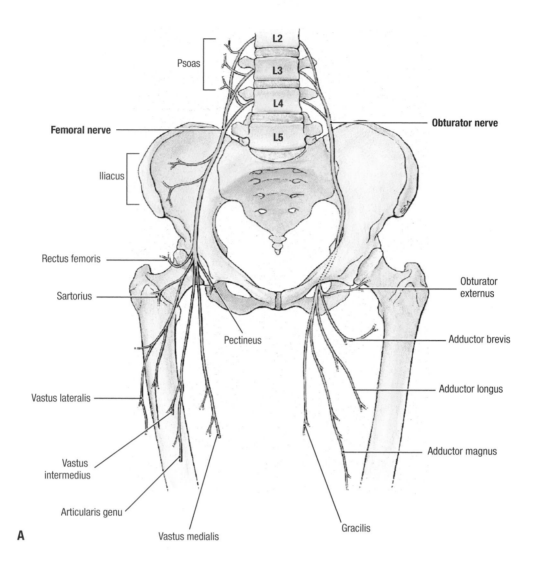

Psoas

Femoral nerve

Obturator nerve

Iliacus

Rectus femoris

Obturator externus

Sartorius

Adductor brevis

Pectineus

Adductor longus

Vastus lateralis

Adductor magnus

Vastus intermedius

Articularis genu

Gracilis

A

Vastus medialis

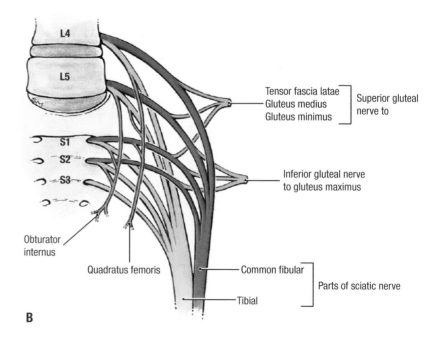

Tensor fascia latae
Gluteus medius
Gluteus minimus

Superior gluteal nerve to

Inferior gluteal nerve to gluteus maximus

Obturator internus

Quadratus femoris

Common fibular

Parts of sciatic nerve

Tibial

B

5.8   Overview of the motor distribution of nerves of lower limb

A. Femoral and obturator nerves, anterior view. The femoral nerve is drawn on the left side of the figure, and the obturator on the right side of the figure, but both nerves are present bilaterally. **B.** Formation of the sciatic nerve in the pelvis, anterior view.

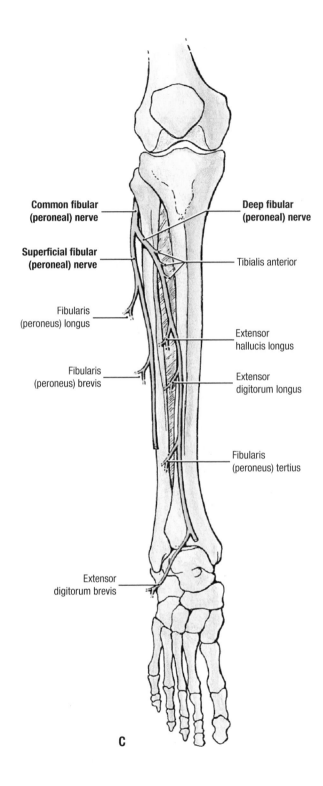

**Common fibular
(peroneal) nerve**

**Superficial fibular
(peroneal) nerve**

Fibularis
(peroneus) longus

Fibularis
(peroneus) brevis

Extensor
digitorum brevis

**Deep fibular
(peroneal) nerve**

Tibialis anterior

Extensor
hallucis longus

Extensor
digitorum longus

Fibularis
(peroneus) tertius

C

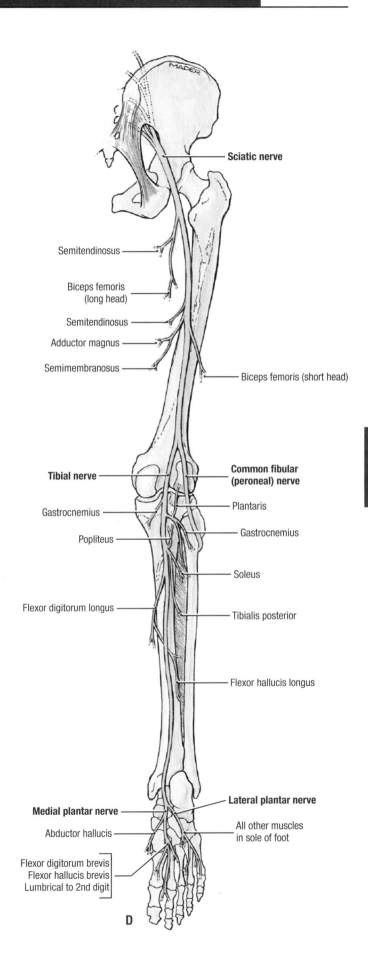

Sciatic nerve

Semitendinosus

Biceps femoris
(long head)

Semitendinosus

Adductor magnus

Semimembranosus

Biceps femoris (short head)

Tibial nerve

Gastrocnemius

Popliteus

Flexor digitorum longus

**Common fibular
(peroneal) nerve**

Plantaris

Gastrocnemius

Soleus

Tibialis posterior

Flexor hallucis longus

Medial plantar nerve

Abductor hallucis

Flexor digitorum brevis
Flexor hallucis brevis
Lumbrical to 2nd digit

Lateral plantar nerve

All other muscles
in sole of foot

D

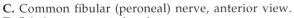

C. Common fibular (peroneal) nerve, anterior view.
D. Sciatic nerve, posterior view.

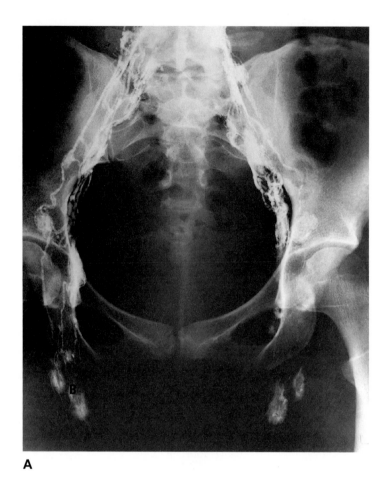

A

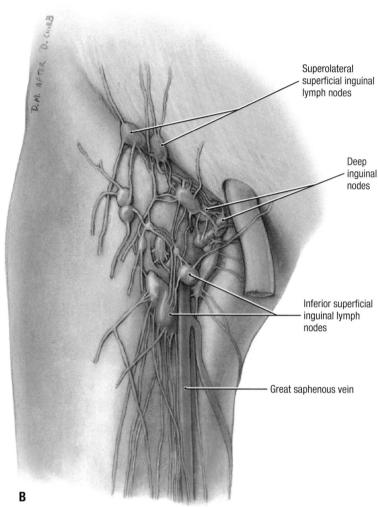

Superolateral superficial inguinal lymph nodes

Deep inguinal nodes

Inferior superficial inguinal lymph nodes

Great saphenous vein

B

5.9   Inguinal lymph nodes

A. Injection, anteroposterior radiograph. **B.** Dissection, anterior view.

OBSERVE:

1. The arrangement of the nodes: (a) a proximal chain parallel to the inguinal ligament (superolateral superficial inguinal nodes); (b) a distal chain on the sides of the great saphenous vein (inferior superficial inguinal nodes); and, proximal to this, (c) a chain of two or three nodes on the medial side of the femoral vein (deep inguinal nodes), one inferior to the femoral canal, and one or two within it;

2. The free anastomosis between the lymph vessels. Approximately 24 efferent vessels leave these nodes and, passing deep to the inguinal ligament, enter the external iliac nodes; of these, fewer than half traverse the femoral canal, and the others ascend alongside the femoral artery and vein, some inside the femoral sheath, and some outside it (see Fig. 5.11 and 5.12).

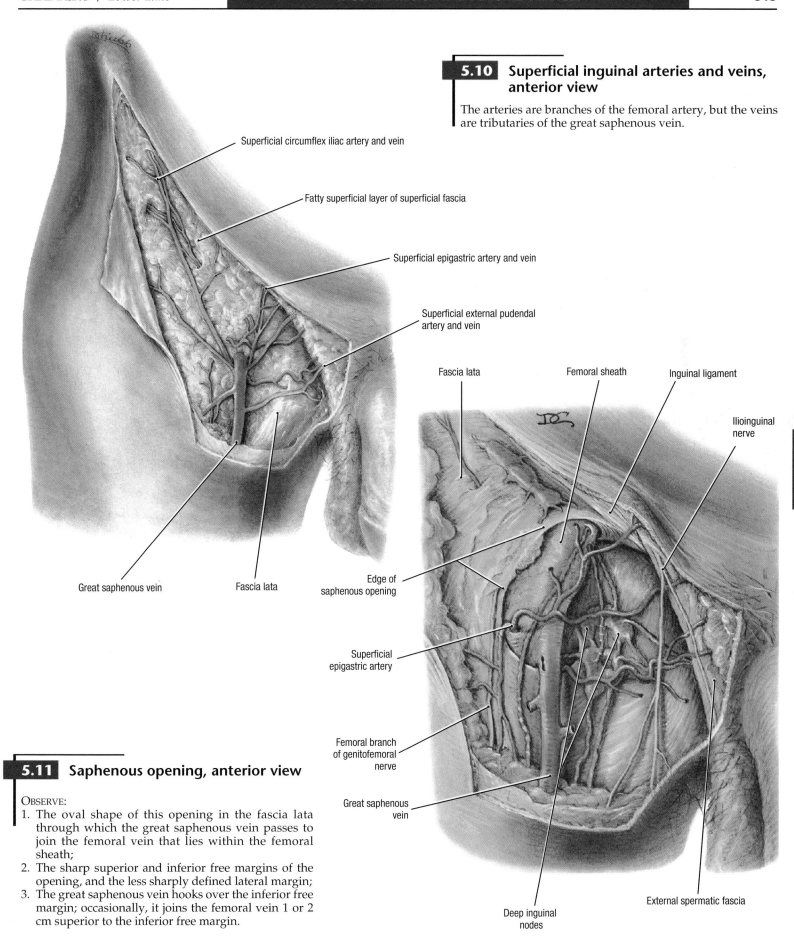

5.10 **Superficial inguinal arteries and veins, anterior view**

The arteries are branches of the femoral artery, but the veins are tributaries of the great saphenous vein.

Superficial circumflex iliac artery and vein

Fatty superficial layer of superficial fascia

Superficial epigastric artery and vein

Superficial external pudendal artery and vein

Great saphenous vein

Fascia lata

Fascia lata

Femoral sheath

Inguinal ligament

Ilioinguinal nerve

Edge of saphenous opening

Superficial epigastric artery

Femoral branch of genitofemoral nerve

Great saphenous vein

Deep inguinal nodes

External spermatic fascia

5.11 **Saphenous opening, anterior view**

OBSERVE:

1. The oval shape of this opening in the fascia lata through which the great saphenous vein passes to join the femoral vein that lies within the femoral sheath;

2. The sharp superior and inferior free margins of the opening, and the less sharply defined lateral margin;

3. The great saphenous vein hooks over the inferior free margin; occasionally, it joins the femoral vein 1 or 2 cm superior to the inferior free margin.

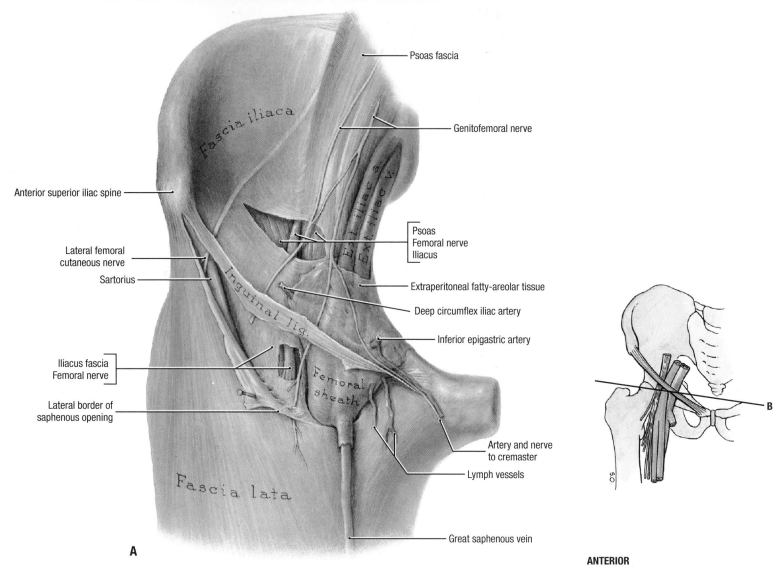

Psoas fascia

Genitofemoral nerve

Fascia iliaca

Anterior superior iliac spine

Psoas
Femoral nerve
Iliacus

Lateral femoral
cutaneous nerve

Sartorius

Inguinal lig.

Extraperitoneal fatty-areolar tissue

Deep circumflex iliac artery

Inferior epigastric artery

Iliacus fascia
Femoral nerve

Lateral border of
saphenous opening

Femoral
sheath

Artery and nerve
to cremaster

Lymph vessels

Fascia lata

Great saphenous vein

A

B

5.12   Femoral sheath

A. Femoral nerve and femoral sheath, anterior view . The three flat muscles of the abdominal wall are cut away from the superior border of the inguinal ligament, and the fascia lata is removed from the inferior border. The lateral margin of the saphenous opening in the fascia lata is cut and reflected, and the inferior epigastric artery is pulled medially. **B.** Transverse section through femoral vessels and nerve. Note that the psoas major tendon separates the femoral artery from the hip joint.

OBSERVE:
1. The iliacus fascia is continuous medially with the psoas fascia and carried inferiorly, anterior to the iliacus muscle, into the thigh; as the iliacus fascia passes posterior to the inguinal ligament, it adheres to the inguinal ligament;
2. The extraperitoneal fatty (areolar) tissue, which lines the abdominal cavity and through which the external iliac vessels run, continues inferiorly around these vessels into the thigh as a delicate, funnel-shaped sac called the femoral sheath;
3. The femoral sheath contains the femoral artery, vein, and lymph vessels; the femoral nerve, lying posterior to the iliacus fascia, is outside the femoral sheath;
4. The lateral margin of the saphenous opening (part of the fascia lata)

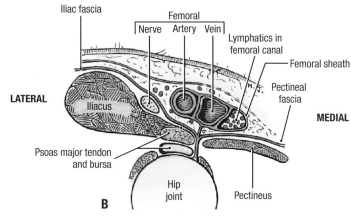

ANTERIOR

Iliac fascia

Femoral

Nerve   Artery   Vein

Lymphatics in
femoral canal

Femoral sheath

Pectineal
fascia

LATERAL

Iliacus

MEDIAL

Psoas major tendon
and bursa

Hip
joint

Pectineus

B

POSTERIOR

lies anterior to the femoral sheath; medially, the fascia passes posterior to the femoral sheath as the pectineal fascia;
5. The genitofemoral nerve pierces the psoas fascia proximally as one or two branches; the lateral femoral cutaneous nerve pierces the iliacus fascia at a variable point, commonly, as here, near the anterior superior iliac spine.

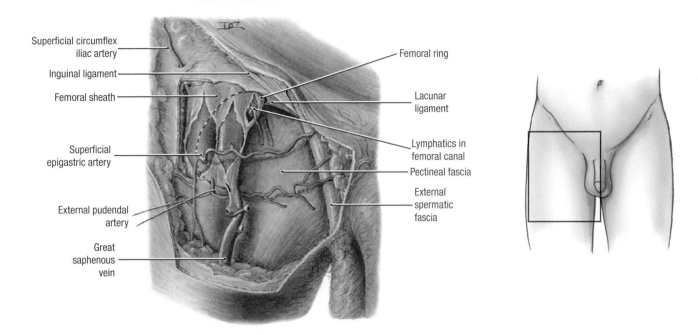

Superficial circumflex iliac artery

Inguinal ligament

Femoral sheath

Superficial epigastric artery

External pudendal artery

Great saphenous vein

Femoral ring

Lacunar ligament

Lymphatics in femoral canal

Pectineal fascia

External spermatic fascia

5.13 Femoral sheath, canal, and ring, anterior view

The lateral margin of the saphenous opening is cut away.

OBSERVE:
1. The superior margin of the opening blends with the inguinal ligament and, in this specimen, with the lacunar ligament;
2. The medial border of the opening is formed by the fascia covering the pectineus muscle and pectineal fascia; the fascia passes posterior to the femoral sheath;

3. The three compartments of the femoral sheath, each incised longitudinally: (a) the lateral compartment for the artery; (b) the middle one for the vein; and (c) the medial one, called the femoral canal, for lymph vessels;
4. The proximal end of the femoral canal, called the femoral ring, is bounded medially by the lacunar ligament, anteriorly by the inguinal ligament, posteriorly by the pectineus muscle and its fascia, and laterally by the femoral vein.

SUPERIOR

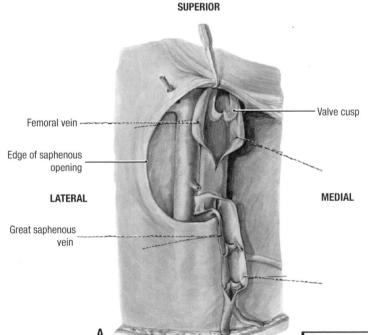

Femoral vein

Edge of saphenous opening

LATERAL

Great saphenous vein

Valve cusp

MEDIAL

A

INFERIOR

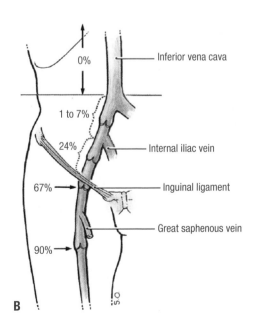

0%

1 to 7%

24%

67%

90%

Inferior vena cava

Internal iliac vein

Inguinal ligament

Great saphenous vein

B

5.14 Valves of proximal part of femoral and great saphenous veins, anterior views

A. Structure of valves. The valve is usually composed of two cusps and permits blood flow toward the heart, but not in the reverse direction. **B.** Percentage incidence of valves between the proximal femoral vein and inferior vena cava.

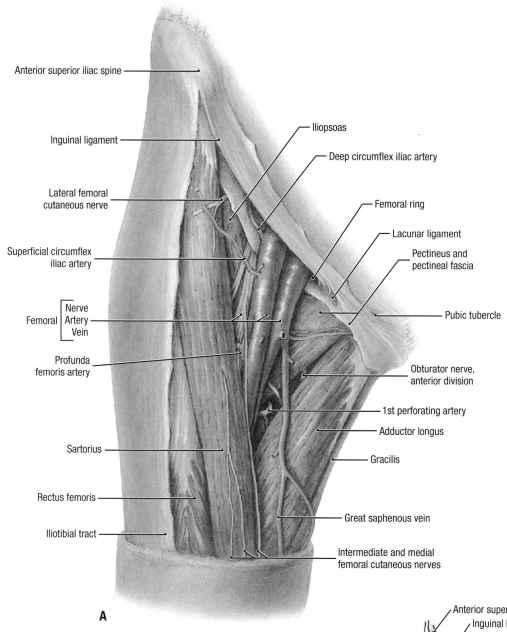

Anterior superior iliac spine

Inguinal ligament

Lateral femoral
cutaneous nerve

Superficial circumflex
iliac artery

Femoral { Nerve
Artery
Vein

Profunda
femoris artery

Sartorius

Rectus femoris

Iliotibial tract

Iliopsoas

Deep circumflex iliac artery

Femoral ring

Lacunar ligament

Pectineus and
pectineal fascia

Pubic tubercle

Obturator nerve,
anterior division

1st perforating artery

Adductor longus

Gracilis

Great saphenous vein

Intermediate and medial
femoral cutaneous nerves

A

5.15   Femoral triangle, anterior views

A. Dissection. **B.** Femoral artery.

OBSERVE:
1. The boundaries of the triangle: (a) the inguinal ligament, which curves from the anterior superior iliac spine to the pubic tubercle, forming the base; (b) the medial border of the sartorius muscle, forming the lateral side; (c) the medial border of the adductor longus muscle, forming the medial side (some authors regard the lateral border of the adductor longus muscle as the medial side of the triangle); and (d) the point at which the two converging sides meet distally, forming the apex;
2. The femoral artery and vein lie anterior to the fascia covering the iliopsoas and pectineus muscles, and the femoral nerve lies posterior to the fascia;
3. The femoral artery appears midway between the anterior superior iliac spine and pubic tubercle, and disappears where the medial border of the sartorius muscle crosses the lateral border of the adductor longus muscle. *Pulsation of the femoral artery can be felt just distal to the inguinal ligament, midway between the anterior superior iliac spine and the pubic tubercle;*
4. When the adjacent borders of the pectineus and adductor longus muscles are not contiguous, as in this specimen, the anterior branch of the obturator nerve is more visible.

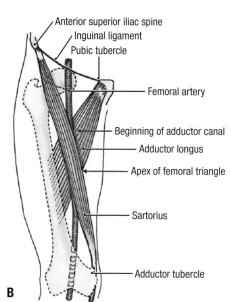

Anterior superior iliac spine
Inguinal ligament
Pubic tubercle

Femoral artery

Beginning of adductor canal

Adductor longus

Apex of femoral triangle

Sartorius

Adductor tubercle

B

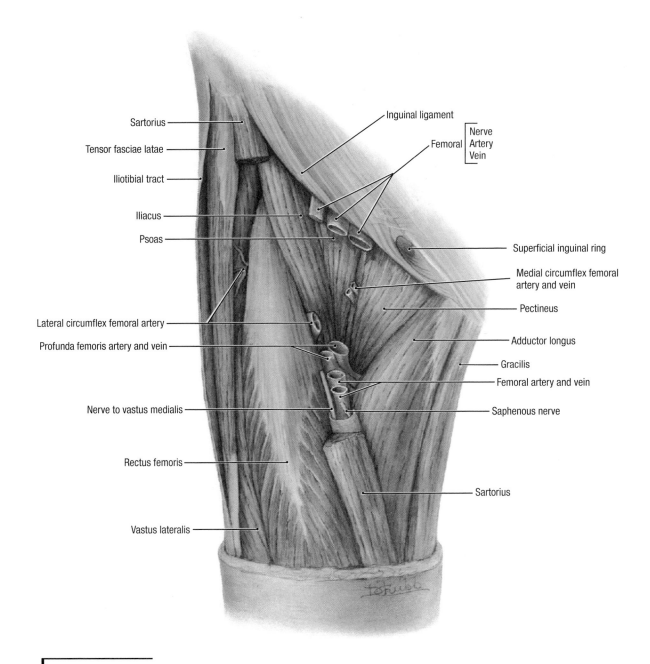

Sartorius

Tensor fasciae latae

Iliotibial tract

Iliacus

Psoas

Lateral circumflex femoral artery

Profunda femoris artery and vein

Nerve to vastus medialis

Rectus femoris

Vastus lateralis

Inguinal ligament

Femoral { Nerve / Artery / Vein }

Superficial inguinal ring

Medial circumflex femoral artery and vein

Pectineus

Adductor longus

Gracilis

Femoral artery and vein

Saphenous nerve

Sartorius

5.16 Floor of femoral triangle, anterior view

Sections are removed from the sartorius muscle, femoral vessels, and femoral nerve.

OBSERVE:
1. The floor of the triangle is a "trough," with sloping lateral and medial walls; the trough is shallow at the base and deep at the apex;
2. At the apex of the femoral triangle, four vessels (the femoral artery and vein and the profunda femoris artery and vein) and two nerves (the nerve to vastus medialis and the saphenous nerve) pass into the adductor (subsartorial) canal, which is located deep to the sartorius muscle.

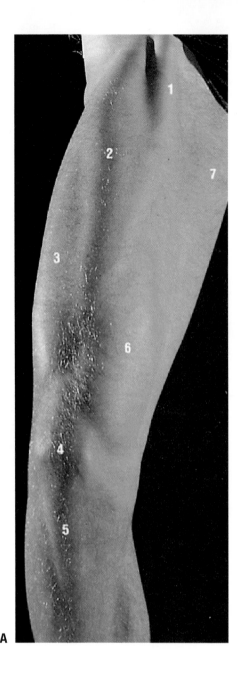

A

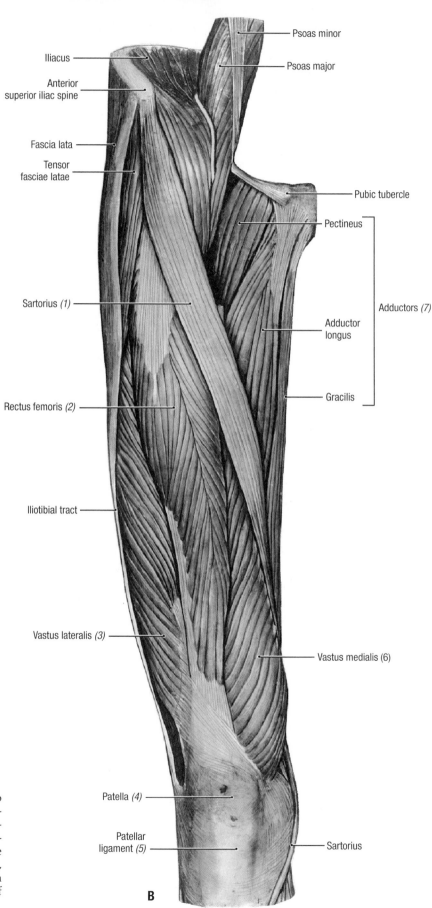

Psoas minor

Iliacus

Psoas major

Anterior
superior iliac spine

Fascia lata

Pubic tubercle

Tensor
fasciae latae

Pectineus

Sartorius *(1)*

Adductors *(7)*

Adductor
longus

Rectus femoris *(2)*

Gracilis

Iliotibial tract

Vastus lateralis *(3)*

Vastus medialis (6)

Patella *(4)*

Patellar
ligament *(5)*

Sartorius

B

5.17   Anterior and medial thigh muscles–I

A. Surface anatomy, anteromedial view. (Numbers refer to structures in **B.**) The quadriceps (consisting of the vastus lateralis, medialis, and intermedius and rectus femoris muscles) insert on the patella and, through the patellar ligament, to the tibial tuberosity. The vastus medialis muscle attaches to the base and proximal two thirds of the medial surface of the patella, and the vastus lateralis attaches mainly to the base of the patella and slightly onto the lateral surface. **B.** Superficial dissection of muscles of anterior and medial aspects of thigh, anterior view.

Table 5.1. Anterior Thigh Muscles

Muscle	Proximal Attachment	Distal Attachment	Innervation[a]	Main Actions
Iliopsoas				
Psoas major	Sides of T12–L5 vertebrae and discs between them; transverse processes of all lumbar vertebrae	Lesser trochanter of femur	Ventral rami of lumbar nerves (**L1**, **L2**, and L3)	Acting jointly in flexing thigh at hip joint and in stabilizing this joint[b]
Iliacus	Iliac crest, iliac fossa, ala of sacrum, and anterior sacroiliac ligaments	Tendon of psoas major, lesser trochanter, and femur distal to it	Femoral nerve (**L2** and L3)	
Tensor fasciae latae	Anterior superior iliac spine and anterior part of iliac crest	Iliotibial tract that attaches to lateral condyle of tibia	Superior gluteal (L4 and L5)	Abducts, medially rotates, and flexes thigh; helps to keep knee extended; steadies trunk on thigh
Sartorius	Anterior superior iliac spine and superior part of notch inferior to it	Superior part of medial surface of tibia	Femoral nerve (L2 and L3)	Flexes, abducts, and laterally rotates thigh at hip joint; flexes leg at knee joint[c]
Quadiceps femoris				
Rectus femoris	Anterior inferior iliac spine and ilium superior to acetabulum	Base of patella and by patellar ligament to tibial tuberosity	Femoral nerve (L2, **L3**, and **L4**)	Extended leg at knee joint; rectus femoris also steadies hip joint and helps iliopsoas to flex thigh
Vastus lateralis	Greater trochanter and lateral lip of linea aspera of femur			
Vastus medialis	Intertrochanteric line and medial lip of linea aspera of femur			
Vastus intermedius	Anterior and lateral surfaces of body of femur			

[a] Numbers indicate spinal cord segmental innervation of nerves (e.g., **L1**, **L2**, and **L3** indicate that nerves supplying psoas major are derived from first three lumbar segments of the spinal cord; boldface type [**L1**, **L2**] indicates main segmental innervation). Damage to one or more of these spinal cord segments or to motor nerve roots arising from these segments results in paralysis of the muscles concerned.

[b] Psoas major is also a postural muscle that helps control deviation of trunk and is active during standing.

[c] Four actions of sartorius (L. sartor, tailor) produce the once common cross-legged sitting position used by tailors—hence the name.

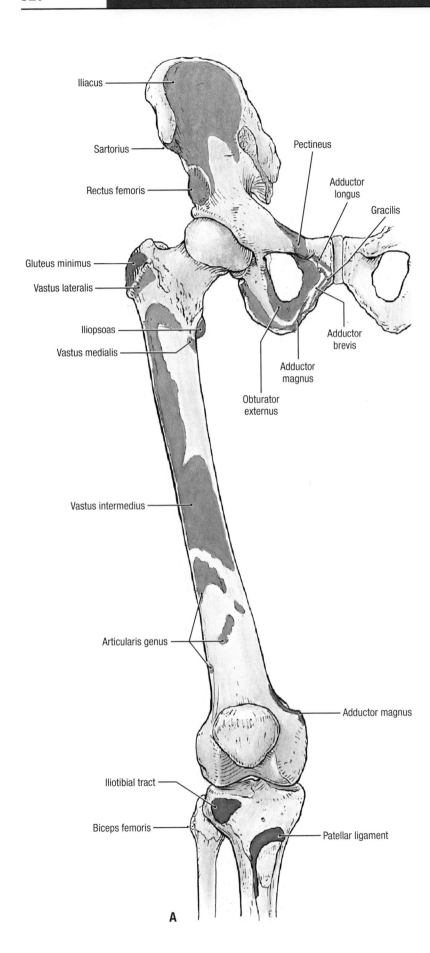

Iliacus

Sartorius

Rectus femoris

Pectineus

Adductor longus

Gracilis

Gluteus minimus

Vastus lateralis

Iliopsoas

Vastus medialis

Adductor brevis

Adductor magnus

Obturator externus

Vastus intermedius

Articularis genus

Adductor magnus

Iliotibial tract

Biceps femoris

Patellar ligament

A

5.18   Bones of lower limb showing muscle attachments

A. Anterior view.

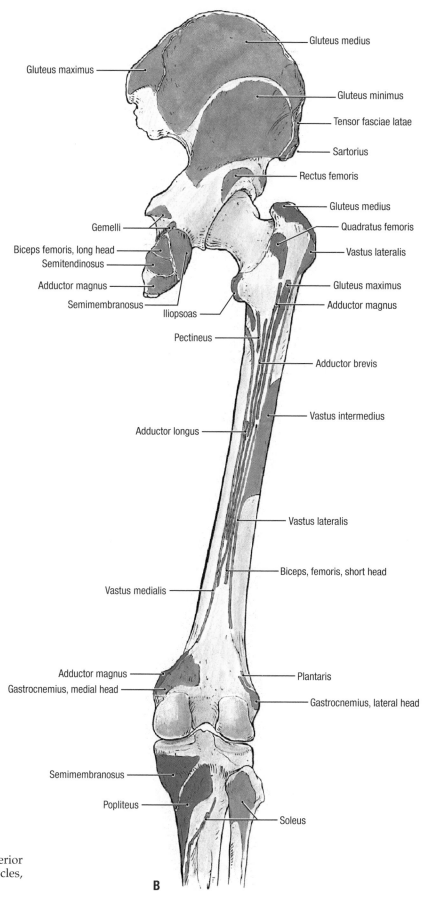

B. Posterior view. This figure illustrates attachments of the anterior (Table 5.1), medial (Table 5.2), and posterior (Table 5.3) thigh muscles, and the gluteal muscles (Table 5.4).

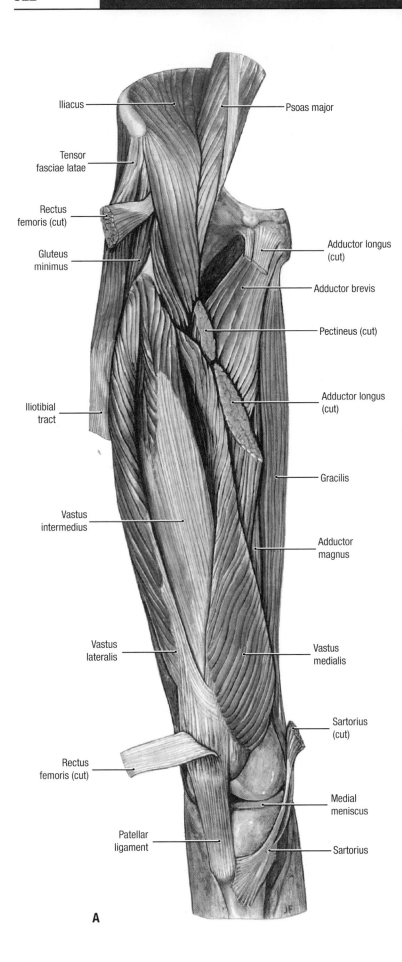

Iliacus

Tensor
fasciae latae

Rectus
femoris (cut)

Gluteus
minimus

Iliotibial
tract

Vastus
intermedius

Vastus
lateralis

Rectus
femoris (cut)

Patellar
ligament

A

Psoas major

Adductor longus
(cut)

Adductor brevis

Pectineus (cut)

Adductor longus
(cut)

Gracilis

Adductor
magnus

Vastus
medialis

Sartorius
(cut)

Medial
meniscus

Sartorius

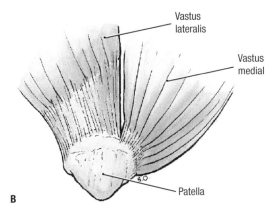

Vastus
lateralis

Vastus
medial

Patella

B

5.19   Anterior and medial thigh muscles–II, anterior views

A. Deep dissection of muscles of the anterior and medial aspects of thigh. Note that the central portions of the muscle bellies of the sartorius, rectus femoris, pectineus, and adductor longus muscles have been removed. **B.** Patellar attachment of vastus medialis and lateralis muscles

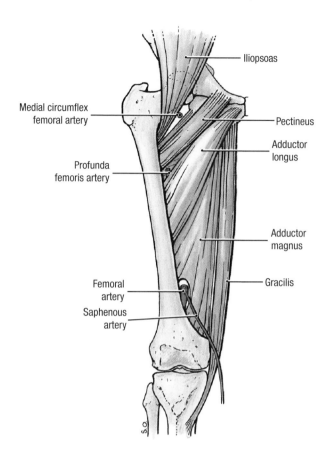

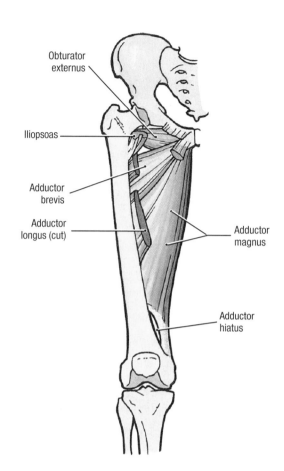

Table 5.2. Medial Thigh Muscles

Muscle	Proximal Attachment	Distal Attachment[a]	Innervation[b]	Main Actions
Pectineus	Superior ramus of pubis	Pectineal line of femur, just inferior to lesser trochanter	Femoral nerve (**L2** and L3); may receive a branch from obturator nerve	Adducts and flexes thigh; assists with medial rotation of thigh
Adductor longus	Body of pubis inferior to pubic rest	Middle third of linea aspera of femur	Obturator nerve, anterior branch (L2, **L3**, and L4)	Adducts thigh
Adductor brevis	Body and inferior ramus of pubis	Pectineal line and proximal part of linea aspera of femur	Obturator nerve (L2, **L3**, and L4)	Adducts thigh and, to some extent, flexes it
Adductor magnus	Inferior ramus of pubis, ramus of ischium (adductor part), and ischial tuberosity	Gluteal tuberosity, linea aspera, medial supracondylar line (adductor part), and adductor tubercle of femur (hamstring part)	*Adductor part:* obturator nerve (L2, **L3**, and **L4**) *Hamstring part:* tibial part of sciatic nerve (**L4**)	Adducts thigh; its adductor part also flexes thigh, and its hamstring part extends it
Gracilis	Body and inferior ramus of pubis	Superior part of medial surface of tibia	Obturator nerve (**L2** and L3)	Adducts thigh, flexes leg, and helps rotate it medially
Obturator externus	Margins of obturator foramen and obturator membrane	Trochanteric fossa of femur	Obturator nerve (L3 and **L4**)	Laterally rotates thigh; steadies head of femur in acetabulum

Collectively, the first five muscles listed are the adductors of the thigh, but their actions are more complex (e.g., they act as flexors of the hip joint during flexion of the knee joint and are active during walking).
[a] See Figure 5.22 for muscle attachments.
[b] See Table 5.1 for explanation of segmental innervation.

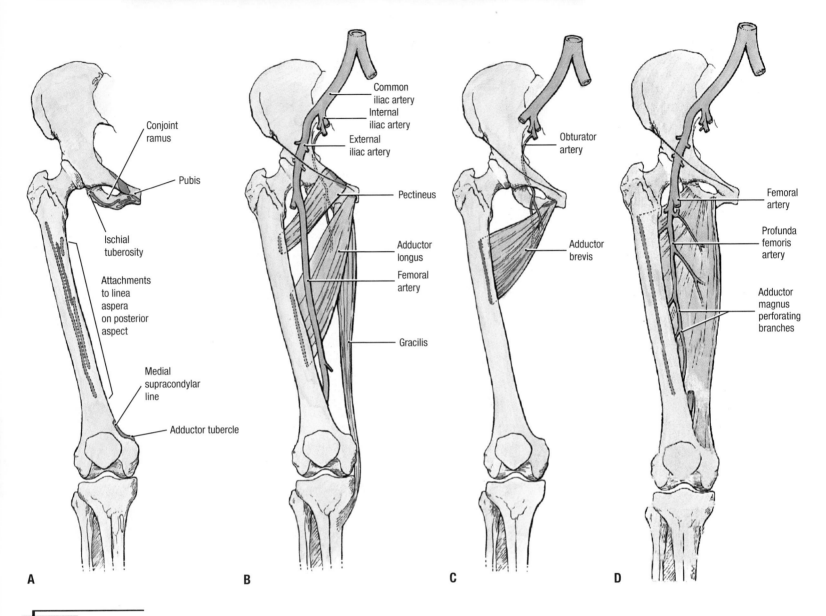

5.20　Adductor muscles of thigh, anterior views

A. Attachments. **B.** Superficial. **C.** Intermediate. **D.** Deep.

OBSERVE:

1. Each of the adductor group of thigh muscles has a linear attachment to the linea aspera on the posterior surface of the femur. While each adducts the thigh, their attachments disclose other actions; for example, the pectineus muscle flexes the thigh, and the gracilis muscle flexes the leg and rotates it medially (see Table 5.2). All contribute to normal gait and posture;

2. In **A,** the distal attachments of the adductor muscles are seen from an anterior view as through a transparent femur. Most medial (green) are the insertions of the pectineus muscle (more proximal) and adductor longus muscle (more distal); the adductor brevis muscle (blue) is intermediate; and the adductor magnus muscle (red) is most lateral, but swings medially to reach the adductor tubercle;

3. In **B,** the superficial layer includes the pectineus, adductor longus, and gracilis muscles; the gracilis alone avoids the femur and attaches on the medial side of the proximal tibia;

4. In **C,** the adductor brevis muscle attaches to the intermediate area of the linea aspera;

5. In **D,** the adductor magnus muscle is deepest, attaches most laterally on the femur, and has the most extensive origin and insertion. Its aponeurosis is punctured by perforating arteries, and the femoral artery passes through the hiatus in its insertion (the adductor hiatus);

Blood supply:

6. In **C,** the obturator artery, a branch of the internal iliac artery, passes through the obturator foramen and divides into anterior and posterior branches, which anastomose with each other and adjacent arteries; the anterior branch supplies the adductor muscles, and the posterior branch supplies hamstring muscles and sends an acetabular branch to the head of the femur;

7. In **B** and **D,** the external iliac artery becomes the femoral artery as it passes posterior to the inguinal ligament; it travels first in the femoral triangle and then in the adductor canal, supplying thigh muscles of the flexor and adductor groups. As the femoral artery passes into the popliteal fossa through the hiatus in the adductor magnus muscle, it becomes the popliteal artery.

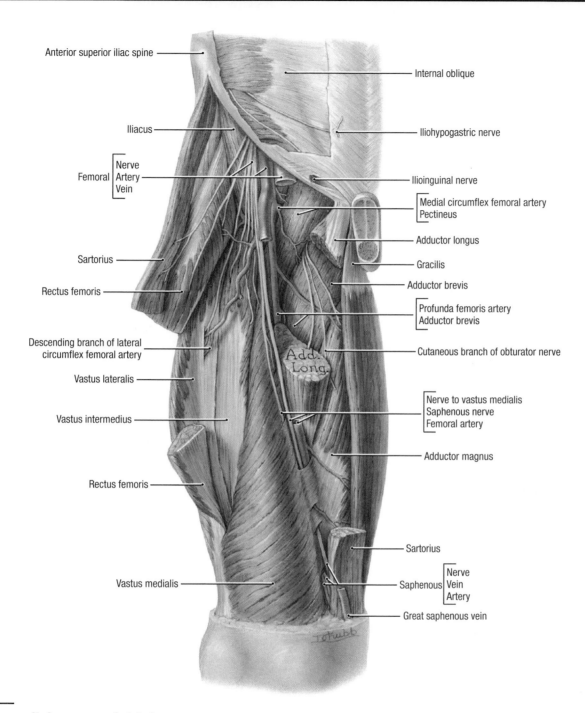

Anterior superior iliac spine

Internal oblique

Iliacus

Iliohypogastric nerve

Femoral { Nerve / Artery / Vein

Ilioinguinal nerve

Medial circumflex femoral artery / Pectineus

Adductor longus

Sartorius

Gracilis

Rectus femoris

Adductor brevis

Profunda femoris artery / Adductor brevis

Descending branch of lateral circumflex femoral artery

Add. Long.

Cutaneous branch of obturator nerve

Vastus lateralis

Vastus intermedius

Nerve to vastus medialis / Saphenous nerve / Femoral artery

Adductor magnus

Rectus femoris

Sartorius

Saphenous { Nerve / Vein / Artery

Vastus medialis

Great saphenous vein

5.21   Anteromedial aspect of thigh

OBSERVE:
1. The limb is rotated laterally;
2. The femoral nerve breaks up into several nerves on entering the thigh;
3. The femoral artery lies between two motor territories: the obturator nerve, which is medial, and the femoral nerve, which is lateral. No motor nerve crosses anterior to the femoral artery, but the twig to the pectineus muscle crosses posterior to the femoral artery;
4. The nerve to the vastus medialis muscle and the saphenous nerve accompany the femoral artery into the adductor canal; the saphenous nerve and artery and their companion anastomotic vein

emerge from the canal distally between the sartorius and gracilis muscles;
5. The profunda femoris artery arises approximately 4 cm inferior to the inguinal ligament, lies posterior to the femoral artery, and disappears posterior to the adductor longus muscle; it supplies the thigh through the medial and lateral circumflex femoral branches and the perforating arteries that pass through the adductor magnus muscle on their way to the posterior aspect of the thigh. Both the femoral and lateral femoral circumflex arteries have descending genicular branches that contribute to the anastomoses around the knee.

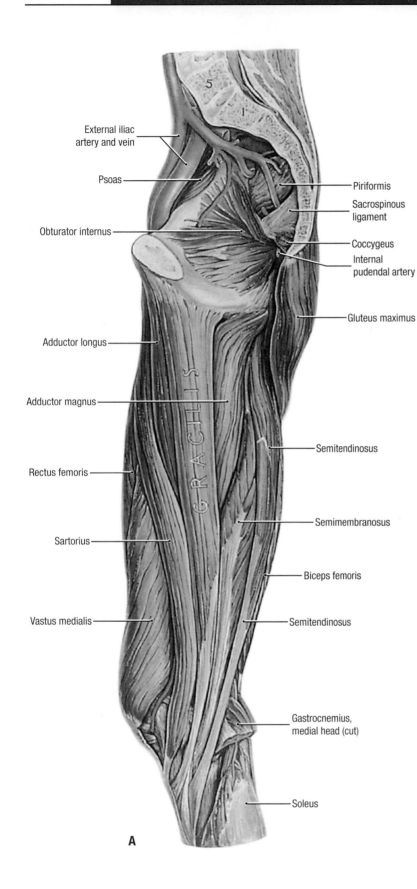

External iliac
artery and vein

Psoas

Obturator internus

Adductor longus

Adductor magnus

Rectus femoris

Sartorius

Vastus medialis

GRACILIS

Piriformis

Sacrospinous
ligament

Coccygeus

Internal
pudendal artery

Gluteus maximus

Semitendinosus

Semimembranosus

Biceps femoris

Semitendinosus

Gastrocnemius,
medial head (cut)

Soleus

A

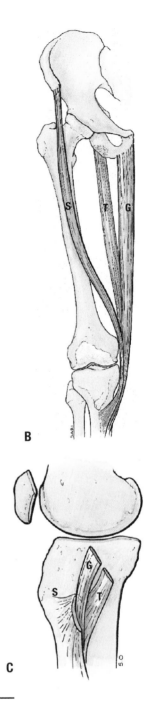

B

C

5.22 Muscles of medial aspect of thigh, medial view

A. Relationships of sartorius, gracilis, and semitendinosus muscles. **B.** Muscular tripod. The sartorius (*S*), gracilis (*G*), and semitendinosus (*T*) muscles form an inverted "tripod," with its base separated at the hip bone and its three legs converging to form an apex on the medial side of the proximal end of the tibia. From examining their attachments, it can be seen that all three muscles flex the knee, but the sartorius is a lateral rotator and abductor, whereas the gracilis is a medial rotator and adductor. **C.** Insertion of tripod to the tibia. All three tendons become thin aponeuroses; the aponeurotic fibers of the sartorius muscle curve posteriorly superior to the insertion of the gracilis muscle.

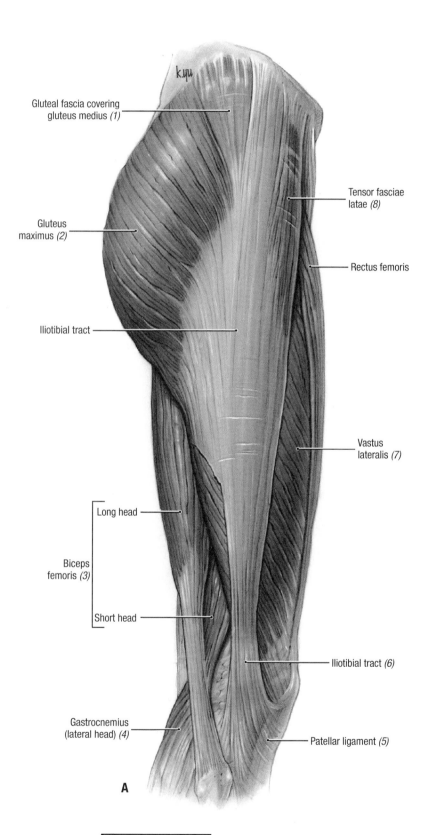

Gluteal fascia covering gluteus medius *(1)*

Gluteus maximus *(2)*

Iliotibial tract

Long head

Biceps femoris *(3)*

Short head

Gastrocnemius (lateral head) *(4)*

Tensor fasciae latae *(8)*

Rectus femoris

Vastus lateralis *(7)*

Iliotibial tract *(6)*

Patellar ligament *(5)*

A

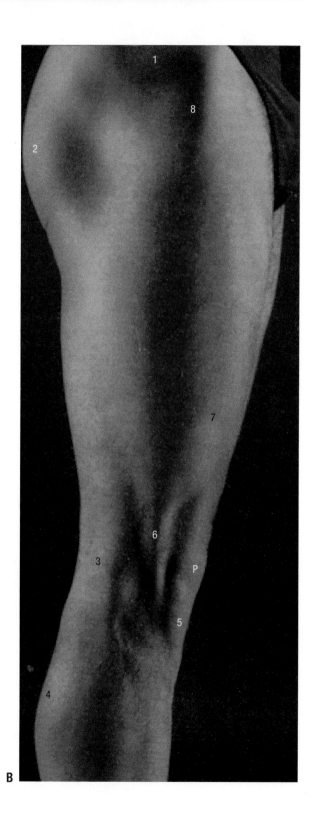

B

5.23   **Lateral aspect of thigh, lateral views**

A. Lateral aspect of thigh. **B.** Surface anatomy of lateral aspect of thigh. (Numbers refer to structures in **A**). The posterior edge of the iliotibial tract (a thickening of the fascia lata) attaches to the lateral condyle of the tibia; the biceps femoris tendon inserts on the head of the fibula; the patella (*P*).

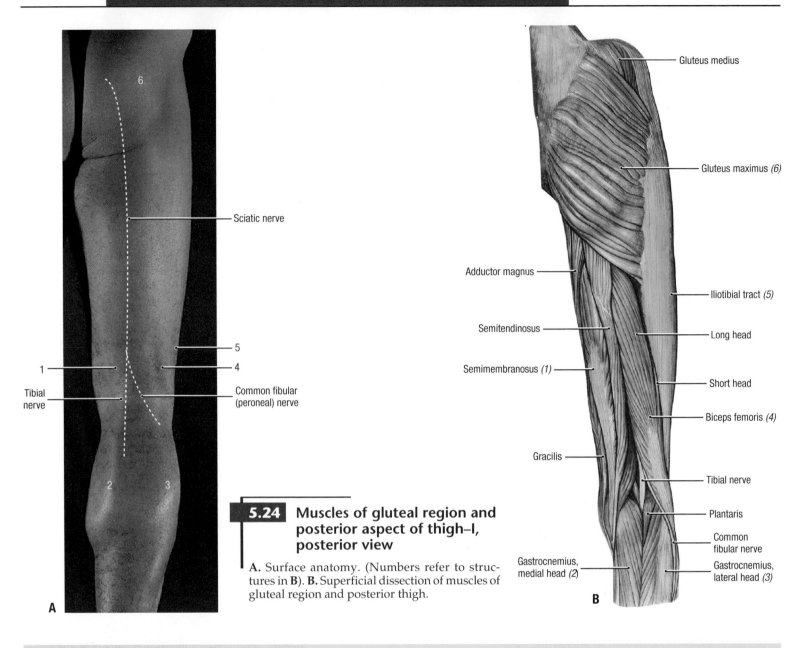

5.24 Muscles of gluteal region and posterior aspect of thigh–I, posterior view

A. Surface anatomy. (Numbers refer to structures in **B**). **B.** Superficial dissection of muscles of gluteal region and posterior thigh.

Table 5.3. Posterior Thigh Muscles

Muscle[a]	Proximal Attachment[b]	Distal Attachment[a]	Innervation[c]	Main Actions
Semitendinosus	Ischial tuberosity	Medial surface of superior part of tibia	Tibial division of sciatic nerve (**L5**, **S1**, and S2)	Extend thigh; flex leg and rotate it medially; when thigh and leg are flexed, they can extend trunk
Semimembranosus	Ischial tuberosity	Posterior part of medial condyle of tibia	Tibial division of sciatic nerve (**L5**, **S1**, and S2)	
Biceps femoris	Long head: ischial tuberosity; Short head: linea aspera and lateral supracondylar line of femur	Lateral side of head of fibula; tendon is split at this site by fibular collateral ligament of knee	*Long head:* tibial division of sciatic nerve (L5, **S1**, and S2); *Short head:* common fibular (peroneal) division of sciatic nerve (L5, **S1**, and S2)	Flexes leg and rotates it laterally; extends thigh (e.g., when starting to walk)

[a]Collectively these three muscles are known as hamstrings.
[b]See Figure 5.18 for muscle attachments.
[c]See Table 5.1 for explanation of segmental innervation.

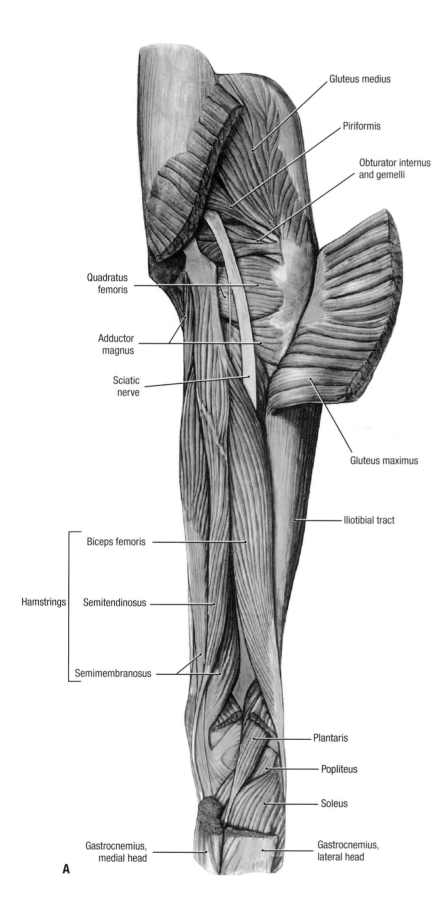

A

Gluteus medius

Piriformis

Obturator internus
and gemelli

Quadratus
femoris

Adductor
magnus

Sciatic
nerve

Gluteus maximus

Iliotibial tract

Biceps femoris

Hamstrings

Semitendinosus

Semimembranosus

Plantaris

Popliteus

Soleus

Gastrocnemius,
medial head

Gastrocnemius,
lateral head

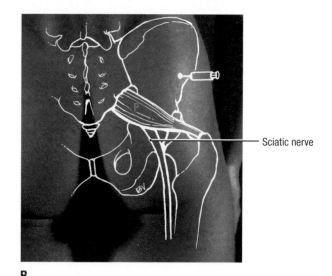

B

Sciatic nerve

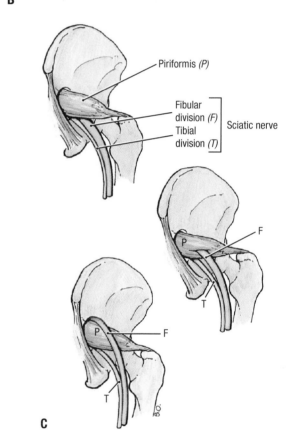

C

Piriformis *(P)*

Fibular
division *(F)*

Tibial
division *(T)*

Sciatic nerve

5.25   **Muscles of gluteal region and posterior aspect of thigh–II, posterior views**

A. Muscles of gluteal region and posterior thigh with gluteus maximus reflected. **B.** Intragluteal injection. *Injections can be made safely only into the superolateral part of the buttock, avoiding injury to the sciatic and gluteal nerves.* **C.** Relationship of sciatic nerve to piriformis muscle. Of 640 limbs studied in our laboratory, in 87% (top), the tibial and fibular (peroneal) divisions passed inferior to the piriformis; in 12.2% (right), the fibular (peroneal) division passed through the piriformis; and in 0.5% (bottom) the fibular (peroneal) division passed superior to the piriformis.

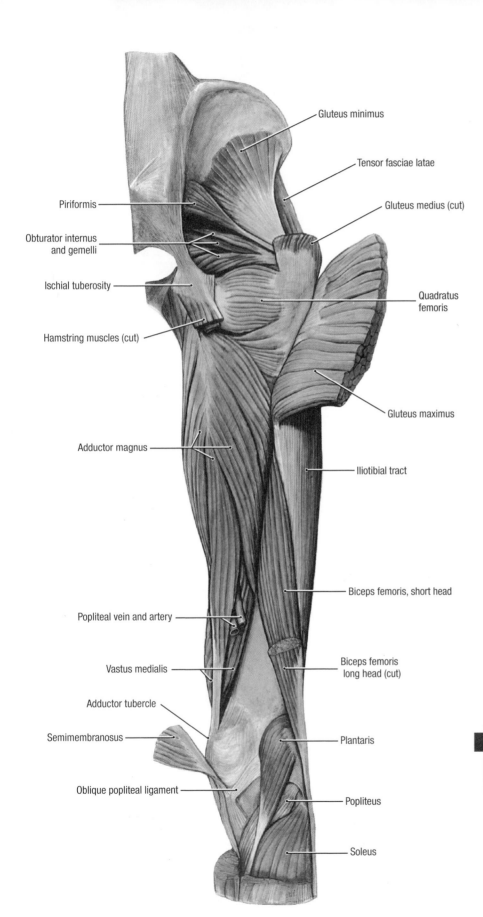

Gluteus minimus

Tensor fasciae latae

Piriformis

Gluteus medius (cut)

Obturator internus
and gemelli

Ischial tuberosity

Quadratus
femoris

Hamstring muscles (cut)

Gluteus maximus

Adductor magnus

Iliotibial tract

Biceps femoris, short head

Popliteal vein and artery

Vastus medialis

Biceps femoris
long head (cut)

Adductor tubercle

Semimembranosus

Plantaris

Oblique popliteal ligament

Popliteus

Soleus

5.26 Adductor magnus muscle, posterior view

The adductor magnus is a large muscle with two parts: one belongs to the adductor group, and the other to the hamstring group. The adductor part is innervated by the obturator nerve and originates from the inferior ramus of the ischium and pubis (conjoint ramus); it inserts on the linea aspera and medial supracondylar line of the femur (see Figure 5.20). The hamstring part originates from the ischial tuberosity and inserts via a palpable tendon into the adductor tubercle; the hamstring part is innervated by the tibial portion of the sciatic nerve.

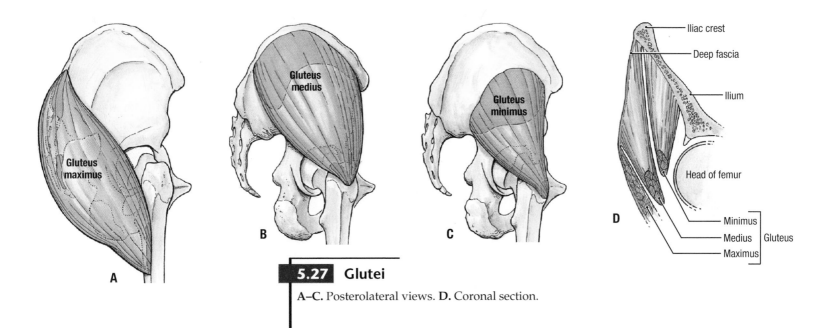

5.27 **Glutei**

A–C. Posterolateral views. **D.** Coronal section.

Table 5.4. Muscles of Gluteal Region

Muscle	Proximal Attachment	Distal Attachment[a]	Innervation[b]	Main Actions
Gluteus maximus	Ilium posterior to posterior gluteal line, dorsal surface of sacrum and coccyx, and sacrotuberous ligament	Most fibers end in iliotibial tract that inserts into lateral condyle of tibia; some fibers insert on gluteal tuberosity of femur	Inferior gluteal nerve (L5, **S1**, and **S2**)	Extends thigh and assists in its lateral rotation; steadies thigh and assists in raising trunk from flexed position
Gluteus medius	External surface of ilium between anterior and posterior gluteal lines	Lateral surface of greater trochanter of femur	Superior gluteal nerve (**L5** and S1)	Abduct and medially rotate thigh; steady pelvis on leg when opposite leg is raised.
Gluteus minimus	External surface of ilium between anterior and inferior gluteal lines	Anterior surface of greater trochanter of femur		
Piriformis	Anterior surface of sacrum and sacrotuberous ligament	Superior border of greater trochanter of femur	Branches of ventral rami of S1 and S2	
Obturator internus	Pelvic surface of obturator membrane and surrounding bones	Medial surface of greater trochanter of femur[c]	Nerve to obturator internus (L5 and S1); *Superior gemellus:* same nerve supply as obturator internus; *Inferior gemellus:* same nerve supply as quadratus femoris	Laterally rotate extended thigh and abduct flexed thigh; steady femoral head in acetabulum
Gemelli, superior, and inferior	Superior, ischial spine; inferior, ischial tuberosity			
Quadratus femoris	Lateral border of ischial tuberosity	Quadrate tubercle on intertrochanteric crest of femur and inferior to it	Nerve to quadratus femoris (L5 and S1)	Laterally rotates thigh[d]; steadies femoral head in acetabulum

[a] See Figure 5.18 for muscle attachments.
[b] See Table 5.1 for explanation of segmental innervation.
[c] Gemelli muscles blend with the tendon of obturator internus muscle as the tendon attaches to greater trochanter of femur.
[d] Three are six lateral rotators of the thigh; piriformis, obturator internus, gemelli (superior and inferior), quadratus femoris, and obturator externus. These muscles also stabilize the hip joint.

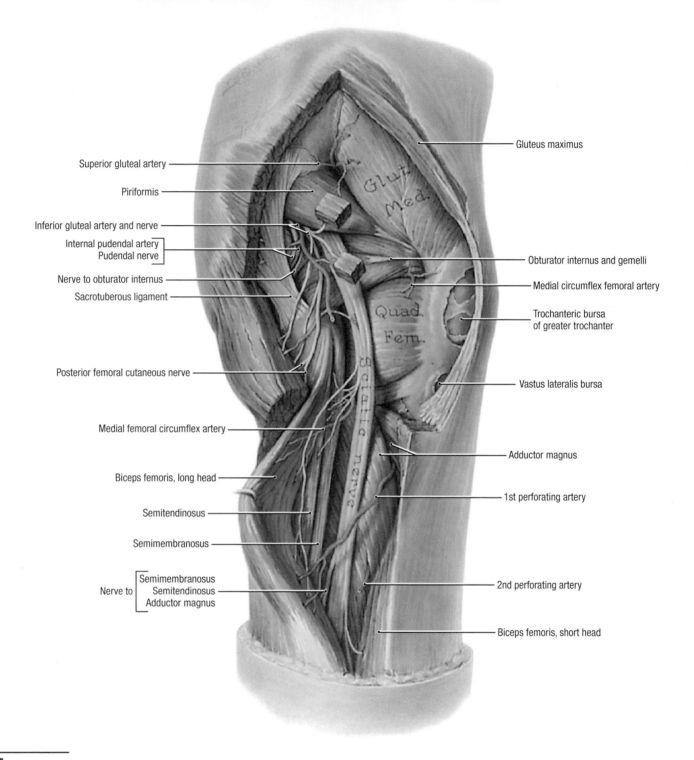

Superior gluteal artery

Piriformis

Inferior gluteal artery and nerve

Internal pudendal artery
Pudendal nerve

Nerve to obturator internus

Sacrotuberous ligament

Posterior femoral cutaneous nerve

Medial femoral circumflex artery

Biceps femoris, long head

Semitendinosus

Semimembranosus

Nerve to [Semimembranosus
Semitendinosus
Adductor magnus]

Gluteus maximus

Obturator internus and gemelli

Medial circumflex femoral artery

Trochanteric bursa
of greater trochanter

Vastus lateralis bursa

Adductor magnus

1st perforating artery

2nd perforating artery

Biceps femoris, short head

5.28   **Muscles of gluteal region and posterior aspect of thigh—III, posterior view**

The gluteus maximus muscle is split superiorly and inferiorly in the direction of its fibers, and the middle part is excised; two cubes remain to identify its nerve.

OBSERVE:

1. The gluteus maximus is the only muscle to cover the greater trochanter; it is aponeurotic and has underlying bursae where it glides on the trochanter and the aponeurosis of the vastus lateralis muscle. A smaller bursa is usually found between the muscle and the ischial tuberosity;

2. The inferior gluteal nerve enters the gluteus maximus muscle in two chief branches near its center;

3. Superior to the piriformis muscle is the gluteus medius muscle, which covers the gluteus minimus muscle;

4. The sciatic nerve appears inferior to the piriformis muscle and crosses, in turn: the dorsal surface of the ischium, obturator internus and gemelli, quadratus femoris, and the adductor magnus. Its branches arise from its medial side at variable levels to supply the hamstrings and part of the adductor magnus muscle; only the branch to the biceps muscle (short head) arises from its lateral side.

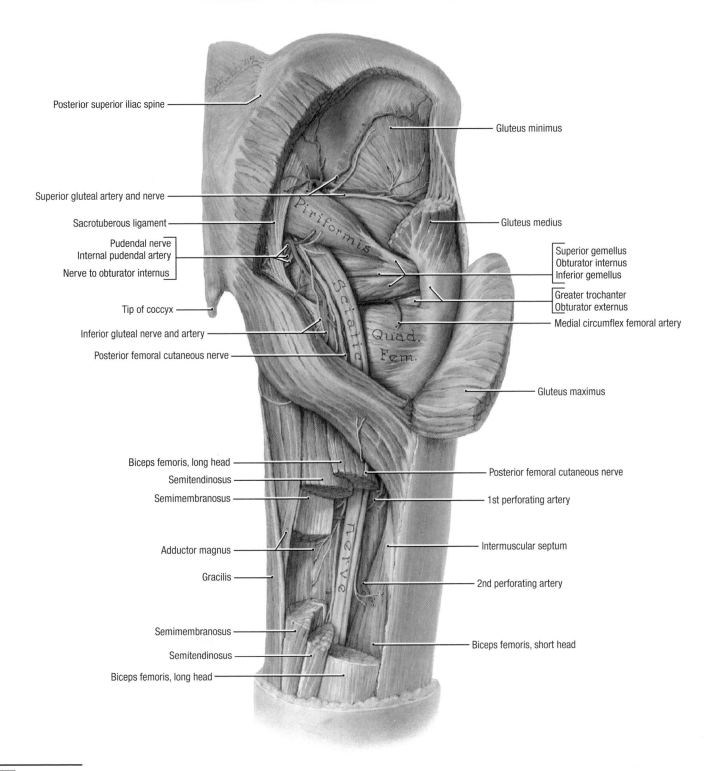

5.29   **Muscles of gluteal region and posterior aspect of thigh–IV, posterior view**

The proximal three quarters of the gluteus maximus muscle is re-flected, and parts of the gluteus medius and three hamstring muscles are excised.

OBSERVE:

1. The superior gluteal vessels and nerves appear superior to the pir-iformis muscle; all other vessels and nerves appear inferior to it;
2. The superior gluteal artery divides into superficial and deep branches; the superficial branch supplies the gluteus maximus

muscle, and the deep branch divides into a superior ramus, which anastomoses with arteries of the region, and an inferior ramus, which supplies the gluteus medius and minimus muscles;

3. The inferior gluteal artery supplies the buttock, proximal part of the thigh, and sciatic nerve;
4. The gluteus maximus muscle consists of bundles of parallel fibers; it is rhomboidal, and the deep fascia covering it is thin;
5. The gluteus medius muscle arises in part from the covering deep fascia, which is strong and thick.

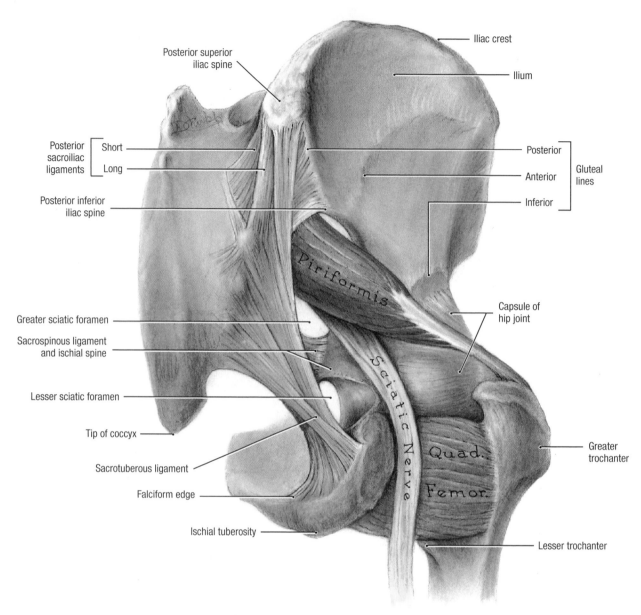

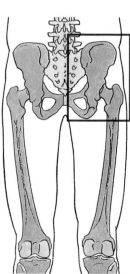

5.30   **Bone and ligaments of gluteal region, posterior view**

OBSERVE:
1. The tip of the coccyx lies superior to the level of the ischial tuberosity and inferior to that of the ischial spine;
2. The inferior border of the quadratus femoris muscle is level with the inferior aspect of the ischial tuberosity, and it crosses the lesser trochanter;
3. The lateral border of the sciatic nerve lies midway between the lateral surface of the greater trochanter and the medial surface of the ischial tuberosity, provided the body is in anatomical position.

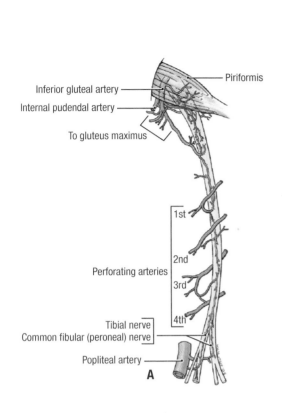

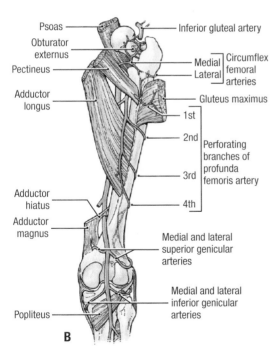

5.31   Blood supply of posterior aspect of the thigh, posterior views

A. Sciatic nerve. **B.** Profunda femoris artery. Observe the continuous anastomotic chain of arteries.

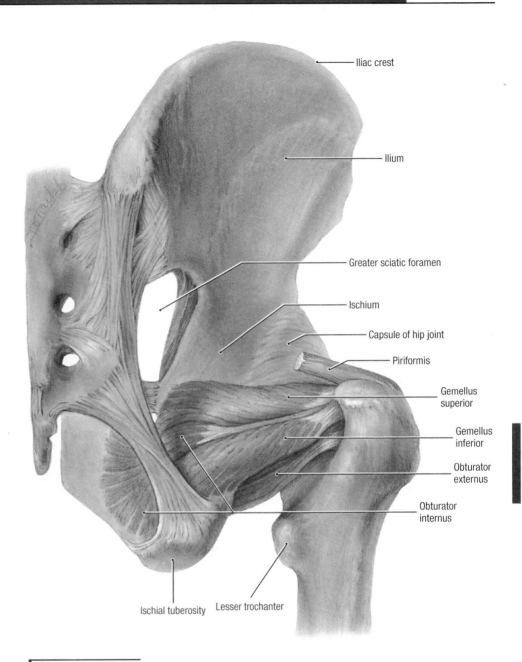

5.32   Obturator muscles, posterior view

OBSERVE:
1. The obturator internus and gemelli muscles fill the gap between the piriformis muscle superiorly and the quadratus femoris muscle inferiorly;
2. The obturator externus muscle passes obliquely, inferior to the neck of femur, to its insertion;
3. The inferior aspect of the ischial tuberosity is on the level of the lesser trochanter.

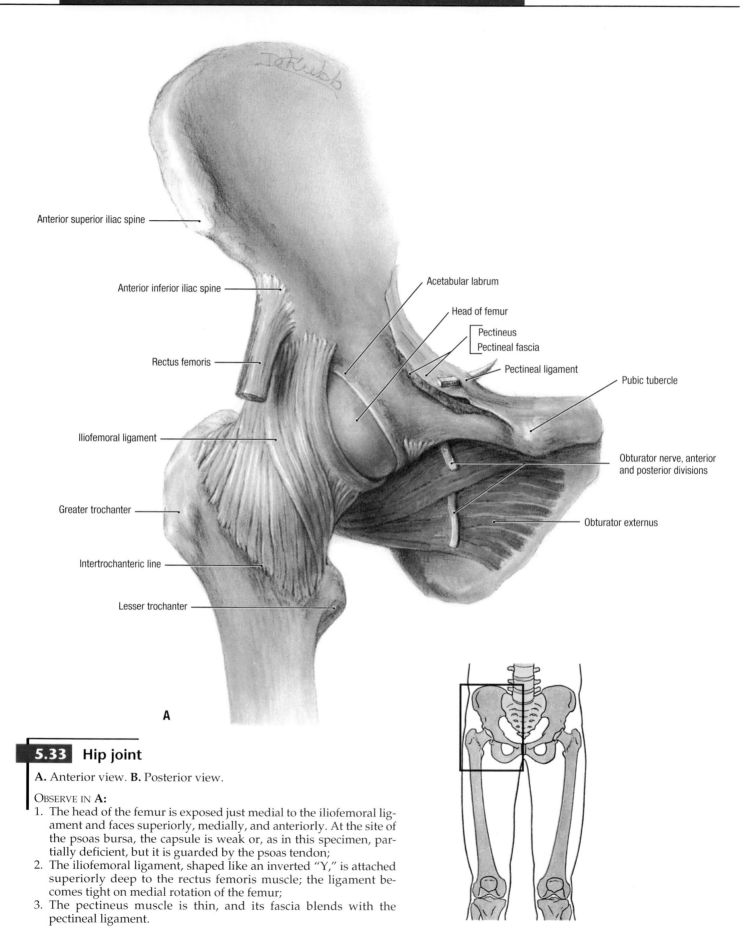

Anterior superior iliac spine

Anterior inferior iliac spine

Rectus femoris

Iliofemoral ligament

Greater trochanter

Intertrochanteric line

Lesser trochanter

Acetabular labrum

Head of femur

Pectineus
Pectineal fascia

Pectineal ligament

Pubic tubercle

Obturator nerve, anterior and posterior divisions

Obturator externus

A

5.33   Hip joint

A. Anterior view. **B.** Posterior view.

OBSERVE IN **A:**
1. The head of the femur is exposed just medial to the iliofemoral lig-ament and faces superiorly, medially, and anteriorly. At the site of the psoas bursa, the capsule is weak or, as in this specimen, par-tially deficient, but it is guarded by the psoas tendon;
2. The iliofemoral ligament, shaped like an inverted "Y," is attached superiorly deep to the rectus femoris muscle; the ligament be-comes tight on medial rotation of the femur;
3. The pectineus muscle is thin, and its fascia blends with the pectineal ligament.

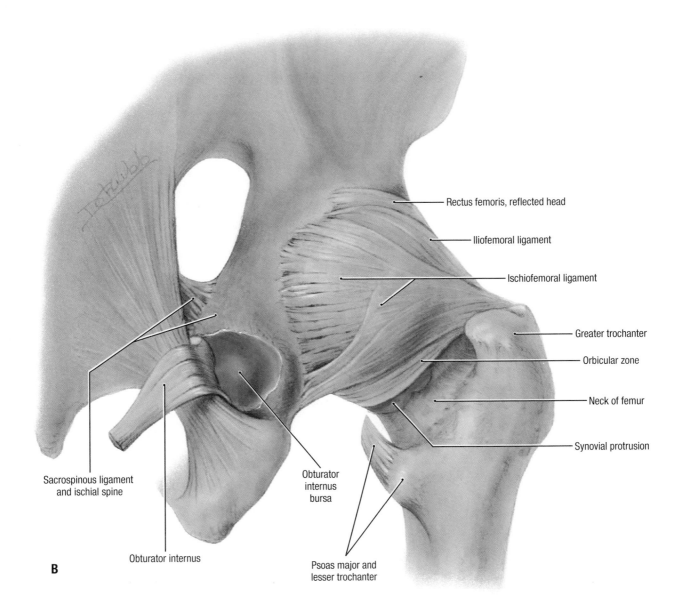

Rectus femoris, reflected head

Iliofemoral ligament

Ischiofemoral ligament

Greater trochanter

Orbicular zone

Neck of femur

Synovial protrusion

Sacrospinous ligament and ischial spine

Obturator internus bursa

Obturator internus

Psoas major and lesser trochanter

B

OBSERVE IN **B**:

4. The fibers of the capsule spiral to become taut during extension and medial rotation of the femur;

5. The synovial membrane protrudes inferior to the fibrous capsule and forms a bursa for the tendon of the obturator externus muscle; note the large obturator internus bursa at the lesser sciatic notch, where the tendon turns at a 900 angle to attach to the greater trochanter;

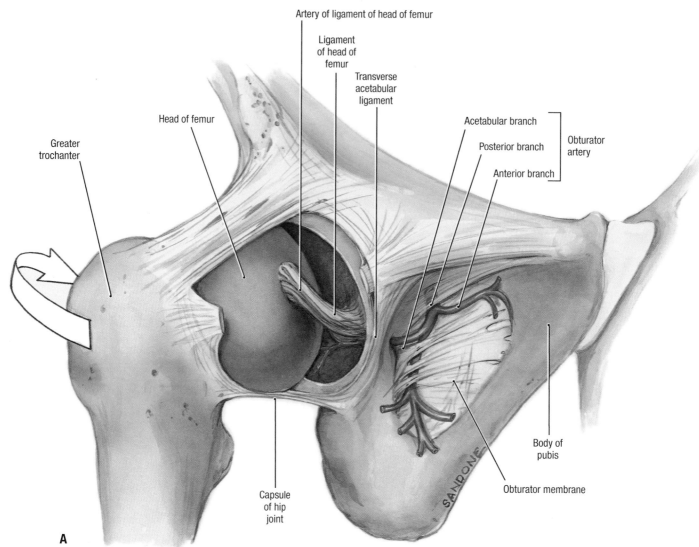

Artery of ligament of head of femur

Ligament of head of femur

Transverse acetabular ligament

Head of femur

Greater trochanter

Acetabular branch

Posterior branch

Anterior branch

Obturator artery

Body of pubis

Obturator membrane

Capsule of hip joint

A

5.34 Blood vessels of acetabular fossa and ligament of head of femur

A. Obturator artery, anterolateral view. The hip joint has been dislocated to reveal the ligament of the head of the femur. Note that the obturator artery divides into anterior and posterior branches, and the acetabular branch arises from the posterior branch. The artery of the ligament of head of femur is a branch of the acetabular artery and can be seen travelling in the ligament to the head of the femur. **B.** Acetabular artery and vein, lateral view. The acetabular branches (an artery and a vein) pass through the acetabular foramen and enter the acetabular fossa, where they diverge in the fatty areolar tissue. The branches radiate to the margin of the fossa, where they enter nutrient foramina. A branch of the acetabular artery and vein runs through the ligament of the head of the femur to the femoral head.

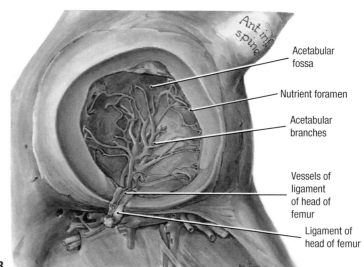

Ant inf spine

Acetabular fossa

Nutrient foramen

Acetabular branches

Vessels of ligament of head of femur

Ligament of head of femur

B

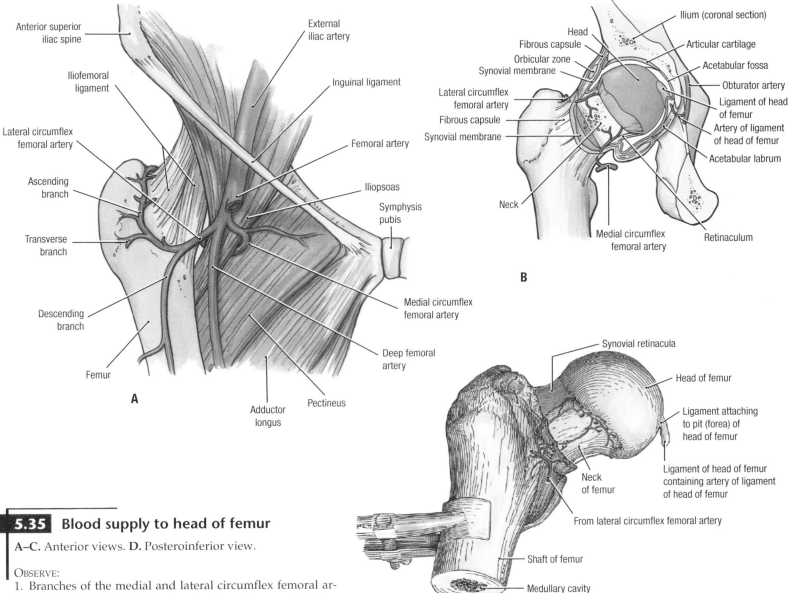

A. Anterior views.

Labels (figure A):
Anterior superior iliac spine; Iliofemoral ligament; Lateral circumflex femoral artery; Ascending branch; Transverse branch; Descending branch; Femur; External iliac artery; Inguinal ligament; Femoral artery; Iliopsoas; Symphysis pubis; Medial circumflex femoral artery; Deep femoral artery; Pectineus; Adductor longus

Labels (figure B):
Head; Fibrous capsule; Orbicular zone; Synovial membrane; Lateral circumflex femoral artery; Fibrous capsule; Synovial membrane; Neck; Medial circumflex femoral artery; Ilium (coronal section); Articular cartilage; Acetabular fossa; Obturator artery; Ligament of head of femur; Artery of ligament of head of femur; Acetabular labrum; Retinaculum

Labels (figure C):
Synovial retinacula; Head of femur; Ligament attaching to pit (forea) of head of femur; Ligament of head of femur containing artery of ligament of head of femur; From lateral circumflex femoral artery; Neck of femur; Shaft of femur; Medullary cavity

5.35　Blood supply to head of femur

A–C. Anterior views. **D.** Posteroinferior view.

OBSERVE:

1. Branches of the medial and lateral circumflex femoral arteries ascend on the posterosuperior and posteroinferior parts of the neck of the femur; the vessels ascend in synovial retinacula. There are reflections of synovial membrane along the neck of the femur; the retinacula have been mostly removed, thus the vessels can be clearly visualized;
2. The branches of the medial and lateral circumflex arteries perforate the bone just distal to the head of the femur where they anastomose with branches from the artery of the ligament of the head of the femur and with medullary branches located within the shaft of the femur;
3. The ligament of the head of the femur usually contains the artery of the ligament of the head of the femur, a branch of the obturator artery. The artery enters the head of the femur only when the center of the ossification has extended to the pit (fovea) for the ligament of the head (12th to 14th year); this anastomosis persists even in advanced age, but in 20% is never established;
4. *Fractures of the femoral neck often disrupt the blood supply to the head of the femur. The medial circumflex femoral artery supplies most of the blood to the head and neck of the femur and is often torn when the femoral neck is fractured. In some cases, the blood supplied by the artery of the ligament of the head may be the only blood received by the proximal fragment of the femoral head. If the blood vessels are ruptured, the fragment of bone may receive no blood and undergo aseptic necrosis.*

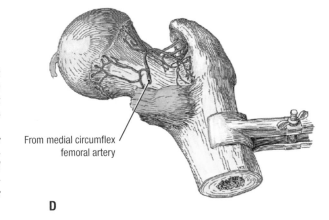

From medial circumflex femoral artery

D

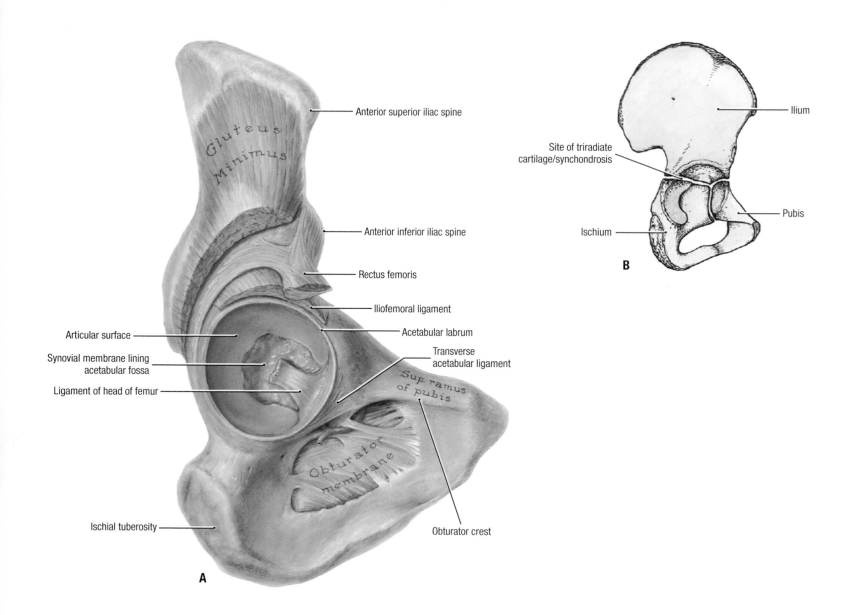

Anterior superior iliac spine

Gluteus Minimus

Anterior inferior iliac spine

Rectus femoris

Iliofemoral ligament

Articular surface

Acetabular labrum

Synovial membrane lining acetabular fossa

Transverse acetabular ligament

Ligament of head of femur

Sup. ramus of pubis

Obturator membrane

Ischial tuberosity

Obturator crest

A

Ilium

Site of triradiate cartilage/synchondrosis

Pubis

Ischium

B

5.36   Socket for head of femur

A. Dissection of acetabulum, lateral view. **B.** Hip bone in youth, lateral view. The three elements of the hip bone (os coxae) meet in the acetabulum at the triradiate synchondrosis. One or more primary centers of ossification appear in the triradiate cartilage at approximately the 12th year. Secondary centers of ossification appear along the length of the iliac crest, at the anterior inferior iliac spine, the ischial tuberosity, and the symphysis pubis at about puberty; fusion is usually complete by age 23.

OBSERVE IN **A**:
1. The transverse acetabular ligament bridges the acetabular notch;
2. The acetabular labrum, attached to the acetabular rim and transverse acetabular ligament, forms a complete ring around the head of the femur;

3. The articular surface is lunate (C-shaped);
4. The synovial membrane is attached to the margin of the articular cartilage and covers the pad of fat and the vessels in the acetabular fossa;
5. The ligament of the head of the femur, which is a hollow cone of synovial membrane compressed between the head of the femur and its socket, envelops ligamentous fibers. These fibers are attached superiorly to the pit (fovea) on the head of the femur and inferiorly to the transverse acetabular ligament and the margins of the acetabular notch; the artery passes through the acetabular notch and into the ligament of the head of the femur (see Figure 5.34).

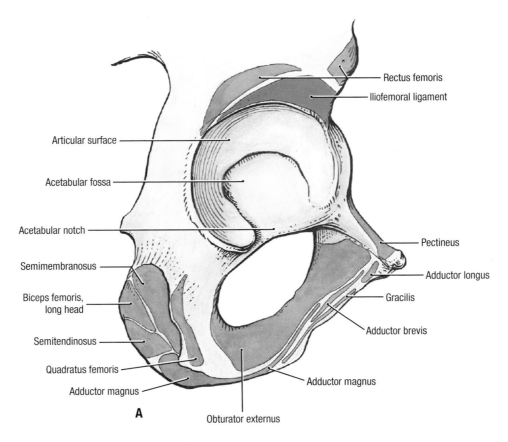

Rectus femoris

Iliofemoral ligament

Articular surface

Acetabular fossa

Acetabular notch

Pectineus

Semimembranosus

Adductor longus

Biceps femoris,
long head

Gracilis

Adductor brevis

Semitendinosus

Quadratus femoris

Adductor magnus

Adductor magnus

A

Obturator externus

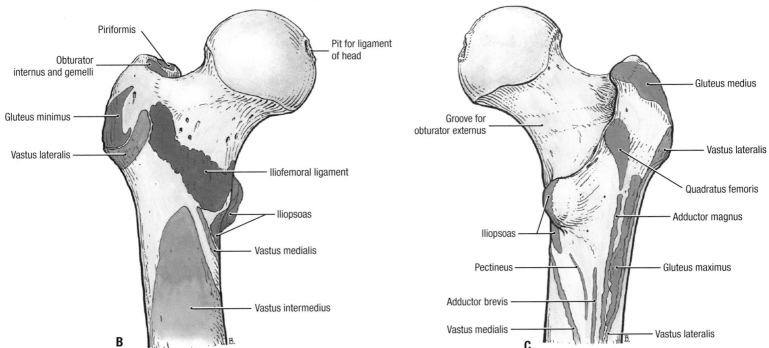

Piriformis

Pit for ligament
of head

Obturator
internus and gemelli

Gluteus medius

Gluteus minimus

Groove for
obturator externus

Vastus lateralis

Vastus lateralis

Iliofemoral ligament

Quadratus femoris

Iliopsoas

Iliopsoas

Adductor magnus

Vastus medialis

Pectineus

Gluteus maximus

Vastus intermedius

Adductor brevis

Vastus lateralis

Vastus medialis

B

C

5.37 **Muscle attachments of acetabular region and proximal femur**

A. Acetabular region, lateral view. **B.** Proximal femur, anterior view. **C.** Proximal femur,
posterior view.

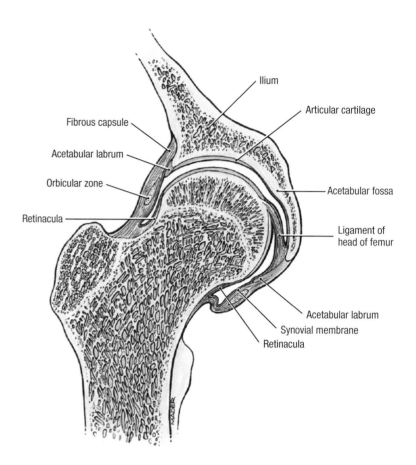

5.38   Hip joint, coronal section

OBSERVE:
1. The bony trabeculae of the ilium project into the head of the femur as lines of pressure; the trabeculae that cross these are lines of tension;
2. The epiphysis of the head of the femur is entirely within the capsule of the joint;
3. The ligament of the head of the femur is a synovial tube that is fixed superiorly at the pit (fovea) on the head of the femur and open inferiorly at the acetabular notch, where it is continuous with the synovial membrane covering the transverse acetabular ligament;
4. The ligament of the head becomes taut during adduction of the hip joint, such as when crossing the legs.

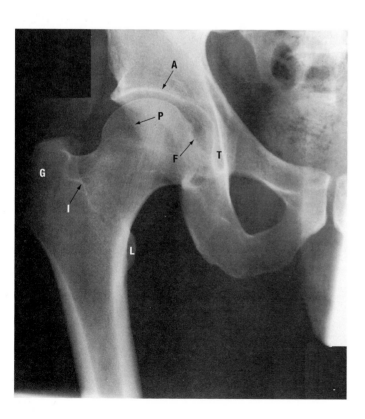

5.39   Anteroposterior radiograph of hip

OBSERVE:
On the femur: the greater (*G*) and lesser (*L*) trochanters, the intertrochanteric crest (*I*), and the pit or fovea (*F*) for the ligament of the head. On the pelvis: the roof (*A*) and posterior rim (*P*) of the acetabulum, and the "teardrop" appearance (*T*) caused by the superimposition of structures at the inferior margin of the acetabulum.

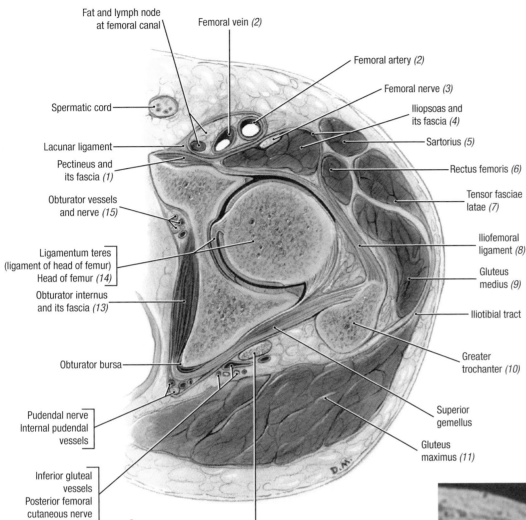

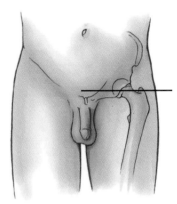

Fat and lymph node at femoral canal
Femoral vein *(2)*
Femoral artery *(2)*
Femoral nerve *(3)*
Iliopsoas and its fascia *(4)*
Spermatic cord
Sartorius *(5)*
Lacunar ligament
Pectineus and its fascia *(1)*
Rectus femoris *(6)*
Obturator vessels and nerve *(15)*
Tensor fasciae latae *(7)*
Ligamentum teres (ligament of head of femur)
Head of femur *(14)*
Iliofemoral ligament *(8)*
Obturator internus and its fascia *(13)*
Gluteus medius *(9)*
Iliotibial tract
Obturator bursa
Greater trochanter *(10)*
Pudendal nerve
Internal pudendal vessels
Superior gemellus
Inferior gluteal vessels
Posterior femoral cutaneous nerve
Gluteus maximus *(11)*
A
Sciatic nerve *(12)*

5.40 **Transverse section through thigh at level of hip joint**

A. Transverse section. **B.** Magnetic resonance image (MRI). (Numbers refer to structures in **A**.)

OBSERVE IN **A**:

1. The fibrous capsule of the joint is thick where it forms the iliofemoral ligament and thin posterior to the psoas bursa and tendon;
2. The femoral sheath, which encloses the femoral artery, vein, lymph node, lymph vessels, and fat, is free, except posteriorly where, between the psoas and pectineus muscles, it is attached to the capsule of the hip joint;
3. The femoral vein is located at the interval between the psoas and pectineus muscles. The femoral nerve lies between the iliacus muscle and fascia.

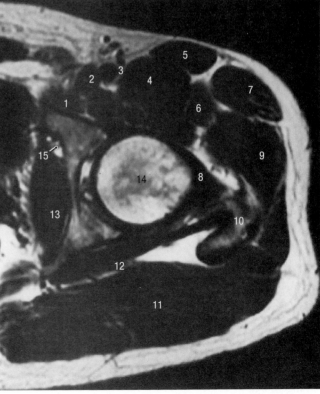

B

SUPERIOR

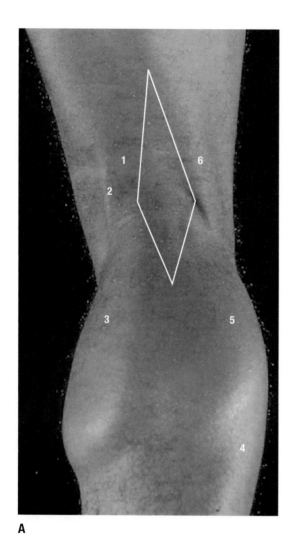

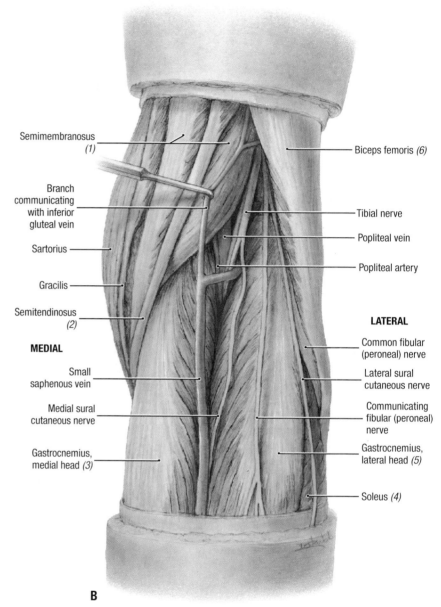

Semimembranosus (1)

Branch communicating with inferior gluteal vein

Sartorius

Gracilis

Semitendinosus (2)

MEDIAL

Small saphenous vein

Medial sural cutaneous nerve

Gastrocnemius, medial head (3)

Biceps femoris (6)

Tibial nerve

Popliteal vein

Popliteal artery

LATERAL

Common fibular (peroneal) nerve

Lateral sural cutaneous nerve

Communicating fibular (peroneal) nerve

Gastrocnemius, lateral head (5)

Soleus (4)

INFERIOR

A   B

5.41   Popliteal fossa, posterior views

A. Surface anatomy. The hamstring muscles diverge: biceps to the fibula, and the semimembranosus and semitendinosus muscles to the tibia. The origins of the medial and lateral heads of the gastrocnemius are deep to the hamstrings. The diamond-shaped popliteal fossa is outlined. (Numbers refer to structures in **B.**) **B.** Superficial dissection.

OBSERVE:

1. The two heads of the gastrocnemius muscle are embraced on the medial side by the semimembranosus muscle, which is overlaid by the semitendinosus muscle, and on the lateral side by the biceps femoris muscle;

2. The small saphenous vein runs between the two heads of the gastrocnemius muscle; deep to this vein is the medial sural cutaneous nerve, which, followed proximally, leads to the tibial nerve. The tibial nerve is superficial to the popliteal vein, which in turn is superficial to the popliteal artery;

3. The common fibular (peroneal) nerve follows the posterior border of the biceps femoris muscle, and, in this specimen, gives off two cutaneous branches.

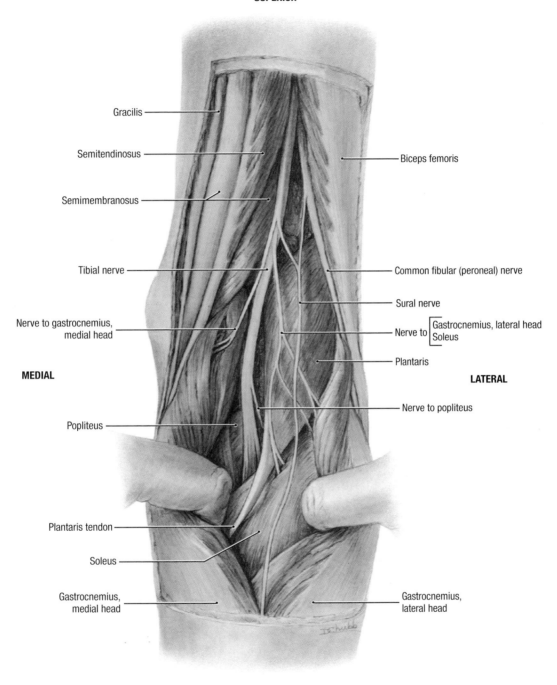

SUPERIOR

Gracilis

Semitendinosus

Semimembranosus

Biceps femoris

Tibial nerve

Common fibular (peroneal) nerve

Sural nerve

Nerve to gastrocnemius, medial head

Nerve to ⎡ Gastrocnemius, lateral head
          ⎣ Soleus

Plantaris

MEDIAL

LATERAL

Nerve to popliteus

Popliteus

Plantaris tendon

Soleus

Gastrocnemius, medial head

Gastrocnemius, lateral head

INFERIOR

5.42 **Nerves of popliteal fossa, posterior view**

The two heads of the gastrocnemius muscle are pulled apart.

OBSERVE:

1. A cutaneous branch of the tibial nerve joins a cutaneous branch of the common fibular (peroneal) nerve to form the sural nerve. In this specimen, the junction is high; usually it is 5 to 8 cm proximal to the ankle;

2. All motor branches in this region emerge from the tibial nerve, one branch from its medial side, and the others from its lateral side; hence, it is safer to dissect on the medial side.

SUPERIOR

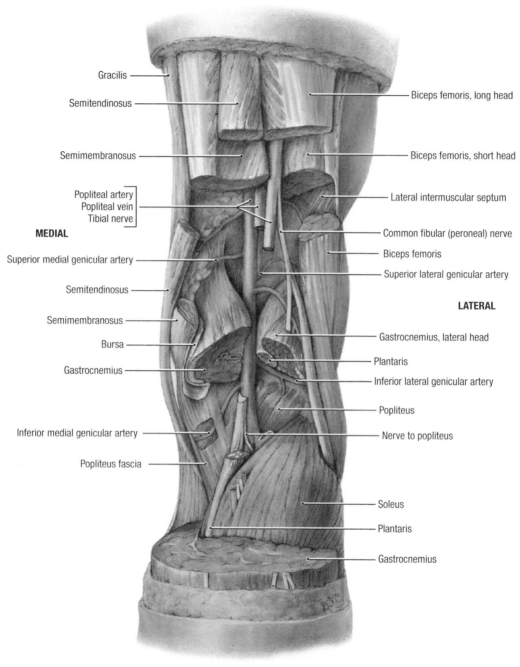

Gracilis

Semitendinosus

Semimembranosus

Popliteal artery
Popliteal vein
Tibial nerve

MEDIAL

Superior medial genicular artery

Semitendinosus

Semimembranosus

Bursa

Gastrocnemius

Inferior medial genicular artery

Popliteus fascia

Biceps femoris, long head

Biceps femoris, short head

Lateral intermuscular septum

Common fibular (peroneal) nerve

Biceps femoris

Superior lateral genicular artery

LATERAL

Gastrocnemius, lateral head

Plantaris

Inferior lateral genicular artery

Popliteus

Nerve to popliteus

Soleus

Plantaris

Gastrocnemius

INFERIOR

5.43   **Deep dissection of popliteal fossa, posterior view**

OBSERVE:
1. The thickness of the muscles varies;
2. The popliteal artery lies on the floor of the fossa formed by the femur, capsule of the knee joint, and popliteus fascia; it gives off genicular branches that also lie on the floor and ends by bifurcating into the anterior and posterior tibial arteries at the proximal border of the soleus muscle.

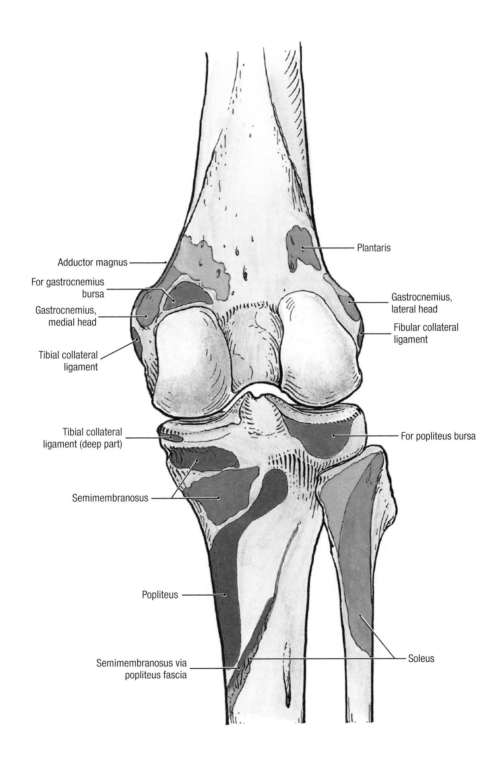

Adductor magnus

For gastrocnemius
bursa

Gastrocnemius,
medial head

Tibial collateral
ligament

Tibial collateral
ligament (deep part)

Semimembranosus

Popliteus

Semimembranosus via
popliteus fascia

Plantaris

Gastrocnemius,
lateral head

Fibular collateral
ligament

For popliteus bursa

Soleus

5.44 **Attachments of muscles of popliteal region, posterior view**

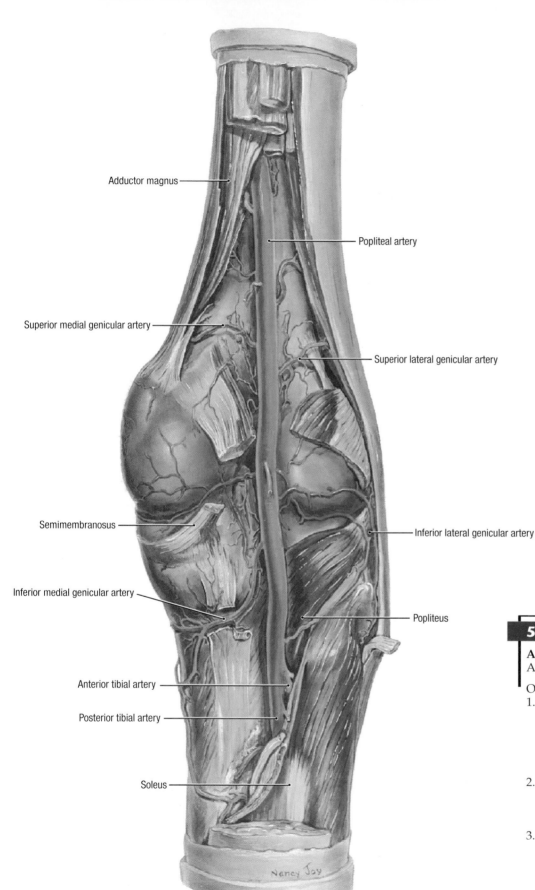

Adductor magnus

Popliteal artery

Superior medial genicular artery

Superior lateral genicular artery

Semimembranosus

Inferior lateral genicular artery

Inferior medial genicular artery

Popliteus

Anterior tibial artery

Posterior tibial artery

Soleus

Nancy Joy

A

5.45   Anastomoses around knee

A. Posterior view. **B.** Anteromedial view. **C.** Anterolateral view.

OBSERVE IN **A:**

1. The popliteal artery (injected with latex) runs from the hiatus in the adductor magnus muscle proximally to the inferior border of the popliteus muscle distally, where it bifurcates into the anterior and posterior tibial arteries;

2. The three anterior relations of the artery: (a) femur (fat intervening); (b) capsule of the joint; and (c) the popliteus muscle (covered with popliteus fascia);

3. The superior and inferior genicular branches of the popliteal artery hug the skeletal plane, with nothing intervening except the popliteus tendon, which the inferior lateral genicular artery must cross; the median genicular artery is not shown.

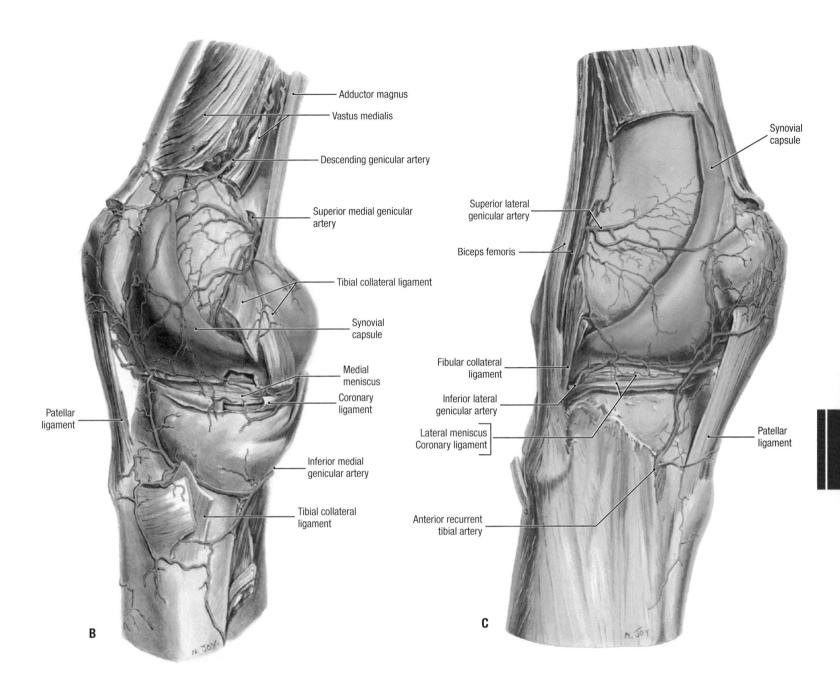

Adductor magnus

Vastus medialis

Descending genicular artery

Superior medial genicular artery

Tibial collateral ligament

Synovial capsule

Medial meniscus

Coronary ligament

Patellar ligament

Inferior medial genicular artery

Tibial collateral ligament

B

Synovial capsule

Superior lateral genicular artery

Biceps femoris

Fibular collateral ligament

Inferior lateral genicular artery

Lateral meniscus
Coronary ligament

Patellar ligament

Anterior recurrent tibial artery

C

OBSERVE IN **B** AND **C**:

4. The descending genicular branch of the femoral artery, superomedially, and the anterior recurrent branch of the anterior tibial artery, inferolaterally;

5. The inferior lateral genicular artery runs along the lateral meniscus; an unnamed artery runs similarly along the medial meniscus.

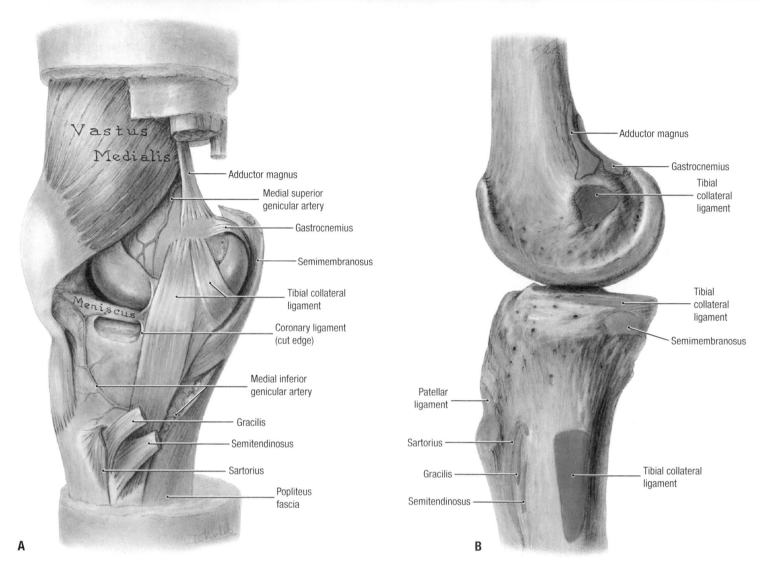

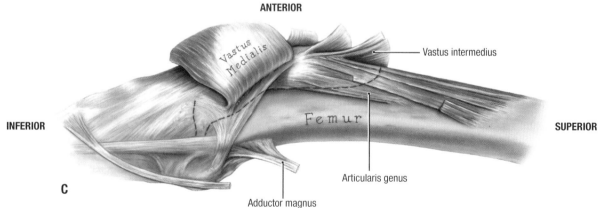

5.46 Medial aspect of knee, medial views

A. Dissection. The band-like part of the tibial collateral ligament attaches to the medial epicondyle of the femur, is almost aligned with the tendon of the adductor magnus muscle, bridges superficial to the insertion of the semimembranosus muscle, crosses the medial inferior genicular artery, and is crossed by three tendons (of the sartorius, gracilis, and semitendinosus muscles). **B.** Bones, showing muscle and ligament attachments. **C.** Articularis genu muscle. This muscle, deep to the vastus intermedius muscle, consists of a few fibers arising from the anterior surface of the femur and inserting into the synovial capsule of the knee joint, which it retracts during extension.

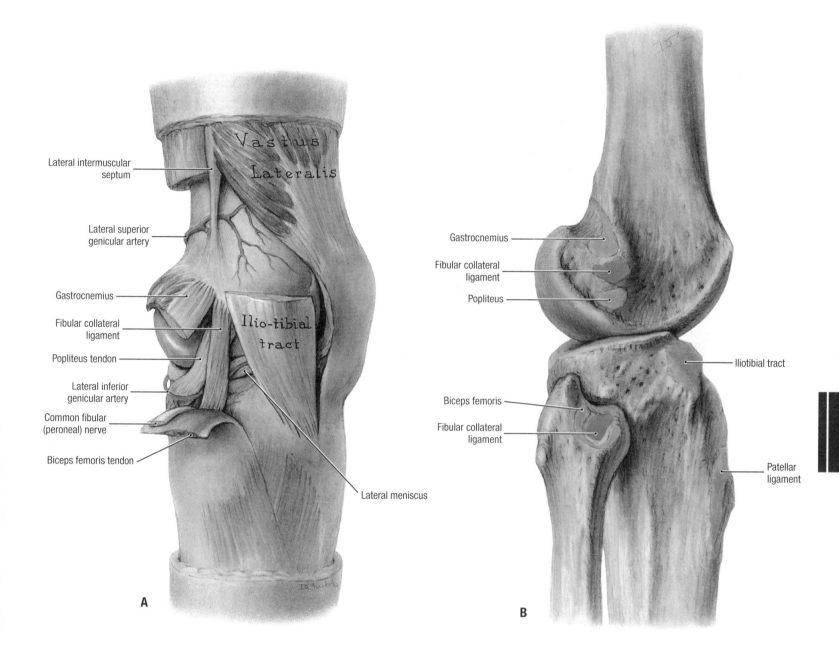

Lateral intermuscular septum

Vastus Lateralis

Lateral superior genicular artery

Gastrocnemius

Fibular collateral ligament

Ilio-tibial tract

Popliteus tendon

Lateral inferior genicular artery

Common fibular (peroneal) nerve

Biceps femoris tendon

Lateral meniscus

A

Gastrocnemius

Fibular collateral ligament

Popliteus

Biceps femoris

Fibular collateral ligament

Iliotibial tract

Patellar ligament

B

5.47   Lateral aspect of knee, lateral views

A. Dissection. **B.** Bones, showing muscle and ligament attachments.

OBSERVE:

1. The iliotibial tract intervenes between the skin and synovial membrane; by virtue of its toughness, it protects this exposed aspect of the joint;
2. Three structures arise from the lateral epicondyle and are uncovered by reflecting the biceps muscle: the gastrocnemius muscle is posterosuperior; the popliteus muscle is anteroinferior; and the fibular collateral ligament is in between, crossing superficial to the popliteus muscle;
3. The lateral inferior genicular artery courses along the lateral meniscus.

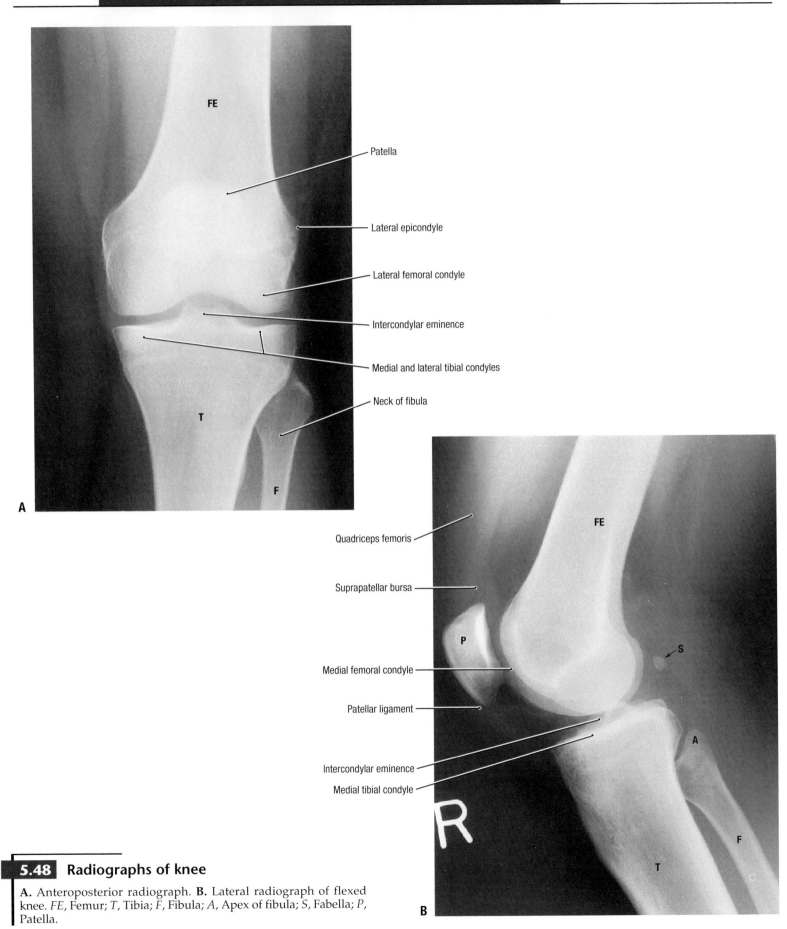

Patella

Lateral epicondyle

Lateral femoral condyle

Intercondylar eminence

Medial and lateral tibial condyles

Neck of fibula

A

Quadriceps femoris

Suprapatellar bursa

Medial femoral condyle

Patellar ligament

Intercondylar eminence

Medial tibial condyle

B

5.48   **Radiographs of knee**

A. Anteroposterior radiograph. **B.** Lateral radiograph of flexed knee. *FE,* Femur; *T,* Tibia; *F,* Fibula; *A,* Apex of fibula; *S,* Fabella; *P,* Patella.

SUPERIOR

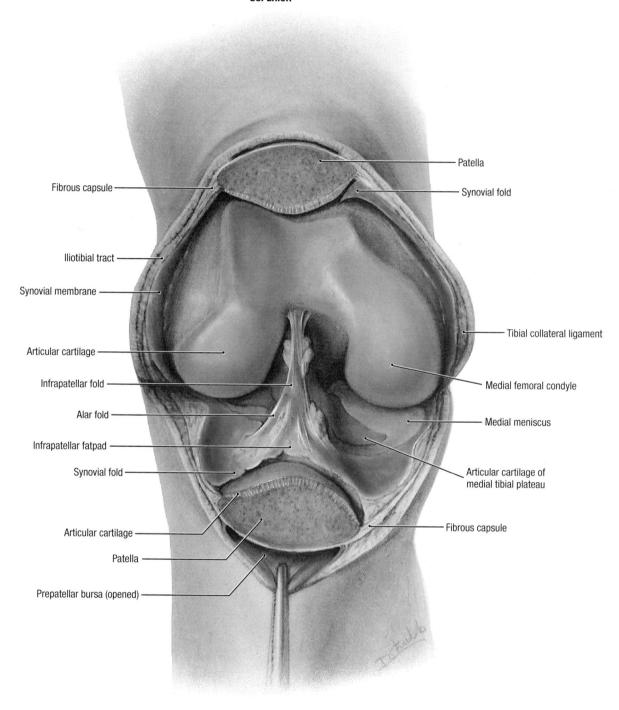

Patella

Fibrous capsule

Synovial fold

Iliotibial tract

Synovial membrane

Tibial collateral ligament

Articular cartilage

Infrapatellar fold

Medial femoral condyle

Alar fold

Medial meniscus

Infrapatellar fatpad

Synovial fold

Articular cartilage of medial tibial plateau

Articular cartilage

Fibrous capsule

Patella

Prepatellar bursa (opened)

INFERIOR

5.49   **Open knee joint, anterior view**

The patella is sawed through, the skin and joint capsule are cut through, and the joint is flexed.

OBSERVE:

1. The articular cartilage of the patella is not of uniform thickness;
2. The infrapatellar synovial fold resembles a partially collapsed tent, with its apex attached to the intercondylar notch of the femur and its base inferior to the patella;
3. *A fracture of the patella would bring the prepatellar bursa into communication with the joint cavity;*
4. The articular cartilage and synovial membrane are continuous with each other on the lateral aspect of the femoral condyle.

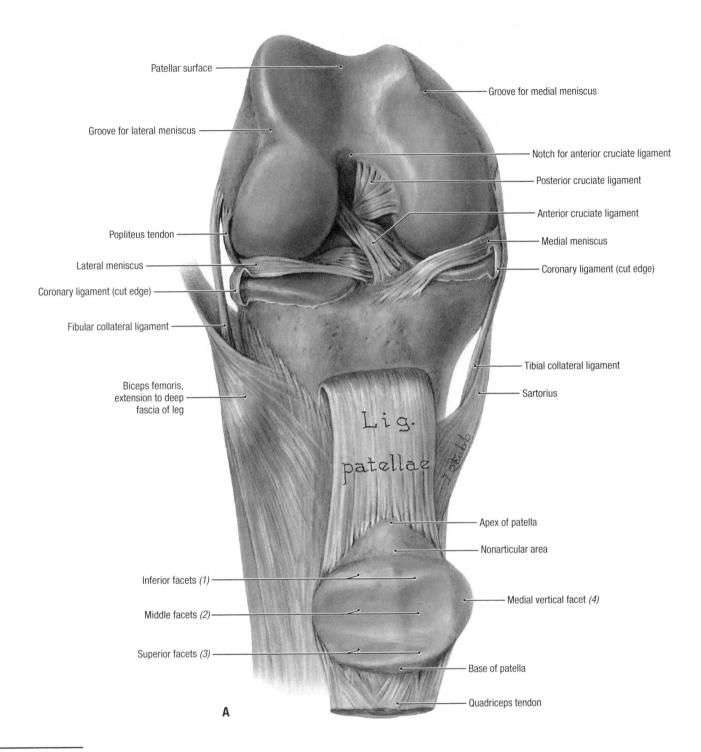

Patellar surface

Groove for medial meniscus

Groove for lateral meniscus

Notch for anterior cruciate ligament

Posterior cruciate ligament

Anterior cruciate ligament

Popliteus tendon

Medial meniscus

Lateral meniscus

Coronary ligament (cut edge)

Coronary ligament (cut edge)

Fibular collateral ligament

Tibial collateral ligament

Biceps femoris, extension to deep fascia of leg

Sartorius

Lig. patellae

Apex of patella

Nonarticular area

Inferior facets (1)

Medial vertical facet (4)

Middle facets (2)

Superior facets (3)

Base of patella

Quadriceps tendon

A

5.50   Articular surfaces and ligaments of knee joint

A. Flexed knee joint with patella reflected, anterior view. **B.** Distal femur, anteroinferior view. **C.** Tibial plateaus, superior view. **D.** Articular surfaces of patella, posterior view. The three paired facets (superior, middle, and inferior) on the posterior surface of the patella articulate with the patellar surface of the femur successively during (1) extension; (2) slight flexion; (3) flexion; and the most medial vertical facet on the patella (4) articulation during full flexion with the crescentic facet that skirts the medial margin of the intercondylar notch of the femur.

OBSERVE:
1. There are indentations on the sides of the femoral condyles at the junction of the patellar and tibial articular areas; the lateral tibial articular area is shorter than the medial one;
2. The subsidiary notch at the anterolateral part of the intercondylar notch receives the anterior cruciate ligament on full extension.

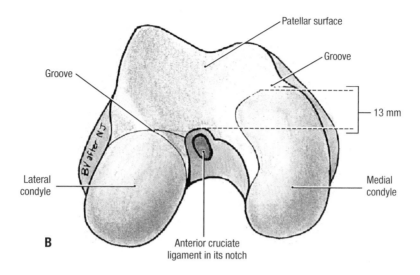

Patellar surface

Groove

Groove

13 mm

Lateral
condyle

Medial
condyle

B

Anterior cruciate
ligament in its notch

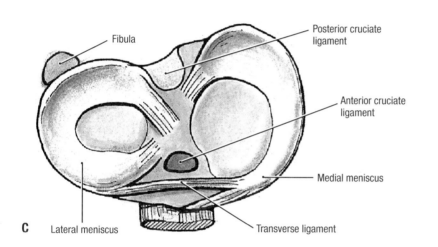

Fibula

Posterior cruciate
ligament

Anterior cruciate
ligament

Medial meniscus

C   Lateral meniscus

Transverse ligament

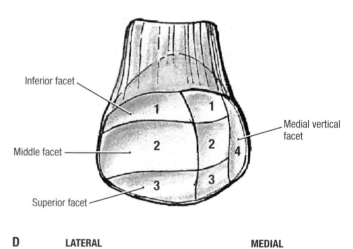

Inferior facet

1   1

Medial vertical
facet

Middle facet

2   2   4

Superior facet

3   3

D   **LATERAL**   **MEDIAL**

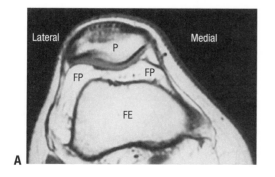

Lateral   Medial

P

FP   FP

FE

A

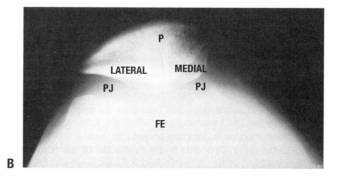

P

LATERAL   MEDIAL

PJ   PJ

FE

B

5.51 Imaging of patellofemoral articulation

A. Transverse MRI. **B.** Radiograph of patella, skyline view (knee joint is flexed). *FE*, Femur; *FP*, Fat pad; *P*, Patella; *PJ*,
Patellofemoral joint.

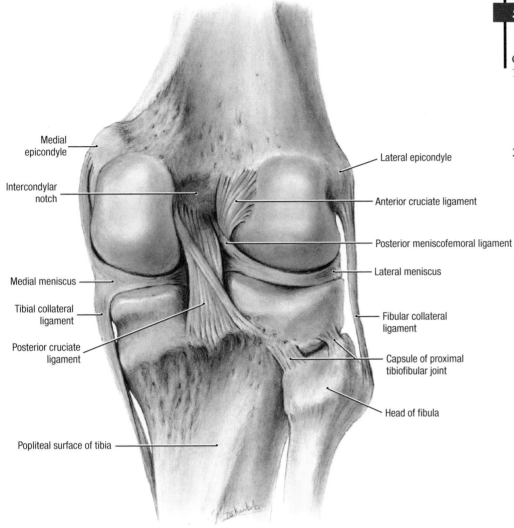

Medial epicondyle

Intercondylar notch

Medial meniscus

Tibial collateral ligament

Posterior cruciate ligament

Popliteal surface of tibia

Lateral epicondyle

Anterior cruciate ligament

Posterior meniscofemoral ligament

Lateral meniscus

Fibular collateral ligament

Capsule of proximal tibiofibular joint

Head of fibula

5.52 Ligaments of knee joint, posterior view

OBSERVE:
1. The band-like medial (tibial) collateral ligament is attached to the medial meniscus (semilunar cartilage); the cord-like lateral (fibular) collateral ligament is separated from the lateral meniscus by the width of the popliteus tendon (removed) (see Fig. 5.50A);
2. The posterior cruciate ligament is joined by a cord from the lateral meniscus; they pass anteriorly to the medial condyle of the femur; the anterior cruciate ligament is the meniscofemoral ligament, attached to the lateral condyle posteriorly.

5.53 Cruciate ligaments

A. Posterior cruciate ligament, lateral view. **B.** Anterior cruciate ligament, medial view. In each illustration, half the femur is sagittally sectioned and removed with the proximal part of the corresponding cruciate ligament.

OBSERVE:
1. In **A,** the posterior cruciate ligament prevents the femur from sliding anteriorly on the tibia, particularly when the knee is flexed;
2. In **B,** the anterior cruciate ligament prevents the femur from sliding posteriorly on the tibia, prevents hyperextension of the knee, and limits medial rotation of the femur when the foot is on the ground, i.e., when the leg is fixed.

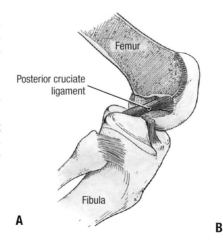

Femur

Posterior cruciate ligament

Fibula

A

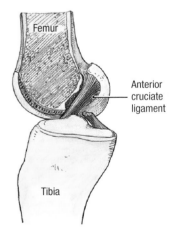

Femur

Anterior cruciate ligament

Tibia

B

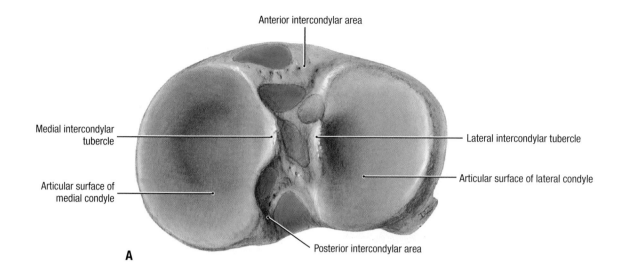

A.

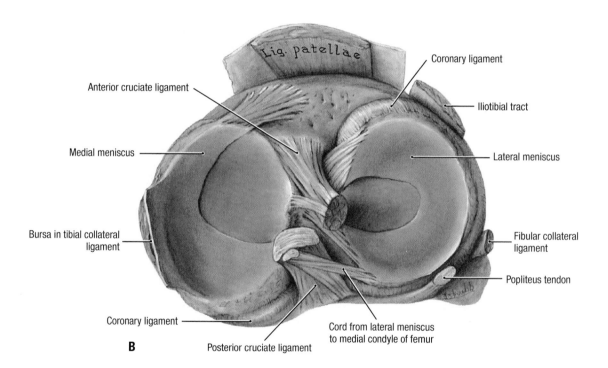

B.

5.54 Cruciate ligaments and menisci

A. Attachments to tibia, superior view. **B.** Menisci in situ, superior view.

OBSERVE:

1. The sites of attachment of the cruciate ligaments are green; those of the medial meniscus are purple; and those of the lateral meniscus are orange;
2. Of the tibial condyles, the lateral is flatter, shorter from anterior to posterior, and more circular; the medial is concave, longer from anterior to posterior, and more oval;
3. The menisci are cartilaginous and tough where compressed be-

tween the femur and tibia, but ligamentous and pliable at their attachments;
4. The menisci conform to the shapes of the surfaces on which they rest. Because the horns of the lateral meniscus are attached close together and its coronary ligament is slack, this meniscus can slide anteriorly and posteriorly on the (flat) condyle; because the horns of the medial meniscus are attached further apart, its movements on the (concave) condyle are restricted;
5. The bursa between the long and short parts of the medial (tibial) collateral ligament of the knee.

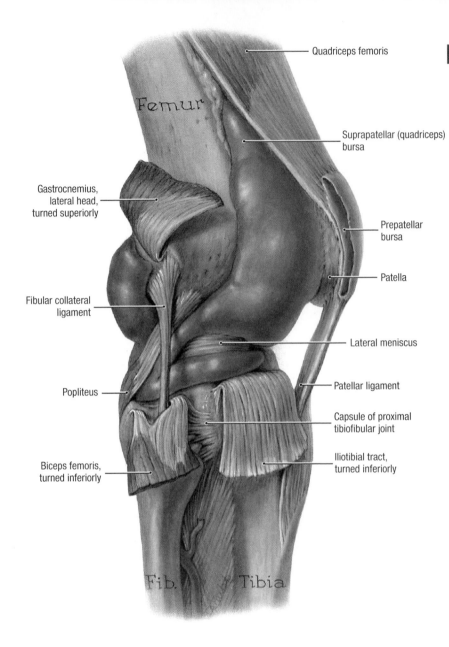

Quadriceps femoris

Femur

Suprapatellar (quadriceps) bursa

Gastrocnemius, lateral head, turned superiorly

Prepatellar bursa

Fibular collateral ligament

Patella

Lateral meniscus

Popliteus

Patellar ligament

Capsule of proximal tibiofibular joint

Biceps femoris, turned inferiorly

Iliotibial tract, turned inferiorly

Fib.   Tibia

5.55 Distended knee joint, lateral view

Latex was injected into the joint cavity and fixed with acetic acid. The distended synovial capsule was exposed and cleaned. The gastrocnemius muscle was reflected proximally, and the biceps femoris muscle and the iliotibial tract were reflected distally. In this specimen, the latex flowed into the proximal tibiofibular joint cavity.

OBSERVE:

1. The extent of the synovial capsule: (a) superiorly, it rises approximately two fingersbreadth superior to the patella, where it rests on a layer of fat that allows it to glide freely within movements of the joint; this superior part is called the suprapatellar bursa; (b) posteriorly, it rises as high as the origin of the gastrocnemius muscle; (c) laterally, it curves inferior to the lateral femoral epicondyle, where the popliteus tendon and fibular collateral ligament are attached; and (d) inferiorly, it bulges inferior to the lateral meniscus, overlapping the tibia (the coronary ligament is removed to show this);
2. The biceps femoris muscle and iliotibial tract protect the joint laterally;
3. The prepatellar bursa, in this specimen more extensive than usual, covers the patella.

5.56 Proximal tibiofibular joint, anterolateral views

A. Oblique form. **B.** Horizontal form. The proximal tibiofibular joint (*arrows*) has important functions: (a) dissipation of torsional stress applied at the ankle; (b) dissipation of lateral tibial bending moments; and (c) tensile weight bearing.

OBSERVE:

1. In **A,** the joint surfaces are inclined at an angle greater than 20%. Generally, the greater the angle, the smaller the surface area of the joint. Rotation at this joint occurs during dorsiflexion of the ankle, especially in horizontal joints. In knee flexion, the fibula moves anteriorly, and in extension, posteriorly;
2. In **B,** two nearly flat surfaces articulate posterior to the lateral edge of the tibia.

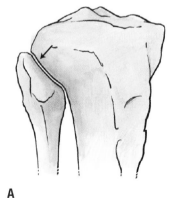

A

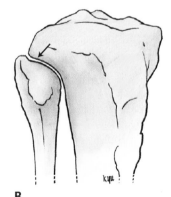

B

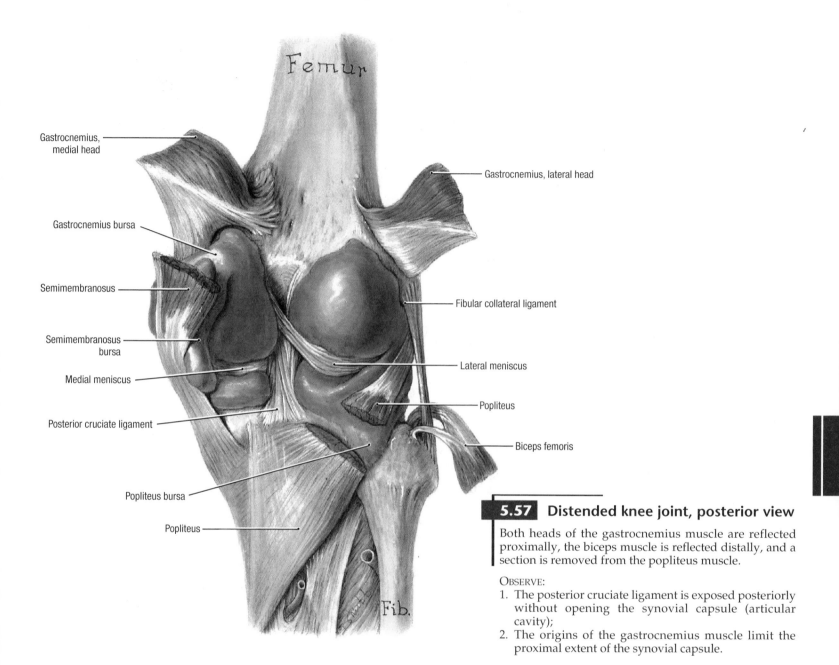

Gastrocnemius, medial head

Gastrocnemius bursa

Semimembranosus

Semimembranosus bursa

Medial meniscus

Posterior cruciate ligament

Popliteus bursa

Popliteus

Femur

Gastrocnemius, lateral head

Fibular collateral ligament

Lateral meniscus

Popliteus

Biceps femoris

Fib.

5.57   **Distended knee joint, posterior view**

Both heads of the gastrocnemius muscle are reflected proximally, the biceps muscle is reflected distally, and a section is removed from the popliteus muscle.

OBSERVE:
1. The posterior cruciate ligament is exposed posteriorly without opening the synovial capsule (articular cavity);
2. The origins of the gastrocnemius muscle limit the proximal extent of the synovial capsule.

Table 5.5. Bursae around Knee

Bursae	Locations	Bursae	Locations
Suprapatellar (Fig. 5.53)	Between femur and tendon of quadriceps femoris	Semimembranosus (Fig. 5.55)	Located between medial head of gastrocnemius and semimembranosus tendon
Popliteus (Fig. 5.55)	Between tendon of popliteus and lateral condyle of tibia	Subcutaneous prepatellar (Fig. 5.53)	Lies between skin and anterior surface of patella
Anserine (Fig. 5.20)	Separates tendons of sartorius, gracilis, and semitendinosus from tibia and tibial collateral ligament	Subcutaneous infrapatellar (Fig. 5.57A)	Located between skin and tibial tuberosity
Gastrocnemius (Fig. 5.55)	Lies deep to proximal attachment of tendon of medial head of gastrocnemius	Deep infrapatellar (Fig. 5.57A)	Lies between patellar ligament and anterior surface of tibia

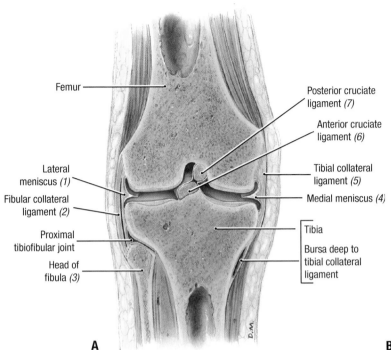

A

Femur

Lateral meniscus *(1)*

Fibular collateral ligament *(2)*

Proximal tibiofibular joint

Head of fibula *(3)*

Posterior cruciate ligament *(7)*

Anterior cruciate ligament *(6)*

Tibial collateral ligament *(5)*

Medial meniscus *(4)*

Tibia

Bursa deep to tibial collateral ligament

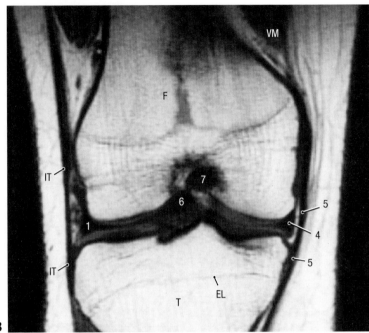

B

VM

F

IT

IT

7

6

1

5

4

5

EL

T

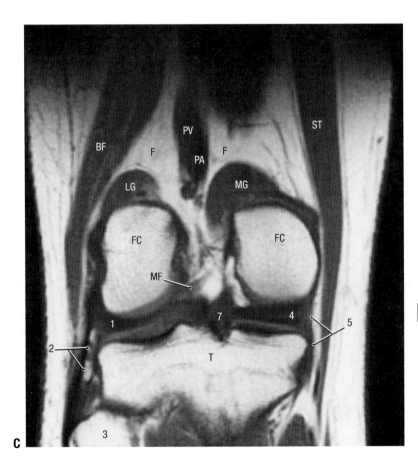

C

BF

PV

ST

F

PA

F

LG

MG

FC

FC

MF

1

7

4

5

2

T

3

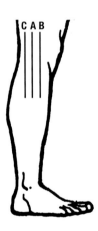

C A B

5.58   Coronal section and MRIs of knee

A. Section through intercondylar notch of femur, tibia, and fibula. **B.** MRI through intercondylar notch of femur and tibia. **C.** MRI through femoral condyles tibia and fibula. Numbers in MRIs refer to structures in **A.** *VM*, Vastus medialis; *EL*, Epiphyseal line; *IT*, Iliotibial tract; *FC*, Femoral condyle; *BF*, Biceps femoris; *ST*, Semitendinosus; *LG*, Lateral head of gastrocnemius; *MG*, Medial head of gastrocnemius; *PV*, Popliteal vein; *PA*, Popliteal artery; *F*, Fat in popliteal fossa; *MF*, Meniscofemoral ligament.

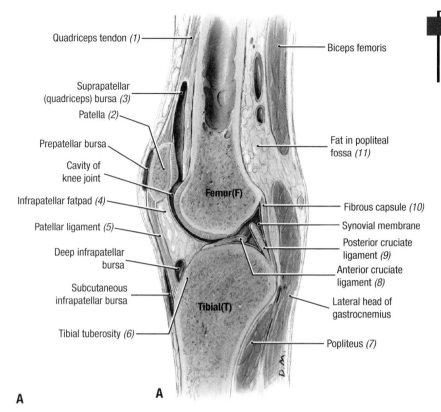

A

Quadriceps tendon *(1)*

Suprapatellar (quadriceps) bursa *(3)*

Patella *(2)*

Prepatellar bursa

Cavity of knee joint

Infrapatellar fatpad *(4)*

Patellar ligament *(5)*

Deep infrapatellar bursa

Subcutaneous infrapatellar bursa

Tibial tuberosity *(6)*

Biceps femoris

Fat in popliteal fossa *(11)*

Femur(F)

Fibrous capsule *(10)*

Synovial membrane

Posterior cruciate ligament *(9)*

Anterior cruciate ligament *(8)*

Lateral head of gastrocnemius

Tibial(T)

Popliteus *(7)*

5.59 Sagittal section and MRIs of knee

A. Section through lateral aspect of intercondylar notch of femur. **B.** MRI through medial aspect of intercondylar notch of femur. **C.** MRI through medial femoral and tibial condyles. Numbers in MRIs refer to structures in **A.** *SM,* Semimembranosus; *ST,* Semitendinosus; *MG,* Medial head of gastrocnemius; *VM,* Vastus medialis; *PF,* Prefemoral fat; *SF,* Suprapatellar fat; *AM,* Anterior horn of medial meniscus; *PM,* Posterior horn of medial meniscus; *PV,* Popliteal vessels.

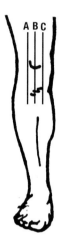

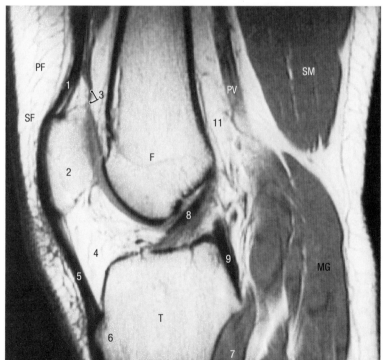

B

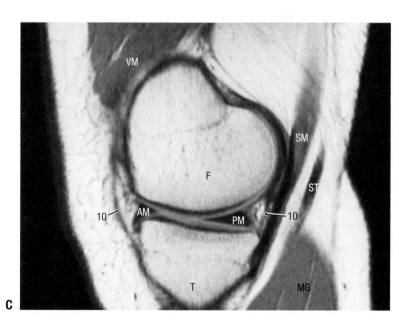

C

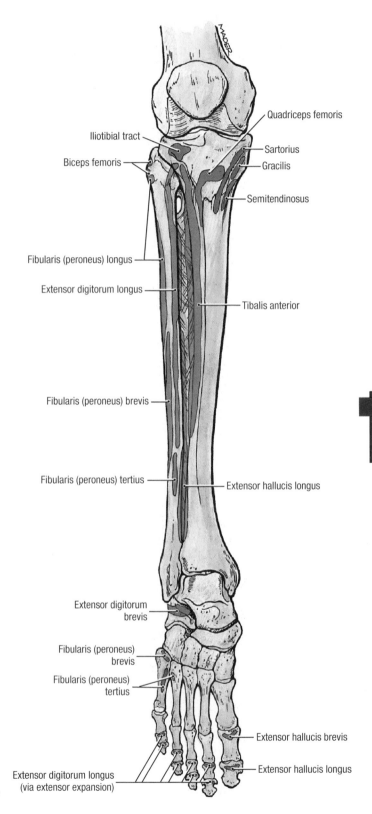

Quadriceps femoris

Iliotibial tract

Biceps femoris

Sartorius

Gracilis

Semitendinosus

Fibularis (peroneus) longus

Extensor digitorum longus

Tibalis anterior

Fibularis (peroneus) brevis

Fibularis (peroneus) tertius

Extensor hallucis longus

Extensor digitorum brevis

Fibularis (peroneus) brevis

Fibularis (peroneus) tertius

Extensor hallucis brevis

Extensor hallucis longus

Extensor digitorum longus (via extensor expansion)

A

5.60 Bones of leg, showing muscle attachments in anterior and lateral compartments

A. Tibia and fibula, and dorsum of foot, anterior view. **B.** Fibula, lateral view. **C.** Disarticulated tibia and fibula, showing opposed aspects.

OBSERVE:
1. The lateral surface of the fibula spirals slightly, thus the proximal end is directed more laterally; the distal end is grooved and faces posteriorly, allowing the lateral malleolus to act as a pulley for the long and short fibularis (peroneal) tendons;
2. The common fibular (peroneal) nerve and its terminal branches are in contact with the fibula;
3. On the fibula, there are two small articular facets for the tibia, one proximally and one distally; inferior to the latter, there is a large, triangular facet for articulation with almost the entire depth of the lateral surface of the body of the talus;
4. The extensor surface of the fibula narrows distally and is almost linear proximally;
5. The interosseous borders of the tibia and fibula, for the attachment of the interosseous membrane, separate the anterior (extensor) surface from the posterior (flexor) surface; each of these borders widens distally into a triangular area for the interosseous ligament. During walking, the fibula moves inferiorly and laterally, stretching the interosseous membrane.

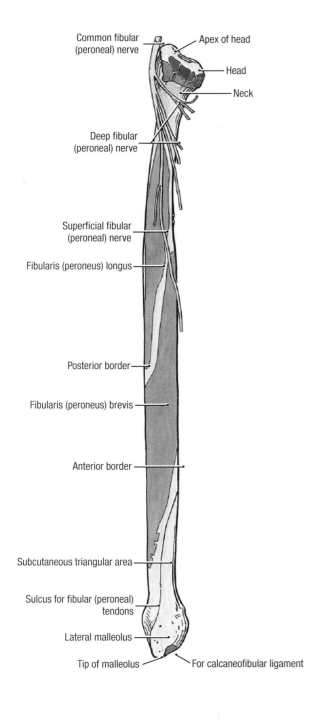

Common fibular (peroneal) nerve

Apex of head

Head

Neck

Deep fibular (peroneal) nerve

Superficial fibular (peroneal) nerve

Fibularis (peroneus) longus

Posterior border

Fibularis (peroneus) brevis

Anterior border

Subcutaneous triangular area

Sulcus for fibular (peroneal) tendons

Lateral malleolus

Tip of malleolus

For calcaneofibular ligament

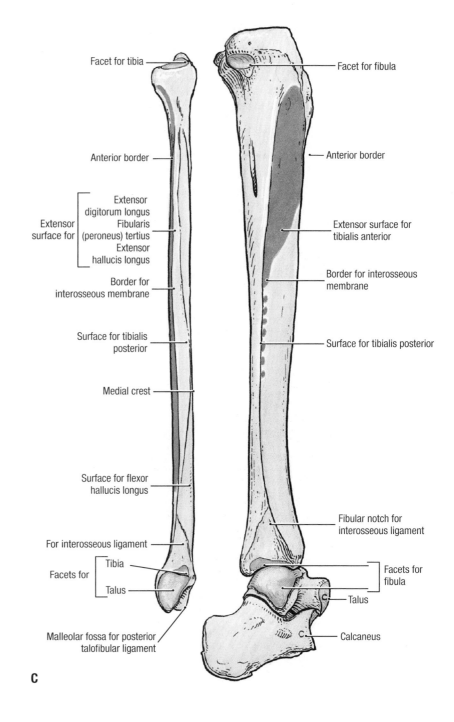

Facet for tibia

Facet for fibula

Anterior border

Anterior border

Extensor surface for

Extensor digitorum longus

Fibularis (peroneus) tertius

Extensor hallucis longus

Extensor surface for tibialis anterior

Border for interosseous membrane

Border for interosseous membrane

Surface for tibialis posterior

Surface for tibialis posterior

Medial crest

Surface for flexor hallucis longus

Fibular notch for interosseous ligament

For interosseous ligament

Facets for | Tibia
Talus

Facets for fibula

Talus

Malleolar fossa for posterior talofibular ligament

Calcaneus

C

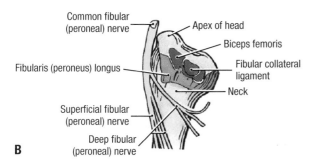

Common fibular (peroneal) nerve

Apex of head

Biceps femoris

Fibular collateral ligament

Fibularis (peroneus) longus

Neck

Superficial fibular (peroneal) nerve

Deep fibular (peroneal) nerve

B

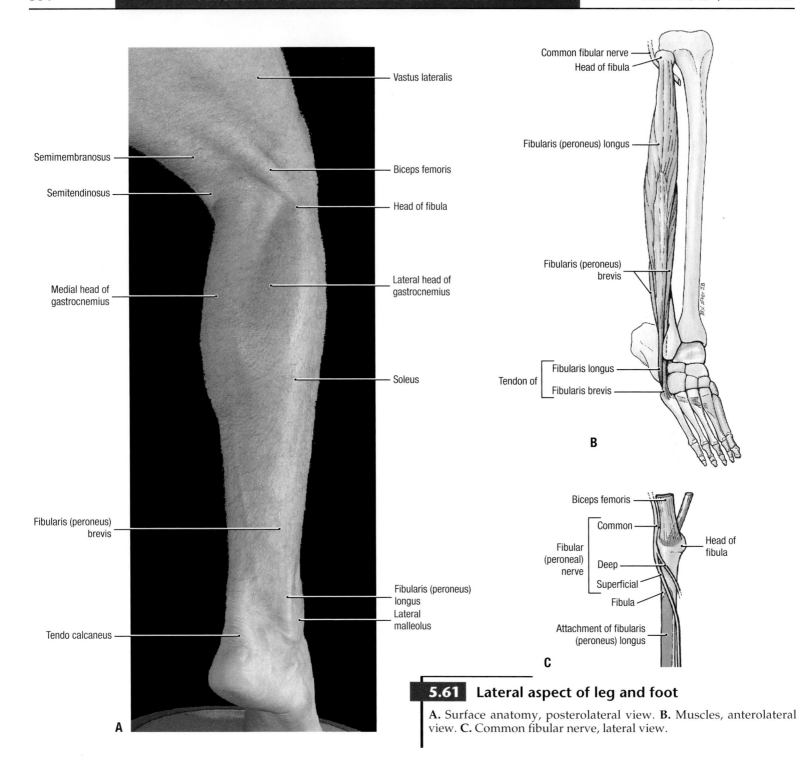

Vastus lateralis

Semimembranosus

Biceps femoris

Semitendinosus

Head of fibula

Medial head of
gastrocnemius

Lateral head of
gastrocnemius

Soleus

Fibularis (peroneus)
brevis

Fibularis (peroneus)
longus
Lateral
malleolus

Tendo calcaneus

A

Common fibular nerve
Head of fibula

Fibularis (peroneus) longus

Fibularis (peroneus)
brevis

Tendon of { Fibularis longus
Fibularis brevis

B

Biceps femoris

Common

Fibular
(peroneal)
nerve

Deep

Superficial

Head of
fibula

Fibula

Attachment of fibularis
(peroneus) longus

C

5.61 **Lateral aspect of leg and foot**

A. Surface anatomy, posterolateral view. **B.** Muscles, anterolateral
view. **C.** Common fibular nerve, lateral view.

Table 5.6. Muscles of the Lateral Compartment of the Leg

Muscle	Proximal Attachment	Distal Attachment	Innervation[a]	Main Actions
Fibularis (peroneus) longus	Head and superior two thirds of lateral surface of fibula	Base of first metatarsal and medial cuneiform	Superficial fibular (peroneal) nerve (**L5**, **S1**, and **S2**)	Evert foot and weakly plantarflex ankle
Fibularis (peroneus) brevis	Inferior two thirds of lateral surface of fibula	Dorsal surface of tuberosity on lateral side of base of fifth metatarsal		

[a] See Table 5.1 for explanation of segmental innervation.

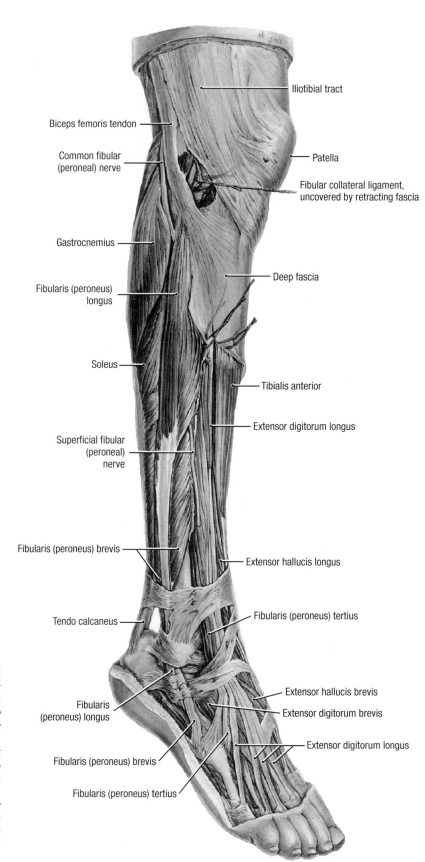

Iliotibial tract

Biceps femoris tendon

Common fibular (peroneal) nerve

Patella

Fibular collateral ligament, uncovered by retracting fascia

Gastrocnemius

Deep fascia

Fibularis (peroneus) longus

Soleus

Tibialis anterior

Extensor digitorum longus

Superficial fibular (peroneal) nerve

Fibularis (peroneus) brevis

Extensor hallucis longus

Fibularis (peroneus) tertius

Tendo calcaneus

Extensor hallucis brevis

Fibularis (peroneus) longus

Extensor digitorum brevis

Extensor digitorum longus

Fibularis (peroneus) brevis

Fibularis (peroneus) tertius

5.62 **Muscles of leg and foot, anterolateral view**

OBSERVE:

1. The attachments of the two fibular (peroneal) muscles: both attach to two thirds of the fibula, the fibularis (peroneus) longus muscle to the proximal two thirds, and the fibularis (peroneus) brevis muscle to the distal two thirds. Where they overlap, the fibularis brevis muscle lies anteriorly;
2. The fibularis (peroneus) longus muscle enters the foot by hooking around the cuboid and traveling medially to the lateral side of the base of the first metatarsal and medial cuneiform;
3. *The common fibular (peroneal) nerve is in contact with the neck of the fibula deep to the fibularis longus muscle. Here it is vulnerable to injury with serious implications; because it supplies the extensor and evertor muscle groups, loss of function results in foot drop and difficulty in everting the foot.*

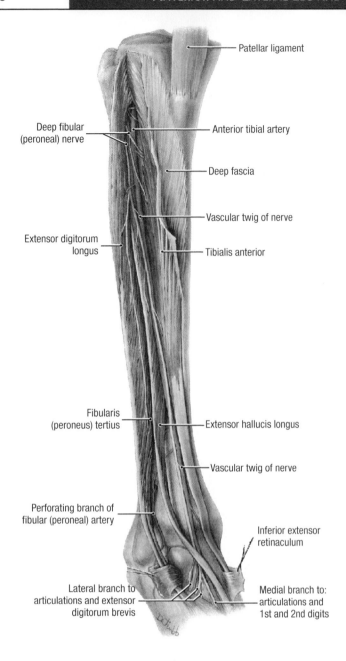

Patellar ligament

Deep fibular (peroneal) nerve

Anterior tibial artery

Deep fascia

Vascular twig of nerve

Extensor digitorum longus

Tibialis anterior

Fibularis (peroneus) tertius

Extensor hallucis longus

Vascular twig of nerve

Perforating branch of fibular (peroneal) artery

Inferior extensor retinaculum

Lateral branch to articulations and extensor digitorum brevis

Medial branch to: articulations and 1st and 2nd digits

5.63 **Leg, anterolateral view**

The muscles are separated to display the anterior tibial artery and deep fibular nerve.

Table 5.7. Muscles of the Anterior Compartment of the Leg

Muscle	Proximal Attachment	Distal Attachment	Innervation[a]	Main Actions
Tibialis anterior	Lateral condyle and superior half of lateral surface of tibia	Medial and inferior surfaces of medial cuneiform and base of first metatarsal	Deep fibular (peroneal) nerve (**L4** and L5)	Dorsiflexes ankle and inverts foot
Extensor hallucis longus	Middle part of anterior surface of fibula and interosseous membrane	Dorsal aspect of base of distal phalanx of great toe (hallux)		Extends great toe and dorsiflexes ankle
Extensor digitorum longus	Lateral condyle of tibia and superior three fourths of anterior surface of interosseous membrane	Middle and distal phalanges of lateral four digits	Deep fibular (peroneal) nerve (L5 and S1)	Extends lateral four digits and dorsiflexes ankle
Fibularis (peroneus) tertius	Interior third of anterior surface of fibula and interosseous membrane	Dorsum of base of fifth metatarsal		Dorsiflexes ankle and aids in eversion of foot

[a] See Table 5.1 for explanation of segmental innervation.

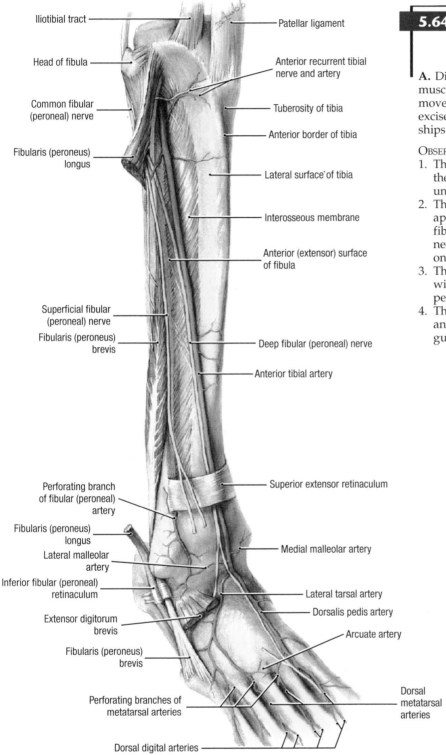

Iliotibial tract

Head of fibula

Common fibular (peroneal) nerve

Fibularis (peroneus) longus

Superficial fibular (peroneal) nerve

Fibularis (peroneus) brevis

Perforating branch of fibular (peroneal) artery

Fibularis (peroneus) longus

Lateral malleolar artery

Inferior fibular (peroneal) retinaculum

Extensor digitorum brevis

Fibularis (peroneus) brevis

Perforating branches of metatarsal arteries

Dorsal digital arteries

Patellar ligament

Anterior recurrent tibial nerve and artery

Tuberosity of tibia

Anterior border of tibia

Lateral surface of tibia

Interosseous membrane

Anterior (extensor) surface of fibula

Deep fibular (peroneal) nerve

Anterior tibial artery

Superior extensor retinaculum

Medial malleolar artery

Lateral tarsal artery

Dorsalis pedis artery

Arcuate artery

Dorsal metatarsal arteries

A

5.64 Arteries and nerves of anterior and lateral aspects of leg and dorsum of foot

A. Dissection, anterolateral view. The anterior crural muscles (muscles of the anterior compartment) were removed, and the fibularis (peroneus) longus muscle was excised. **B.** Tibiofibular articulations and their relationships to arteries of the leg, anterior view.

OBSERVE:

1. The anterior tibial artery, common fibular nerve, and their named branches lie strictly on the skeletal plane, undisturbed by the removal of muscles;
2. The common fibular (peroneal) nerve is exposed. It is applied to the posterior aspect of the head of the fibula, and its branches are applied directly to the neck and body of the fibula deep to the fibularis (peroneus) longus muscle;
3. The anterior tibial artery enters the region in contact with the medial side of the neck of the fibula; the deep peroneal nerve is in contact with the lateral side;
4. The superficial fibular (peroneal) nerve follows the anterior border of the peroneus brevis muscle, which guides it to the surface to become cutaneous.

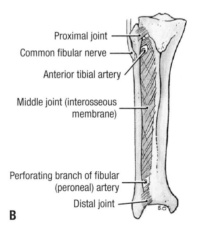

Proximal joint

Common fibular nerve

Anterior tibial artery

Middle joint (interosseous membrane)

Perforating branch of fibular (peroneal) artery

Distal joint

B

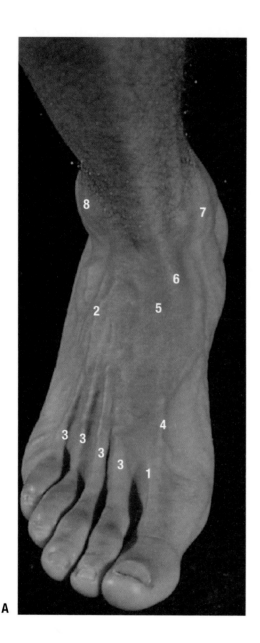

A

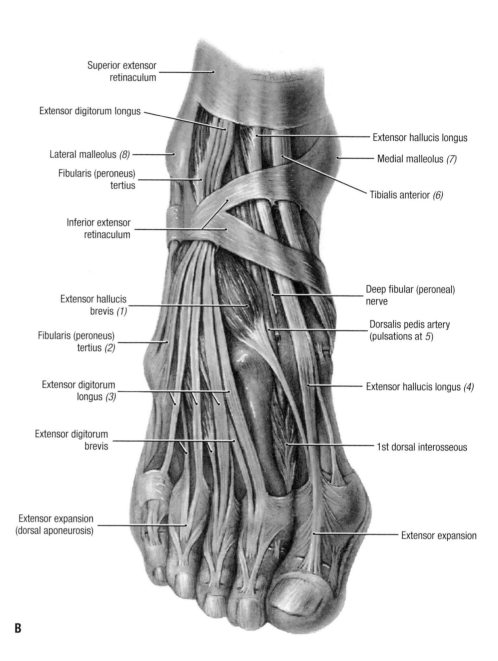

Superior extensor retinaculum

Extensor digitorum longus

Lateral malleolus *(8)*

Fibularis (peroneus) tertius

Inferior extensor retinaculum

Extensor hallucis brevis *(1)*

Fibularis (peroneus) tertius *(2)*

Extensor digitorum longus *(3)*

Extensor digitorum brevis

Extensor expansion (dorsal aponeurosis)

Extensor hallucis longus

Medial malleolus *(7)*

Tibialis anterior *(6)*

Deep fibular (peroneal) nerve

Dorsalis pedis artery (pulsations at *5*)

Extensor hallucis longus *(4)*

1st dorsal interosseous

Extensor expansion

B

| **5.65** | **Dorsum of foot, superior views** |

A. Surface anatomy. (Numbers refer to structures labeled in **B.**) Follow the tendon of the extensor hallucis longus (4) to its insertion into the base of the distal phalanx of the great toe; the tendon of tibialis anterior (6) disappears as it moves to its insertion on the medial cuneiform and base of the first metatarsal. *The pulsations of the dorsalis pedis artery (5) can be palpated on the dorsum of the foot midway between the two malleoli (medial [7] and lateral [8]), just lateral to the tendon of the extensor hallucis longus over the navicular bone.* **B.** Dorsalis pedis vein and deep fibular nerve, cut short. **C.** Bones. **D.** Arterial supply. The dorsal arterial arch is formed by the dorsalis pedis artery, which also contributes to the plantar arch formed by the medial and lateral plantar arteries.

OBSERVE:
1. At the ankle, the dorsalis pedis artery and deep fibular nerve lie midway between the malleoli;
2. On the dorsum of the foot, the dorsalis pedis artery is crossed by the extensor hallucis brevis muscle and disappears between the two heads of the first dorsal interosseous muscle;
3. The inferior extensor retinaculum crosses the tendons of the anterior compartment anteromedially.

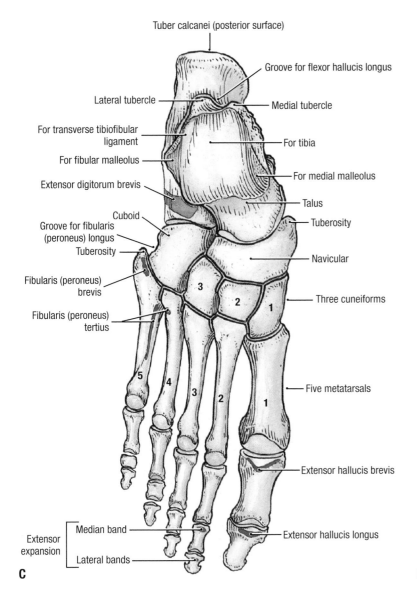

C

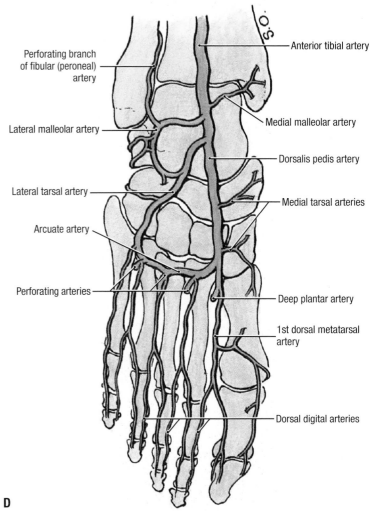

D

5.66 **Anomalous dorsalis pedis artery, lateral view**

The anomalous dorsalis pedis artery is rarely a continuation of the perforating branch of the fibular (peroneal) artery; when it is a continuation, the anterior tibial artery does not reach the ankle or is a slender vessel.

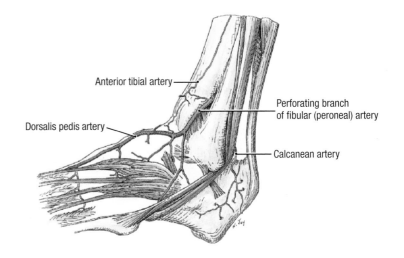

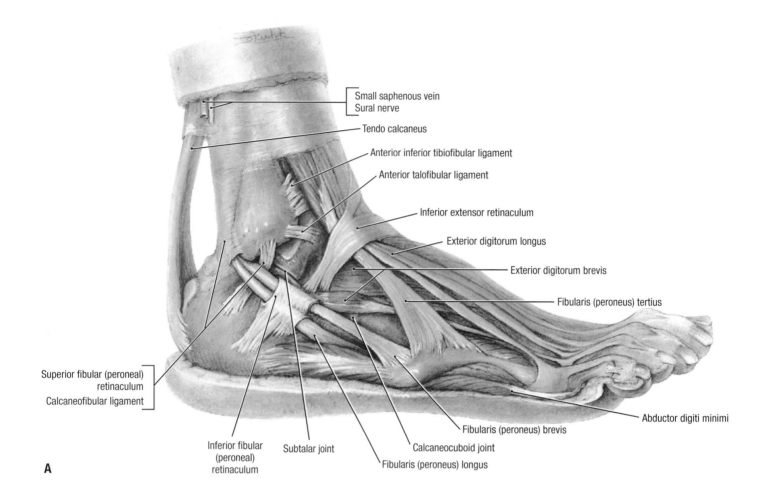

Small saphenous vein
Sural nerve
Tendo calcaneus
Anterior inferior tibiofibular ligament
Anterior talofibular ligament
Inferior extensor retinaculum
Exterior digitorum longus
Exterior digitorum brevis
Fibularis (peroneus) tertius
Abductor digiti minimi
Fibularis (peroneus) brevis
Calcaneocuboid joint
Fibularis (peroneus) longus
Subtalar joint
Inferior fibular (peroneal) retinaculum
Superior fibular (peroneal) retinaculum
Calcaneofibular ligament

A

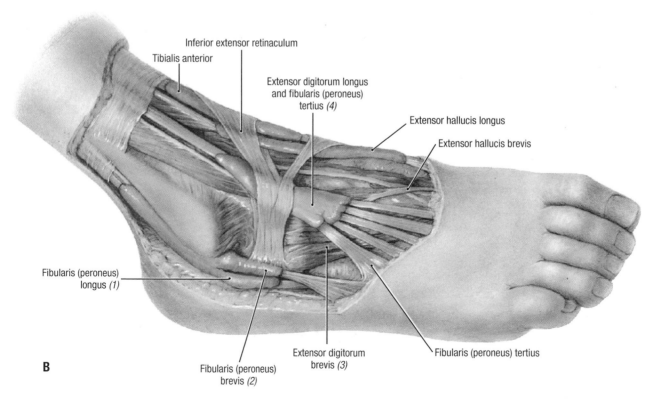

Inferior extensor retinaculum
Tibialis anterior
Extensor digitorum longus and fibularis (peroneus) tertius *(4)*
Extensor hallucis longus
Extensor hallucis brevis
Fibularis (peroneus) longus *(1)*
Fibularis (peroneus) brevis *(2)*
Extensor digitorum brevis *(3)*
Fibularis (peroneus) tertius

B

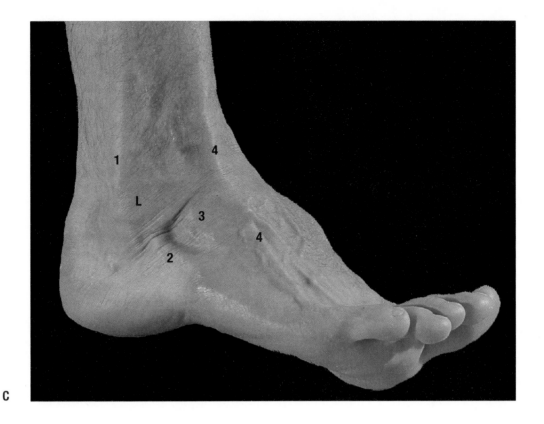

C

5.67   Synovial sheaths and tendons at ankle

A. Tendons at the ankle, lateral view. The ankle, subtalar, and calcaneocuboid joints are exposed to reveal their positions. **B.** Synovial sheaths of tendons at the ankle, anterolateral view. The tendons of the fibularis (peroneus) longus and fibularis (peroneus) brevis muscles are enclosed in a common synovial sheath posterior to the lateral malleolus; this sheath splits into two, one for each tendon, posterior to the fibular (peroneal) trochlea. (Numbers refer to landmarks in **C.**) **C.** Surface anatomy of ankle and foot, lateral view. Observe the swelling of the fleshy belly of the extensor digitorum brevis muscle *(3)*; the location of the synovial sheath, distal to which the tendons of the extensor digitorum longus muscle *(4)* fan out to reach the digits; and the

tendons of the fibularis (peroneus) longus *(1)* and brevis *(2)*, hooking around the lateral malleolus *(L)*.

OBSERVE:
1. The calcaneofibular ligament is attached anterior to the tip of the lateral malleolus, thereby allowing the tip of the lateral malleolus to flap over the fibularis (peronei) tendons to prevent them from slipping anteriorly;
2. The inferior fibular (peroneal) retinaculum, attached to the lateral surface of the calcaneus, is in line with the inferior extensor retinaculum, which is attached to the superior surface of the calcaneus.

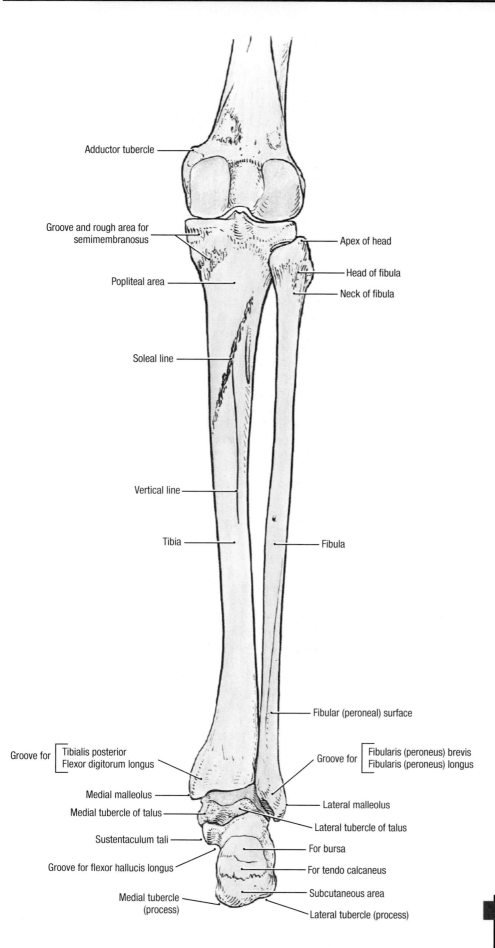

Adductor tubercle

Groove and rough area for semimembranosus

Apex of head

Head of fibula

Popliteal area

Neck of fibula

Soleal line

Vertical line

Tibia

Fibula

Fibular (peroneal) surface

Groove for [Tibialis posterior / Flexor digitorum longus]

Groove for [Fibularis (peroneus) brevis / Fibularis (peroneus) longus]

Medial malleolus

Lateral malleolus

Medial tubercle of talus

Lateral tubercle of talus

Sustentaculum tali

For bursa

Groove for flexor hallucis longus

For tendo calcaneus

Medial tubercle (process)

Subcutaneous area

Lateral tubercle (process)

5.68 Bones of leg, posterior view

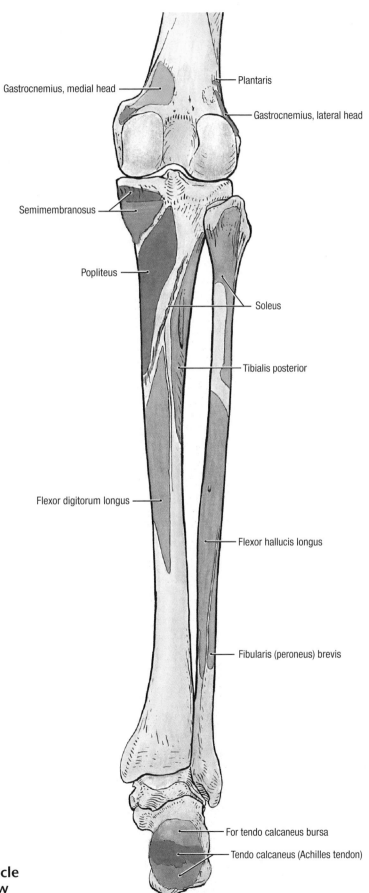

Gastrocnemius, medial head

Plantaris

Gastrocnemius, lateral head

Semimembranosus

Popliteus

Soleus

Tibialis posterior

Flexor digitorum longus

Flexor hallucis longus

Fibularis (peroneus) brevis

For tendo calcaneus bursa

Tendo calcaneus (Achilles tendon)

5.69 **Bones of leg, showing muscle attachments, posterior view**

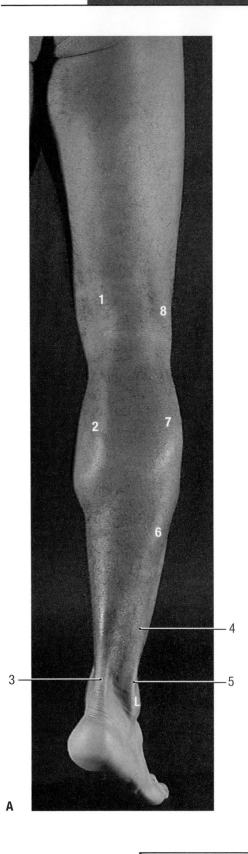

A

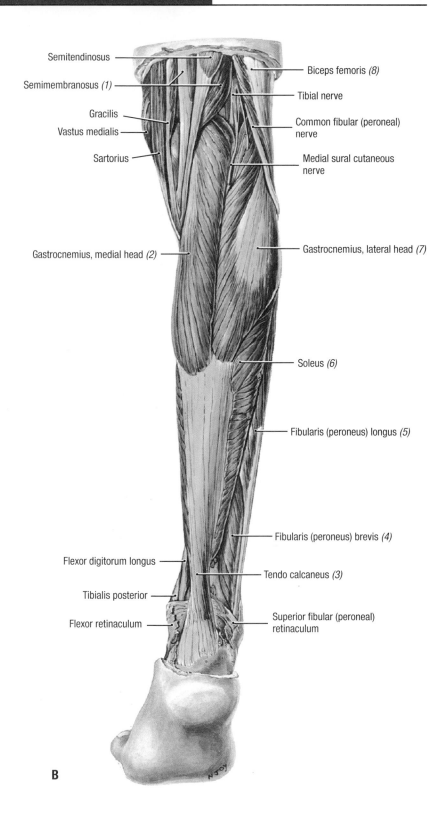

Semitendinosus

Semimembranosus (1)

Gracilis

Vastus medialis

Sartorius

Gastrocnemius, medial head (2)

Flexor digitorum longus

Tibialis posterior

Flexor retinaculum

Biceps femoris (8)

Tibial nerve

Common fibular (peroneal) nerve

Medial sural cutaneous nerve

Gastrocnemius, lateral head (7)

Soleus (6)

Fibularis (peroneus) longus (5)

Fibularis (peroneus) brevis (4)

Tendo calcaneus (3)

Superior fibular (peroneal) retinaculum

B

5.70   **Posterior leg, superficial compartment, posterior views**

A. Surface anatomy. *L,* Lateral malleolus. (Numbers refer to labeled structures in **B.**)
B. Superficial dissection.

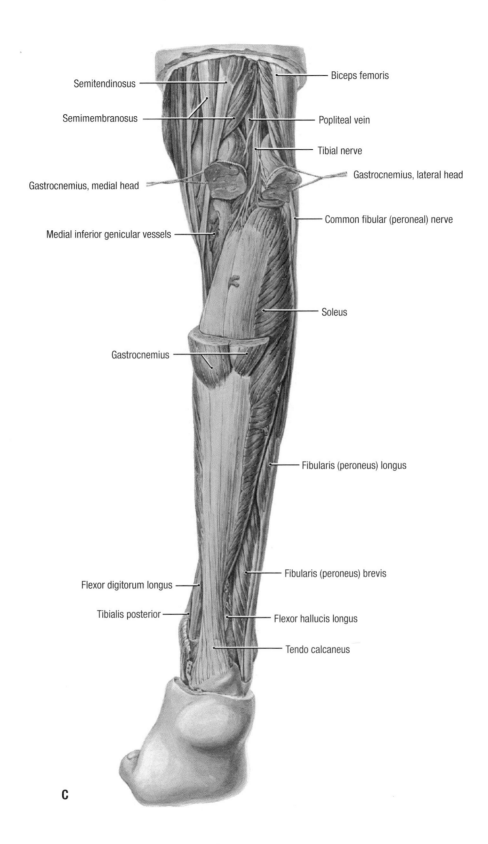

Semitendinosus

Semimembranosus

Gastrocnemius, medial head

Medial inferior genicular vessels

Gastrocnemius

Flexor digitorum longus

Tibialis posterior

Biceps femoris

Popliteal vein

Tibial nerve

Gastrocnemius, lateral head

Common fibular (peroneal) nerve

Soleus

Fibularis (peroneus) longus

Fibularis (peroneus) brevis

Flexor hallucis longus

Tendo calcaneus

C

C. Deeper dissection. The fleshy bellies of the gastrocnemius muscle are largely excised, and the proximal attachment of the soleus muscle is thereby exposed; the plantaris muscle is absent from this specimen.

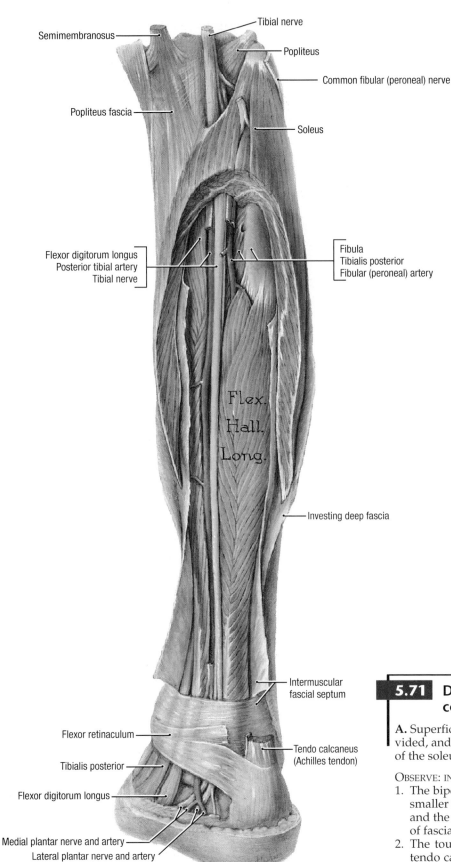

Semimembranosus

Tibial nerve

Popliteus

Common fibular (peroneal) nerve

Popliteus fascia

Soleus

Flexor digitorum longus
Posterior tibial artery
Tibial nerve

Fibula
Tibialis posterior
Fibular (peroneal) artery

Flex.
Hall.
Long.

Investing deep fascia

Intermuscular
fascial septum

Flexor retinaculum

Tendo calcaneus
(Achilles tendon)

Tibialis posterior

Flexor digitorum longus

Medial plantar nerve and artery
Lateral plantar nerve and artery

A

5.71 **Dissection of posterior leg, deep compartment, posterior views**

A. Superficial dissection. The tendo calcaneus (Achilles tendon) is divided, and the gastrocnemius muscle and a horseshoe-shaped section of the soleus muscle are removed.

OBSERVE: IN **A**:
1. The bipennate structure of the large flexor hallucis longus and the smaller flexor digitorum longus muscles; the posterior tibial artery and the tibial nerve descend between these two muscles on a layer of fascia that covers the tibialis posterior;
2. The tough, intermuscular fascial septum deep to the soleus and tendo calcaneus acts as a restraining anklet at the ankle and there blends medially with the weaker investing deep fascia to form the flexor retinaculum.

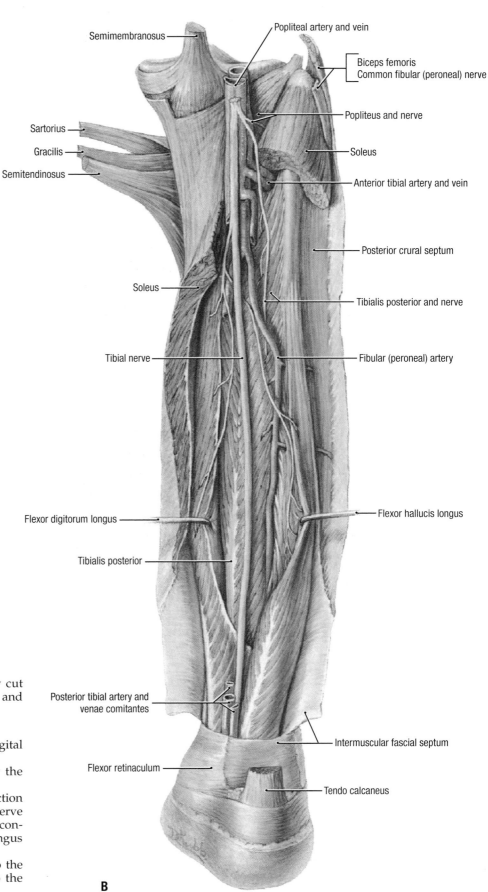

Semimembranosus

Popliteal artery and vein

Biceps femoris
Common fibular (peroneal) nerve

Popliteus and nerve

Sartorius

Gracilis

Soleus

Semitendinosus

Anterior tibial artery and vein

Posterior crural septum

Soleus

Tibialis posterior and nerve

Tibial nerve

Fibular (peroneal) artery

Flexor digitorum longus

Flexor hallucis longus

Tibialis posterior

Posterior tibial artery and
venae comitantes

Intermuscular fascial septum

Flexor retinaculum

Tendo calcaneus

B

B. Deeper dissection. The soleus muscle is largely cut away, the two long digital flexors are pulled apart, and the posterior tibial artery is partly excised.

OBSERVE: IN **B:**

1. The tibialis posterior lies deep to the two long digital flexors;
2. The fibular (peroneal) artery is overlapped by the flexor hallucis longus muscle;
3. The nerve to the tibialis posterior arises in conjunction with the nerve to the popliteus muscle, and the nerve to the flexor digitorum longus muscle arises in conjunction with the nerve to the flexor hallucis longus muscle;
4. In the popliteal fossa, the nerve is superficial to the artery; at the ankle, the artery is superficial to the nerve.

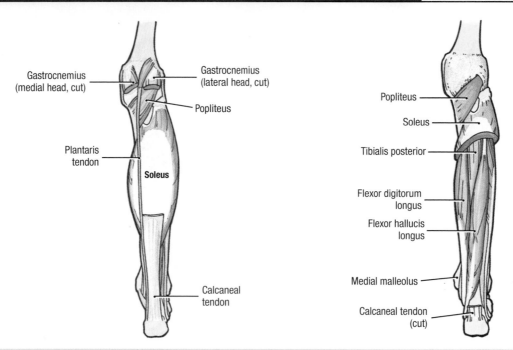

Table 5.8. Muscles of the Posterior Compartment of the Leg

Muscle	Proximal Attachment	Distal Attachment	Innervation[a]	Main Actions
Superficial muscles				
Gastrocnemius	Lateral head: lateral aspect of lateral condyle of femur; Medial head: popliteal surface of femur, superior to medial condyle	Posterior surface of calcaneus with calcaneal tendon (tendocalcaneus)	Tibial nerve (S1 and **S2**)	Plantarflexes ankle, raises heel during walking, and flexes leg at knee joint
Soleus	Posterior aspect of head of fibula, superior fourth of posterior surface of fibula, soleal line and medial border of tibia			Plantarflexes ankle and steadies leg on foot
Plantaris	Inferior end of lateral supracondylar line of femur and oblique popliteal ligament			Weakly assists gastrocnemius in plantarflexing ankle and flexing knee
Deep muscles				
Popliteus	Lateral surface of lateral condyle of femur and lateral meniscus	Posterior surface of tibia, superior to soleal line	Tibial nerve (**L4, L5,** and S1)	Weakly flexes knee and unlocks it
Flexor hallucis longus	Inferior two thirds of posterior surface of fibula and inferior part of interosseous membrane	Base of distal phalanx of great toe (hallux)	Tibial nerve (**S2** and S3)	Flexes great toe at all joints and plantarflexes ankle; supports medial longitudinal arch of foot
Flexor digitorum longus	Medial part of posterior surface of tibia inferior to soleal line, and by a broad tendon to fibula	Bases of distal phalanges of lateral four digits		Flexes lateral four digits and plantarflexes ankle; supports longitudinal arches of foot
Tibialis posterior	Interosseous membrane, posterior surface of tibia inferior to soleal line, and posterior surface of fibula	Tuberosity of navicular, cuneiform, and cuboid and bases of second, third, and fourth metatarsals	Tibial nerve (L4 and L5)	Plantarflexes ankle and inverts foot

[a] See Table 5.1 for explanation of segmental innervation.

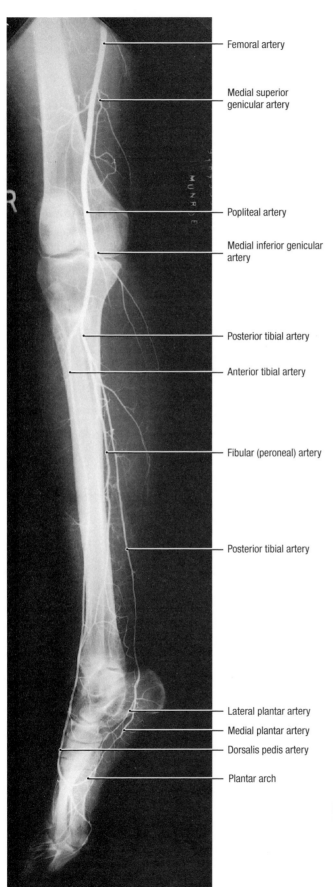

Femoral artery

Medial superior genicular artery

Popliteal artery

Medial inferior genicular artery

Posterior tibial artery

Anterior tibial artery

Fibular (peroneal) artery

Posterior tibial artery

Lateral plantar artery

Medial plantar artery

Dorsalis pedis artery

Plantar arch

5.72 Popliteal arteriogram, oblique view

OBSERVE:
1. The femoral artery becomes the popliteal artery at the tendinous opening in the adductor magnus muscle, the adductor hiatus;
2. The branches of the popliteal artery supply skin, muscles, and the knee joint; the popliteal artery successively lies on the femur, the capsule of the knee joint, and the popliteus muscle before dividing into anterior and posterior tibial arteries at the inferior angle of the popliteal fossa;
3. The anterior tibial artery supplies the anterior compartment of the leg and the ankle; it continues as the dorsalis pedis artery into the foot;
4. The posterior tibial artery supplies the posterior compartment of the leg and terminates as the medial and lateral plantar arteries; its major branch is the fibular (peroneal) artery, which supplies the posterior and lateral compartments of the leg.

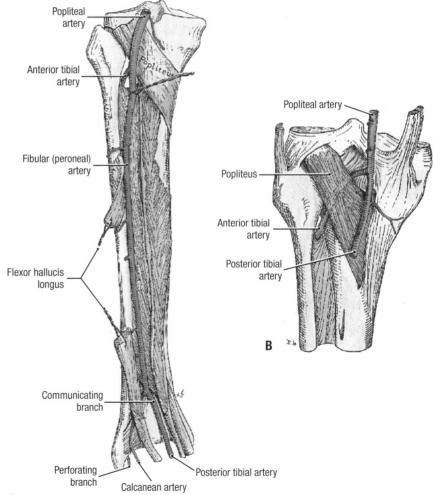

Popliteal artery

Anterior tibial artery

Fibular (peroneal) artery

Flexor hallucis longus

Communicating branch

Perforating branch

Calcanean artery

Posterior tibial artery

Popliteal artery

Popliteus

Anterior tibial artery

Posterior tibial artery

A

B

5.73 Arterial anomalies of posterior leg, posterior views

A. Absence of posterior tibial artery. Compensatory enlargement of the fibular (peroneal) artery was found to occur in approximately 5% of limbs. **B.** High division of popliteal artery. Along with the anterior tibial artery descending anterior to the popliteus muscle, this anomaly was found to occur in approximately 2% of limbs.

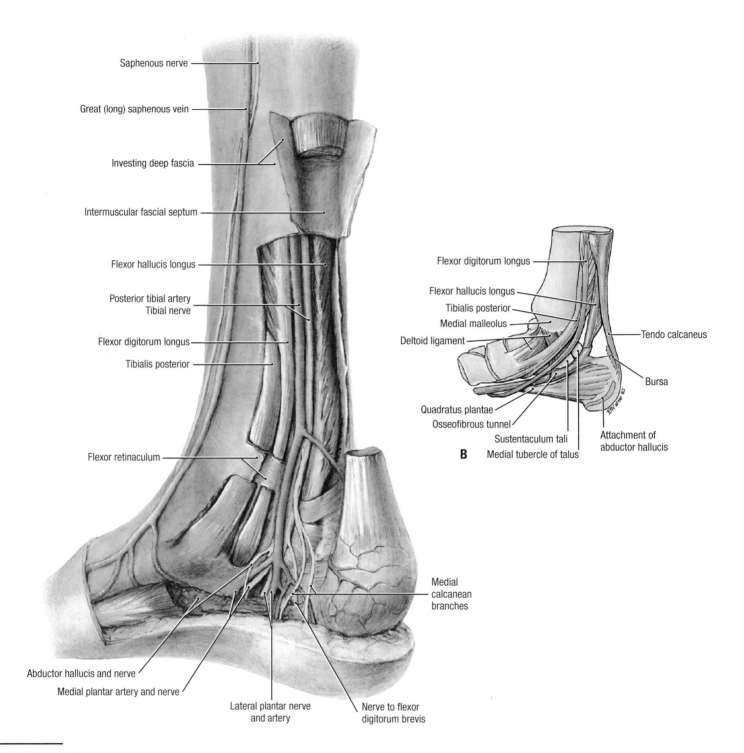

Saphenous nerve

Great (long) saphenous vein

Investing deep fascia

Intermuscular fascial septum

Flexor hallucis longus

Posterior tibial artery
Tibial nerve

Flexor digitorum longus

Tibialis posterior

Flexor retinaculum

Abductor hallucis and nerve

Medial plantar artery and nerve

Lateral plantar nerve
and artery

Nerve to flexor
digitorum brevis

Medial
calcanean
branches

A

Flexor digitorum longus

Flexor hallucis longus

Tibialis posterior

Medial malleolus

Deltoid ligament

Tendo calcaneus

Bursa

Quadratus plantae

Osseofibrous tunnel

Sustentaculum tali

Medial tubercle of talus

Attachment of
abductor hallucis

B

5.74   Medial ankle

A. Medial view. The posterior part of the abductor hallucis was excised. **B.** Schematic of tendons passing posterior to medial malleolus, medial view.

OBSERVE IN **A** and **B**:
1. The posterior tibial artery and the tibial nerve lie between the flexor digitorum longus and flexor hallucis longus muscles, and divide into medial and lateral plantar branches on the surface of the osseofibrous tunnel of the flexor hallucis longus muscle;

2. The tibialis posterior and flexor digitorum longus tendons occupy separate osseofibrous tunnels posterior to the medial malleolus. *The pulsations of the posterior tibial artery are palpated just posterior to the medial malleolus and to these two tendons;*
3. The tibialis posterior and flexor digitorum longus tendons use the medial malleolus as a pulley; only the flexor hallucis longus muscle uses the sustentaculum tali as a pulley;
4. The medial and lateral plantar nerves lie within the fork of the medial and lateral plantar arteries.

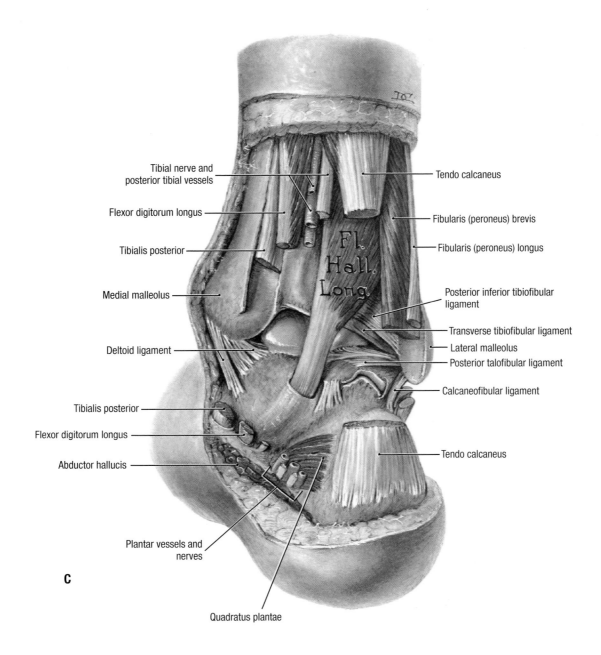

Tibial nerve and posterior tibial vessels

Flexor digitorum longus

Tibialis posterior

Medial malleolus

Deltoid ligament

Tibialis posterior

Flexor digitorum longus

Abductor hallucis

Plantar vessels and nerves

Fl. Hall. Long.

Tendo calcaneus

Fibularis (peroneus) brevis

Fibularis (peroneus) longus

Posterior inferior tibiofibular ligament

Transverse tibiofibular ligament

Lateral malleolus

Posterior talofibular ligament

Calcaneofibular ligament

Tendo calcaneus

C

Quadratus plantae

C. Posterior view.

OBSERVE IN **C:**

5. The flexor hallucis longus muscle is midway between the medial and lateral malleoli; the tendons of the flexor digitorum and tibialis posterior are medial to it; and the tendons of fibularis longus and brevis are lateral to it;

6. The entrance to the sole of the foot lies deep to the abductor hallucis muscle; the plantar vessels and nerves, two long digital flexors,

and part of the tibialis posterior enter here. The quadratus plantae serves as a soft pad for the vessel and nerves;

7. The posterior tibial artery and the tibial nerve lie medial to the flexor hallucis longus muscle proximally and distally, after bifurcating posterolateral to it;

8. The strongest parts of the ligaments of the ankle are those that prevent anterior displacement of the leg bones, namely, the posterior part of the deltoid (posterior tibiotalar), the posterior talofibular, the tibiocalcanean, and the calcaneofibular.

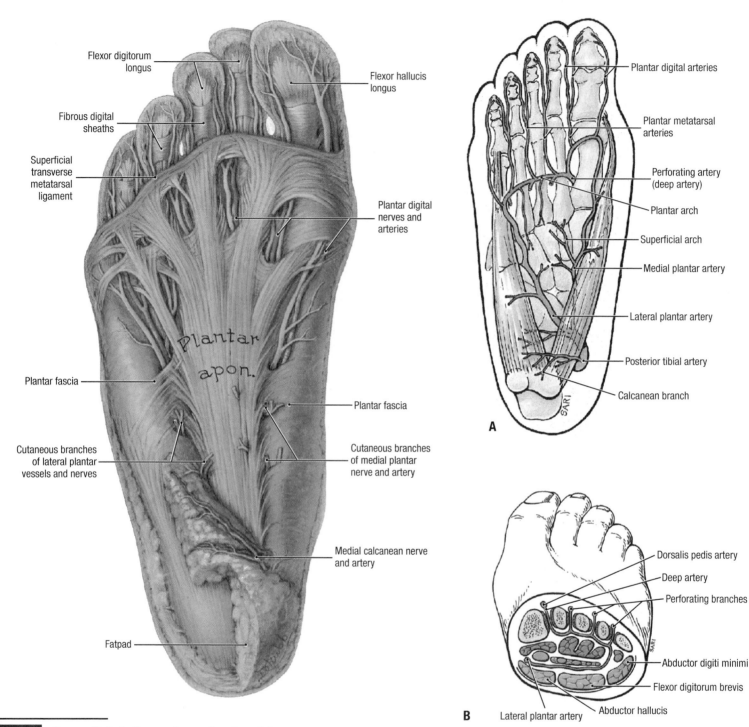

Flexor digitorum
longus

Flexor hallucis
longus

Fibrous digital
sheaths

Superficial
transverse
metatarsal
ligament

Plantar digital
nerves and
arteries

Plantar fascia

Plantar fascia

Cutaneous branches
of lateral plantar
vessels and nerves

Cutaneous branches
of medial plantar
nerve and artery

Medial calcanean nerve
and artery

Fatpad

Plantar apon.

Plantar digital arteries

Plantar metatarsal
arteries

Perforating artery
(deep artery)

Plantar arch

Superficial arch

Medial plantar artery

Lateral plantar artery

Posterior tibial artery

Calcanean branch

A

Dorsalis pedis artery

Deep artery

Perforating branches

Abductor digiti minimi

Flexor digitorum brevis

Abductor hallucis

B   Lateral plantar artery

5.75   **Superficial dissection of sole of foot**

Compare and contrast the plantar aponeurosis, the medial
and lateral parts of the plantar fascia, and the digital vessels and nerves with the corresponding structures in the
palm (Figures 6.61 and 6.62).

5.76   **Blood supply of foot**

A. Plantar arteries of sole of foot. **B.** Transverse section near
bases of metatarsals. The lateral plantar artery courses first
between the first and second layers of muscles, and then between the third and fourth layers. *Green*, first layer; *orange
and gray*, second layer; *brown*, third layer; *purple*, fourth layer.

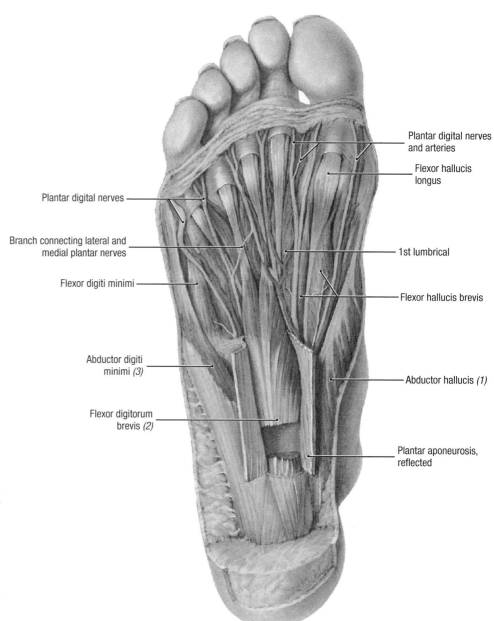

Plantar digital nerves and arteries

Flexor hallucis longus

Plantar digital nerves

Branch connecting lateral and medial plantar nerves

1st lumbrical

Flexor digiti minimi

Flexor hallucis brevis

Abductor digiti minimi *(3)*

Abductor hallucis *(1)*

Flexor digitorum brevis *(2)*

Plantar aponeurosis, reflected

5.77   **First layer of muscles of sole of foot, digital nerves, and arteries**

OBSERVE:

1. The muscles of this layer are: abductor digiti minimi, flexor digitorum brevis, and abductor hallucis;
2. The plantar aponeurosis and fascia are reflected or removed, and a section is removed from the flexor digitorum brevis muscle to show the fibrous tissue encasing it;
3. The lateral and medial plantar digital nerves, like the corresponding palmar digital branches of the ulnar and median nerves, supply 1½ and 3½ digits, respectively.

Table 5.9. Muscles in Sole of Foot—First Layer

Muscle	Proximal Attachment	Distal Attachment	Innervation	Main Actions
Abductor hallucis *(1)*	Medial tubercle of tuberosity of calcaneus, flexor retinaculum, and plantar aponeurosis	Medial side of base of proximal phalanx of first digit	Medial plantar nerve (S2 and **S3**)	Abducts and flexes
Flexor digitorum brevis *(2)*	Medial tubercle of tuberosity of calcaneus, plantar aponeurosis, and intermuscular septa	Both sides of middle phalanges of lateral four digits		Flexes lateral four digits
Abductor digiti minimi *(3)*	Medial and lateral tubercles of tuberosity of calcaneus, plantar aponeurosis, and intermuscular septa	Lateral side of base of proximal phalanx of fifth digit	Lateral plantar nerve (S2 and **S3**)	Abducts and flexes fifth digit

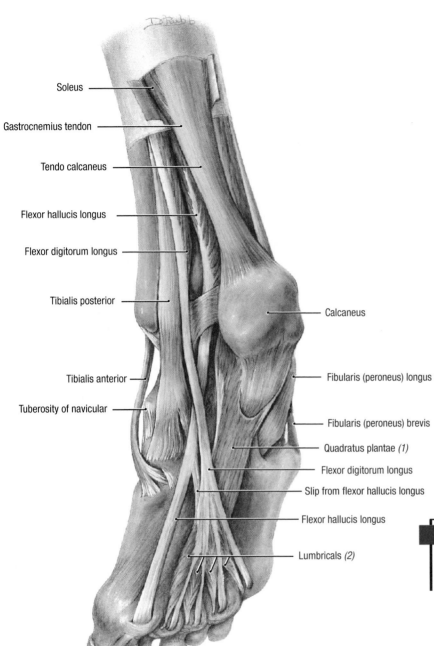

Soleus

Gastrocnemius tendon

Tendo calcaneus

Flexor hallucis longus

Flexor digitorum longus

Tibialis posterior

Tibialis anterior

Tuberosity of navicular

Calcaneus

Fibularis (peroneus) longus

Fibularis (peroneus) brevis

Quadratus plantae *(1)*

Flexor digitorum longus

Slip from flexor hallucis longus

Flexor hallucis longus

Lumbricals *(2)*

5.78   **Second layer of muscles of sole of foot**

OBSERVE:
1. The muscles of this layer are: flexor hallucis longus, flexor digitorum longus, four lumbricals, and quadratus plantae;
2. The flexor digitorum longus muscle crosses superficial to the tibialis posterior to the medial malleolus and superficial to the flexor hallucis longus muscle at the tuberosity of the navicular bone;
3. The four lumbrical muscles pass to the hallux (great toe) side of the toes.

Table 5.10. Muscles in Sole of Foot—Second Layer

Muscle	Proximal Attachment	Distal Attachment	Innervation	Main Actions
Quadratus plantae *(1)*	Medial surface and lateral margin of plantar surface of calcaneus	Posterolateral margin of tendon of flexor digitorum longus	Lateral plantar nerve (S2 and **S3**)	Assists flexor digitorum longus in flexing lateral four digits
Lumbricals *(2)*	Tendons of flexor digitorum longus	Medial aspect of expansion over lateral four digits	*Medial one:* medial plantar nerve (S2 and **S3**); *Lateral three:* lateral plantar nerve (S2 and **S3**)	Flex proximal phalanges and extend middle and distal phalanges of lateral four digits

5.79 Medial ankle and foot

A. Sesamoids of hallux, plantar surface. The sesamoid bones of the hallux are bound together and located on each side of a bony ridge on the first metatarsal. **B.** Foot raised as in walking, medial view.

OBSERVE:

1. The heel is raised, but the toes remain on the ground;
2. The sesamoid bones are a "footstool" for the first metatarsal, giving it increased height;
3. The quadratus plantae muscle lines the concave medial surface of the calcaneus;
4. By inserting into the flexor digitorum longus muscle, the quadratus plantae muscle acts as a guy wire, modifying the oblique pull of the flexor tendons;
5. The flexor hallucis longus muscle uses three pulleys: a groove on the posterior aspect of the distal end of the tibia, a groove on the posterior aspect of the talus, and a groove inferior to the sustentaculum tali.

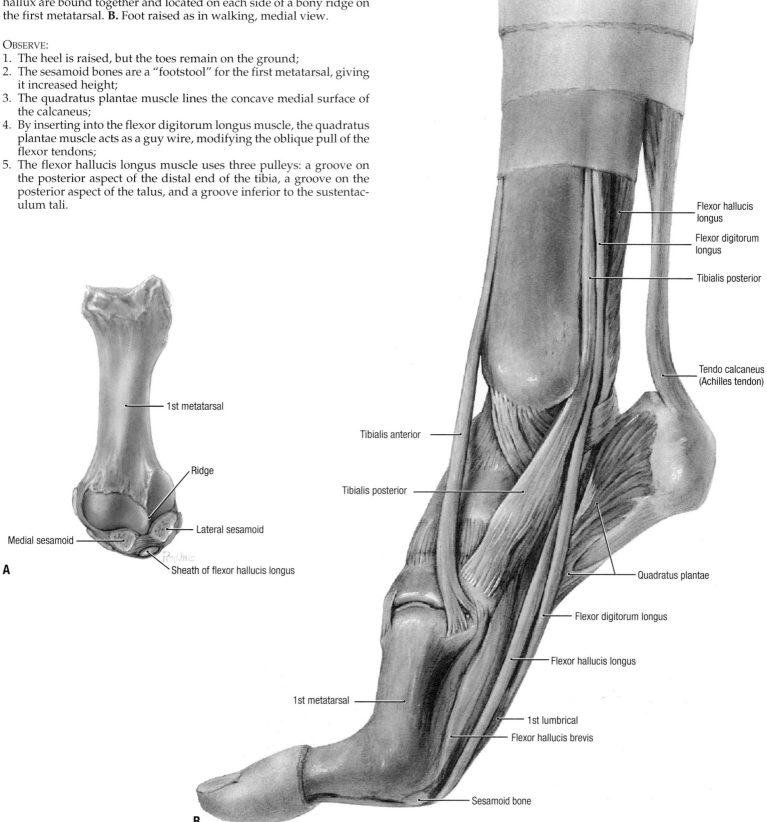

A.
- 1st metatarsal
- Ridge
- Lateral sesamoid
- Medial sesamoid
- Sheath of flexor hallucis longus

B.
- Flexor hallucis longus
- Flexor digitorum longus
- Tibialis posterior
- Tendo calcaneus (Achilles tendon)
- Tibialis anterior
- Tibialis posterior
- Quadratus plantae
- Flexor digitorum longus
- Flexor hallucis longus
- 1st metatarsal
- 1st lumbrical
- Flexor hallucis brevis
- Sesamoid bone

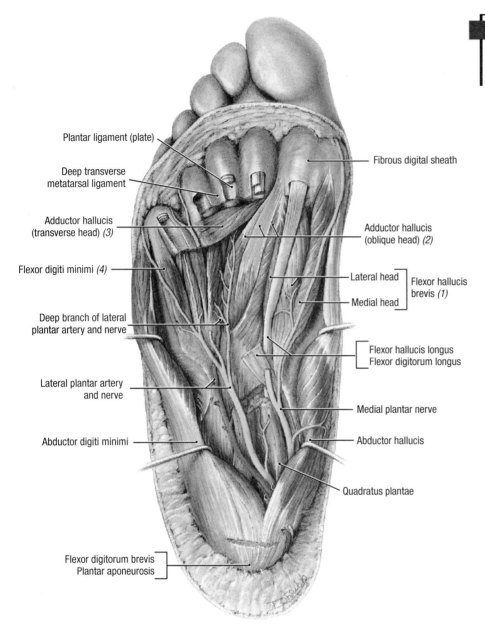

Plantar ligament (plate)

Deep transverse
metatarsal ligament

Adductor hallucis
(transverse head) *(3)*

Flexor digiti minimi *(4)*

Deep branch of lateral
plantar artery and nerve

Lateral plantar artery
and nerve

Abductor digiti minimi

Flexor digitorum brevis
Plantar aponeurosis

Fibrous digital sheath

Adductor hallucis
(oblique head) *(2)*

Lateral head ⎤ Flexor hallucis
Medial head ⎦ brevis *(1)*

Flexor hallucis longus
Flexor digitorum longus

Medial plantar nerve

Abductor hallucis

Quadratus plantae

5.80 Third layer of muscles of sole of foot

OBSERVE:

1. The muscles of this layer are: flexor digiti minimi, adductor hallucis, and flexor hallucis brevis;
2. Of the first layer, the abductor digiti minimi and abductor hallucis muscles are pulled aside and the flexor digitorum brevis muscle is cut short. Of the second layer, the flexor digitorum longus and lumbrical muscles are excised and the quadratus plantae muscle is cut;
3. The lateral plantar nerve and artery course laterally between the muscles of the first and second layers; their deep branches then course medially between the muscles of the third and fourth layers.

Table 5.11. Muscles in Sole of Foot—Third Layer

Muscle	Proximal Attachment	Distal Attachment	Innervation	Main Actions
Flexor hallucis brevis *(1)*	Plantar surfaces of cuboid and lateral cuneiforms	Both sides of base of proximal phalanx of first digit	Medial plantar nerve (S2 and **S3**)	Flexes proximal phalanx of first digit
Adductor hallucis	*Oblique head (2):* bases of metatarsals 2–4; *Transverse head (3):* plantar ligaments of metatarsophalangeal joints	Tendons of both heads attach to lateral side of base of proximal phalanx of first digit	Deep branch of lateral plantar nerve (S2 and **S3**)	Adducts first digit; assists in maintaining transverse arch of foot
Flexor digiti minimi *(4)*	Base of fifth metatarsal	Base of proximal phalanx of fifth digit	Superficial branch of lateral plantar nerve (S2 and **S3**)	Flexes proximal phalanx of fifth digit, thereby assisting with its flexion

5.81 Fourth layer of muscles of sole of foot

OBSERVE:

1. The muscles of this layer are the three plantar and four dorsal interossei in the anterior half of the foot, and the tendons of fibularis (peroneus) longus and of tibialis posterior in the posterior half;
2. Of the first three layers, the abductor and flexor brevis muscles of the fifth toe and the abductor and flexor brevis muscles of the big toe remain for purposes of orientation;
3. The plantar interossei adduct the three lateral toes toward an axial line that passes through the second metatarsal bone and second toe, whereas the dorsal interossei abduct from this line.

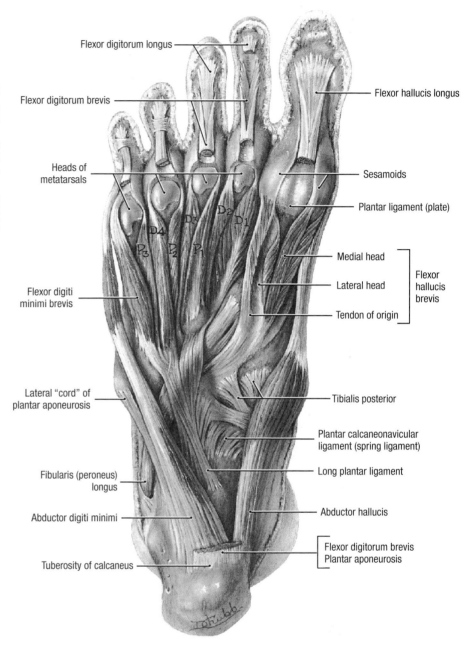

Flexor digitorum longus

Flexor digitorum brevis

Heads of metatarsals

D4 D3 D2 D1

P3 P2 P1

Flexor digiti minimi brevis

Lateral "cord" of plantar aponeurosis

Fibularis (peroneus) longus

Abductor digiti minimi

Tuberosity of calcaneus

Flexor hallucis longus

Sesamoids

Plantar ligament (plate)

Medial head

Lateral head Flexor hallucis brevis

Tendon of origin

Tibialis posterior

Plantar calcaneonavicular ligament (spring ligament)

Long plantar ligament

Abductor hallucis

Flexor digitorum brevis
Plantar aponeurosis

Table 5.12. Muscles in Sole of Foot—Fourth Layer

Muscle	Proximal Attachment	Distal Attachment	Innervation	Main Actions
Plantar interossei (three muscles, P1–P3)	Bases and medial sides of metatarsals 3–5	Medial sides of bases of proximal phalanges of third to fifth digits	Lateral plantar nerve (S2 and S3)	Adduct digits (2–4) and flex metatarsophalangeal joints
Dorsal interossei (four muscles, D1–D4)	Adjacent sides of metatarsals 1–5	First: medial side of proximal phalanx of second digit; Second to fourth: lateral sides of second to fourth digits		Abduct digits (2–4) and flex metatarsophalangeal joints

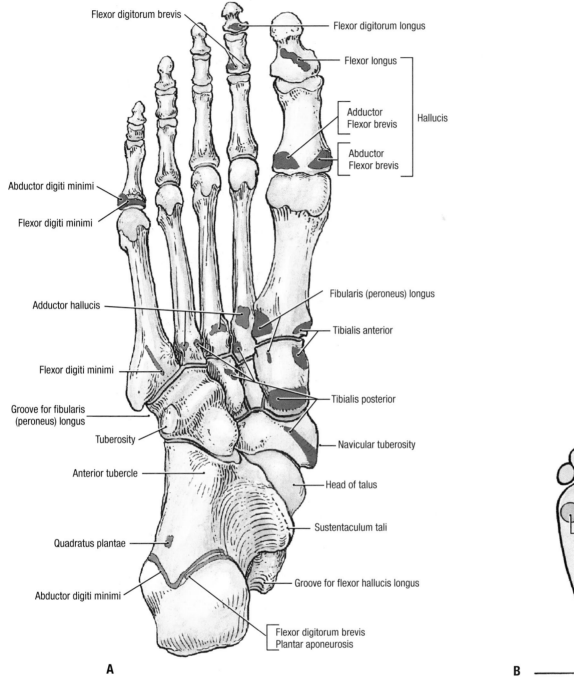

Flexor digitorum brevis

Flexor digitorum longus

Flexor longus

Adductor
Flexor brevis

Hallucis

Abductor
Flexor brevis

Abductor digiti minimi

Flexor digiti minimi

Adductor hallucis

Fibularis (peroneus) longus

Tibialis anterior

Flexor digiti minimi

Groove for fibularis
(peroneus) longus

Tuberosity

Tibialis posterior

Navicular tuberosity

Anterior tubercle

Head of talus

Quadratus plantae

Sustentaculum tali

Abductor digiti minimi

Groove for flexor hallucis longus

Flexor digitorum brevis
Plantar aponeurosis

A

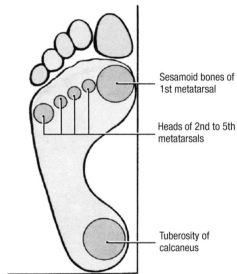

Sesamoid bones of
1st metatarsal

Heads of 2nd to 5th
metatarsals

Tuberosity of
calcaneus

B

5.82   Bones of foot, plantar view

A. Muscle attachments. **B.** Weight-bearing areas. The weight of the body is transmitted to the talus from the tibia and fibula; it is then transmitted to the tuberosity of the calcaneus, the heads of the second to fifth metatarsals, and the sesamoid bones of the first digit.

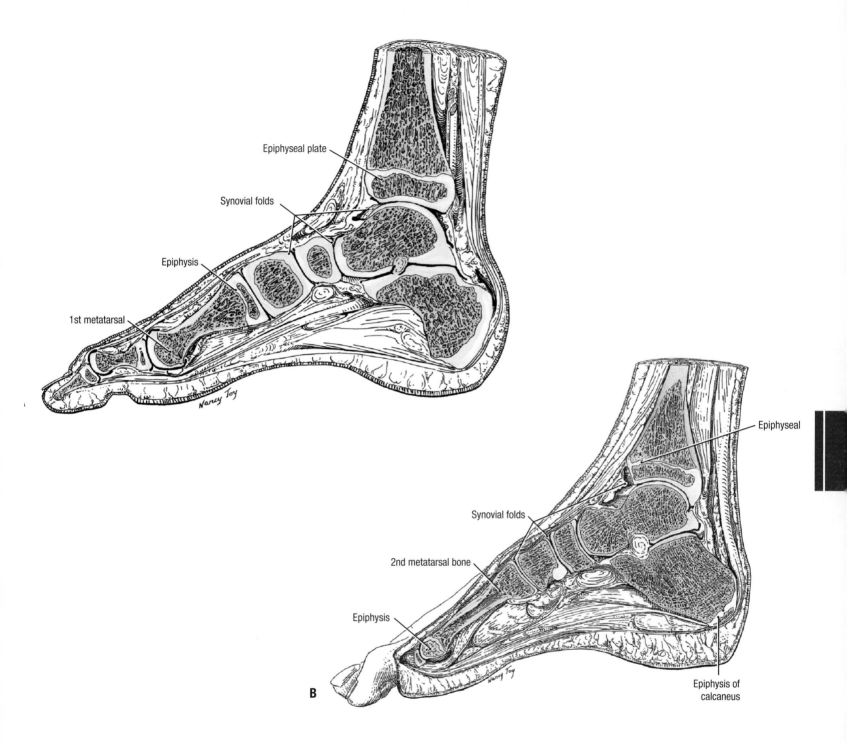

5.83 Sagittal sections through the foot

A. Foot of child age 4. **B.** Foot of child age 10.

OBSERVE:

1. In the foot of the younger child **(A)**, epiphyses of long bones (tibia, metatarsals, and phalanges) ossify like short bones, with the ossific centers being enveloped in cartilage. Ossification has already extended to the surface of the larger tarsal bones;
2. In the foot of the older child **(B)**, ossification has spread to the dorsal and plantar surfaces of all tarsal bones in view, and cartilage persists on the articular surfaces only;

3. The traction epiphysis of the calcaneus for the tendo calcaneus and plantar aponeurosis begins to ossify from the ages of 6 to 10 years;
4. The first metatarsal bone is similar to a phalanx in that its epiphysis is at the base versus the head, as in the second and other metatarsal bones;
5. The tuberosity of the calcaneus and the sesamoid bones of the first and the heads of the second to fifth metatarsals (here the second) support the longitudinal arch of the foot; the medial part of the longitudinal arch is higher and more mobile than the lateral.

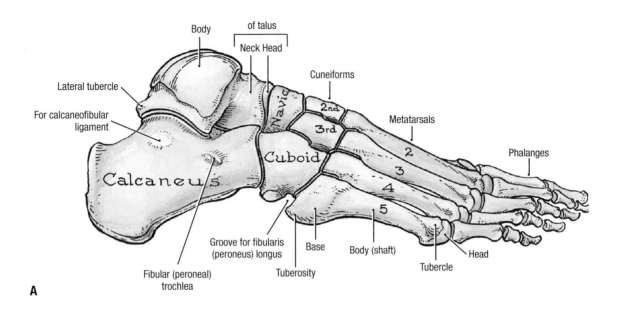

A. Lateral view.

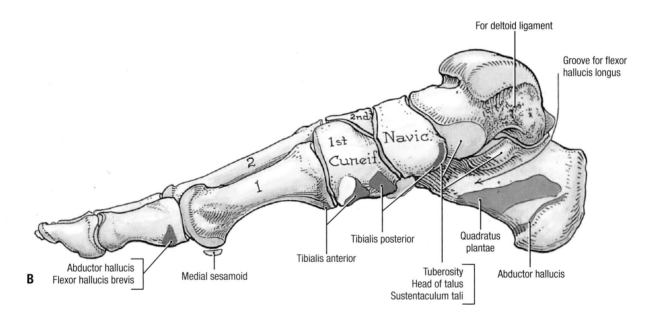

5.84 Bones of foot, medial and lateral views

A. Lateral view. The lateral part of the longitudinal arch of the foot consists of the calcaneus, cuboid, and fourth and fifth metatarsals. **B.** Medial view. The medial part of the longitudinal arch of the foot consists of the calcaneus, talus, navicular, three cuneiforms, and first, second, and third metatarsals.

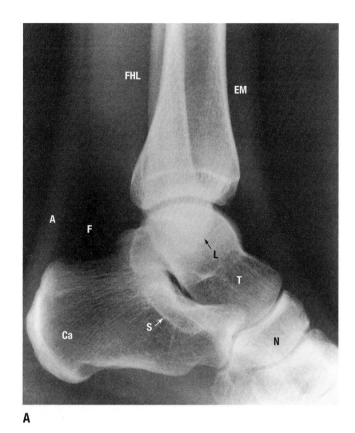

A

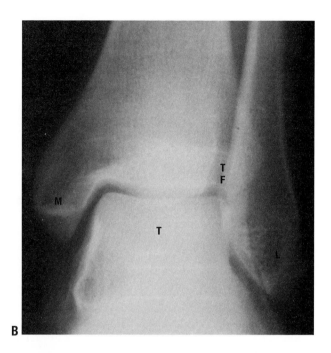

B

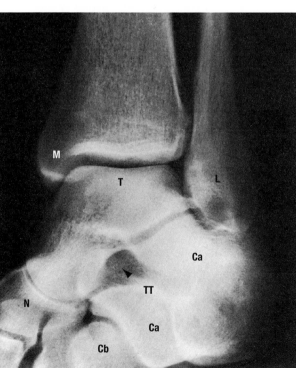

C

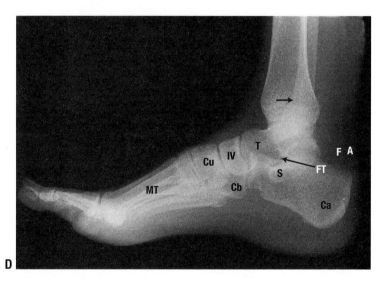

D

5.85 Radiographs of foot and ankle

A. Medial view of ankle region. **B.** Anterior view of ankle. **C.** Lateral view of ankle region. **D.** Lateral view of foot. *M,* Medial malleolus; *L,* Lateral malleolus; *T,* Talus; *Ca,* Calcaneus; *S,* Sustentaculum tali; *N,* Navicular; *Cu,* Cuneiforms; *Cb,* Cuboid; *Mt,* Metatarsal; *TT,* Tarsal tunnel; *A,* Achilles tendon; *F,* Fat; *Arrowhead,* Superimposed tibia and fibula; *TF,* Inferior tibiofibular joint; *FHL,* Flexor hallucis longus; *EM,* Extensor muscles.

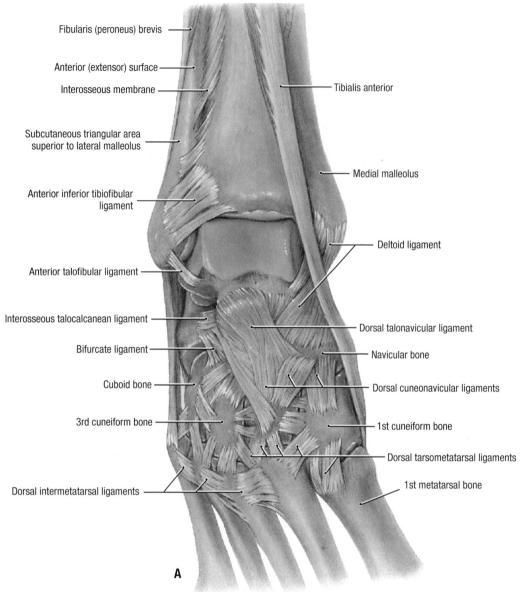

Fibularis (peroneus) brevis

Anterior (extensor) surface

Interosseous membrane

Subcutaneous triangular area
superior to lateral malleolus

Anterior inferior tibiofibular
ligament

Anterior talofibular ligament

Interosseous talocalcanean ligament

Bifurcate ligament

Cuboid bone

3rd cuneiform bone

Dorsal intermetatarsal ligaments

Tibialis anterior

Medial malleolus

Deltoid ligament

Dorsal talonavicular ligament

Navicular bone

Dorsal cuneonavicular ligaments

1st cuneiform bone

Dorsal tarsometatarsal ligaments

1st metatarsal bone

A

5.86   Ankle joint and joints of dorsum of foot

A. Ligaments, anterosuperior view. The ankle joint is plantar flexed, and its anterior capsular fibers are removed. **B.** Distended ankle joint, anterior view.

OBSERVE IN **A**:
1. The fibers of the interosseous membrane and ligaments uniting the fibula to the tibia are so directed as to resist the inferior pull of the muscles, but allow the fibula to be forced superiorly;
2. The anterior talofibular ligament is a weak band that is easily torn;

OBSERVE IN **B**:
3. The extension of the synovial membrane on the neck of the talus;
4. The anterior articular surfaces of the talus and calcaneus, each convex from side to side, thus the foot can be inverted and everted at the transverse tarsal joint;
5. The relations of the tendons to the sustentaculum tali: the flexor hallucis longus inferior to it, flexor digitorum longus along its medial aspect, and tibialis posterior superior to it and in contact with the deltoid ligament.

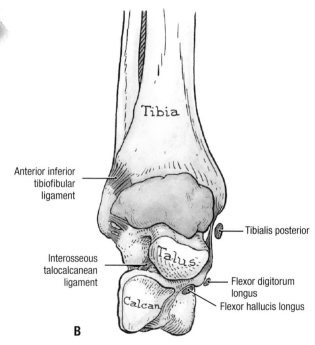

Tibia

Anterior inferior
tibiofibular
ligament

Interosseous
talocalcanean
ligament

Tibialis posterior

Talus

Flexor digitorum
longus

Flexor hallucis longus

Calcan

B

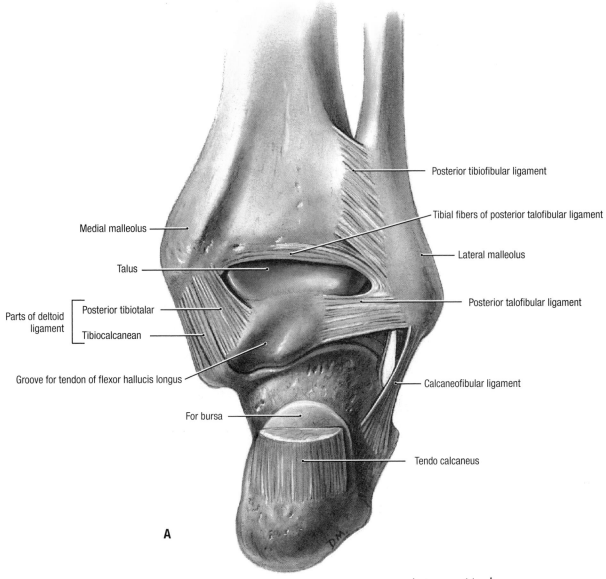

Posterior tibiofibular ligament

Tibial fibers of posterior talofibular ligament

Medial malleolus

Talus

Lateral malleolus

Parts of deltoid ligament
- Posterior tibiotalar
- Tibiocalcanean

Posterior talofibular ligament

Groove for tendon of flexor hallucis longus

Calcaneofibular ligament

For bursa

Tendo calcaneus

A

5.87 Ankle joint, posterior views

A. Dissection. **B.** Distended ankle joint. Observe the grooves for the flexor hallucis longus muscle, which crosses the middle of the ankle joint posteriorly, the two tendons posterior to the medial malleolus, and the two tendons posterior to the lateral malleolus.

OBSERVE:

1. The posterior aspect of the ankle joint is strengthened by the transversely oriented posterior tibiofibular and posterior talofibular ligaments;
2. The calcaneofibular ligament stabilizes the joint laterally, and the posterior tibiotalar and tibiocalcanean parts of the deltoid ligament stabilize it medially;
3. The groove for the flexor hallucis tendon is between the medial and lateral tubercles of the talus and continues inferior to the sustentaculum tali.

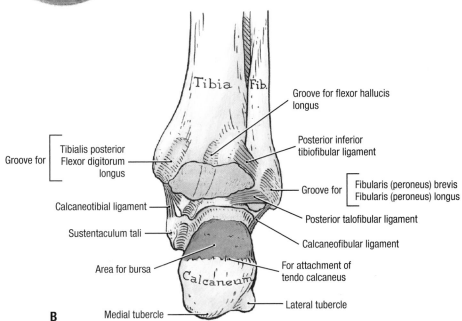

Tibia   Fib.

Groove for flexor hallucis longus

Groove for
- Tibialis posterior
- Flexor digitorum longus

Posterior inferior tibiofibular ligament

Calcaneotibial ligament

Groove for
- Fibularis (peroneus) brevis
- Fibularis (peroneus) longus

Sustentaculum tali

Posterior talofibular ligament

Calcaneofibular ligament

Area for bursa

For attachment of tendo calcaneus

Calcaneum

Lateral tubercle

Medial tubercle

B

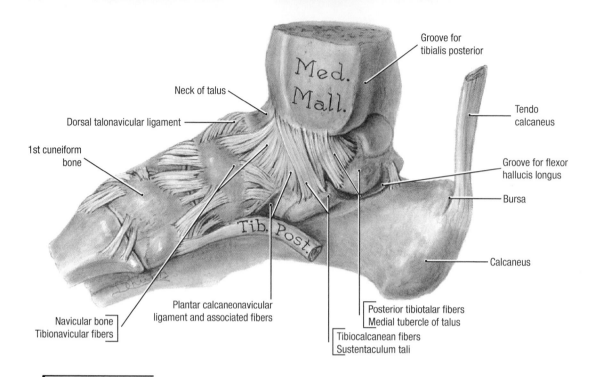

Groove for
tibialis posterior

Neck of talus

Dorsal talonavicular ligament

Med. Mall.

Tendo
calcaneus

1st cuneiform
bone

Groove for flexor
hallucis longus

Bursa

Tib. Post.

Calcaneus

Navicular bone
Tibionavicular fibers

Plantar calcaneonavicular
ligament and associated fibers

Posterior tibiotalar fibers
Medial tubercle of talus

Tibiocalcanean fibers
Sustentaculum tali

5.88 **Ligaments of ankle, medial view**

OBSERVE:
1. The tibialis posterior is displaced from its "bed" of the medial malleolus, deltoid ligament, and plantar calcaneonavicular (spring) ligament;
2. The deltoid ligament is attached superiorly to the medial malleolus of the tibia and inferiorly to the talus, navicular, and calcaneus.

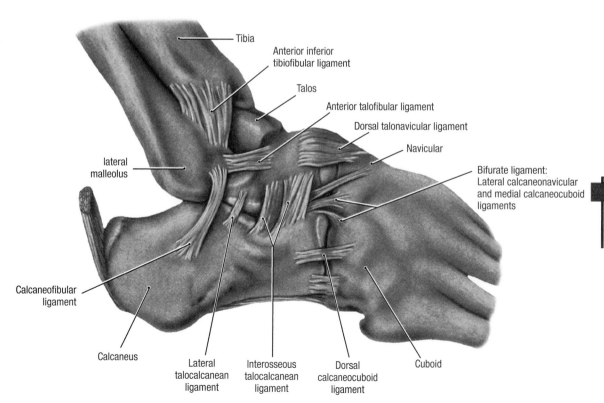

Tibia

Anterior inferior
tibiofibular ligament

Talos

Anterior talofibular ligament

Dorsal talonavicular ligament

Navicular

lateral
malleolus

Bifurate ligament:
Lateral calcaneonavicular
and medial calcaneocuboid
ligaments

Calcaneofibular
ligament

Calcaneus

Lateral
talocalcanean
ligament

Interosseous
talocalcanean
ligament

Dorsal
calcaneocuboid
ligament

Cuboid

5.89 **Ligaments of ankle, lateral view**

OBSERVE:
1. The ankle is plantar flexed, thus part of the body of the talus is exposed, and the foot is inverted;
2. The direction of the ligaments that unite the calcaneus to the navicular, talus, and fibula prevents the calcaneus from being driven posteriorly.

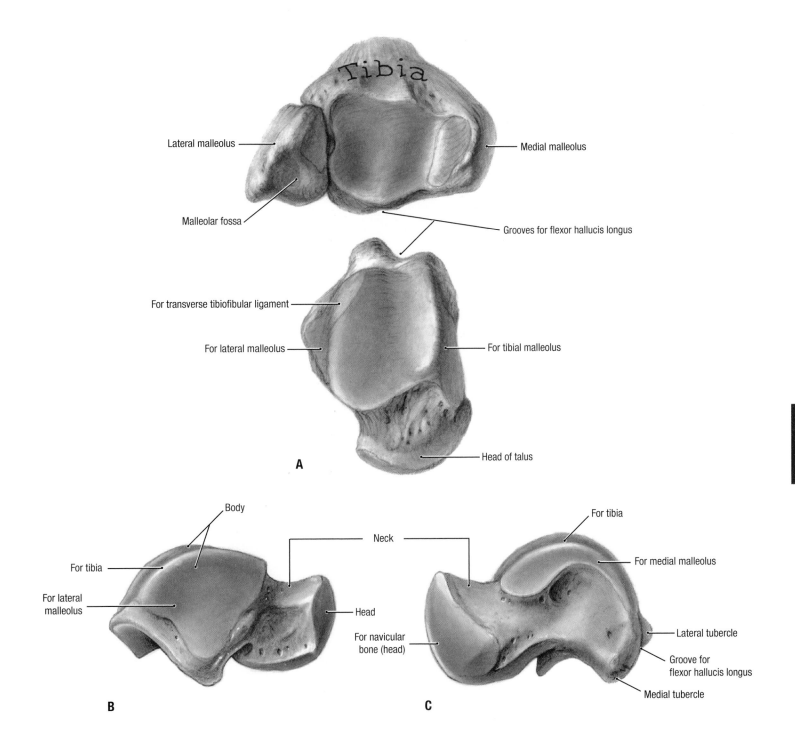

5.90 Articular surfaces of ankle joint

A. Talus separated from tibia and fibula (inferior view of the articular surfaces of the tibia and fibula, and superior view of the articular surface of the talus). The superior articular surface of the talus is broader anteriorly than posteriorly; hence the medial and lateral malleoli, which grasp the sides of the talus tend to be forced apart in dorsiflexion. The fully dorsiflexed position is stable compared to the fully plantar flexed position; in plantar flexion, when the tibia and fibula ar-

ticulate with the narrower posterior part of the superior articular surface of the talus, some side- to-side movement of the joint is allowed, accounting for the instability of the joint in this position. **B.** Talus, lateral view. Observe the lateral, triangular area for articulation with the lateral malleolus. **C.** Talus, medial view. Observe the comma-shaped area for articulation with the medial malleolus.

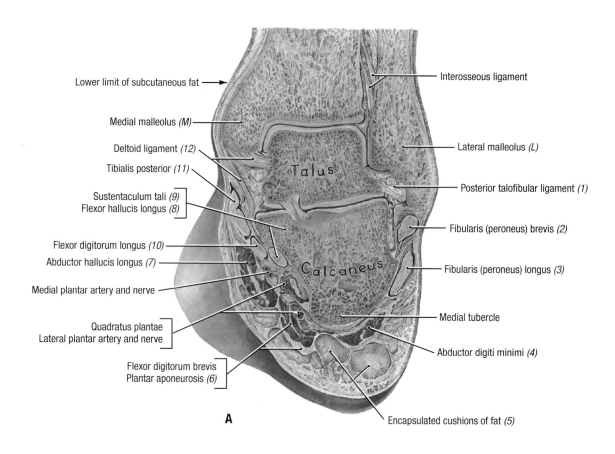

Lower limit of subcutaneous fat →

Medial malleolus *(M)*

Deltoid ligament *(12)*

Tibialis posterior *(11)*

Sustentaculum tali *(9)*
Flexor hallucis longus *(8)*

Flexor digitorum longus *(10)*

Abductor hallucis longus *(7)*

Medial plantar artery and nerve

Quadratus plantae
Lateral plantar artery and nerve

Flexor digitorum brevis
Plantar aponeurosis *(6)*

Interosseous ligament

Lateral malleolus *(L)*

Posterior talofibular ligament *(1)*

Fibularis (peroneus) brevis *(2)*

Fibularis (peroneus) longus *(3)*

Medial tubercle

Abductor digiti minimi *(4)*

Encapsulated cushions of fat *(5)*

Talus

Calcaneus

A

5.91   Coronal section and MRI through ankle

A. Coronal section. **B.** Coronal MRI. (Numbers in **B** refer to structures labeled in **A**.)

OBSERVE:
1. The tibia rests on the talus, and the talus rests on the calcaneus; between the calcaneus and the skin are several encapsulated cushions of fat;
2. The lateral malleolus descends much farther in-feriorly than the medial malleolus;
3. The interosseous tibiofibular ligament is weak;
4. The interosseous band between the talus and calcaneus separates the subtalar, or posterior, talocalcanean joint from the talocalcaneonavicu-lar joint;
5. The sustentaculum tali acts as a pulley for the flexor hallucis longus muscle and gives attach-ment to the calcaneotibial band of the deltoid ligament.

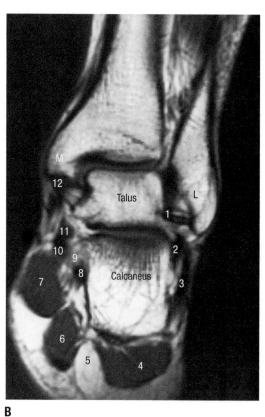

B

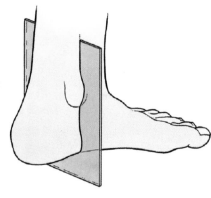

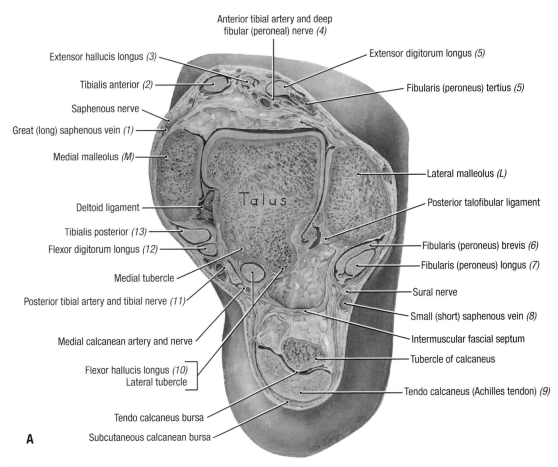

Anterior tibial artery and deep fibular (peroneal) nerve (4)

Extensor hallucis longus (3)

Tibialis anterior (2)

Saphenous nerve

Great (long) saphenous vein (1)

Medial malleolus (M)

Deltoid ligament

Tibialis posterior (13)

Flexor digitorum longus (12)

Medial tubercle

Posterior tibial artery and tibial nerve (11)

Medial calcanean artery and nerve

Flexor hallucis longus (10)
Lateral tubercle

Tendo calcaneus bursa

Subcutaneous calcanean bursa

Extensor digitorum longus (5)

Fibularis (peroneus) tertius (5)

Lateral malleolus (L)

Posterior talofibular ligament

Fibularis (peroneus) brevis (6)

Fibularis (peroneus) longus (7)

Sural nerve

Small (short) saphenous vein (8)

Intermuscular fascial septum

Tubercle of calcaneus

Tendo calcaneus (Achilles tendon) (9)

Talus

A

5.92　Transverse section and MRI through ankle

A. Transverse section. **B.** Transverse MRI. (Numbers in **B** refer to structures labeled in **A**.)

OBSERVE:

1. The body of the talus is wedge-shaped and grasped by the malleoli, which are bound to it by the deltoid and posterior talofibular ligaments and thereby prevented from sliding anteriorly;

2. The flexor hallucis longus muscle lies within its fibroosseous sheath between the medial and lateral tubercles of the talus;

3. Two tendons, each within a separate sheath (fibrous and synovial), lie posterior to the medial malleolus, and two tendons within a common sheath lie posterior to the lateral malleolus;

4. Because of the intervening fibrous sheath, the posterior tibial vessels and the tibial nerve are undisturbed by the excursions of the flexor hallucis longus muscle;

5. There is a small, inconstant bursa superficial to the tendo calcaneus and a large, constant bursa deep to it that contains a long synovial fold;

6. The anterior tibial artery and its companion nerve are at the midpoint of the anterior aspect of the ankle, with two tendons medial to it and two tendons lateral to it.

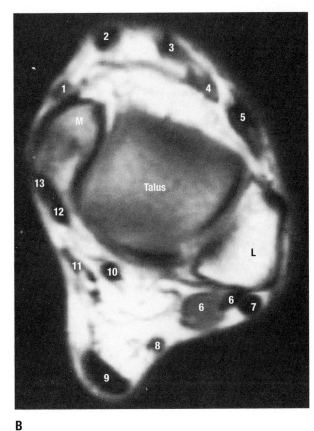

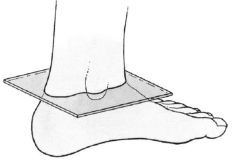

B

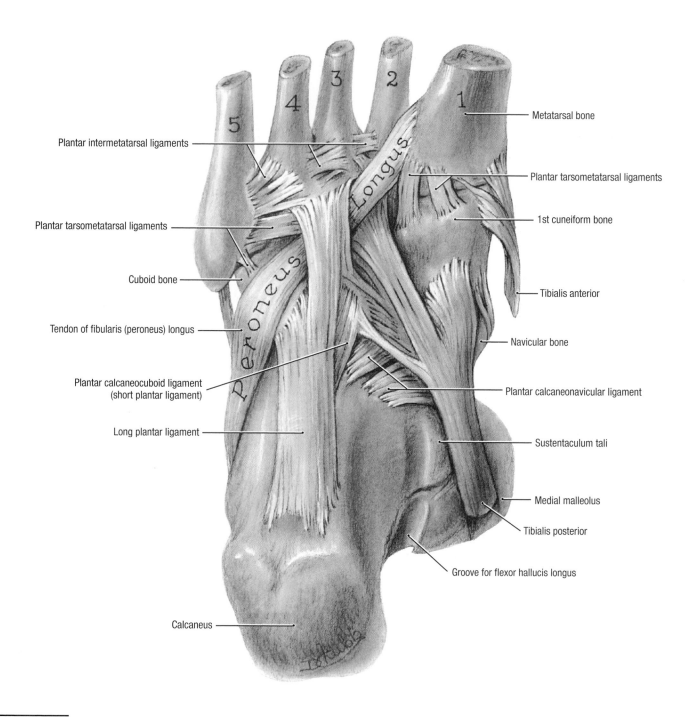

Metatarsal bone

Plantar intermetatarsal ligaments

Plantar tarsometatarsal ligaments

Plantar tarsometatarsal ligaments

1st cuneiform bone

Cuboid bone

Tibialis anterior

Tendon of fibularis (peroneus) longus

Navicular bone

Plantar calcaneocuboid ligament (short plantar ligament)

Plantar calcaneonavicular ligament

Long plantar ligament

Sustentaculum tali

Medial malleolus

Tibialis posterior

Groove for flexor hallucis longus

Calcaneus

5.93   Ligaments of sole of foot–I, plantar view

OBSERVE:

1. The insertions of three long tendons: fibularis (peroneus) longus, tibialis anterior, and tibialis posterior;
2. The tendon of the fibularis (peroneus) longus muscle crosses the sole of the foot in the groove anterior to the ridge of the cuboid, is bridged by some fibers of the long plantar ligament, and inserts into the base of the first metatarsal. Usually, like the tibialis an-

terior, it also inserts into the first cuneiform. It is an evertor of the foot; the tendon of fibularis longus has a synovial sheath that accompanies it across the sole of the foot;

3. Slips of the tibialis posterior tendon extend like the fingers of an open hand to grasp the bones anterior to the transverse tarsal joint; the tibialis posterior tendon is an invertor of the foot.

5.94 Ligaments of sole of foot–II, plantar views

A. Deep dissection. **B.** Support for head of talus. Bones, plantar view (left). Bones and ligaments, plantar view (right). The head of the talus is supported by the plantar calcaneonavicular ligament (spring ligament) and the tendon of tibialis posterior.

OBSERVE:

1. The plantar calcaneocuboid (short plantar) and plantar calcaneonavicular (spring) ligaments are the inferior ligaments of the transverse tarsal joint;
2. The ligaments in the anterior of the foot diverge posteriorly from each side of the long axis of the third metatarsal and third cuneiform; hence a backward thrust to the first metatarsal, as when rising on the big toe while in walking, is transmitted directly to the navicular and talus by the first cuneiform, and indirectly by the second metatarsal, second cuneiform, third metatarsal, and third cuneiform;
3. A posterior thrust to the fourth and fifth metatarsals is transmitted directly to the cuboid and calcaneus;
4. Posterior displacement of the bones of the lateral longitudinal arch is prevented by the adjoining ligaments.

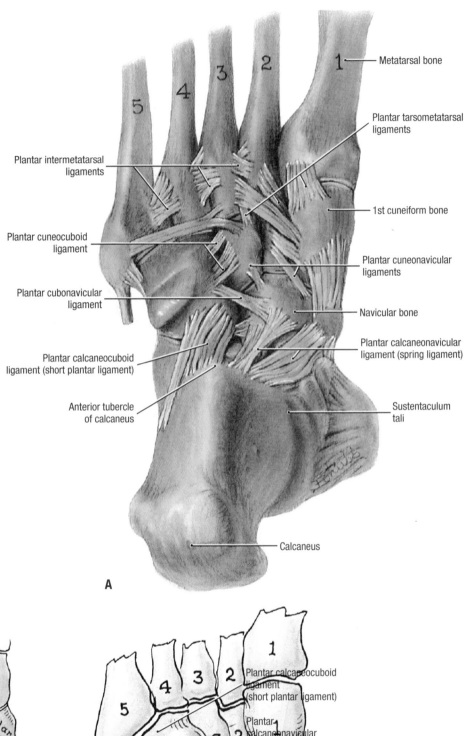

A

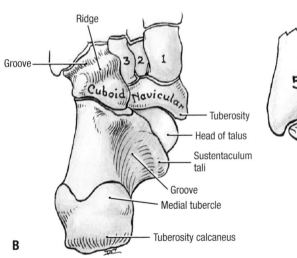

B

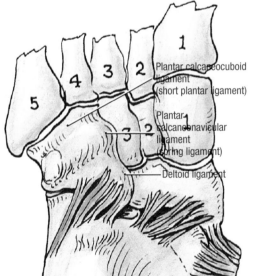

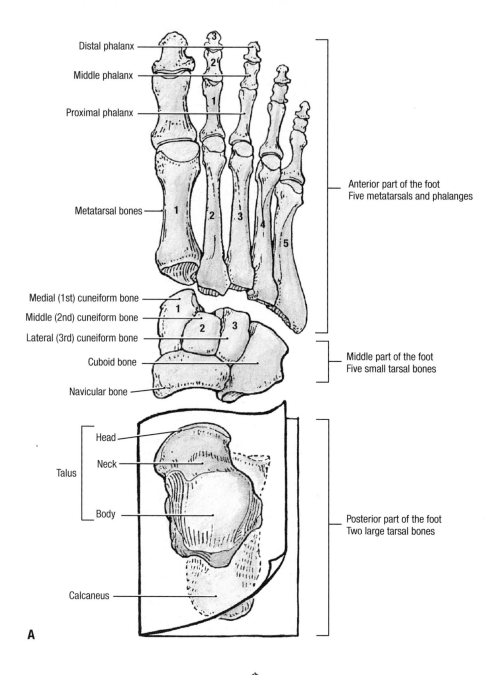

Distal phalanx

Middle phalanx

Proximal phalanx

Metatarsal bones

Anterior part of the foot
Five metatarsals and phalanges

Medial (1st) cuneiform bone

Middle (2nd) cuneiform bone

Lateral (3rd) cuneiform bone

Cuboid bone

Navicular bone

Middle part of the foot
Five small tarsal bones

Head

Neck

Talus

Body

Posterior part of the foot
Two large tarsal bones

Calcaneus

A

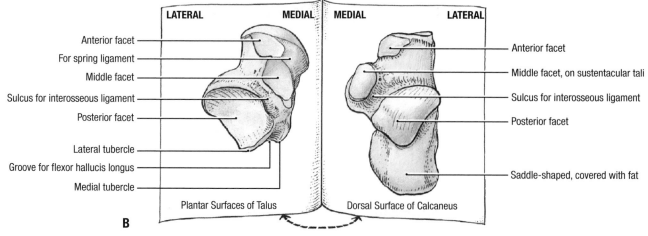

LATERAL   MEDIAL   MEDIAL   LATERAL

Anterior facet

For spring ligament

Middle facet

Sulcus for interosseous ligament

Posterior facet

Lateral tubercle

Groove for flexor hallucis longus

Medial tubercle

Anterior facet

Middle facet, on sustentacular tali

Sulcus for interosseous ligament

Posterior facet

Saddle-shaped, covered with fat

Plantar Surfaces of Talus   Dorsal Surface of Calcaneus

B

Table 5.13. Joints of Foot

Joint	Type	Articular Surface	Articular Capsule	Ligaments	Movements
Subtalar	Plane type of synovial joint	Inferior surface of body of talus articulates with superior surface of calcaneus	Fibrous capsule is attached to margins of articular surfaces	Medial, lateral, and posterior talocalcaneal ligaments support capsule; interosseous talocalcaneal ligament binds bones together	Inversion and eversion of foot
Talocalcaneo-navicular	Synovial joint; talonavicular part is ball and socket type	Head of talus articulates with calcaneus and navicular bones	Fibrous capsule incompletely encloses joint	Plantar calcaneonav-icular ("spring") ligament supports head of talus	Gliding and rotary movements are possible
Calcaneocuboid	Plane type of synovial joint	Anterior end of calcaneus articulates with posterior surface of cuboid	Fibrous capsule encloses joint	Dorsal calcaneocu-boid ligament, plantar calcaneocu-boid ligament, and long plantar ligament support fibrous capsule	Inversion and eversion of foot
Tarsometatarsal	Plane type of synovial joint	Anterior tarsal bones articulate with bases of metatarsal bones	Fibrous capsule encloses joint	Dorsal, plantar, and interosseous ligaments	Gliding or sliding
Intermetatarsal	Plane type of synovial joint	Bases of metatarsal bones articulate with each other	Fibrous capsule encloses each joint	Dorsal, plantar, and interosseous ligaments bind bones together	Little individual movement of bones possible
Metatarso-phalangeal	Condyloid type of synovial joint	Heads of metatarsal bones articulate with bases of proximal phalanges	Fibrous capsule encloses each joint	Collateral ligaments support capsule on each side; plantar ligament supports plantar part of capsule	Flexion, extension, and some abduction, adduction, and circumduction
Interphalangeal	Hinge type of synovial joint	Head of one phalanx articulates with base of one distal to it	Fibrous capsule encloses each joint	Collateral and plantar ligaments support joints	Flexion and extension

5.95 Bones of foot and talocalcanean joint

A. Bones of foot, dorsal view. **B.** Bony surfaces of talocalcanean joints. The plantar surface of the talus and dorsal surface of the calcaneus are displayed as pages in a book.

OBSERVE IN **B:**

1. The joints are synovial gliding joints; therefore, the apposed, or cor-responding, facets are not exact counterparts of each other, i.e., one is more extensive than the other;
2. The talus is part of: (a) the ankle (supratalar) joint; (b) the posterior talocalcanean (subtalar) and anterior talocalcanean (infratalar) joints; and the (c) talonavicular (pretalar) joint;
3. At the supratalar joint, only flexion and extension are usually per-mitted; at the infratalar and pretalar joints, inversion and eversion occur;
4. The two parts of the infratalar joint are separated from each other by the sulcus tali and sulcus calcanei, which, when the talus and calca-neus are in articulation, become the tarsal sinus, or tunnel;
5. The convex posterior talar facet of the calcaneus, the concave mid-dle and anterior talar facets, and the concave talar facet of the nav-icular all have their counterparts on the talus.

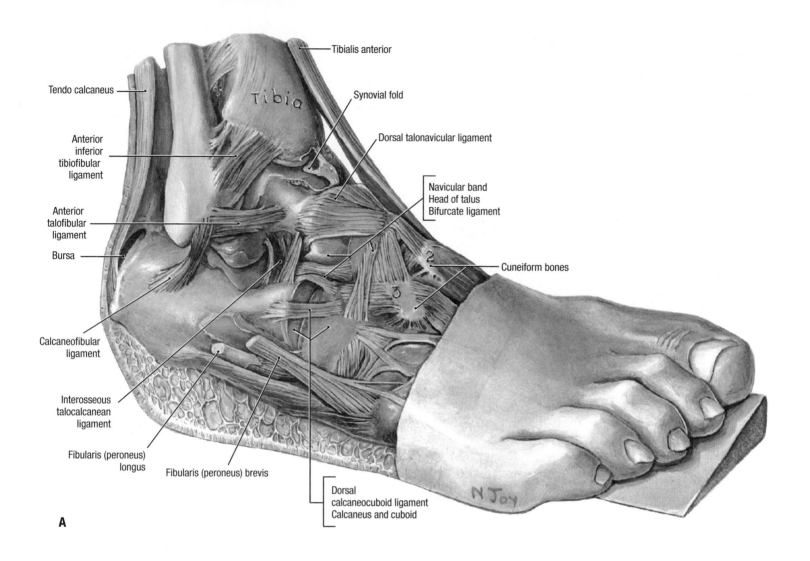

Tibialis anterior

Tendo calcaneus

Synovial fold

Anterior
inferior
tibiofibular
ligament

Dorsal talonavicular ligament

Navicular band
Head of talus
Bifurcate ligament

Anterior
talofibular
ligament

Bursa

Cuneiform bones

Calcaneofibular
ligament

Interosseous
talocalcanean
ligament

Fibularis (peroneus)
longus

Fibularis (peroneus) brevis

Dorsal
calcaneocuboid ligament
Calcaneus and cuboid

A

5.96 Joints of inversion and eversion

The joints of inversion and eversion are: the subtalar (posterior talo-calcanean) joint, talocalcaneonavicular joint, and transverse tarsal (combined calcaneocuboid and talonavicular) joint. **A.** Foot, supero-lateral view. The foot has been inverted to facilitate observation of the articular surfaces and tightened ligaments. **B.** Posterior and middle parts of foot with talus removed, superior view. **C.** Posterior part of foot with talus removed, superolateral view. Note the posterior, middle, and anterior calcaneus facets, the spring ligament, and the facet on the navicular constitute the socket for the talus.

OBSERVE IN **A**:
1. The exposed articular surfaces include: (a) the posterior talar facet of the calcaneus; (b) the anterior surface of the calcaneus; and (c) the head of the talus, all of which are palpable. Because inversion of the foot is commonly associated with plantar flexion of the ankle joint, (d) the superior and lateral articular surfaces of the body of the talus are also commonly uncovered;
2. The anterior talofibular and dorsal calcaneocuboid ligaments are weak and easily torn, and the bifurcate and talonavicular ligaments are under strain. The strong calcaneofibular ligament is not attached to the tip of the malleolus, but to a facet anterior to the tip; hence, the free projecting tip, helps to retain the fibularis (peroneal) tendons.

OBSERVE IN **B**:
3. The convex posterior talar facet is separated from the concave, middle, and anterior facets by the ligamentous structures within the tarsal sinus;
4. At the wide lateral end of the sinus: (a) the strong interosseous talo-calcanean ligament; and (b) the attachments of the extensor retinaculum, which extend medially between the posterior ligament of the anterior talocalcanean joint and the anterior ligament of the posterior talocalcanean, or subtalar, joint;
5. The subtalar joint has its own synovial cavity, whereas the talonavicular and anterior talocalcanean joints share a common synovial cavity;
6. The angular space between the navicular bone and the middle talar facet on the sustentaculum tali is bridged by the plantar calcaneonavicular ligament, the central part of which is fibrocartilaginous;
7. The socket for the head of the talus is deepened medially by the part of the deltoid ligament that blends into the spring ligament, and laterally by the calcaneonavicular part of the bifurcate ligament;
8. Various synovial folds lie over the margins of the articular cartilage, some of these containing fat.

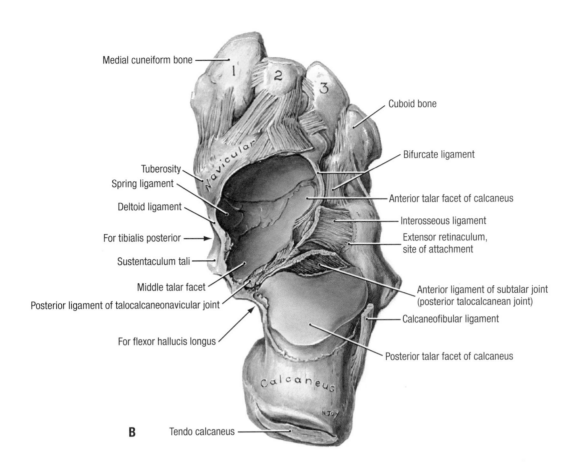

Medial cuneiform bone

Cuboid bone

Bifurcate ligament

Tuberosity

Spring ligament

Deltoid ligament

Anterior talar facet of calcaneus

Interosseous ligament

For tibialis posterior

Extensor retinaculum,
site of attachment

Sustentaculum tali

Middle talar facet

Posterior ligament of talocalcaneonavicular joint

Anterior ligament of subtalar joint
(posterior talocalcanean joint)

Calcaneofibular ligament

For flexor hallucis longus

Posterior talar facet of calcaneus

B   Tendo calcaneus

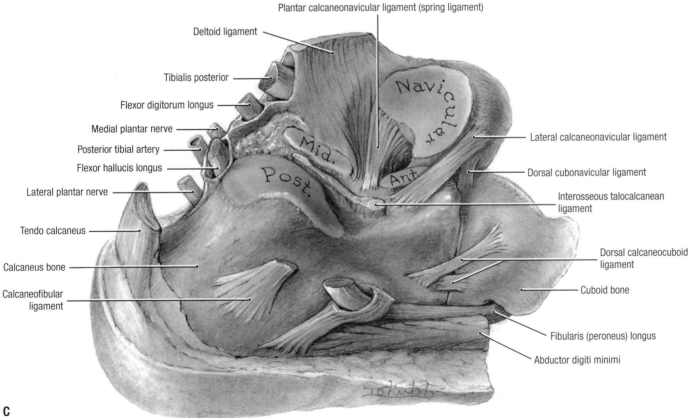

Plantar calcaneonavicular ligament (spring ligament)

Deltoid ligament

Tibialis posterior

Flexor digitorum longus

Medial plantar nerve

Posterior tibial artery

Lateral calcaneonavicular ligament

Flexor hallucis longus

Dorsal cubonavicular ligament

Lateral plantar nerve

Interosseous talocalcanean
ligament

Tendo calcaneus

Calcaneus bone

Dorsal calcaneocuboid
ligament

Calcaneofibular
ligament

Cuboid bone

Fibularis (peroneus) longus

Abductor digiti minimi

C

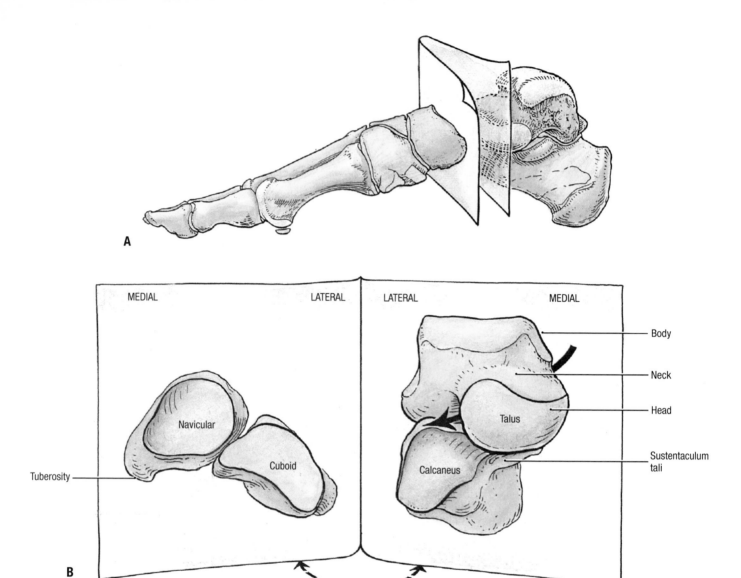

5.97 Transverse tarsal joint

A. Bones of foot, medial view. **B.** Bony surface of transverse tarsal joint. This joint includes the talonavicular and calcaneocuboid articulations. The posterior surfaces of the navicular and cuboid bones, and the anterior surfaces of the talus and calcaneus are displayed as pages in a book. The *black arrow* traverses the tarsal sinus (tunnel), in which the interosseous talocalcanean ligament is located.

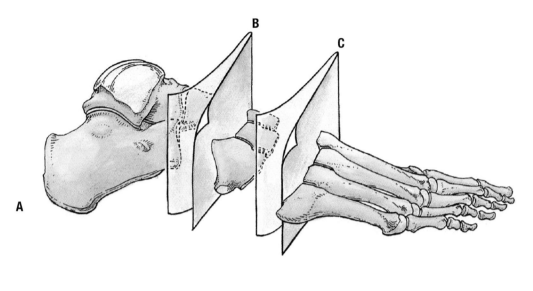

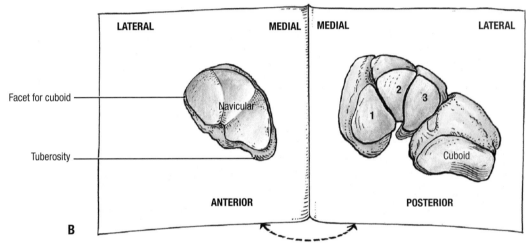

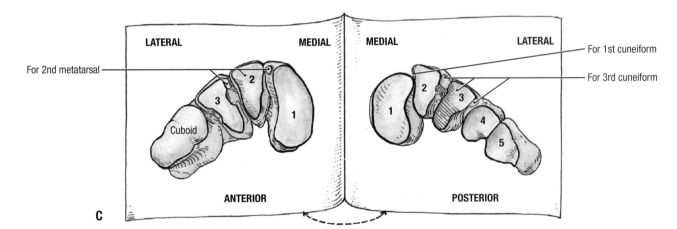

5.98　Cuneonavicular, cubonavicular, and tarsometatarsal joints

A. Bones of foot, lateral view. **B.** Bony surfaces of the cuneonavicular and cubonavicular joints. The anterior surface of the navicular bone, posterior surfaces of the three cuneiform bones, and medial and posterior surfaces of the cuboid bone are displayed as pages in a book. **C.** Bony surfaces of the tarsometatarsal joints. The anterior surfaces of the cuboid and three cuneiform bones, and the posterior surfaces of the bases of the five metatarsal bones are displayed as pages in a book.

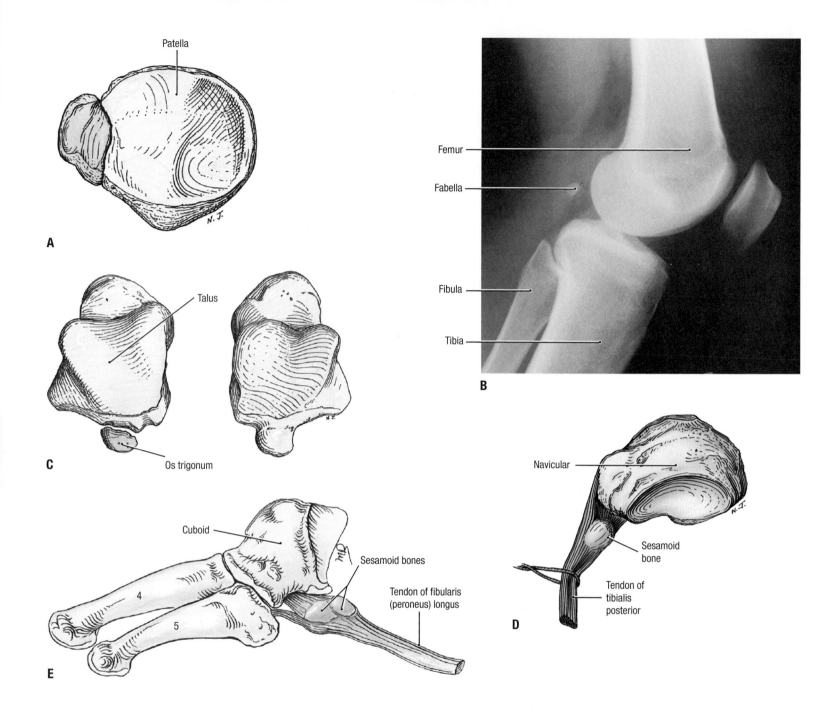

Patella

A

Talus

C   Os trigonum

Cuboid

4

5

E   Sesamoid bones

Tendon of fibularis (peroneus) longus

Femur

Fabella

Fibula

Tibia

B

Navicular

Sesamoid bone

Tendon of tibialis posterior

D

5.99   Bony anomalies

A. Bipartite patella, posterior view. Occasionally, the superolateral angle of the patella ossifies independently and remains discrete. **B.** Fabella, lateral view. A sesamoid bone (fabella) on the lateral head of the gastrocnemius muscle was present in 21.6% of 116 limbs. **C.** Os trigonum, superior view. The lateral (posterior) tubercle of the talus has a separate center of ossification, which appears from the ages of 7 to 13 years; when this fails to fuse with the body of the talus, as in the left bone of this pair, it is called an os trigonum. It was found in 7.7% of 558 adult feet; 22 were paired, and 21 were unpaired. **D.** Sesamoid bone in tibialis posterior, posterior view. A sesamoid bone was found in 23% of 348 adults. **E.** Sesamoid bone in fibularis (peroneus) longus, lateral view. A sesamoid bone was found in 26% of 92 feet. In this specimen, it is bipartite, and the fibularis (peroneus) longus muscle has an additional attachment to the fifth metatarsal bone.

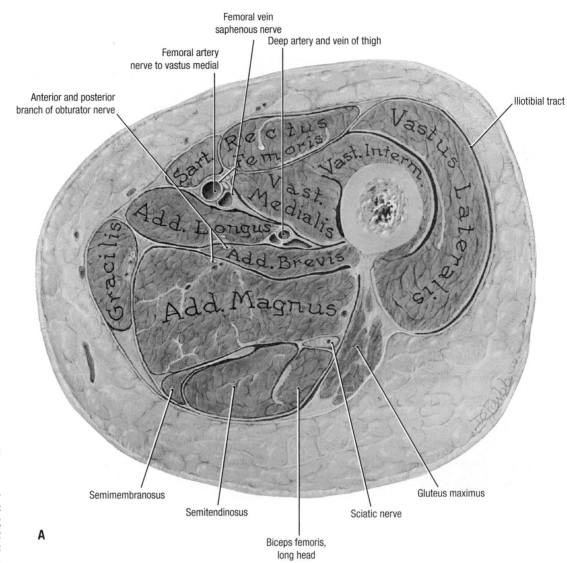

Femoral vein
saphenous nerve

Deep artery and vein of thigh

Femoral artery
nerve to vastus medial

Anterior and posterior
branch of obturator nerve

Iliotibial tract

Sart. Rectus femoris

Vast. Intern.

Vast. Medialis

Vastus Lateralis

Gracilis

Add. Longus

Add. Brevis

Add. Magnus

Semimembranosus

Semitendinosus

Biceps femoris,
long head

Sciatic nerve

Gluteus maximus

A

5.100   Transverse section of thigh

A. Dissection. **B.** Diagram. (*AB*, adductor brevis; *AL*, adductor longus; *AM*, adductor magnus; *BFL*, long head of biceps femoris; *BFS*, short head of biceps femoris; *G*, gracilis; *RF*, rectus femoris; *S*, sartorius; *SM*, semimembranosus, *ST*, semitendinosus; *VI*, vastus intermedius; *VL*, vastus lateralis; *VM*, vastus medialis)

OBSERVE IN **A**:
1. The level of the section is just inferior to the apex of the femoral triangle, about 10 to 15 cm down the femur;
2. The gracilis muscle abuts against the free, medial borders of the adductor muscles;
3. The adductor longus muscle intervenes between the femoral and deep vessels of thigh;
4. The adductor brevis muscle intervenes between the anterior and posterior divisions of the obturator nerve;
5. The vastus intermedius muscle arises from the anterior and lateral surfaces of the shaft of the femur. The vastus medialis muscle covers the medial surface, but does not arise from it, i.e., the vastus intermedius muscle alone arises from the surfaces, and the other muscles attach to the linea aspera or to its extensions; proximally, the vastus lateralis muscle is large.

OBSERVE IN **B**:

6. The muscles of the thigh are divided into three groups, each with its own nerve supply and primary functions;
7. The anterior group is supplied by the femoral nerve and functions to extend the knee.
8 The medial group is supplied by the obturator nerve and functions to adduct the hip;
9. The posterior group is supplied by the sciatic nerve and functions to flex the knee.

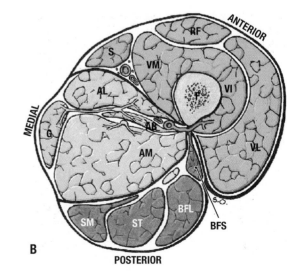

B

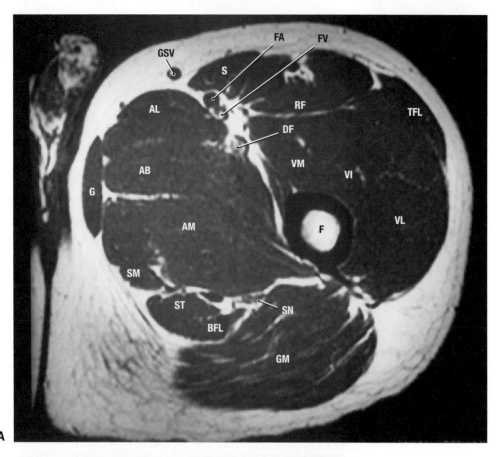

A

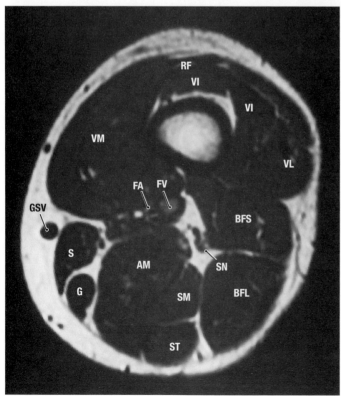

B

AB	Adductor brevis
AL	Adductor longus
AM	Adductor magnus
BFL	Long head of biceps femoris
BFS	Short head of biceps femoris
DF	Deep vessels of thigh
F	Femur
FA	Femoral artery
FV	Femoral vein
G	Gracilis
GM	Gluteus maximus
GSV	Great saphenous vein
RF	Rectus femoris
S	Sartorius
SM	Semimembranosus
SN	Sciatic nerve
ST	Semitendinosus
TFL	Tensor fasciae latae
VI	Vastus intermedius
VL	Vastus lateralis
VM	Vastus medialis

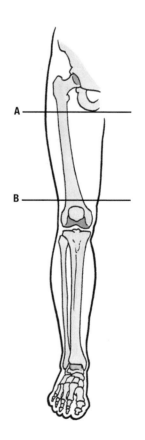

5.101 T1 axial (transverse) MRIs of thigh

A. Proximal. **B.** Distal.

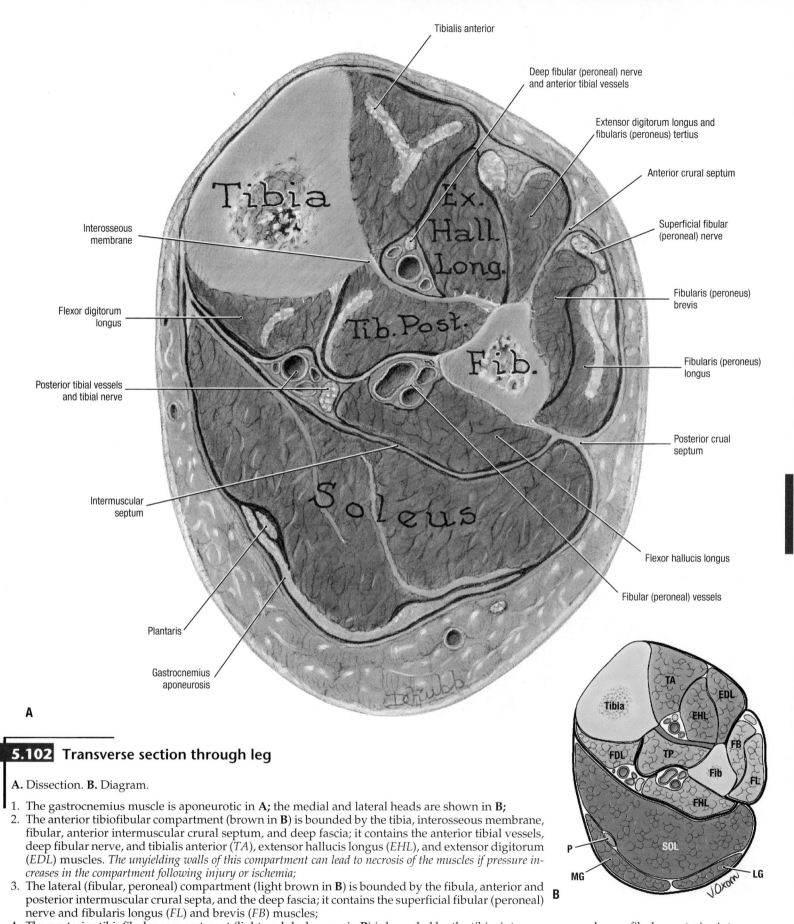

Tibialis anterior

Deep fibular (peroneal) nerve
and anterior tibial vessels

Extensor digitorum longus and
fibularis (peroneus) tertius

Anterior crural septum

Superficial fibular
(peroneal) nerve

Interosseous
membrane

Fibularis (peroneus)
brevis

Flexor digitorum
longus

Fibularis (peroneus)
longus

Posterior tibial vessels
and tibial nerve

Posterior crual
septum

Intermuscular
septum

Flexor hallucis longus

Fibular (peroneal) vessels

Plantaris

Gastrocnemius
aponeurosis

Tibia · **Ex. Hall. Long.** · **Tib. Post.** · **Fib.** · **Soleus**

A

5.102 Transverse section through leg

A. Dissection. **B.** Diagram.

1. The gastrocnemius muscle is aponeurotic in **A;** the medial and lateral heads are shown in **B;**
2. The anterior tibiofibular compartment (brown in **B**) is bounded by the tibia, interosseous membrane, fibular, anterior intermuscular crural septum, and deep fascia; it contains the anterior tibial vessels, deep fibular nerve, and tibialis anterior (*TA*), extensor hallucis longus (*EHL*), and extensor digitorum (*EDL*) muscles. *The unyielding walls of this compartment can lead to necrosis of the muscles if pressure increases in the compartment following injury or ischemia;*
3. The lateral (fibular, peroneal) compartment (light brown in **B**) is bounded by the fibula, anterior and posterior intermuscular crural septa, and the deep fascia; it contains the superficial fibular (peroneal) nerve and fibularis longus (*FL*) and brevis (*FB*) muscles;
4. The posterior tibiofibular compartment (light and dark green in **B**) is bounded by the tibia, interosseous membrane, fibula, posterior intermuscular crural septum, and deep fascia; this compartment is subdivided by two coronal septa into three subcompartments. The deepest subcompartment contains the tibialis posterior (*TP*); the intermediate contains the flexor hallucis longus (*FHL*), flexor digitorum longus (*FDL*), and posterior tibial vessels and tibial nerve; and the most superficial contains the soleus (*SOL*), gastrocnemius (*MG*, medial head; *LG*, lateral head), and plantaris (*P*) muscles.

B

TA · EDL · Tibia · EHL · FB · FDL · TP · Fib · FL · FHL · P · SOL · MG · LG

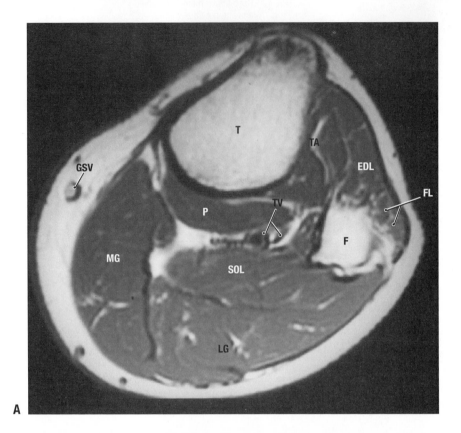

A

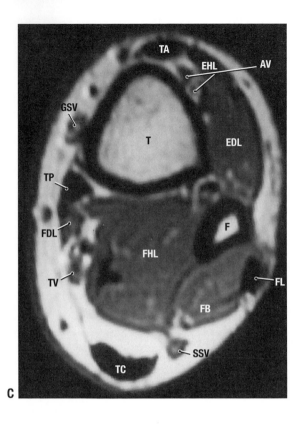

C

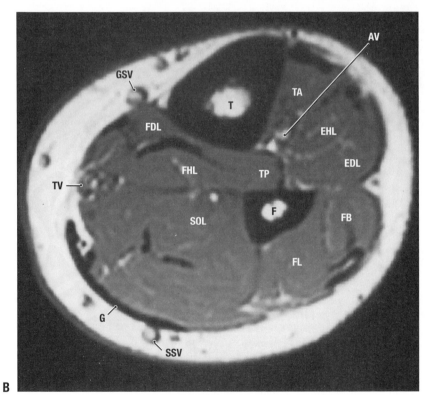

B

AV	Anterior tibial vessels and deep fibular nerve
EDL	Extensor digitorum longus
EHL	Extensor hallucis longus
F	Femur
FB	Fibularis brevis
FDL	Flexor digitorum longus
FHL	Flexor hallucis longus
FL	Fibularis longus
G	Gracilis
GSV	Great saphenous vein
LG	Lateral head of gastrocnemius
MG	Medial head of gastrocnemius
P	Popliteus
SOL	Soleus
SSV	Small saphenous vein
T	Tibia
TA	Tibialis anterior
TC	Tendo calcaneous
TP	Tibialis posterior
TV	Tibial nerve and posterior tibial vessels

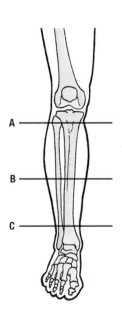

5.103 T1 axial (transverse) MRIs of leg

A. Proximal. **B.** Middle. **C.** Distal.

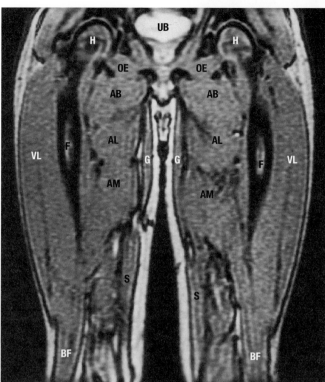

A

AB	Adductor brevis
AL	Adductor longus
AM	Adductor magnus
BF	Biceps femoris
F	Femur
G	Gracilis
H	Head of femur
OE	Obturator externus
S	Sartorius
UB	Urinary bladder
VL	Vastus lateralis

HF	Head of fibula
MG	Medial head of gastrocnemius
MM	Medial malleolus
P	Popliteus
Sol	Soleus
T	Tibia
Ta	Talus

B

5.104 **T1 coronal MRIs of lower limb**

A. Thigh. **B.** Leg.

CHAPTER 6

Upper Limb

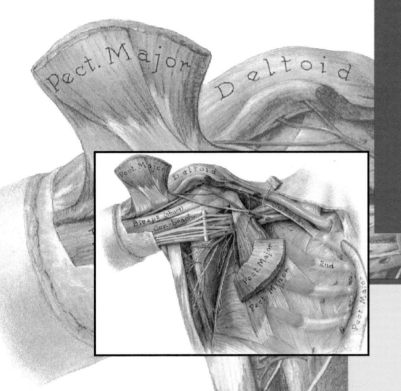

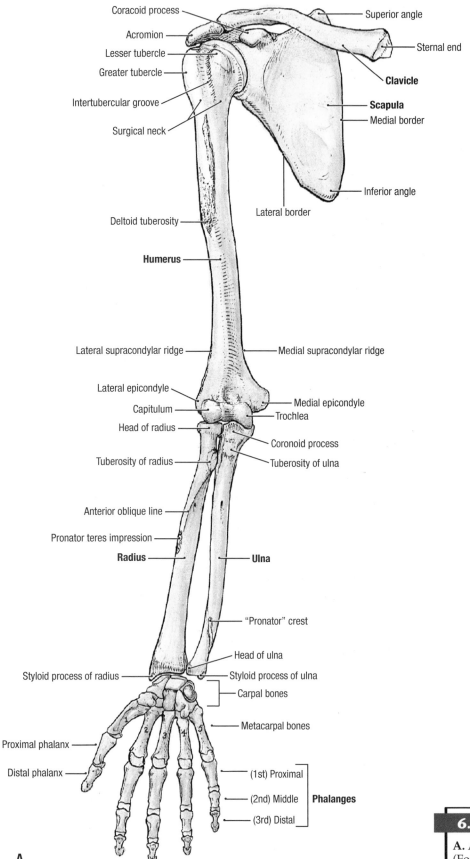

Coracoid process

Acromion

Lesser tubercle

Greater tubercle

Intertubercular groove

Surgical neck

Superior angle

Sternal end

Clavicle

Scapula

Medial border

Deltoid tuberosity

Inferior angle

Lateral border

Humerus

Lateral supracondylar ridge

Medial supracondylar ridge

Lateral epicondyle

Capitulum

Head of radius

Tuberosity of radius

Medial epicondyle

Trochlea

Coronoid process

Tuberosity of ulna

Anterior oblique line

Pronator teres impression

Radius

Ulna

"Pronator" crest

Head of ulna

Styloid process of radius

Styloid process of ulna

Carpal bones

Metacarpal bones

Proximal phalanx

Distal phalanx

(1st) Proximal

(2nd) Middle

(3rd) Distal

Phalanges

6.1   **Bones of upper limb**

A. Anterior view. **B.** Posterior view
(For bones of the hand, see Fig. 6.82.)

A

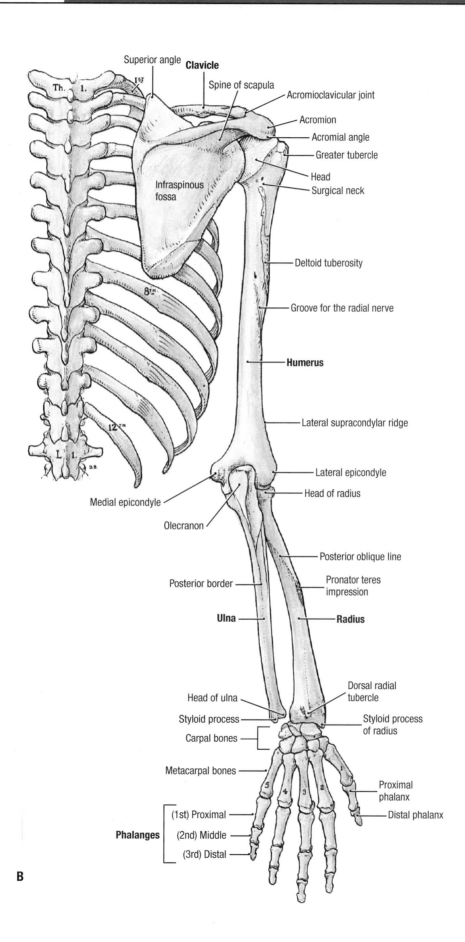

Superior angle **Clavicle**

Spine of scapula

Th. 1.

1ˢᵗ

Acromioclavicular joint

Acromion

Acromial angle

Greater tubercle

Head

Surgical neck

Infraspinous fossa

8ᵀᴴ

Deltoid tuberosity

Groove for the radial nerve

Humerus

12ᵀᴴ

L 1.

Lateral supracondylar ridge

Lateral epicondyle

Head of radius

Medial epicondyle

Olecranon

Posterior oblique line

Posterior border

Pronator teres impression

Ulna

Radius

Head of ulna

Dorsal radial tubercle

Styloid process

Styloid process of radius

Carpal bones

Metacarpal bones

Proximal phalanx

Distal phalanx

(1st) Proximal

Phalanges

(2nd) Middle

(3rd) Distal

B

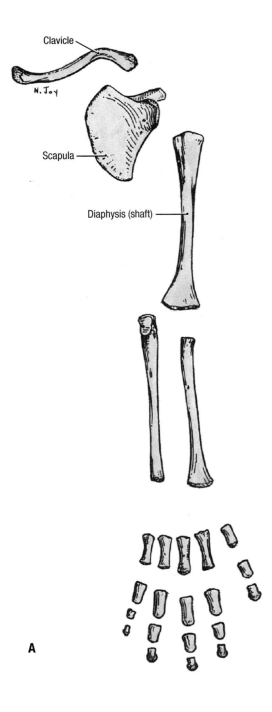

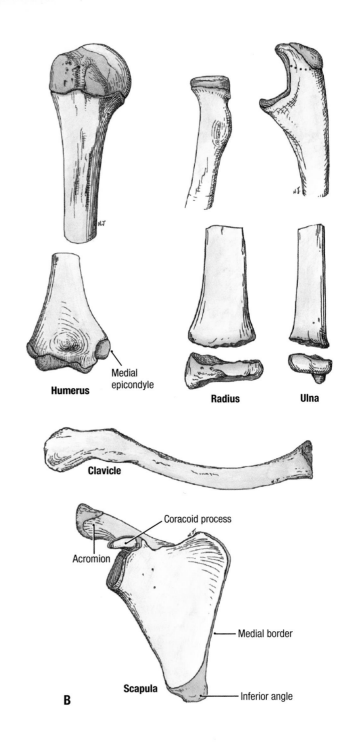

6.2   Ossification of bones of upper limb, anterior views

A. At birth. The diaphyses of the long bones and scapula are ossified. The epiphyses, carpal bones, coracoid process, medial border of the scapula, and acromion are cartilaginous (not shown in **A**). **B.** Epiphyses. The epiphyses are shown as darker orange regions.

OBSERVE IN **B**:
1. The ends of the long bones are ossified by the formation of one or more secondary centers of ossification; these epiphyses develop from birth to approximately 20 years of age in the clavicle, humerus, radius, ulna, metacarpals, and phalanges;

2. When the epiphysis and diaphysis join (fuse), active bone growth stops. Sometimes, as in the proximal humerus, many epiphyses fuse to form a single mass that later fuses with the diaphysis, i.e., three centers of ossification develop (for the head, greater tubercle, and lesser tubercle) and fuse into a single mass by the 7th year and to the diaphysis by the 24th year;

3. The epiphysis of the clavicle is the last of the long bone epiphyses to fuse (by 31 years), but the clavicle is one of the first bones to begin ossification; the acromial epiphysis of the scapula may persist into adult life.

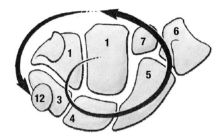

Sequence of ossification

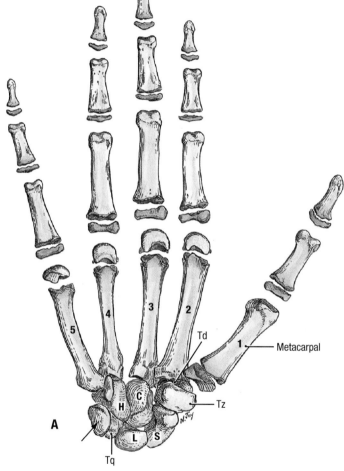

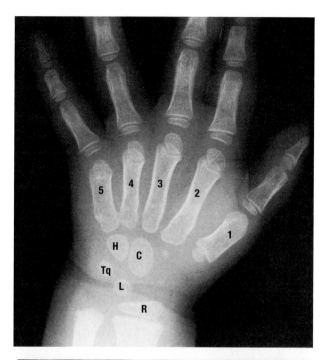

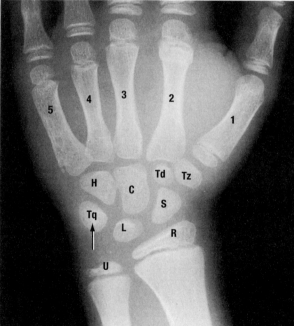

A

B

6.3   Epiphyses of hand and wrist

A. Ossification of bones of hand, anterior view. **B.** Anteroposterior radiographs of stages of ossification of wrist and hand.

in years. There are individual and gender differences in sequence and timing.

OBSERVE IN **A**:

1. Phalanges have a single proximal epiphysis;
2. Metacarpals 2, 3, 4, and 5 have single distal epiphyses; the 1st metacarpal behaves as a phalanx by having a proximal epiphysis. Short-lived epiphyses may appear at the other ends of metacarpals 1 and/or 2;
3. The capitate starts to ossify soon after birth; the arrows show the spiral sequence of ossification of the carpals with approximate age

OBSERVE IN **B**:

4. *Radiographs of the hand and wrist are commonly used to assess skeletal age.*
5. Top: a 2½-year-old child; lunate are ossifying, and the distal radial epiphysis (*R*) is present (*C*, Capitate; *H*, Hamate; *Tq*, Triquetrum; *L*, Lunate);
6. Bottom: an 11 year old; all carpal bones are ossified (*S*, Scapnoid; *Td*, Trapezoid; *Tz*, Trapezium; *Arrowhead*, Pisiform), and the distal epiphysis of the ulna (*U*) has ossified.

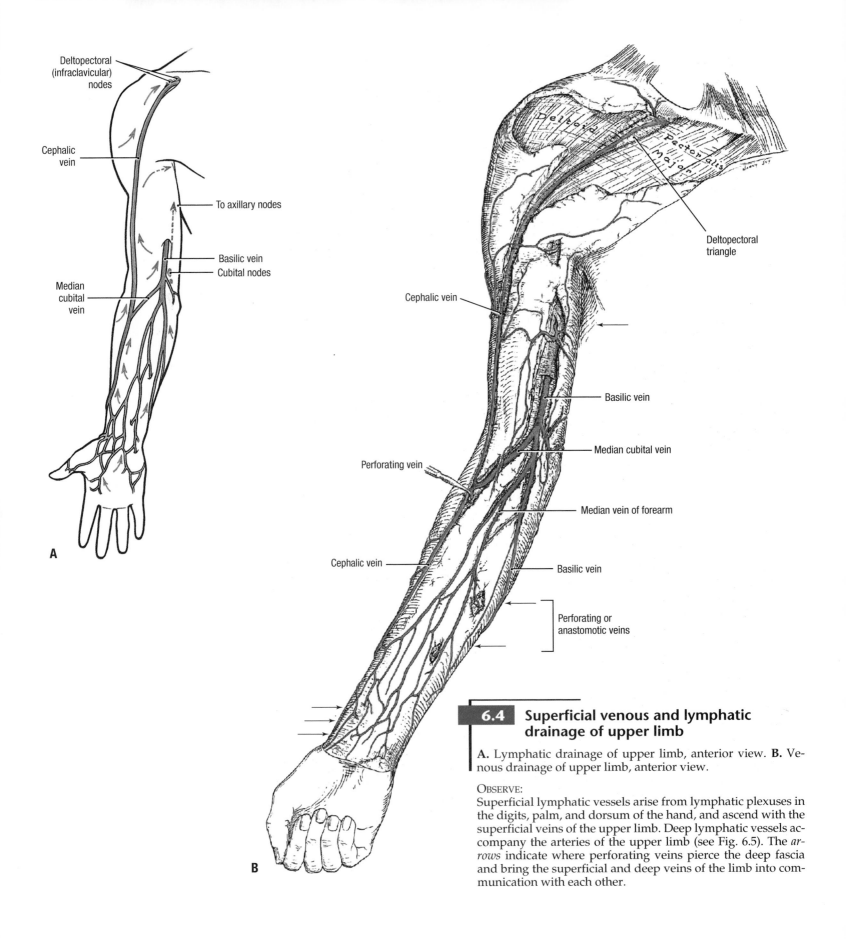

Deltopectoral (infraclavicular) nodes

Cephalic vein

To axillary nodes

Basilic vein
Cubital nodes

Median cubital vein

A

Deltopectoral triangle

Cephalic vein

Basilic vein

Median cubital vein

Perforating vein

Median vein of forearm

Cephalic vein

Basilic vein

Perforating or anastomotic veins

B

6.4 Superficial venous and lymphatic drainage of upper limb

A. Lymphatic drainage of upper limb, anterior view. **B.** Venous drainage of upper limb, anterior view.

OBSERVE:
Superficial lymphatic vessels arise from lymphatic plexuses in the digits, palm, and dorsum of the hand, and ascend with the superficial veins of the upper limb. Deep lymphatic vessels accompany the arteries of the upper limb (see Fig. 6.5). The *arrows* indicate where perforating veins pierce the deep fascia and bring the superficial and deep veins of the limb into communication with each other.

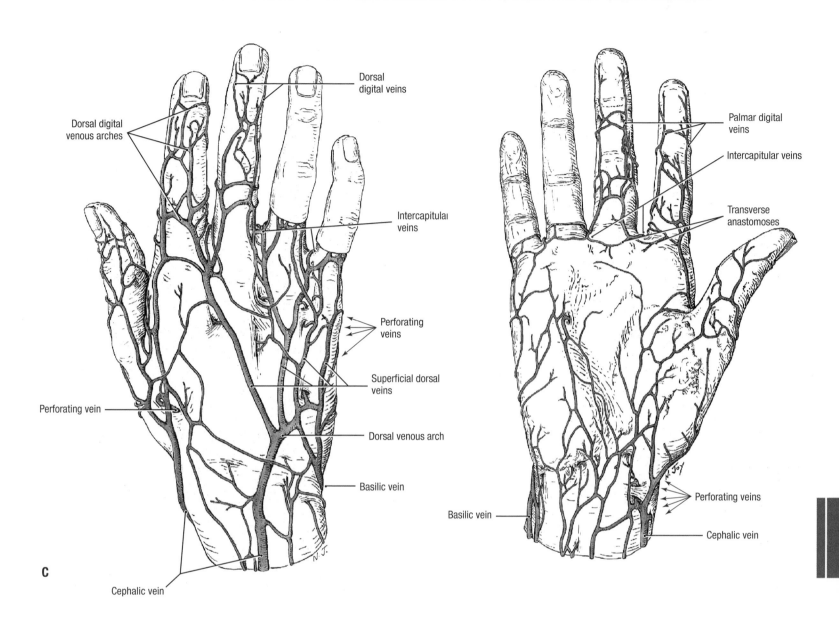

C. Venous drainage of hand (left, dorsal view; right, palmar view). **D.** Lymphatic drainage of hand, dorsal view.

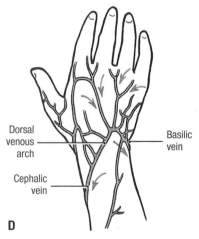

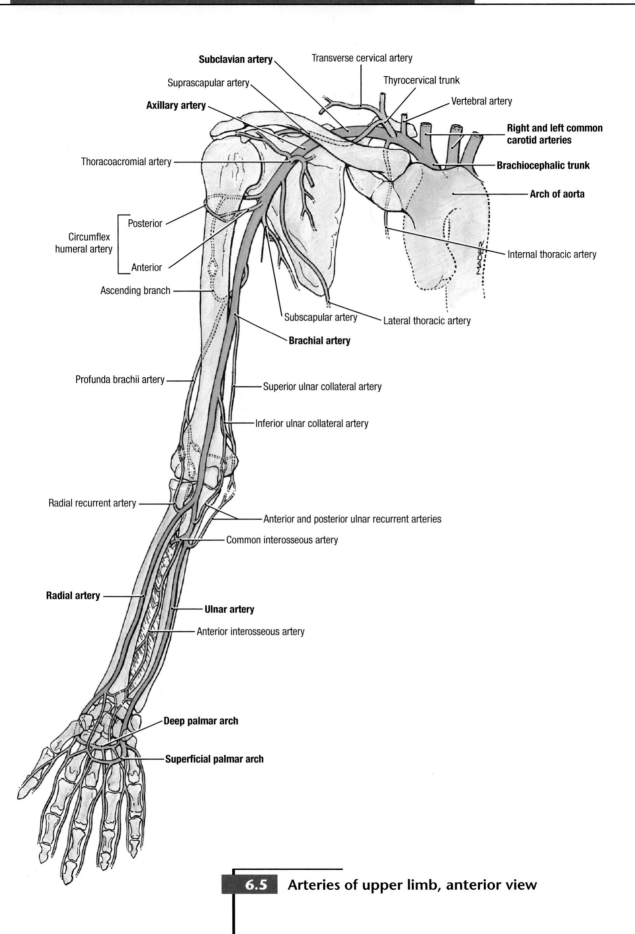

Subclavian artery

Transverse cervical artery

Suprascapular artery

Thyrocervical trunk

Vertebral artery

Axillary artery

Right and left common carotid arteries

Thoracoacromial artery

Brachiocephalic trunk

Arch of aorta

Posterior

Circumflex humeral artery

Internal thoracic artery

Anterior

Ascending branch

Subscapular artery

Lateral thoracic artery

Brachial artery

Profunda brachii artery

Superior ulnar collateral artery

Inferior ulnar collateral artery

Radial recurrent artery

Anterior and posterior ulnar recurrent arteries

Common interosseous artery

Radial artery

Ulnar artery

Anterior interosseous artery

Deep palmar arch

Superficial palmar arch

6.5   Arteries of upper limb, anterior view

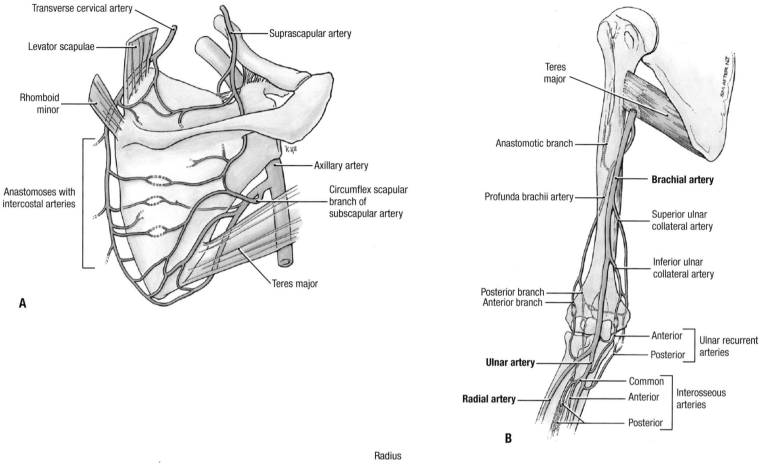

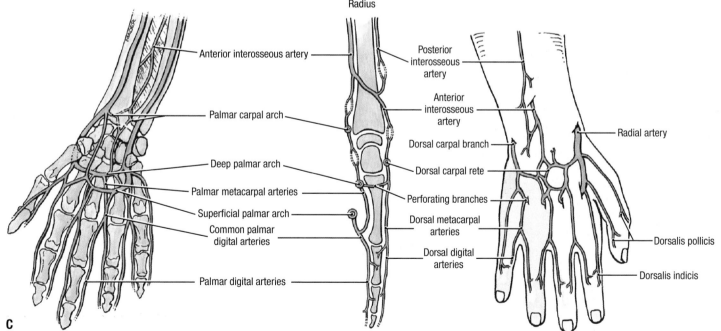

6.6 **Arterial anastomoses**

A. Of the scapula, posterior view. **B.** Of the elbow, anterior view. **C.** Of the hand (left, anterior view; middle, lateral view; right, posterior view).

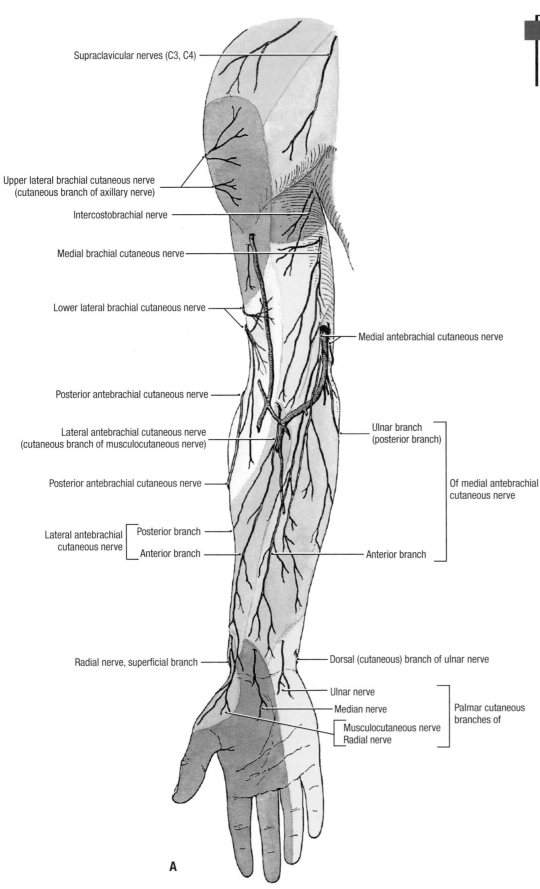

Supraclavicular nerves (C3, C4)

Upper lateral brachial cutaneous nerve
(cutaneous branch of axillary nerve)

Intercostobrachial nerve

Medial brachial cutaneous nerve

Lower lateral brachial cutaneous nerve

Posterior antebrachial cutaneous nerve

Lateral antebrachial cutaneous nerve
(cutaneous branch of musculocutaneous nerve)

Posterior antebrachial cutaneous nerve

Lateral antebrachial
cutaneous nerve
   Posterior branch
   Anterior branch

Radial nerve, superficial branch

Medial antebrachial cutaneous nerve

Ulnar branch
(posterior branch)

Of medial antebrachial
cutaneous nerve

Anterior branch

Dorsal (cutaneous) branch of ulnar nerve

Ulnar nerve

Median nerve

Musculocutaneous nerve
Radial nerve
   Palmar cutaneous
   branches of

A

6.7   Cutaneous nerves of upper limb

A. Anterior view. **B.** Posterior view. Of the five terminal branches of the brachial plexus (musculocutaneous, median, ulnar, radial, and axillary nerves), the first four contribute cutaneous branches to the hand. The posterior cord of the plexus is represented by five cutaneous nerves. One of these, the upper lateral brachial cutaneous nerve, is a branch of the axillary nerve. The other branches of the posterior cord are the posterior brachial cutaneous nerve, lower lateral brachial cutaneous nerve, posterior antebrachial cutaneous nerve, and superficial branch of the radial nerve.

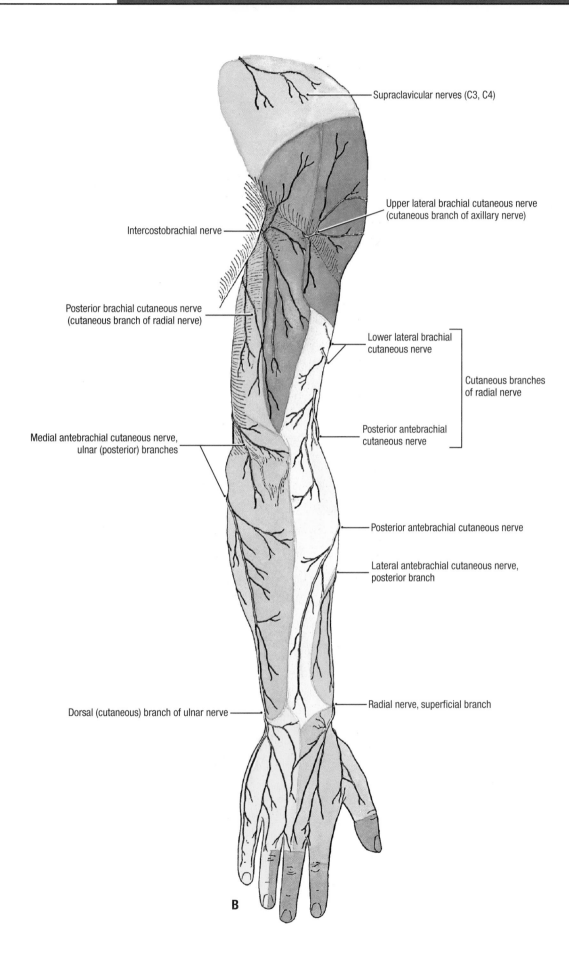

Supraclavicular nerves (C3, C4)

Upper lateral brachial cutaneous nerve
(cutaneous branch of axillary nerve)

Intercostobrachial nerve

Posterior brachial cutaneous nerve
(cutaneous branch of radial nerve)

Lower lateral brachial
cutaneous nerve

Cutaneous branches
of radial nerve

Posterior antebrachial
cutaneous nerve

Medial antebrachial cutaneous nerve,
ulnar (posterior) branches

Posterior antebrachial cutaneous nerve

Lateral antebrachial cutaneous nerve,
posterior branch

Dorsal (cutaneous) branch of ulnar nerve

Radial nerve, superficial branch

B

6.8   Innervation of muscles of upper limb

A. Median and musculocutaneous nerves, anterior view. **B.** Ulnar nerve, anterior view.

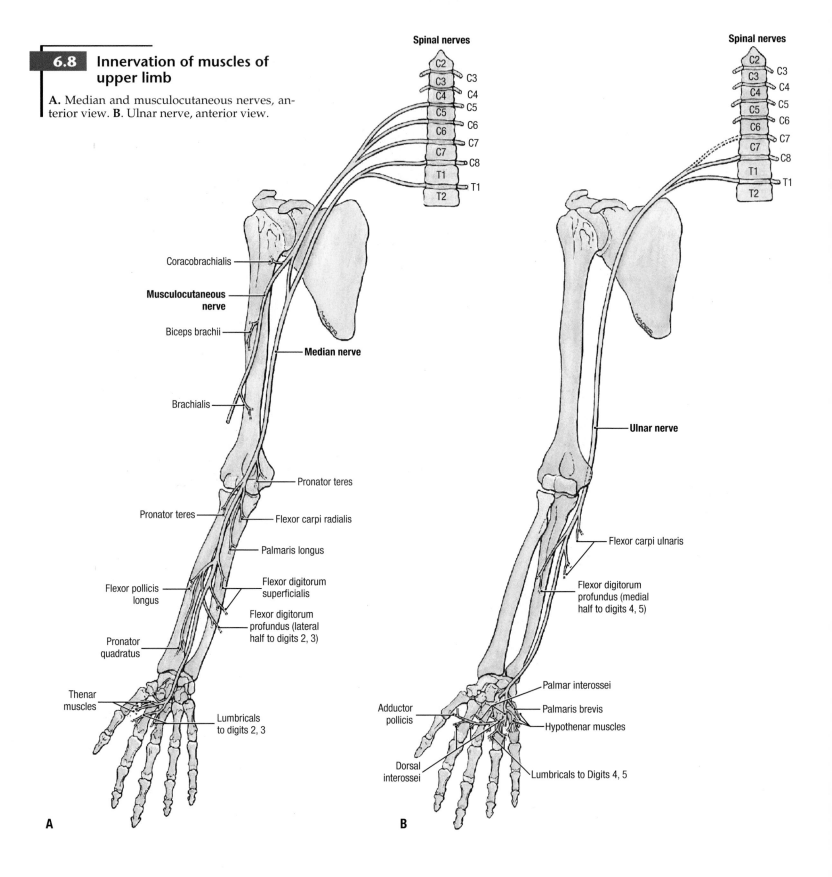

Spinal nerves

C2
C3
C4
C5
C6
C7
C8
T1
T2

Coracobrachialis

Musculocutaneous nerve

Biceps brachii

Median nerve

Brachialis

Pronator teres

Pronator teres

Flexor carpi radialis

Palmaris longus

Flexor pollicis longus

Flexor digitorum superficialis

Flexor digitorum profundus (lateral half to digits 2, 3)

Pronator quadratus

Thenar muscles

Lumbricals to digits 2, 3

A

Spinal nerves

C2
C3
C4
C5
C6
C7
C8
T1
T2

Ulnar nerve

Flexor carpi ulnaris

Flexor digitorum profundus (medial half to digits 4, 5)

Palmar interossei

Adductor pollicis

Palmaris brevis

Hypothenar muscles

Dorsal interossei

Lumbricals to Digits 4, 5

B

C. Nerves to pectoralis major and minor (medial and lateral pectoral nerves), anterior view. **D.** Radial nerve, posterior view.

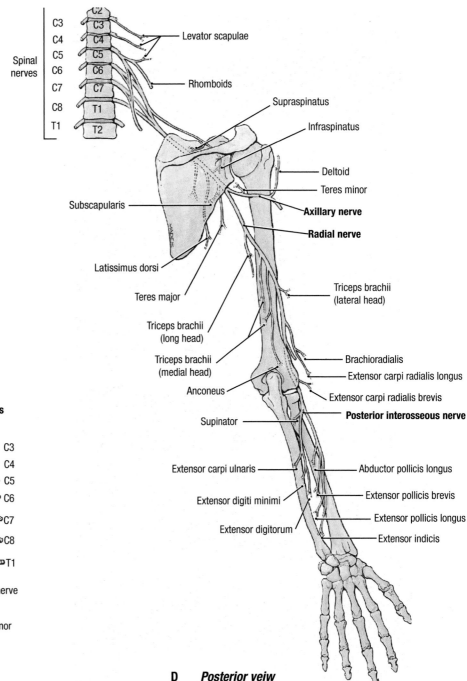

D   *Posterior veiw*

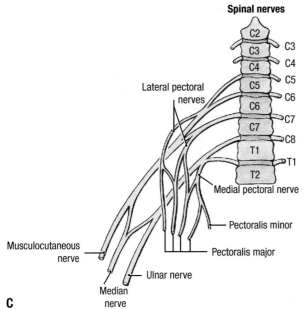

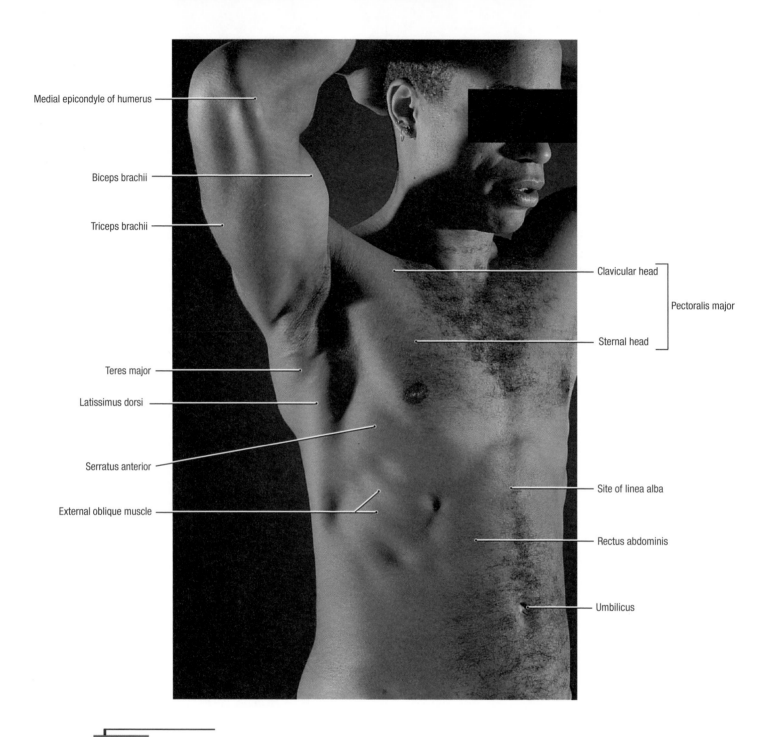

Medial epicondyle of humerus

Biceps brachii

Triceps brachii

Clavicular head

Pectoralis major

Sternal head

Teres major

Latissimus dorsi

Serratus anterior

Site of linea alba

External oblique muscle

Rectus abdominis

Umbilicus

6.9 **Surface anatomy of axilla and anterolateral aspect of trunk**

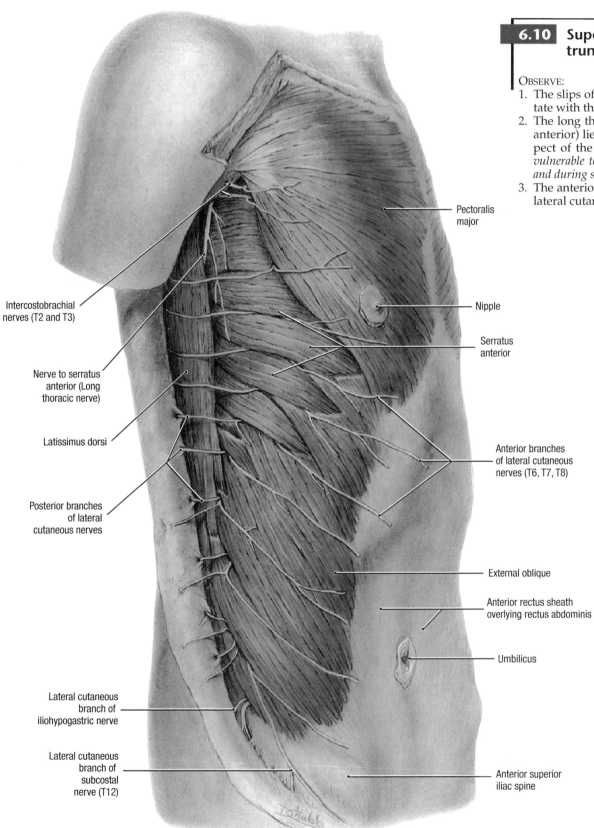

6.10 **Superficial dissection of trunk, lateral view**

OBSERVE:
1. The slips of the serratus anterior interdigitate with the external oblique;
2. The long thoracic nerve (nerve to serratus anterior) lies on the lateral (superficial) aspect of the serratus anterior; *this nerve is vulnerable to damage from puncture wounds and during surgery (e.g., radical mastectomy);*
3. The anterior and posterior branches of the lateral cutaneous nerves.

Pectoralis major

Intercostobrachial nerves (T2 and T3)

Nerve to serratus anterior (Long thoracic nerve)

Latissimus dorsi

Posterior branches of lateral cutaneous nerves

Nipple

Serratus anterior

Anterior branches of lateral cutaneous nerves (T6, T7, T8)

External oblique

Anterior rectus sheath overlying rectus abdominis

Umbilicus

Lateral cutaneous branch of iliohypogastric nerve

Lateral cutaneous branch of subcostal nerve (T12)

Anterior superior iliac spine

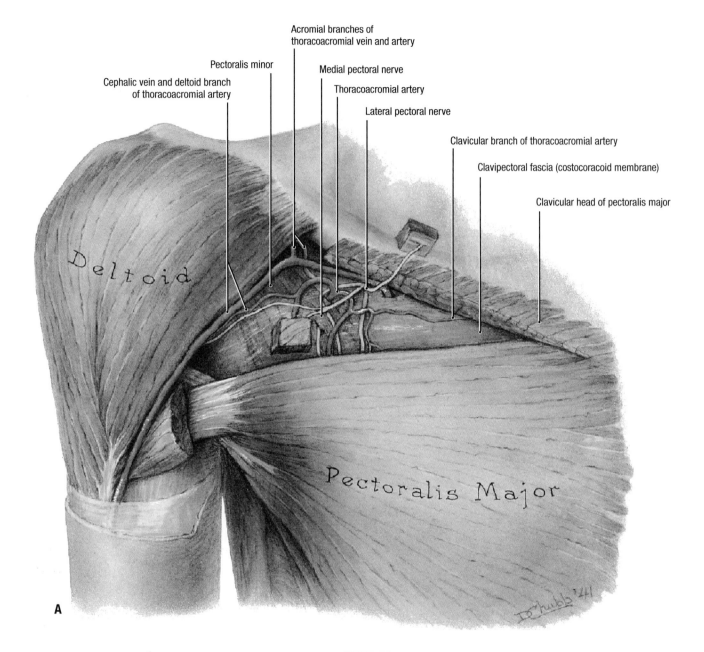

Acromial branches of
thoracoacromial vein and artery

Pectoralis minor

Medial pectoral nerve

Cephalic vein and deltoid branch
of thoracoacromial artery

Thoracoacromial artery

Lateral pectoral nerve

Clavicular branch of thoracoacromial artery

Clavipectoral fascia (costocoracoid membrane)

Clavicular head of pectoralis major

Deltoid

Pectoralis Major

A

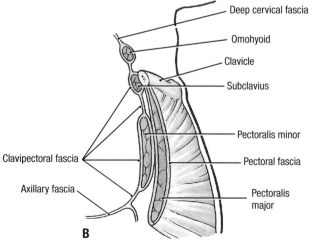

Deep cervical fascia

Omohyoid

Clavicle

Subclavius

Clavipectoral fascia

Pectoralis minor

Pectoral fascia

Axillary fascia

Pectoralis
major

B

6.11 Anterior wall of axilla and clavipectoral fascia

A. Anterior view. The clavicular head of pectoralis major is excised, except for two cubes that remain to identify its nerves. **B.** Sagittal section.

OBSERVE:

1. The part of the clavipectoral fascia superior to the pectoralis minor (the costocoracoid membrane) is pierced by the lateral pectoral nerve and its companion vessels;
2. The cephalic vein courses through the deltopectoral triangle and costocoracoid membrane;
3. The pectoralis minor and clavipectoral fascia are pierced by the medial pectoral nerve;
4. The trilaminar insertion of pectoralis major.
5. In **B**, the clavipectoral fascia encloses the pectoralis minor and subclavius muscles and then attaches to the clavicle.

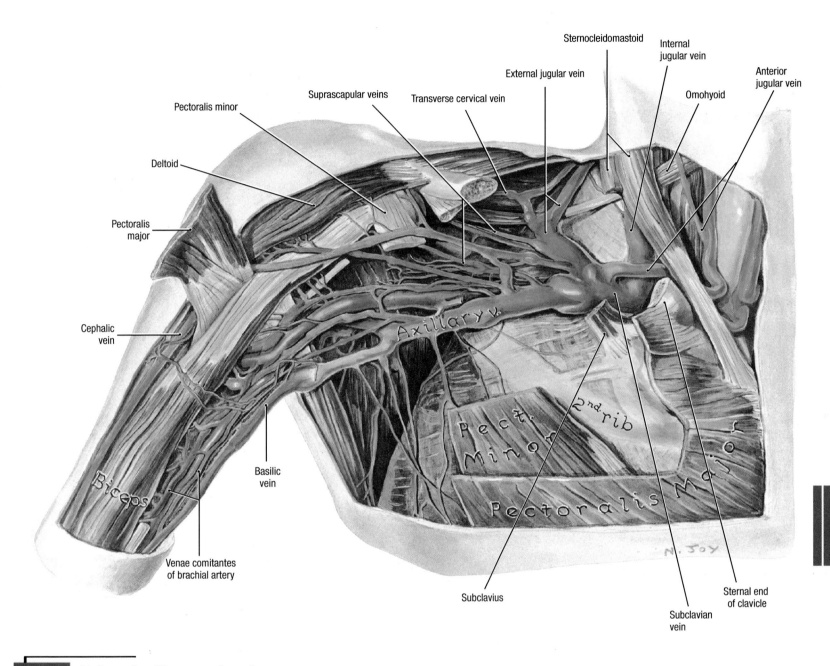

6.12 Veins of axilla, anterior view

OBSERVE:
1. The basilic vein becomes the axillary vein, the axillary vein becomes the subclavian vein, and the subclavian joins the internal jugular to become the brachiocephalic vein posterior to the sternal end of the clavicle;
2. More than 40 venous valves (swellings in the vein) are shown; note three in the axillary and one in the subclavian, which is the last valve before the heart;

3. Venae comitantes of the brachial artery unite and join the axillary vein near the middle of the axilla;
4. The cephalic vein in this specimen bifurcates to end in the axillary and external jugular veins;
5. Three suprascapular veins: one from inferior to the suprascapular ligament to the axillary vein, and two superior to the ligament to the external jugular vein;
6. The many veins in the axilla.

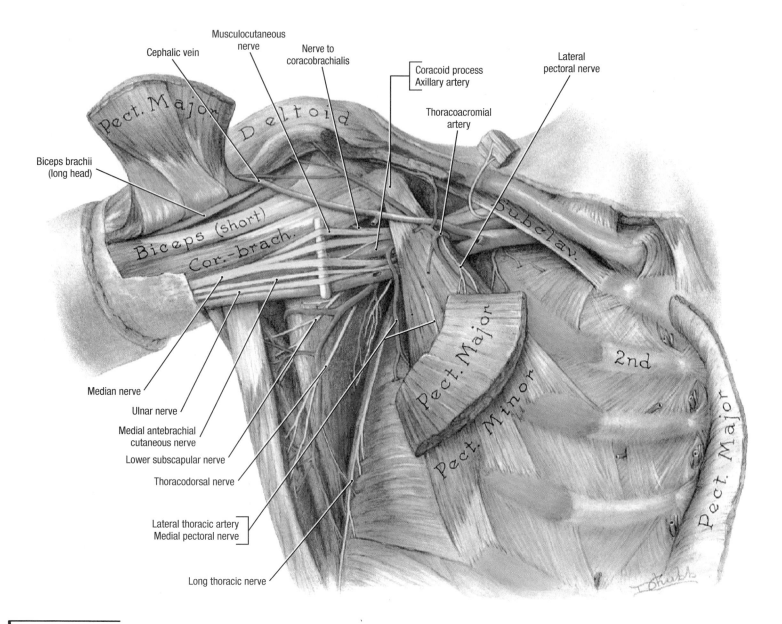

6.13   Structures of axilla, anterior view

The pectoralis major muscle is reflected, and the clavipectoral fascia is removed.

OBSERVE:

1. The subclavius and pectoralis minor are the two deep muscles of the anterior wall;
2. The axillary artery passes posterior to the pectoralis minor muscle, a fingerbreath from the tip of the coracoid process;
3. The axillary vein lies medial to the axillary artery;
4. The median nerve, followed proximally, leads by its lateral root to the lateral cord and musculocutaneous nerve, and by its medial root to the medial cord and ulnar nerve. These four nerves and the medial antebrachial cutaneous nerve are raised on a stick. The lateral root of the median nerve may be in several strands;
5. The nerve to coracobrachialis arises within the axilla;
6. The cube of muscle superior to the clavicle is cut from the clavicular head of the pectoralis major muscle.

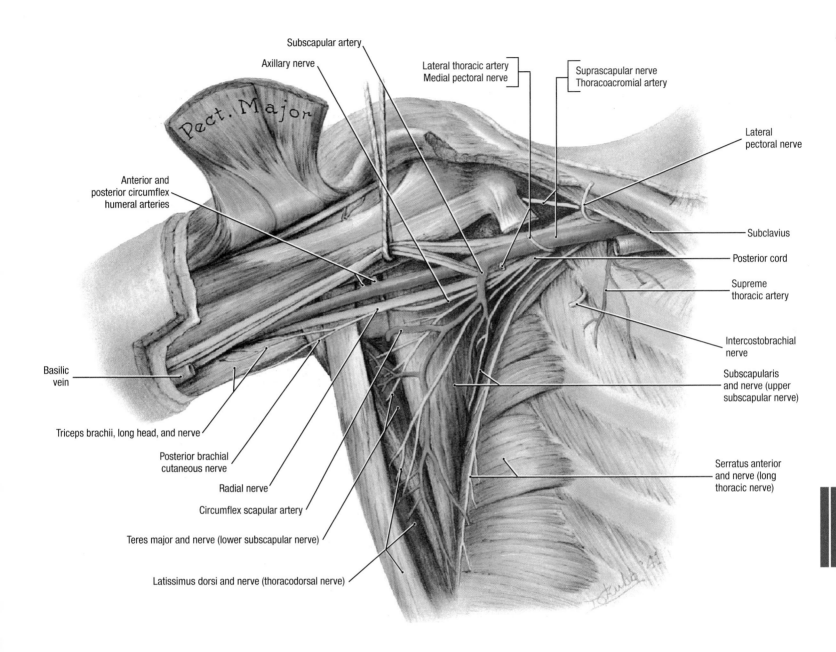

Subscapular artery

Axillary nerve

Lateral thoracic artery
Medial pectoral nerve

Suprascapular nerve
Thoracoacromial artery

Pect. Major

Anterior and
posterior circumflex
humeral arteries

Lateral
pectoral nerve

Subclavius

Posterior cord

Supreme
thoracic artery

Basilic
vein

Intercostobrachial
nerve

Subscapularis
and nerve (upper
subscapular nerve)

Triceps brachii, long head, and nerve

Posterior brachial
cutaneous nerve

Serratus anterior
and nerve (long
thoracic nerve)

Radial nerve

Circumflex scapular artery

Teres major and nerve (lower subscapular nerve)

Latissimus dorsi and nerve (thoracodorsal nerve)

6.14   Posterior and medial walls of axilla, anterior view

The pectoralis minor muscle is excised, the lateral and medial cords
are retracted, and the axillary vein is removed.

OBSERVE:

1. The posterior cord and its two terminal branches (the radial and axillary nerves) lie posterior to the axillary artery;
2. The nerves to the three posterior muscles: (a) the nerve to the latissimus dorsi muscle enters its deep surface 1 cm from its free lateral
   border at a point midway between the thoracic wall and the abducted arm; (b) the upper nerve to subscapularis lies parallel to (a),

but superior to it; and (c) the lower nerve to the subscapularis and
teres major muscles lies parallel to (a), but inferior to it;

3. The nerve to serratus anterior clings to its muscle throughout; superiorly, some fat may intervene;
4. The suprascapular nerve passes toward the base of the coracoid
   process;
5. The subscapular artery, the largest branch of the axillary artery, in
   this specimen arises more proximally; usually it arises at the inferior border of subscapularis;

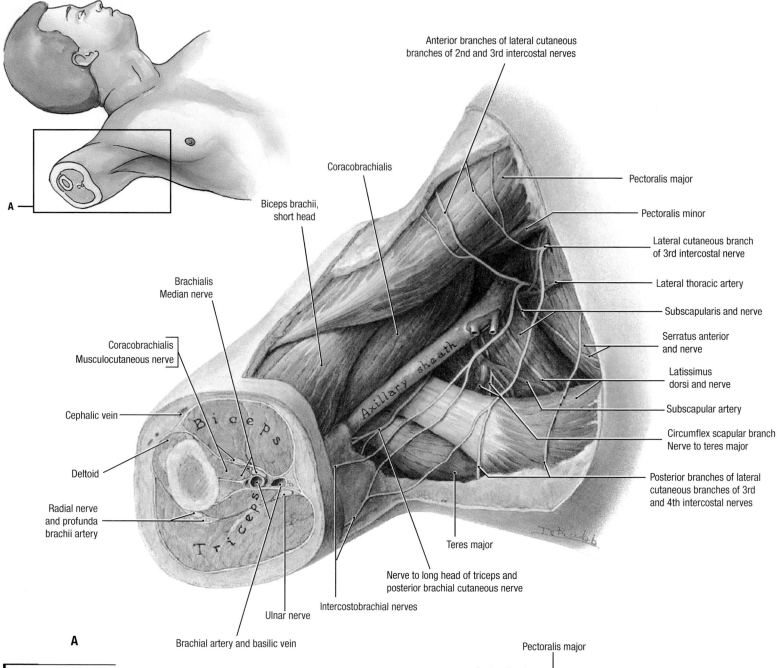

Anterior branches of lateral cutaneous branches of 2nd and 3rd intercostal nerves

Coracobrachialis

Biceps brachii, short head

Brachialis
Median nerve

Coracobrachialis
Musculocutaneous nerve

Cephalic vein

Deltoid

Radial nerve and profunda brachii artery

Pectoralis major

Pectoralis minor

Lateral cutaneous branch of 3rd intercostal nerve

Lateral thoracic artery

Subscapularis and nerve

Serratus anterior and nerve

Latissimus dorsi and nerve

Subscapular artery

Circumflex scapular branch
Nerve to teres major

Posterior branches of lateral cutaneous branches of 3rd and 4th intercostal nerves

Teres major

Nerve to long head of triceps and posterior brachial cutaneous nerve

Intercostobrachial nerves

Ulnar nerve

Brachial artery and basilic vein

A

Axillary sheath

Biceps

Triceps

6.15   Axilla

A. Inferior view. **B.** Transverse section

OBSERVE:
1. The walls of the axilla: (a) anterior wall: pectoralis major, pectoralis minor, and subclavius muscles (only the pectoral muscles are in view); (b) posterior wall: subscapularis, latissimus dorsi, and teres major muscles; (c) medial wall: serratus anterior muscle; and (d) lateral wall: intertubercular (bicipital) groove of the humerus, concealed by the biceps and coracobrachialis muscles;
2. In A, the axillary sheath and cutaneous nerves cross the latissimus dorsi muscle; the most lateral of these nerves is also the sole nerve supply of the long head of the triceps muscle;
3. In A, the axillary sheath transmits the nerves and vessels of the limb; it is a neurovascular bundle.

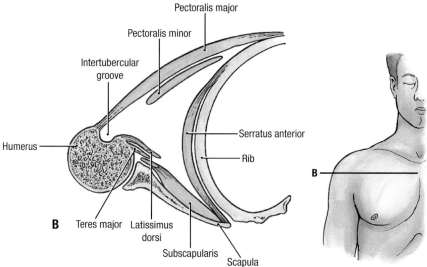

Pectoralis major

Pectoralis minor

Intertubercular groove

Humerus

B   Teres major   Latissimus dorsi

Subscapularis

Scapula

Serratus anterior

Rib

B

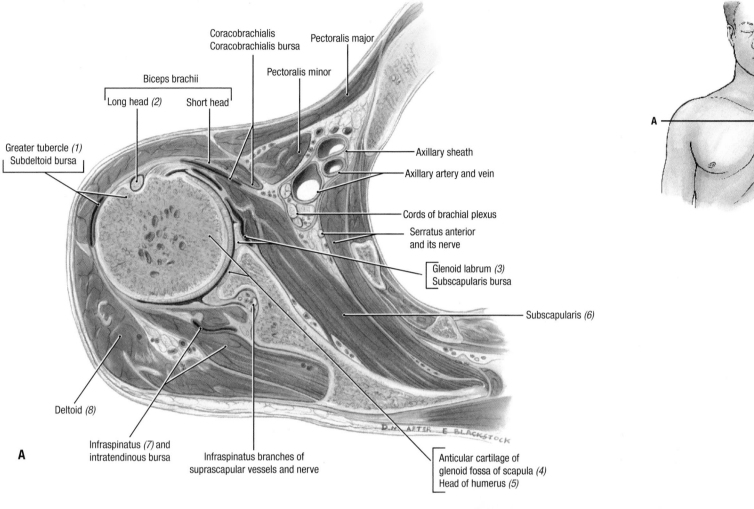

A. Transverse section (numbers in parentheses refer to labeled structures in **B**).

Coracobrachialis
Coracobrachialis bursa

Pectoralis major

Pectoralis minor

Biceps brachii

Long head *(2)*   Short head

Greater tubercle *(1)*
Subdeltoid bursa

Axillary sheath

Axillary artery and vein

Cords of brachial plexus

Serratus anterior
and its nerve

Glenoid labrum *(3)*
Subscapularis bursa

Subscapularis *(6)*

Deltoid *(8)*

Infraspinatus *(7)* and
intratendinous bursa

Infraspinatus branches of
suprascapular vessels and nerve

Articular cartilage of
glenoid fossa of scapula *(4)*
Head of humerus *(5)*

A

6.16 **Transverse section and magnetic resonance imaging (MRI) through shoulder joint and axilla**

A. Transverse section (numbers in parentheses refer to labeled structures in **B**). **B.** Transverse MRI.

OBSERVE:

1. The tendon of the long head of the biceps brachii muscle faces anteriorly; the short head of the biceps muscle and the coracobrachialis and pectoralis minor muscles are sectioned just inferior to their attachments to the coracoid process;
2. The fibrous capsule of the shoulder joint is thin posteriorly and partly fused with the tendon of infraspinatus; it is thicker anteriorly;
3. The small glenoid cavity is deepened by the glenoid labrum;
4. Bursae: (a) subdeltoid (subacromial) bursa, between the deltoid and greater tubercle; (b) subscapular bursa, between the subscapularis tendon and scapula; and (c) coracobrachialis bursa, between the coracobrachialis and subscapularis;
5. The walls of the axilla near its apex are formed by the subscapularis and scapula posteriorly, the serratus anterior, ribs, and intercostals medially, and the pectoralis major and minor muscles anteriorly; there is no bone in the anterior wall;
6. The axillary sheath encloses the axillary artery and vein and the three cords of the brachial plexus to form a neurovascular bundle, surrounded by axillary fat.

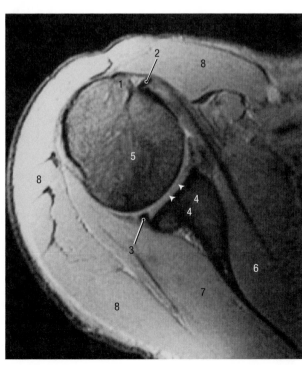

B

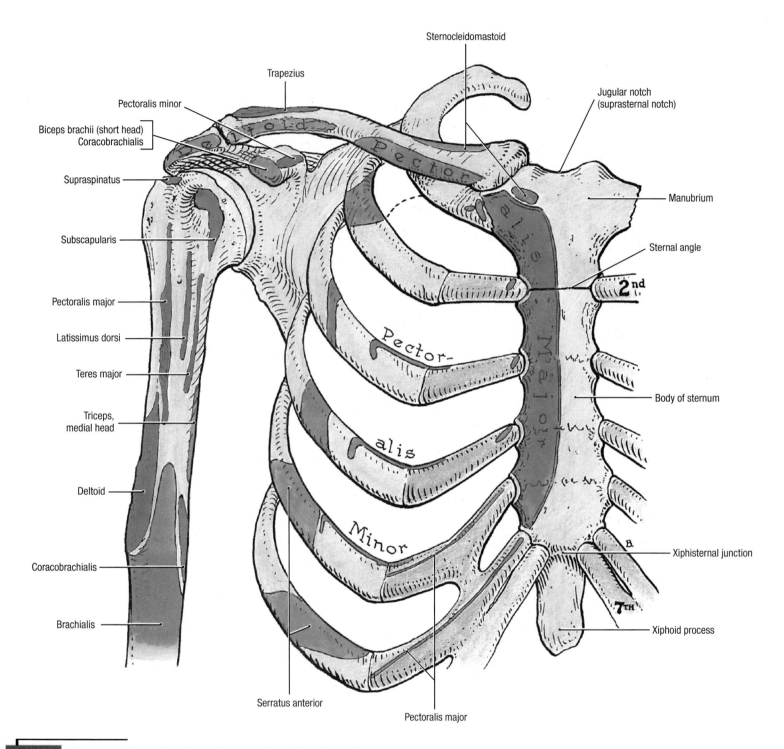

6.17 **Bones of pectoral region and axilla, showing muscle attachments, anterior view**

OBSERVE:
1. The following muscles are attached in line with one another horizontally on the clavicle: anteriorly, the trapezius and sternocleidomastoid; posteriorly, the deltoid and clavicular head of the pectoralis major;
2. The following muscles are attached longitudinally on the humerus: laterally, the supraspinatus, pectoralis major, and anterior fibers of the deltoid; medially, the subscapularis and latissimus dorsi and teres major;
3. The pectoralis major muscle has a crescentic attachment from the clavicle, sternum, and 5th and/or 6th costal cartilages;
4. The pectoralis minor muscle in this specimen attaches to the 3rd, 4th, and 5th ribs; it commonly arises from the 2nd or 6th rib.

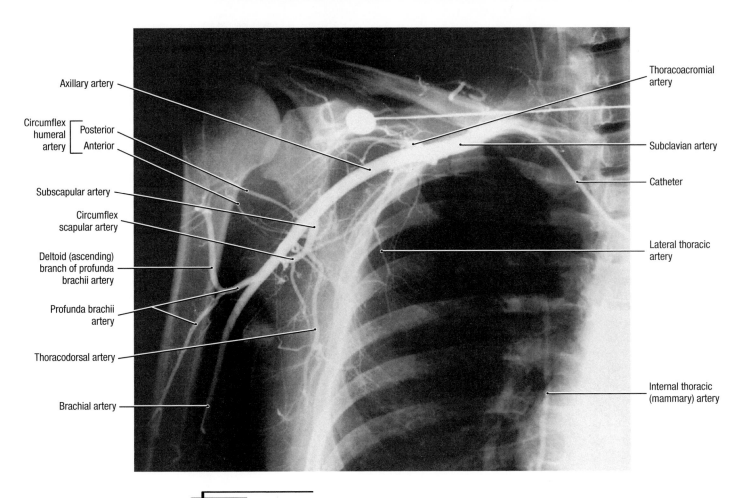

6.18 **Anteroposterior axillary arteriogram**

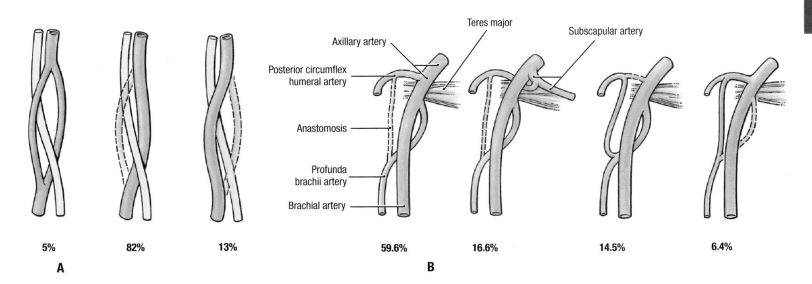

| 5% | 82% | 13% | | 59.6% | 16.6% | 14.5% | 6.4% |
| **A** | | | | **B** | | | |

6.19 **Arterial anomalies, anterior views**

A. Median nerve and brachial artery. The variable relationship of these two structures can be explained developmentally. In a study of 307 limbs, both primitive brachial arteries persisted in 5%, the posterior in 82%, and the anterior in 13%. **B.** Posterior circumflex humeral and profunda brachii arteries. Four variations in origin of the posterior humeral circumflex and profunda brachii arteries are shown; in 2.9%, the arteries were otherwise irregular. Percentages are based on 235 specimens.

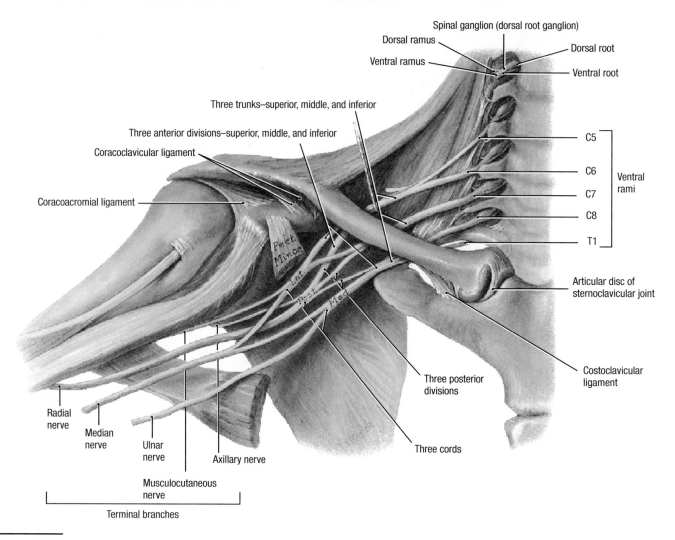

Spinal ganglion (dorsal root ganglion)
Dorsal ramus
Ventral ramus
Dorsal root
Ventral root

Three trunks—superior, middle, and inferior

Three anterior divisions—superior, middle, and inferior

Coracoclavicular ligament

Coracoacromial ligament

C5
C6
C7
C8
T1

Ventral rami

Articular disc of sternoclavicular joint

Costoclavicular ligament

Three posterior divisions

Three cords

Radial nerve
Median nerve
Ulnar nerve
Axillary nerve

Musculocutaneous nerve

Terminal branches

6.20 Brachial plexus, anterior view

OBSERVE:

1. The dorsal and ventral roots unite beyond the ganglion to form a short, "mixed" spinal nerve; the spinal nerve divides into a small dorsal ramus and large ventral ramus; five ventral rami form the brachial plexus;

2. These five rami unite to form the three trunks of the plexus;

3. Each trunk divides into two divisions: anterior and posterior;

4. The six divisions become three cords: lateral, medial, and posterior;

5. The three cords (lateral, medial and posterior) lie posterior to the pectoralis minor and form the terminal branches.

1. Dorsal scapular nerve
2. Suprascapular nerve
3. Nerve to subclavius
4. Long thoracic nerve
5. Lateral pectoral nerve
6. Medial pectoral nerve
7. Medial brachial cutaneous nerve
8. Medial antebrachial cutaneous nerve
9. Upper subscapular nerve
10. Thoracodorsal nerve
11. Lower subscapular nerve

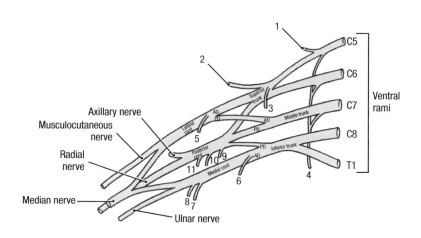

Observe that three nerves (musculocutaneous, median, and ulnar) are arranged like limbs of an uppercase M. Also observe anterior divisions (AD) and posterior divisions (PD).

Table 6.1. Branches of Brachial Plexus

Nerve	Origin	Course	Distribution
Supraclavicular branches			
Dorsal scapular (*1*)	Ventral ramus of C5 with a frequent contribution from C4	Pierces scalenus medius, descends deep to levator scapulae, and enters deep surface of rhomboids	Innervates rhomboids and occasionally supplies levator scapulae
Long thoracic (*4*)	Ventral rami of C5–C7	Descends posterior to C8 and T1 rami and passes distally on external surface of serratus anterior	Innervates serratus anterior
Nerve to subclavius (*3*)	Superior trunk receiving fibers from C5 and C6 and often C4	Descends posterior to clavicle and anterior to brachial plexus and subclavian artery	Innervates subclavius and sternoclavicular joint
Suprascapular (*2*)	Superior trunk receiving fibers from C5 and C6 and often C4	Passes laterally across posterior triangle of neck, through scapular notch under superior transverse scapular ligament	Innervates supraspinatus, infraspinatus, and shoulder joint
Infraclavicular branches			
Lateral pectoral (*5*)	Lateral cord receiving fibers from C5–C7	Pierces clavipectoral fascia to reach deep surface of pectoral muscles	Primarily supplies pectoralis major but sends a loop to medial pectoral nerve that innervates pectoralis minor
Musculocutaneous	Lateral cord receiving fibers from C5–C7	Enters deep surface of coracobrachialis and descends between biceps brachii and brachialis	Innervates coracobrachialis, biceps brachii, and brachialis; continues as lateral antebrachial cutaneous nerve
Median	Lateral root is a continuation of lateral cord, receiving fibers from C6 and C7; medial root is a continuation of medial cord receiving fibers from C8 and T1	Lateral root joins medial root to form median nerve lateral to axillary artery	Innervates flexor muscles in forearm (except flexor carpi ulnaris, ulnar half of flexor digitorum profundus, and five hand muscles)
Medial pectoral (*6*)	Medial cord receiving fibers from C8 and T1	Passes between axillary artery and vein and enters deep surface of pectoralis minor	Innervates the pectoralis minor and part of pectoralis major
Medial brachial cutaneous (*7*)	Medial cord receiving fibers from C8 and T1	Runs along the medial side of axillary vein and communicates with intercostobrachial nerve	Supplies skin on medial side of arm
Medial antebrachial cutaneous (*8*)	Medial cord receiving fibers from C8 and T1	Runs between axillary artery and vein	Supplies skin over medial side of forearm
Ulnar	A terminal branch of medial cord receiving fibers from C8 and T1 and often C7	Passes down medial aspect of arm and runs posterior to medial epicondyle to enter forearm	Innervates one and one-half flexor muscles in forearm, most small muscles in hand, and skin of hand medial to a line bisecting fourth digit (ring finger)
Upper subscapular (*9*)	Branch of posterior cord receiving fibers from C5 and C6	Passes posteriorly and enters subscapularis	Innervates superior portion of subscapularis
Thoracodorsal (*10*)	Branch of posterior cord receiving fibers from C6–C8	Arises between upper and lower subscapular nerves and runs inferolaterally to latissimus dorsi	Innervates latissimus dorsi
Lower subscapular (*11*)	Branch of posterior cord receiving fibers from C5 and C6	Passes inferolaterally, deep to subscapular artery and vein, to subscapularis and teres major	Innervates inferior portion of subscapularis and teres major
Axillary	Terminal branch of posterior cord receiving fibers from C5 and C6	Passes to posterior aspect of arm through quadrangular space[a] in company with posterior circumflex humeral artery and then winds around surgical neck of humerus; gives rise to lateral brachial cutaneous nerve	Innervates teres minor and deltoid, shoulder joint, and skin over inferior part of deltoid
Radial	Terminal branch of posterior cord receiving fibers from C5–C8 and C11	Descends posterior to axillary artery; enters radial groove with deep brachial artery to pass between long and medial heads of triceps	Innervates triceps brachii, anconeus, brachioradialis, and extensor muscles of forearm; supplies skin on posterior aspect of arm and forearm through posterior cutaneous nerves of arm and forearm

a Quadrangular space is bounded superiorly by subscapularis and teres minor, inferiorly by teres major, medially by long head of triceps, and laterally by humerus.

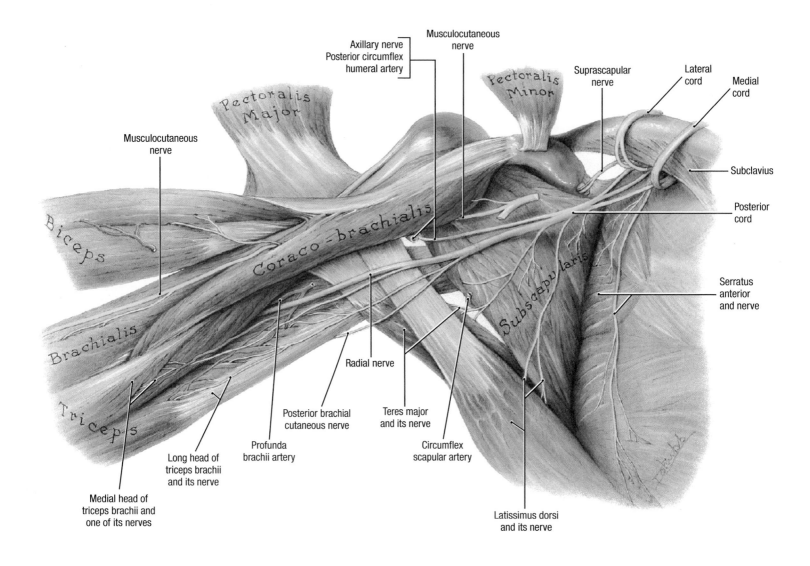

6.21 Posterior wall of axilla, musculocutaneous nerve, and posterior cord, anterior view

The pectoralis major and minor muscles are reflected laterally, the lateral and medial cords are reflected superiorly, and the arteries, veins, and median and ulnar nerves are removed.

OBSERVE:

1. Coracobrachialis arises with the short head of the biceps brachii muscle from the tip of the coracoid process and attaches halfway down the humerus;
2. The musculocutaneous nerve pierces the coracobrachialis muscle and supplies it, the biceps, and the brachialis before becoming cutaneous;
3. The posterior cord of the plexus, formed by the union of the three posterior divisions, supplies the three muscles of the posterior wall of the axilla and soon ends as the radial and axillary nerves;

4. In the axilla, the radial nerve gives off the nerve to the long head of the triceps brachii muscle and a cutaneous branch; in this specimen, it also gives off a branch to the medial head of the triceps. It then enters the radial (spiral) groove of the humerus with the profunda brachii artery;
5. The axillary nerve traverses the quadrangular space with the posterior circumflex humeral artery. The borders of the quadrilateral space: superiorly, the lateral border of the scapula; inferiorly, the teres major; laterally, the humerus; and medially, the long head of triceps brachii. The circumflex scapular artery traverses the triangular space.

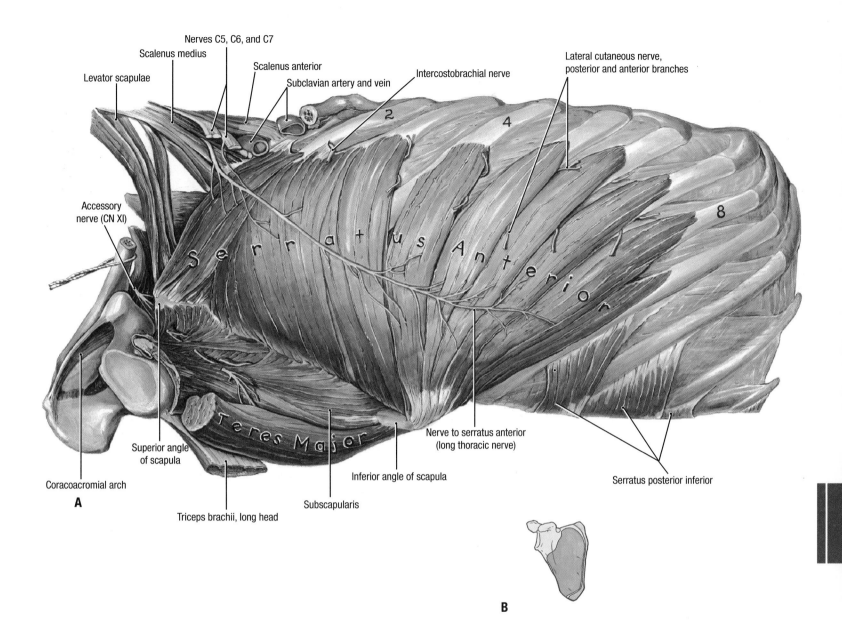

6.22 **Serratus anterior and subscapularis**

A. Supine position, lateral view. **B.** Scapular attachments of subscapularis (*red*) and serratus anterior (*blue*), anterior view.

OBSERVE IN **A**:
1. The serratus anterior muscle, which forms the medial wall of the axilla, has an extensive, fleshy span from the superior eight (here nine) ribs in the midclavicular line to the medial border of the scapula. The fibers from the 1st rib and the arch between the 1st and 2nd ribs converge on the superior angle of the scapula; those from the 2nd and 3rd ribs diverge to spread thinly along the medial border, and the remainder (from the 4th to 9th ribs), which form the bulk of the muscle, converge on the inferior angle and have a tendinous insertion;

2. The nerve to serratus anterior arises from C5, C6, and C7 and is applied to the whole length of the muscle; the fibers from C5 and C6 pierce the scalenus medius and appear lateral to the brachial plexus, and those from C7 descend posterior to the plexus;
3. The teres major muscle is applied to the lateral border of the subscapularis muscle; the nerve to the teres major muscle helps to supply subscapularis;
4. The brachial plexus and subclavian artery appear between the scalenus anterior and scalenus medius muscles; the subclavian vein is separated from the artery by the scalenus anterior muscle.

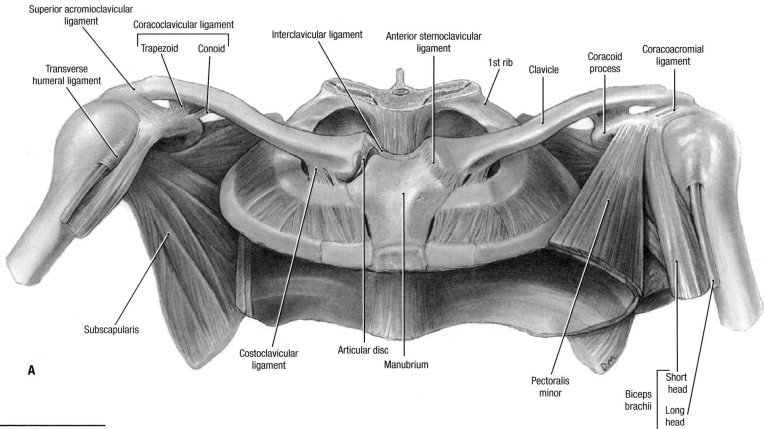

6.23   Pectoral girdle

A. Pectoral girdle, anterosuperior view. **B.** Acromioclavicular joint, superior view.

OBSERVE:
1. The pectoral (shoulder) girdle consists of the sternoclavicular, acromioclavicular, and shoulder (glenohumeral) joints; the mobility of the clavicle is essential to the free movement of the upper limb;
2. The sternoclavicular joint is the only joint connecting the upper limb to the trunk. The articular disc of the sternoclavicular joint divides the joint cavity into two parts and attaches superiorly to the clavicle and inferiorly to the first costal cartilage; the disc resists superior and medial displacement of the clavicle;
3. The strong coracoclavicular ligament, consisting of the conoid and trapezoid ligaments, provides stability to the acromioclavicular joint and prevents the scapula from being driven medially and the acromion from being driven inferior to the clavicle;
4. The coracoacromial ligament, together with the acromion and coracoid process, forms the coracoacromial arch; the arch prevents superior displacement of the head of the humerus.
5. In B, the medial border of the acromion has a small oval facet that articulates with a similar small facet on the lateral end of the clavicle.

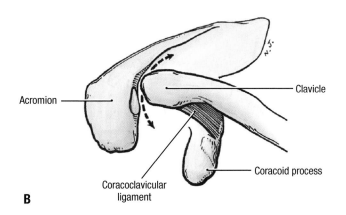

6.24   Scapular movements

A. Elevation. **B.** Depression. **C.** Protraction. **D.** Retraction. **E.** Elevation with superior (upward) rotation of glenoid fossa. **F.** Depression with inferior (downward) rotation of glenoid fossa. The dotted outlines represent the starting position for each movement.

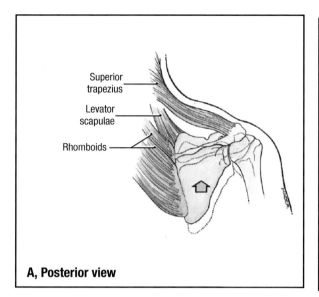

Superior
trapezius

Levator
scapulae

Rhomboids

A, Posterior view

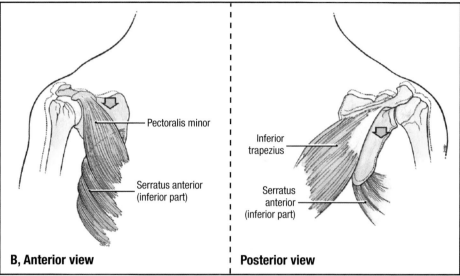

Pectoralis minor

Serratus anterior
(inferior part)

Inferior
trapezius

Serratus
anterior
(inferior part)

B, Anterior view   **Posterior view**

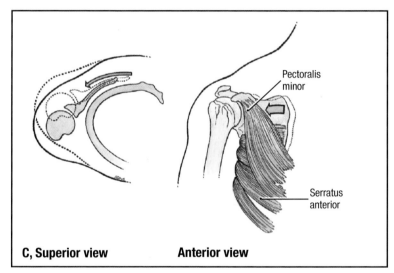

Pectoralis
minor

Serratus
anterior

C, Superior view   **Anterior view**

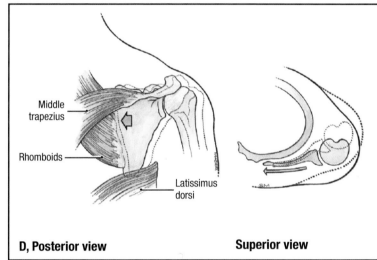

Middle
trapezius

Rhomboids

Latissimus
dorsi

D, Posterior view   **Superior view**

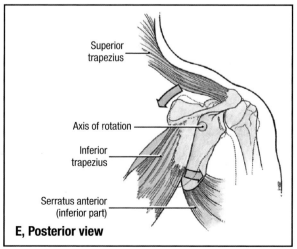

Superior
trapezius

Axis of rotation

Inferior
trapezius

Serratus anterior
(inferior part)

E, Posterior view

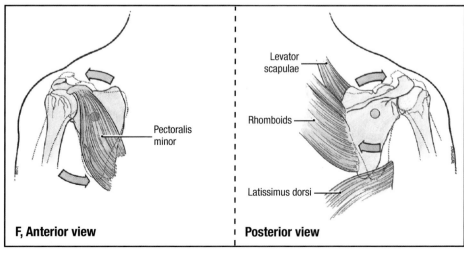

Pectoralis
minor

Levator
scapulae

Rhomboids

Latissimus dorsi

F, Anterior view   **Posterior view**

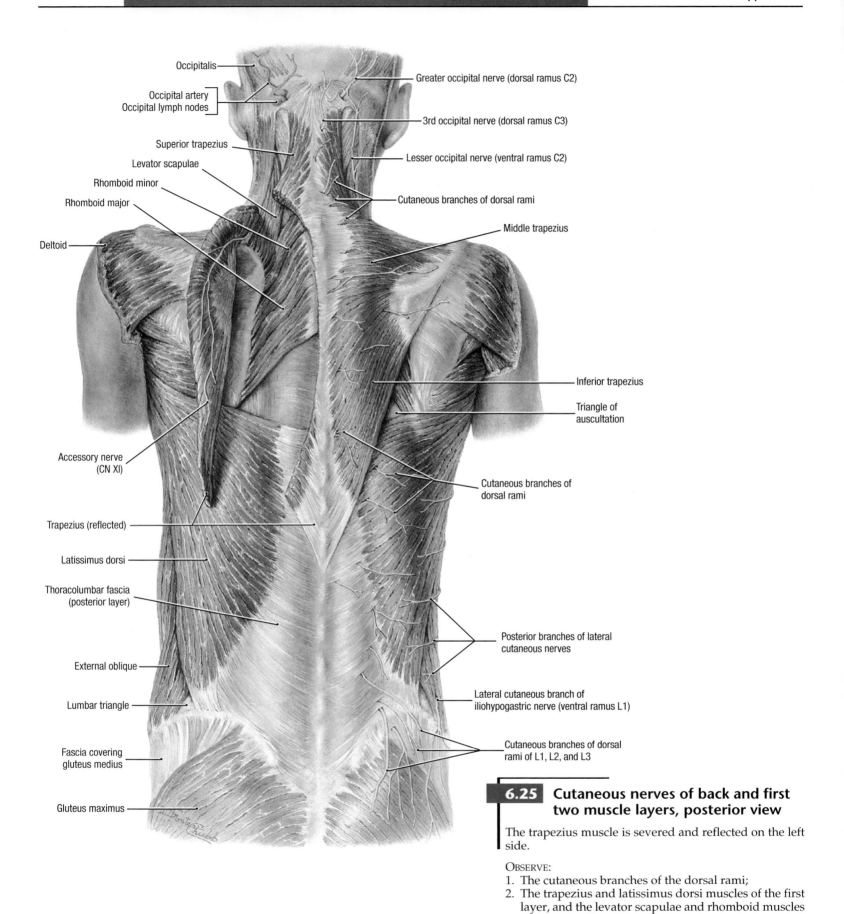

Occipitalis

Occipital artery
Occipital lymph nodes

Superior trapezius

Levator scapulae

Rhomboid minor

Rhomboid major

Deltoid

Accessory nerve
(CN XI)

Trapezius (reflected)

Latissimus dorsi

Thoracolumbar fascia
(posterior layer)

External oblique

Lumbar triangle

Fascia covering
gluteus medius

Gluteus maximus

Greater occipital nerve (dorsal ramus C2)

3rd occipital nerve (dorsal ramus C3)

Lesser occipital nerve (ventral ramus C2)

Cutaneous branches of dorsal rami

Middle trapezius

Inferior trapezius

Triangle of
auscultation

Cutaneous branches of
dorsal rami

Posterior branches of lateral
cutaneous nerves

Lateral cutaneous branch of
iliohypogastric nerve (ventral ramus L1)

Cutaneous branches of dorsal
rami of L1, L2, and L3

6.25 Cutaneous nerves of back and first two muscle layers, posterior view

The trapezius muscle is severed and reflected on the left side.

OBSERVE:
1. The cutaneous branches of the dorsal rami;
2. The trapezius and latissimus dorsi muscles of the first layer, and the levator scapulae and rhomboid muscles of the second layer.

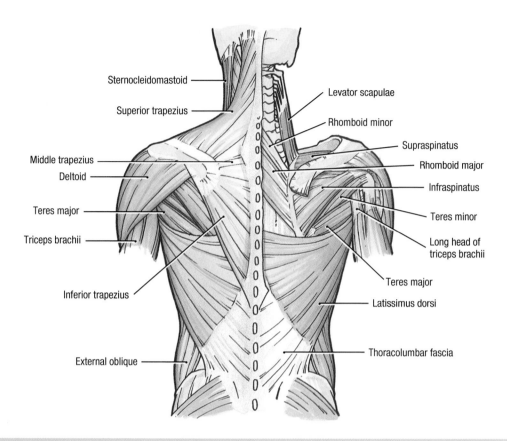

Table 6.2. Superficial Back Muscles

Muscle	Proximal Attachment	Distal Attachment	Innervation	Main Actions
Trapezius	Medial third of superior nuchal line; external occipital protuberance, ligamentum nuchae, and spinous processes of C7–T12 vertebrae	Lateral third of clavicle, acromion, and spine of scapula	Spinal root of accessory nerve (CN XI) and cervical nerves (C3 and C4)	Elevates, retracts, and rotates scapula; superior fibers elevate, middle fibers retract, and inferior fibers depress scapula; superior and inferior fibers act together in superior rotation of scapula
Latissimus dorsi	Spinous processes of inferior six thoracic vertebrae, thoracolumbar fascia, iliac crest, and inferior three or four ribs	Floor of intertubercular groove of humerus	Thoracodorsal nerves (C6, C7, and C8)	Extends, adducts, and medially rotates humerus; raises body toward arms during climbing
Levator scapulae	Posterior tubercles of transverse processes of C1–C4 vertebrae	Superior part of medial border of scapula	Dorsal scapular (C5) and cervical (C3 and C4) nerves	Elevates scapula and tilts its glenoid cavity inferiorly by rotating scapula
Rhomboid minor and major	*Minor:* ligamentum nuchae and spinous processes of C7 and T1 vertebrae *Major:* spinous processes of T2–T5 vertebrae	Medial border of scapula from level of spine to inferior angle	Dorsal scapular nerve (C4 and **C5**) rotate	Retracts scapula and rotates it to depress glenoid cavity; fixes scapula to thoracic wall
Deltoid	Lateral third of clavicle, acromion, and spine of scapula	Deltoid tuberosity of humerus	Axillary nerve (C5 and C6)	*Anterior part:* flexes and medially rotates arm; *Middle part:* abducts arm; *Posterior part:* extends and laterally rotates arm.

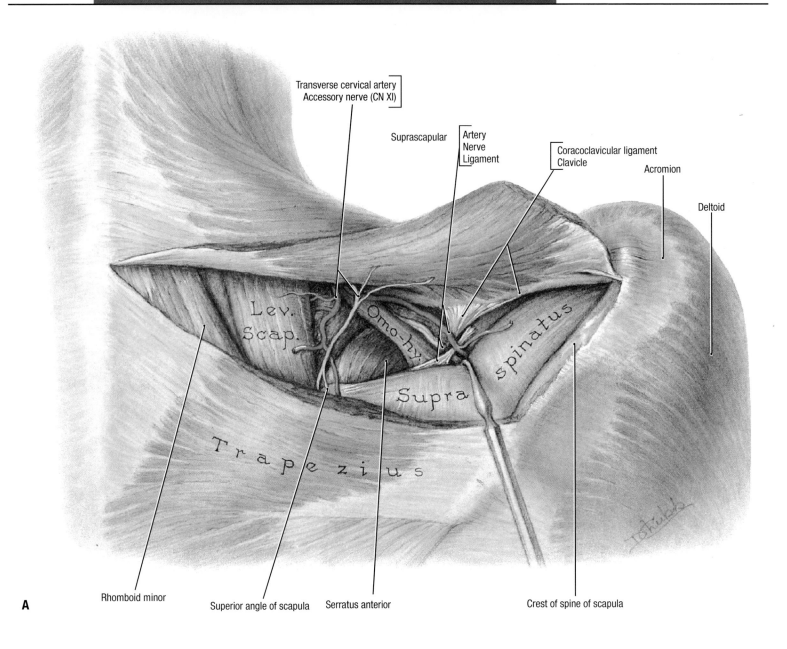

A

Transverse cervical artery
Accessory nerve (CN XI)

Suprascapular

Artery
Nerve
Ligament

Coracoclavicular ligament
Clavicle

Acromion

Deltoid

Lev.
Scap.

Omo-hy.

Supra spinatus

Trapezius

Rhomboid minor

Superior angle of scapula

Serratus anterior

Crest of spine of scapula

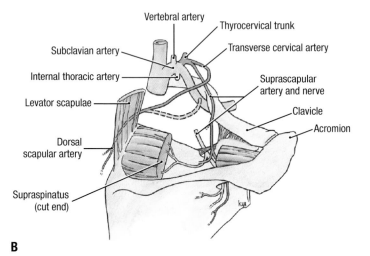

B

Vertebral artery

Thyrocervical trunk

Subclavian artery

Transverse cervical artery

Internal thoracic artery

Suprascapular
artery and nerve

Levator scapulae

Clavicle

Acromion

Dorsal
scapular artery

Supraspinatus
(cut end)

6.26   Suprascapular region, posterosuperior views

A. Dissection. At the level of the superior angle of the scapula, the middle fibers of the trapezius muscle are separated, and the incision is carried laterally along the crest of the spine of the scapula. **B.** Suprascapular and dorsal scapular arteries.

OBSERVE:
1. The accessory nerve (CN XI) crosses the superior angle of the scapula;
2. The transverse cervical artery is split by the levator scapulae muscle into superficial and deep branches; one follows the accessory nerve, and the other (not shown) follows the dorsal scapular nerve (nerve to rhomboid muscles);
3. The suprascapular artery runs posterior to the clavicle before crossing superior to the suprascapular ligament;
4. The suprascapular nerve crosses inferior to the ligament.

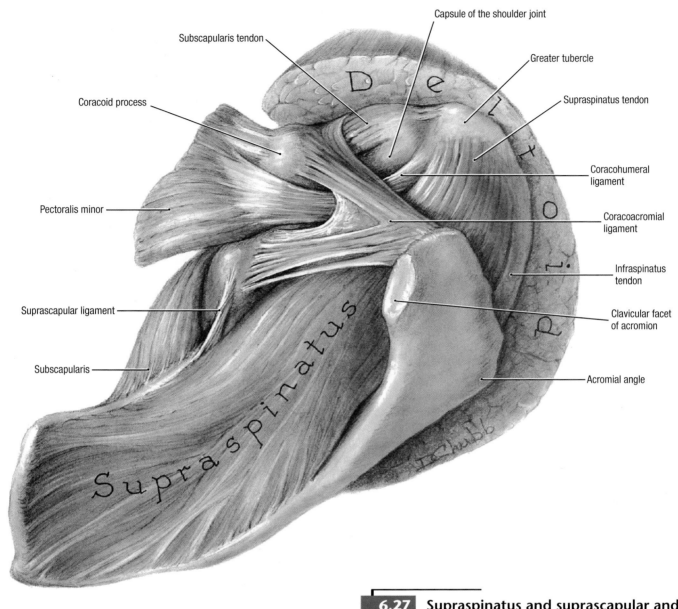

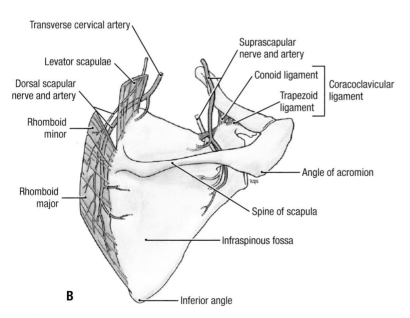

6.27 Supraspinatus and suprascapular and dorsal scapular nerves

A. Supraspinatus, superior view. **B.** Suprascapular and dorsal scapular nerves, posterior view.

OBSERVE:

1. The clavicular facet on the acromion is small, oval, and obliquely set;
2. The triangular coracoacromial ligament arches from the lateral border of the coracoid process to the acromion between the articular facet and tip;
3. Part of the pectoralis minor tendon divides the coracoacromial ligament into two limbs and continues as the anterior part of the coracohumeral ligament to the greater tubercle of the humerus;
4. The supraspinatus muscle passes inferior to the coracoacromial arch and then lies between the deltoid muscle superiorly and the capsule of the shoulder joint inferiorly; the supraspinatus muscle and the middle fibers of the deltoid muscle are the abductors of the joint. Although the middle part of the deltoid muscle is thin, it is multipennate and powerful.

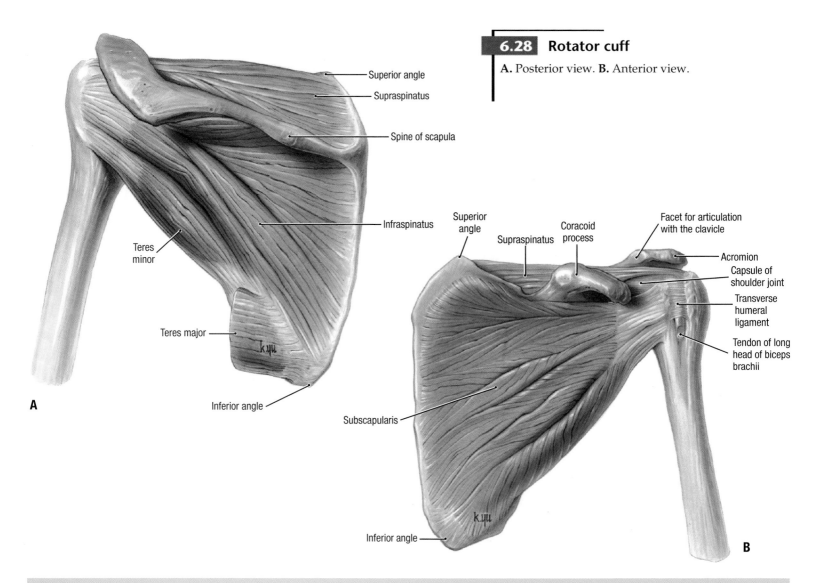

6.28 **Rotator cuff**

A. Posterior view. **B.** Anterior view.

Table 6.3. Rotator Cuff Muscles

Muscle	Proximal Attachment	Distal Attachment	Innervation	Main Actions
Supraspinatus	Supraspinous fossa of scapula	Superior facet on greater tubercle of humerus	Suprascapular nerve (C4, **C5**, and C6)	Helps deltoid to abduct arm and acts with rotator cuff muscles[a]
Infraspinatus	Infraspinous fossa of scapula	Middle facet on greater tubercle of humerus	Suprascapular nerve (**C5** and C6)	Laterally rotate arm; help to hold humeral head in glenoid cavity of scapula
Teres minor	Superior part of lateral border of scapula	Inferior facet on greater tubercle of humerus	Axillary nerve (**C5** and C6)	
Teres major	Dorsal surface of inferior angle of scapula	Medial lip of intertubercular groove of humerus	Lower subscapular nerve (**C6** and C7)	Adducts and medially rotates arm
Subscapularis	Subscapular fossa	Lesser tubercle of humerus Upper and lower	subscapular nerves (C5, **C6**, and C7)	Medially rotates arm and adducts it; helps to hold humeral head in glenoid cavity

[a] Collectively, the supraspinatus, infraspinatus, teres minor, and subscapularis muscles are referred to as the rotator cuff muscles. Their prime function during all movements of should joint is to hold head of humerus in glenoid cavity of scapula.

6.29　Arm, lateral views

A. Surface anatomy. **B.** Dissection (numbers in parentheses refer to structures in **A**).

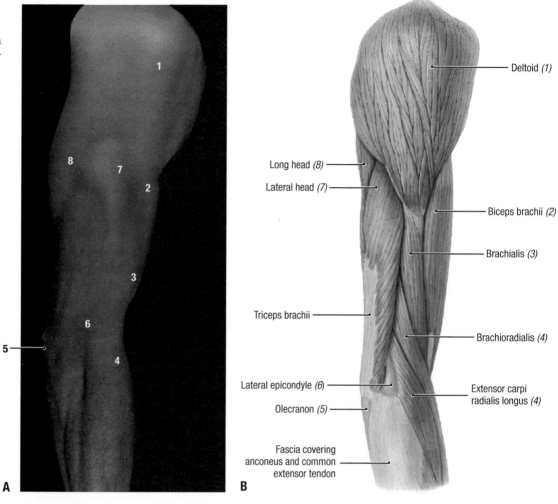

Deltoid *(1)*

Long head *(8)*

Lateral head *(7)*

Biceps brachii *(2)*

Brachialis *(3)*

Triceps brachii

Brachioradialis *(4)*

Lateral epicondyle *(6)*

Extensor carpi radialis longus *(4)*

Olecranon *(5)*

Fascia covering anconeus and common extensor tendon

A　　　　B

Table 6.4. Arm Muscles

Muscle	Proximal Attachment	Distal Attachment	Innervation	Main Actions
Biceps brachii	*Short head:* tip of coracoid process of scapula; *Long head:* supraglenoid tubercle of scapula	Tuberosity of radius and fascia of forearm through bicipital aponeurosis	Musculocutaneous nerve (C5 and **C6**)	Supinates forearm and, when supine, flexes forearm
Brachialis	Distal half of anterior surface of humerus	Coronoid process and tuberosity of ulna		Flexes forearm in all positions
Coracobrachialis	Tip of coracoid process of scapula	Middle third of medial surface of humerus	Musculocutaneous nerve (C5, **C6**, and C7)	Helps to flex and adduct arm
Triceps brachii	Long head: infraglenoid tubercle of scapula; Lateral head: posterior surface of humerus, superior to radial groove; Medial head: posterior surface of humerus, inferior to radial groove	Proximal end of olecranon of ulna and fascia of forearm	Radial nerve (C6, **C7**, and **C8**)	Extends the forearm; it is chief extensor of forearm; long head steadies head of abducted humerus
Anconeus	Lateral epicondyle of humerus	Lateral surface of olecranon and superior part of posterior surface of ulna	Radial nerve (C7, C8, and T1)	Assists triceps in extending forearm; stabilizes elbow joint; abducts ulna during pronation

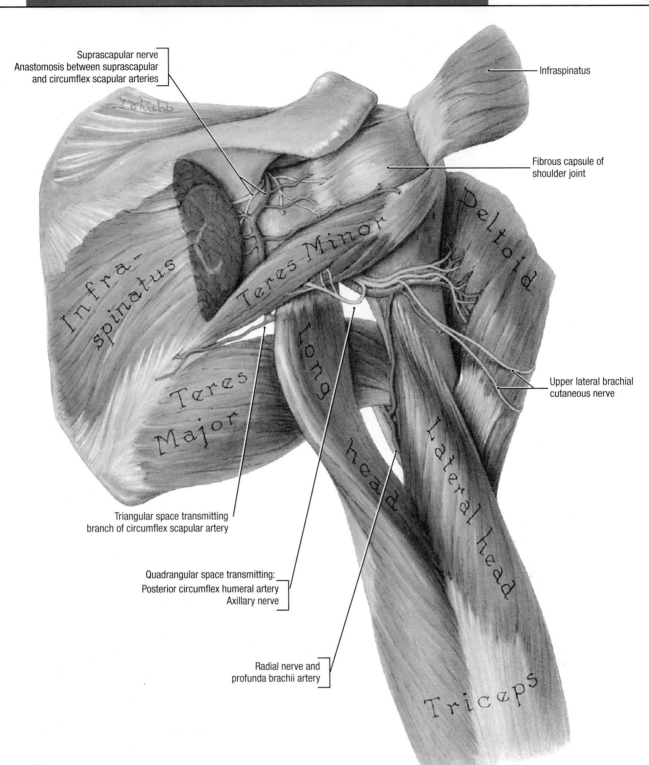

Suprascapular nerve
Anastomosis between suprascapular
and circumflex scapular arteries

Infraspinatus

Fibrous capsule of
shoulder joint

Upper lateral brachial
cutaneous nerve

Triangular space transmitting
branch of circumflex scapular artery

Quadrangular space transmitting:
Posterior circumflex humeral artery
Axillary nerve

Radial nerve and
profunda brachii artery

6.30   Dorsal scapular and subdeltoid regions, posterior view

OBSERVE:

1. The thickness of the infraspinatus muscle, aided by the teres minor and posterior fibers of the deltoid, rotates the humerus laterally;
2. The long head of the triceps muscle passes between the teres minor (a lateral rotator) and teres major (a medial rotator) muscles;
3. The long head of the triceps muscle separates the quadrangular space from the triangular space;

4. The distribution of the suprascapular and axillary nerves: each comes from C5 and C6; each supplies two muscles; the suprascapular nerve innervates the supraspinatus and infraspinatus; the axillary nerve innervates the teres minor and deltoid muscles; each supplies the shoulder joint; and only the axillary nerve has cutaneous branches.

6.31   Triceps brachii, posterior view

A. Triceps and related nerves. **B.** Surface anatomy. (*R*, Rhomboids, *TM*, Teres major, *LD*, Latissimus dorsi. Numbers in parentheses refer to structures in **A**.)

OBSERVE:

1. The long head is most medial and attaches to the infraglenoid tubercle of the scapula. The lateral head is divided and reflected laterally to reveal its attachment to the humerus. The medial head is attached to the deep surface of the triceps tendon, which attaches to the olecranon and deep fascia of the forearm;
2. The radial nerve travels in the gap between the origins of the lateral and medial heads of the triceps muscle;
3. The axillary nerve, passing through the quadrangular space, supplies the deltoid and teres minor muscles;
4. The ulnar nerve follows the medial border of triceps.

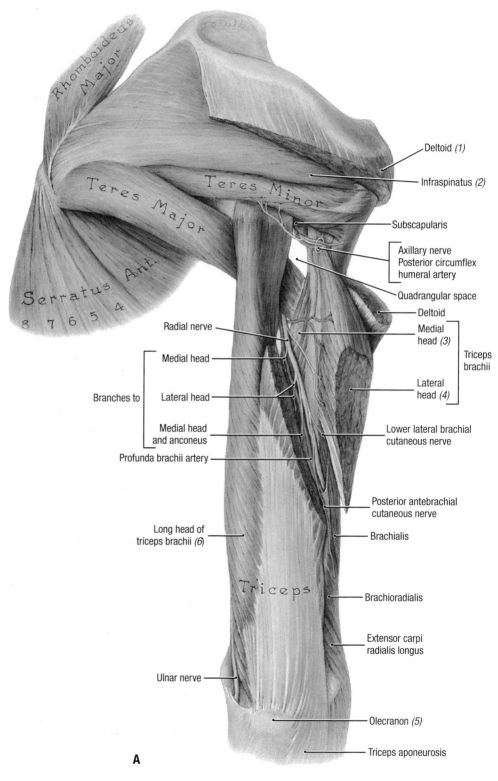

A

Deltoid *(1)*
Infraspinatus *(2)*
Subscapularis
Axillary nerve
Posterior circumflex humeral artery
Quadrangular space
Deltoid
Medial head *(3)*
Triceps brachii
Lateral head *(4)*
Lower lateral brachial cutaneous nerve
Posterior antebrachial cutaneous nerve
Brachialis
Brachioradialis
Extensor carpi radialis longus
Olecranon *(5)*
Triceps aponeurosis

Radial nerve
Branches to — Medial head
Lateral head
Medial head and anconeus
Profunda brachii artery
Long head of triceps brachii *(6)*
Ulnar nerve

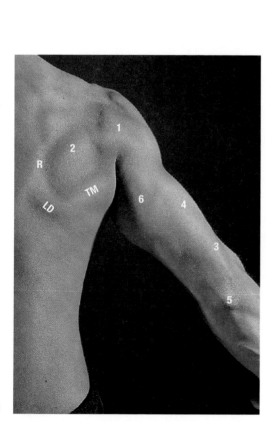

B

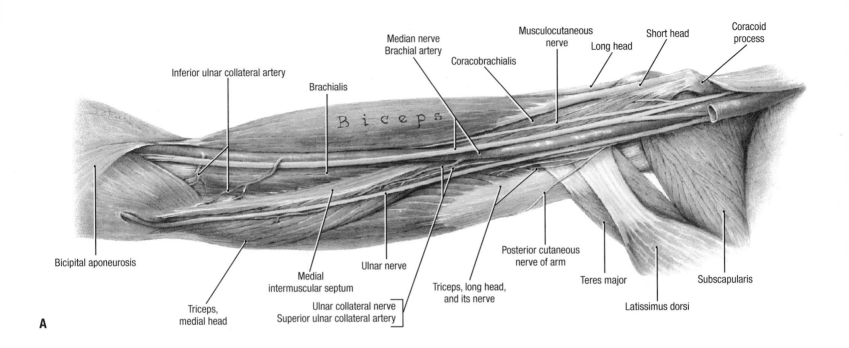

Inferior ulnar collateral artery

Brachialis

Median nerve
Brachial artery

Coracobrachialis

Musculocutaneous nerve

Long head

Short head

Coracoid process

Bicipital aponeurosis

Triceps, medial head

Medial intermuscular septum

Ulnar nerve

Ulnar collateral nerve
Superior ulnar collateral artery

Triceps, long head, and its nerve

Posterior cutaneous nerve of arm

Teres major

Latissimus dorsi

Subscapularis

A

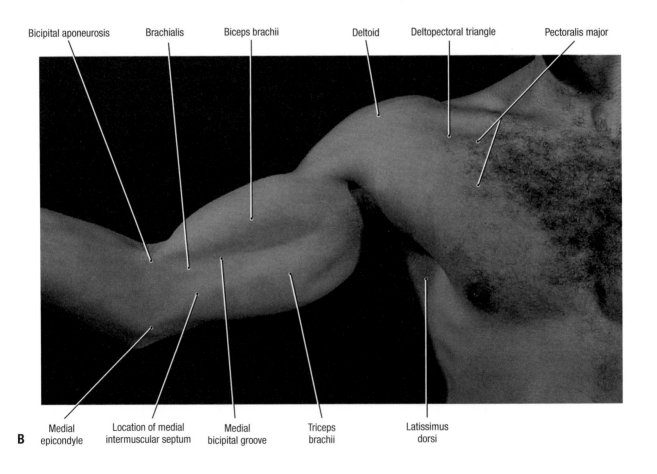

Bicipital aponeurosis

Brachialis

Biceps brachii

Deltoid

Deltopectoral triangle

Pectoralis major

Medial epicondyle

Location of medial intermuscular septum

Medial bicipital groove

Triceps brachii

Latissimus dorsi

B

6.32   Arm, medial views

A. Dissection. **B.** Surface anatomy.

OBSERVE:
1. Three muscles, the biceps, brachialis, and coracobrachialis, lie in the anterior compartment of the arm, and triceps brachii lies in the posterior compartment; the medial intermuscular septum separates these two muscle groups in the distal two-thirds of the arm;
2. The great artery of the limb (axillary/brachial) passes a finger-breath medial to the tip of the coracoid process, and is applied to the medial side of coracobrachialis proximally and to the anterior aspect of brachialis distally;
3. The median nerve is adjacent to the artery throughout and crosses the artery from lateral to medial;

4. The ulnar nerve is adjacent to the medial side of the artery, passes posterior to the medial intermuscular septum, and descends on the medial head of triceps to pass posterior to the medial epicondyle; *here, the ulnar nerve is palpable;*
5. The superior ulnar collateral artery and ulnar collateral branch of the radial nerve (to medial head of the triceps) accompany the ulnar nerve;
6. The musculocutaneous nerve supplies the coracobrachialis muscle, follows the lateral side of the brachial artery, and disappears between the biceps and brachialis; more commonly, it pierces the coracobrachialis muscle.

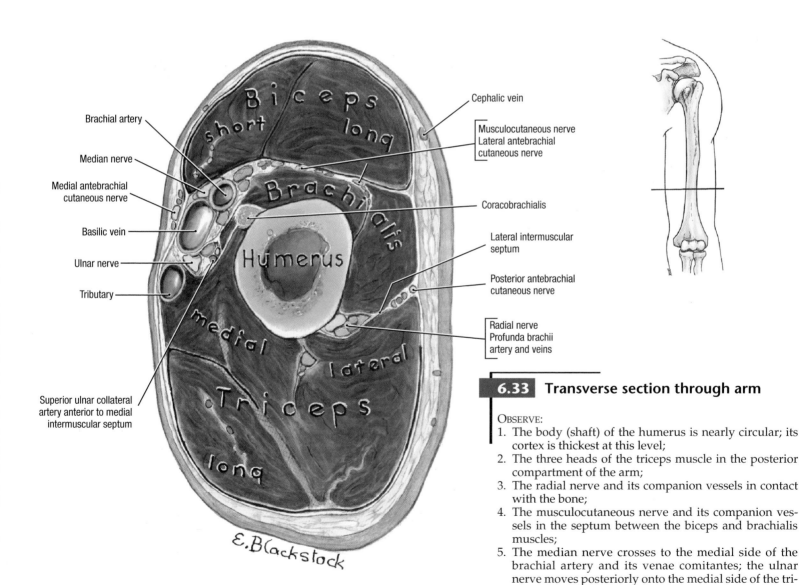

6.33   Transverse section through arm

OBSERVE:
1. The body (shaft) of the humerus is nearly circular; its cortex is thickest at this level;
2. The three heads of the triceps muscle in the posterior compartment of the arm;
3. The radial nerve and its companion vessels in contact with the bone;
4. The musculocutaneous nerve and its companion vessels in the septum between the biceps and brachialis muscles;
5. The median nerve crosses to the medial side of the brachial artery and its venae comitantes; the ulnar nerve moves posteriorly onto the medial side of the triceps muscle, and the basilic vein (here as two vessels) has pierced the deep fascia;

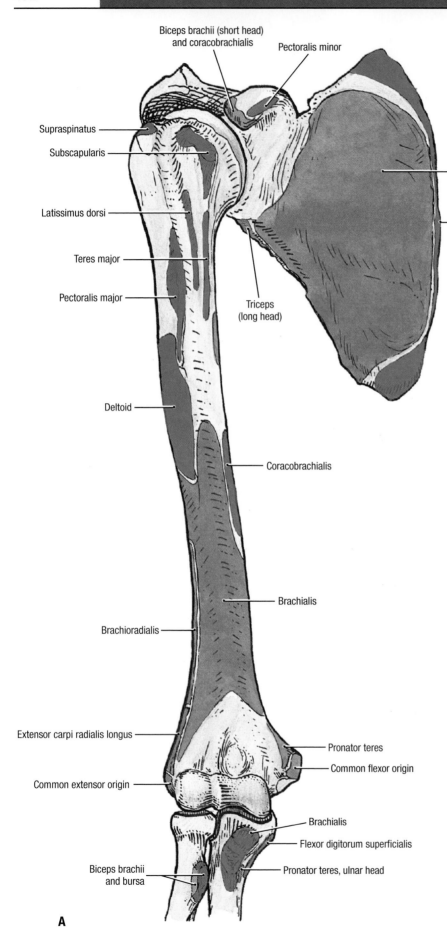

Biceps brachii (short head) and coracobrachialis

Pectoralis minor

Supraspinatus

Subscapularis

Latissimus dorsi

Teres major

Pectoralis major

Triceps (long head)

Deltoid

Coracobrachialis

Subscapularis

Serratus anterior

Brachialis

Brachioradialis

Extensor carpi radialis longus

Pronator teres

Common flexor origin

Common extensor origin

Brachialis

Flexor digitorum superficialis

Biceps brachii and bursa

Pronator teres, ulnar head

A

6.34 **Bones of upper limb, showing muscle attachments**

A. Anterior view. (For anterior view of bones of the forearm, see Fig. 6.55.)

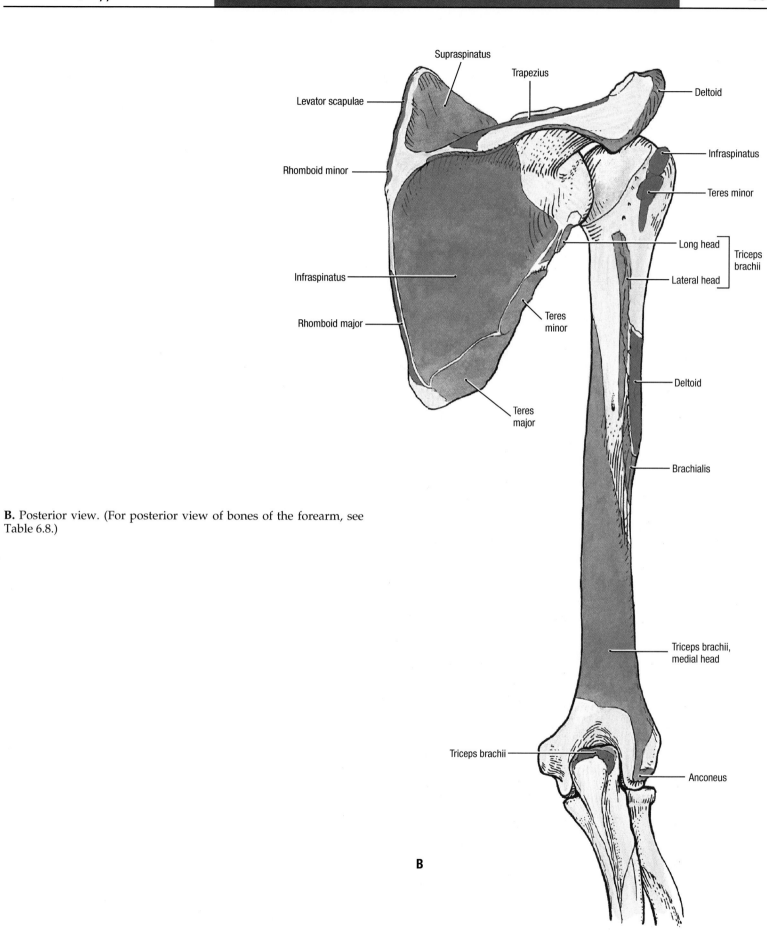

B. Posterior view. (For posterior view of bones of the forearm, see Table 6.8.)

B

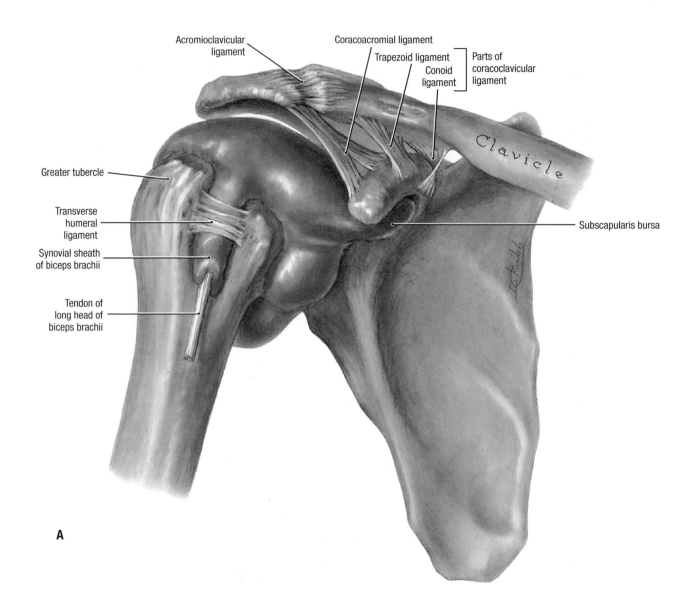

Acromioclavicular ligament

Coracoacromial ligament

Trapezoid ligament

Conoid ligament — Parts of coracoclavicular ligament

Clavicle

Greater tubercle

Transverse humeral ligament

Synovial sheath of biceps brachii

Tendon of long head of biceps brachii

Subscapularis bursa

A

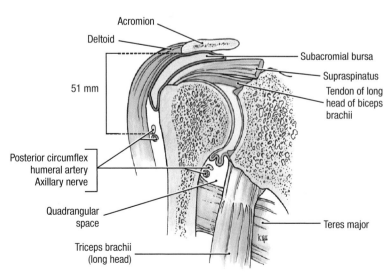

Acromion

Deltoid

Subacromial bursa

Supraspinatus

Tendon of long head of biceps brachii

51 mm

Posterior circumflex humeral artery
Axillary nerve

Quadrangular space

Teres major

Triceps brachii (long head)

B

6.35   Shoulder joint

A. Synovial capsule and ligaments at lateral end of clavicle, anterolateral view. **B.** Coronal section, posterior view.

OBSERVE:
1. The attachments of the four rotator cuff muscles prevent the capsule (purple) from extending onto the lesser and greater tubercles of the humerus, but it extends inferiorly onto the surgical neck of the humerus;
2. The capsule has two prolongations: (a) where it forms a synovial sheath for the tendon of the long head of the biceps muscle in its osseofibrous tunnel, and (b) inferior to the coracoid process, where it forms a bursa between the subscapularis tendon and margin of the glenoid cavity.

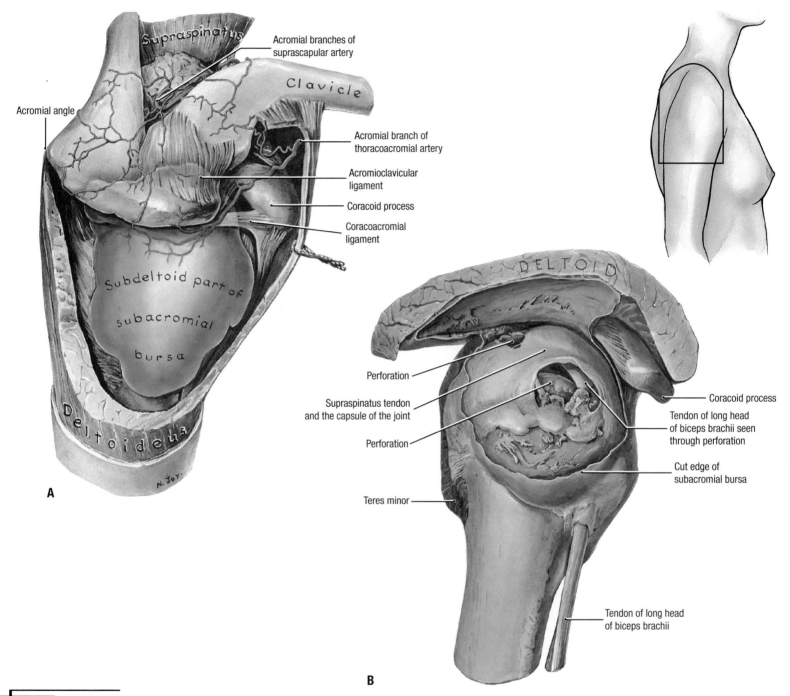

6.36 Subacromial bursa, lateral views

A. Subacromial bursa. **B.** Attrition of supraspinatus tendon.

OBSERVE:

1. The bursa has been injected with purple latex;
2. The term "subacromial bursa" usually includes the subdeltoid bursa because the two bursae are usually combined;
3. Parts of the deltoid, acromion, coracoacromial ligament, and acromioclavicular joint are superficial to the bursa;
4. The greater tubercle of the humerus and the supraspinatus tendon are deep to the bursa;
5. The bursa can extend more widely under the acromion and can, through attrition, communicate with the shoulder joint and acromioclavicular joint (**B**);

6. The acromial branches of the thoracoacromial (acromiothoracic) and suprascapular arteries contribute to the acromial rete network.
7. In **B**, *as a result of wearing away of the supraspinatus tendon and underlying capsule, the subacromial bursa and shoulder joint come into wide open communication; the intracapsular part of the long tendon of the biceps muscle becomes frayed (even worn away), leaving it adherent to the intertubercular groove; Of 95 dissecting room subjects, none of the 18 younger than 50 years of age had a perforation, but 4 of the 19 who were 50 to 60 years and 23 of the 57 older than 60 years had perforations. The perforation was bilateral in 11 subjects and unilateral in 14.*

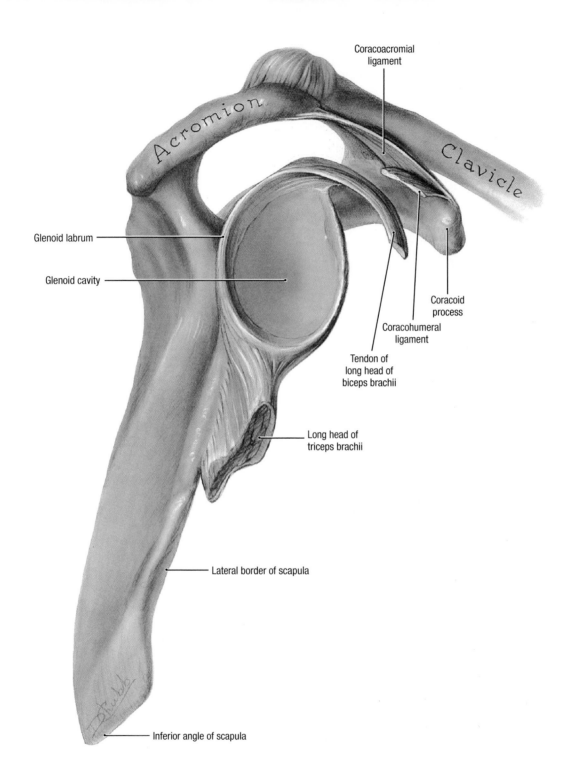

Coracoacromial
ligament

Acromion

Clavicle

Glenoid labrum

Glenoid cavity

Coracoid
process

Coracohumeral
ligament

Tendon of
long head of
biceps brachii

Long head of
triceps brachii

Lateral border of scapula

Inferior angle of scapula

6.37   Glenoid cavity, lateral view

OBSERVE:
1. The glenoid cavity is overhung by the resilient coracoacromial arch (coracoid process, coracoacromial ligament, and acromion), which prevents superior displacement of the head of the humerus;
2. The long head of the triceps brachii muscle arises just inferior to the glenoid cavity;
3. The long head of the biceps brachii muscle arises just superior to the

glenoid cavity; proximally, it continues as the posterior lip of the glenoid labrum, and distally, it curves anterior to the front of the head of the humerus, not superior to it;
4. The orientation of the scapula ensures that, should the head of the humerus be dislocated inferiorly, it would pass onto the costal surface of the scapula.

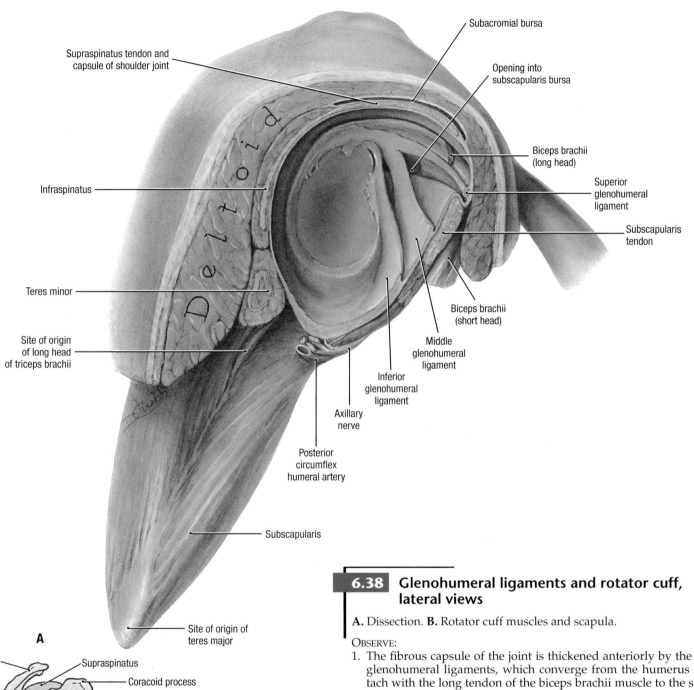

Subacromial bursa

Supraspinatus tendon and
capsule of shoulder joint

Opening into
subscapularis bursa

Biceps brachii
(long head)

Superior
glenohumeral
ligament

Infraspinatus

Subscapularis
tendon

Teres minor

Biceps brachii
(short head)

Site of origin
of long head
of triceps brachii

Middle
glenohumeral
ligament

Inferior
glenohumeral
ligament

Axillary
nerve

Posterior
circumflex
humeral artery

Subscapularis

Site of origin of
teres major

A

Acromion

Supraspinatus

Coracoid process

Glenoid cavity

Infraspinatus

Subscapularis

Teres minor

Inferior angle

B

6.38 Glenohumeral ligaments and rotator cuff, lateral views

A. Dissection. **B.** Rotator cuff muscles and scapula.

OBSERVE:

1. The fibrous capsule of the joint is thickened anteriorly by the three glenohumeral ligaments, which converge from the humerus to attach with the long tendon of the biceps brachii muscle to the supraglenoid tubercle;
2. The subacromial bursa is between the acromion and deltoid superiorly and the tendon of supraspinatus inferiorly;
3. The four short rotator cuff muscles (supraspinatus, infraspinatus, teres minor, and subscapularis) cross the joint, blend with the capsule, and secure the head of the humerus in its socket;
4. The axillary nerve and posterior circumflex humeral artery are in contact with the capsule inferiorly;
5. The subscapularis bursa opens superior and inferior to the middle glenohumeral ligament; several synovial folds overlap the glenoid cavity.

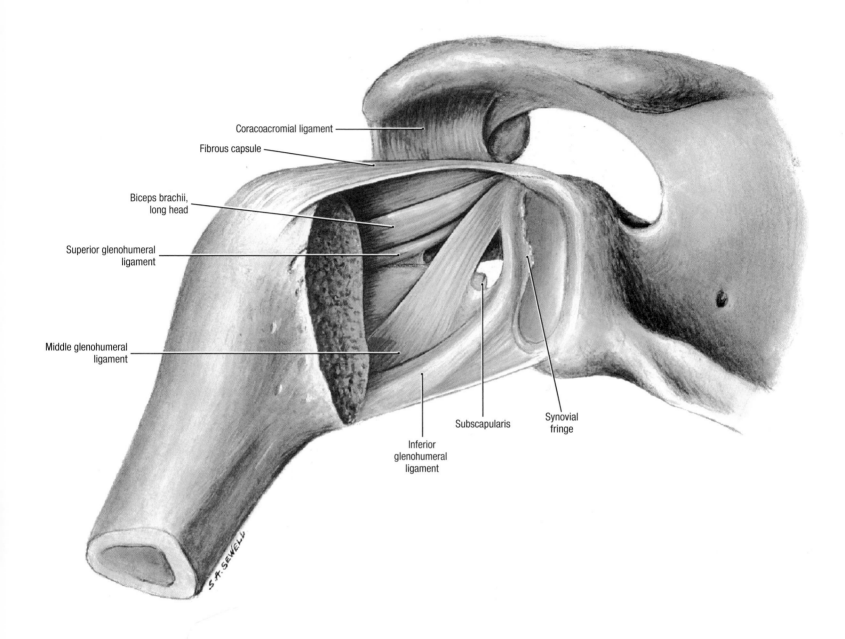

Coracoacromial ligament

Fibrous capsule

Biceps brachii, long head

Superior glenohumeral ligament

Middle glenohumeral ligament

Inferior glenohumeral ligament

Subscapularis

Synovial fringe

6.39   Interior of shoulder joint, posterior view

The joint is exposed from the posterior aspect by cutting away the posterior part of the capsule and sawing off the head of the humerus.

OBSERVE:

1. The glenohumeral ligaments are visible from within the joint, but are not easily seen from outside of the joint;
2. The glenohumeral ligaments and long tendon of the biceps brachii muscle converge on the supraglenoid tubercle;

3. The slender superior glenohumeral ligament lies parallel to the biceps tendon; the middle ligament is free medially because the subscapularis bursa communicates with the joint cavity superior and inferior to this ligament. The inferior ligament contributes largely to the anterior lip of the glenoid labrum;

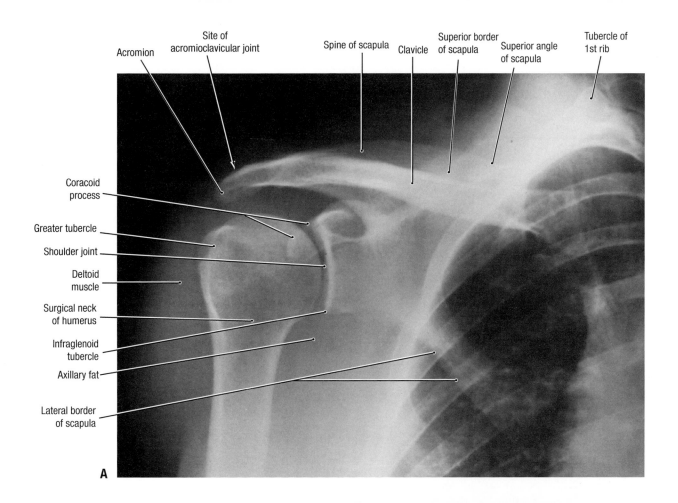

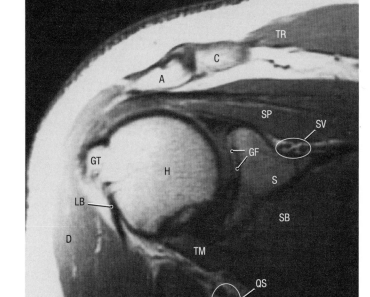

6.40   Imaging of shoulder

A. Radiograph. **B.** Coronal MRI. *A*, Acromion; *C*, Clavicle; *GT*, Greater tubercle; *H*, Head of humerus; *TR*, Trapezius, *SP*, Supraspinatus; *SV*, Suprascapular vessels and nerve; *GF*, Glenoid fossa; *S*, Scapula; *SB*, Subscapularis; *TM*, Teres minor; *LB*, Long head of biceps brachii; *D*, Deltoid; *QS*, Quadrilateral space.

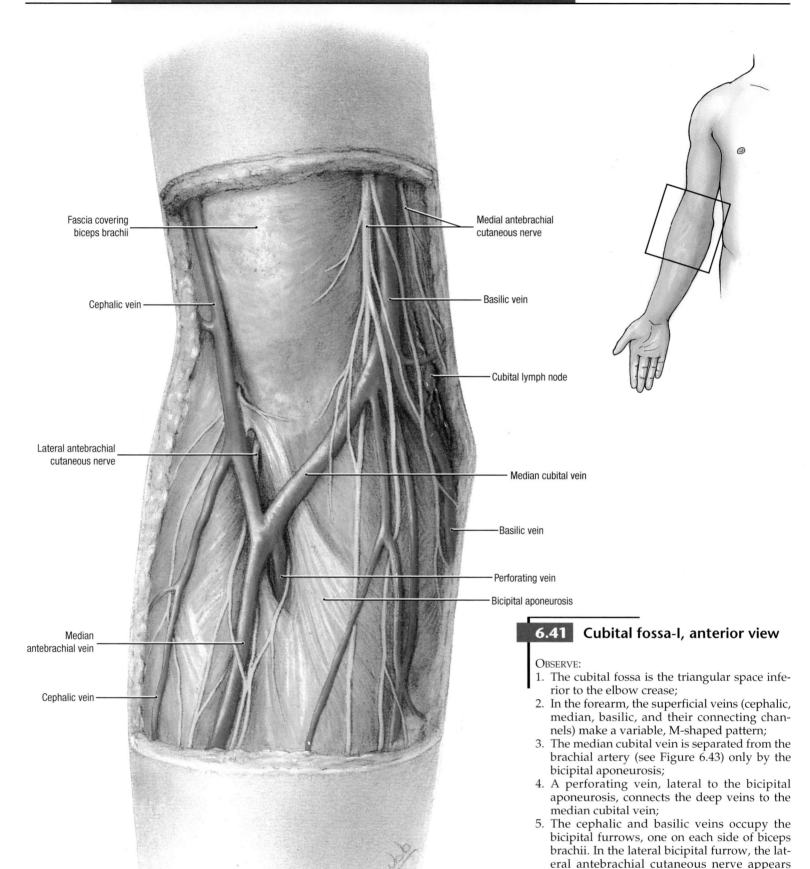

Fascia covering
biceps brachii

Medial antebrachial
cutaneous nerve

Cephalic vein

Basilic vein

Cubital lymph node

Lateral antebrachial
cutaneous nerve

Median cubital vein

Basilic vein

Perforating vein

Bicipital aponeurosis

Median
antebrachial vein

Cephalic vein

6.41   Cubital fossa-I, anterior view

OBSERVE:
1. The cubital fossa is the triangular space inferior to the elbow crease;
2. In the forearm, the superficial veins (cephalic,
   median, basilic, and their connecting channels) make a variable, M-shaped pattern;
3. The median cubital vein is separated from the
   brachial artery (see Figure 6.43) only by the
   bicipital aponeurosis;
4. A perforating vein, lateral to the bicipital
   aponeurosis, connects the deep veins to the
   median cubital vein;
5. The cephalic and basilic veins occupy the
   bicipital furrows, one on each side of biceps
   brachii. In the lateral bicipital furrow, the lateral antebrachial cutaneous nerve appears
   just superior to the elbow crease; in the medial
   bicipital furrow, the medial antebrachial cutaneous nerve becomes cutaneous at approximately the midpoint of the arm.

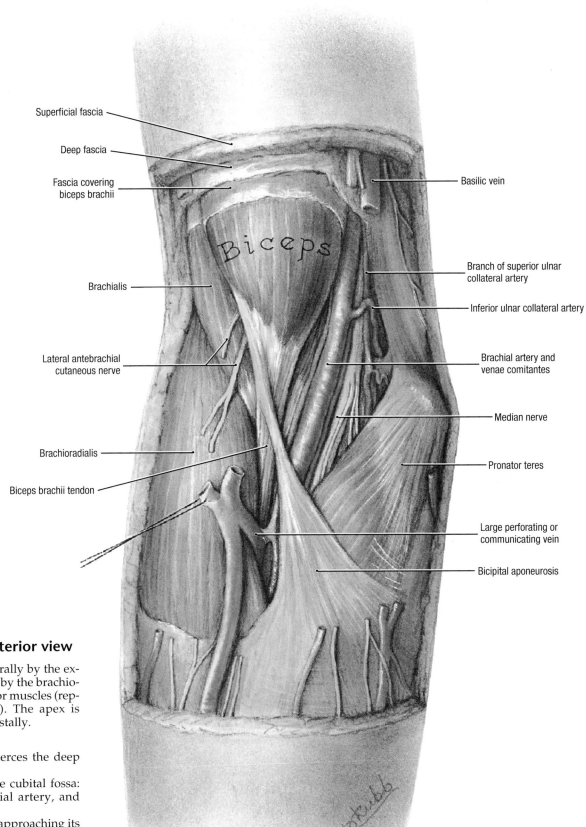

Superficial fascia

Deep fascia

Fascia covering biceps brachii

Basilic vein

Brachialis

Branch of superior ulnar collateral artery

Inferior ulnar collateral artery

Lateral antebrachial cutaneous nerve

Brachial artery and venae comitantes

Median nerve

Brachioradialis

Pronator teres

Biceps brachii tendon

Large perforating or communicating vein

Bicipital aponeurosis

6.42   Cubital fossa-II, anterior view

The cubital fossa is bounded laterally by the extensor muscles (represented here by the brachioradialis) and medially by the flexor muscles (represented by the pronator teres). The apex is where these two muscles meet distally.

OBSERVE:
1. The large perforating vein pierces the deep fascia at the apex of the fossa;
2. The three chief contents of the cubital fossa: biceps brachii tendon, brachial artery, and median nerve;
3. The biceps brachii tendon, on approaching its insertion, rotates through a right angle, and the bicipital aponeurosis springs from the tendon.

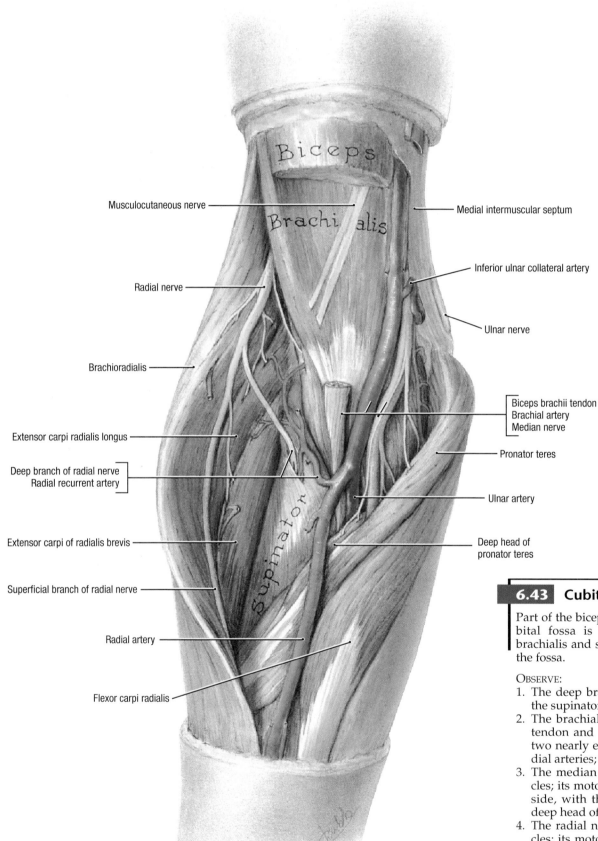

Musculocutaneous nerve

Radial nerve

Brachioradialis

Extensor carpi radialis longus

Deep branch of radial nerve
Radial recurrent artery

Extensor carpi of radialis brevis

Superficial branch of radial nerve

Radial artery

Flexor carpi radialis

Biceps

Brachialis

Supinator

Medial intermuscular septum

Inferior ulnar collateral artery

Ulnar nerve

Biceps brachii tendon
Brachial artery
Median nerve

Pronator teres

Ulnar artery

Deep head of
pronator teres

6.43 Cubital fossa-III, anterior view

Part of the biceps muscle is excised, and the cubital fossa is opened widely, exposing the
brachialis and supinator muscles in the floor of
the fossa.

OBSERVE:
1. The deep branch of the radial nerve pierces
   the supinator;
2. The brachial artery lies between the biceps
   tendon and median nerve, and divides into
   two nearly equal branches, the ulnar and radial arteries;
3. The median nerve supplies the flexor muscles; its motor branches arise from its medial
   side, with the exception of the twig to the
   deep head of pronator teres;
4. The radial nerve supplies the extensor muscles; its motor branches arise from its lateral
   side, with the exception of the twig to brachioradialis. In this specimen, the radial nerve
   has been displaced laterally, so its lateral
   branches appear to run medially.

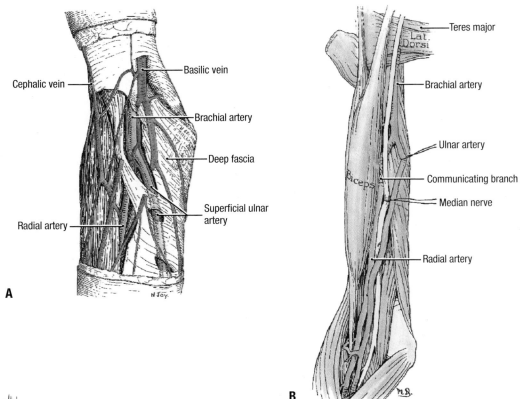

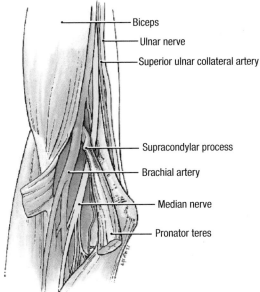

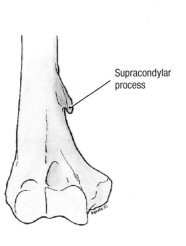

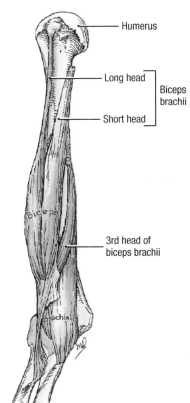

6.44　**Anomalies, anteromedial views**

A. Superficial ulnar artery. The ulnar artery may descend superficial to the flexor muscles. *This must be kept in mind when doing intravenous injections in the cubital area.* **B.** Anomalous division of brachial artery. In this case, the median nerve passes between the radial and ulnar arteries, which arise high in the arm. The musculocutaneous and median nerves commonly communicate, as shown here. **C.** Supracondylar process of humerus. A fibrous band joins this supracondylar process to the medial epicondyle; the median nerve passes through the foramen so-formed, and the brachial artery may go with it. **D.** Third head of biceps brachii. In this case, there is also attrition of the biceps tendon.

6.45 Posterior aspect of elbow-I

OBSERVE:
1. The triceps brachii is inserted into the superior surface of the olecranon and, through the deep fascia covering anconeus (tricipital aponeurosis), into the lateral border of olecranon;
2. The subcutaneous, palpable posterior surfaces of the medial epicondyle, lateral epicondyle, and olecranon;
3. The ulnar nerve, also palpable, runs subfascially posterior to the medial epicondyle; distal to this point, it disappears deep to the two heads of flexor carpi ulnaris;
4. The two heads of flexor carpi ulnaris; one arises from the common flexor tendon, and the other from the medial border of the olecranon and posterior border of the shaft of the ulna;

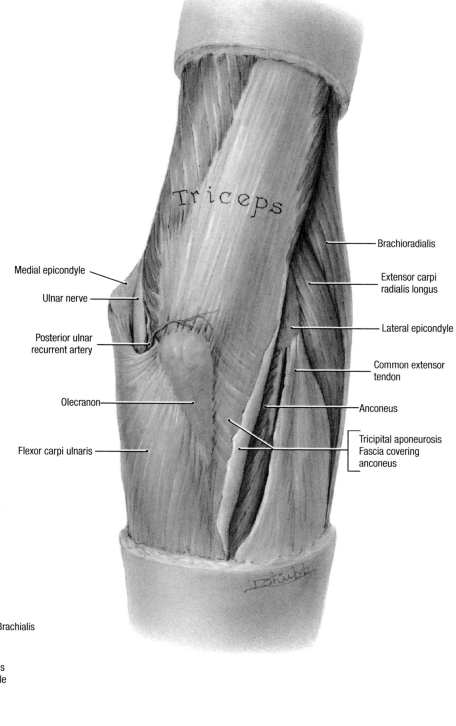

Medial epicondyle
Ulnar nerve
Posterior ulnar recurrent artery
Olecranon
Flexor carpi ulnaris

Brachioradialis
Extensor carpi radialis longus
Lateral epicondyle
Common extensor tendon
Anconeus
Tricipital aponeurosis
Fascia covering anconeus

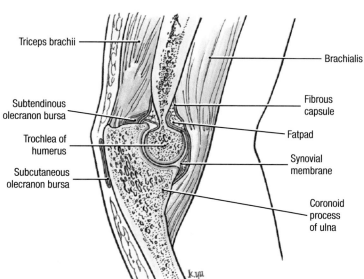

Triceps brachii
Subtendinous olecranon bursa
Trochlea of humerus
Subcutaneous olecranon bursa

Brachialis
Fibrous capsule
Fatpad
Synovial membrane
Coronoid process of ulna

6.46 Olecranon bursa, sagittal section

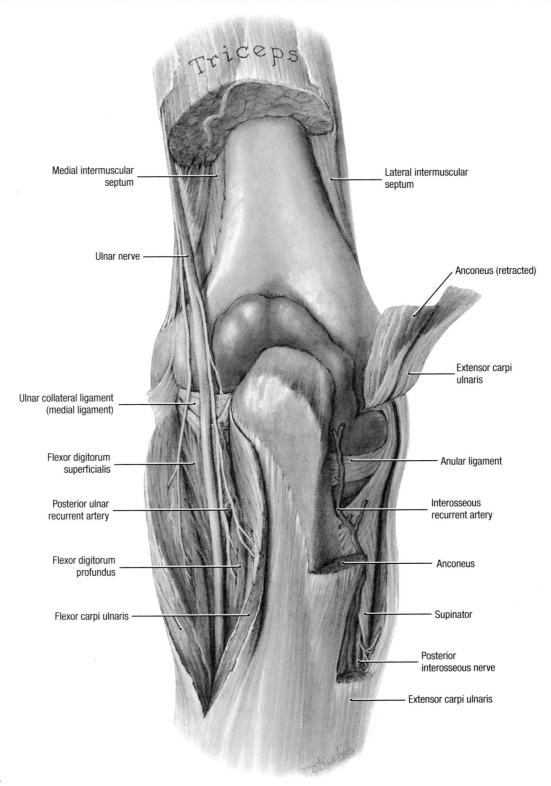

Triceps

Medial intermuscular septum

Lateral intermuscular septum

Ulnar nerve

Anconeus (retracted)

Extensor carpi ulnaris

Ulnar collateral ligament (medial ligament)

Flexor digitorum superficialis

Anular ligament

Posterior ulnar recurrent artery

Interosseous recurrent artery

Flexor digitorum profundus

Anconeus

Flexor carpi ulnaris

Supinator

Posterior interosseous nerve

Extensor carpi ulnaris

6.47   **Posterior aspect of elbow-II**

The distal portion of the triceps brachii muscle was removed.

OBSERVE:

1. The ulnar nerve descends subfascially within the posterior compartment of the arm and is applied to the triceps muscle and posterior to the medial epicondyle. It is then applied to the ulnar collateral ligament of the elbow joint and, finally, between the flexor carpi ulnaris and flexor digitorum profundus muscles;

2. The proximal branches of the ulnar nerve are distributed to the flexor carpi ulnaris muscle, half of the profundus, and the elbow joint;

3. Laterally, the synovial membrane protrudes inferior to the anular ligament; at this location, the joint is covered, with the anconeus and the common extensor tendon, including extensor carpi ulnaris;

4. The posterior interosseous nerve (continuation of the deep branch of the radial nerve) appears through the supinator inferior to the head of the radius.

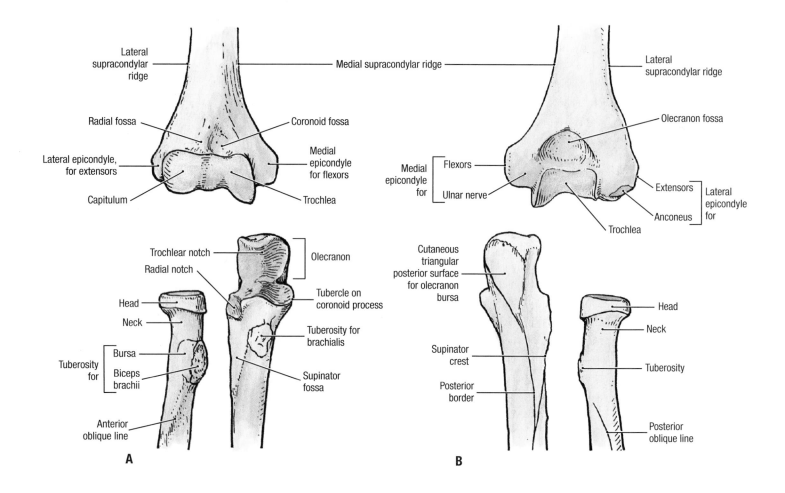

Lateral supracondylar ridge
Medial supracondylar ridge
Lateral supracondylar ridge
Radial fossa
Coronoid fossa
Olecranon fossa
Lateral epicondyle, for extensors
Medial epicondyle for flexors
Medial epicondyle for {
Flexors
Ulnar nerve
Capitulum
Trochlea
Extensors
Lateral epicondyle for
Anconeus
Trochlea

Trochlear notch
Olecranon
Radial notch
Head
Tubercle on coronoid process
Neck
Tuberosity for brachialis
Tuberosity for {
Bursa
Biceps brachii
Supinator fossa
Anterior oblique line

Cutaneous triangular posterior surface for olecranon bursa
Head
Neck
Supinator crest
Tuberosity
Posterior border
Posterior oblique line

A   **B**

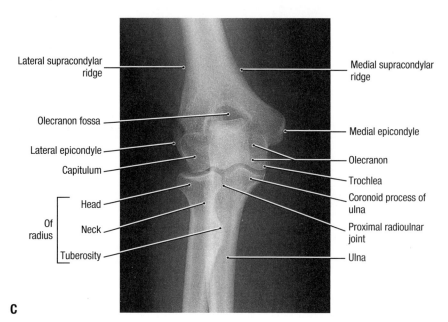

Lateral supracondylar ridge
Medial supracondylar ridge
Olecranon fossa
Medial epicondyle
Lateral epicondyle
Olecranon
Capitulum
Trochlea
Coronoid process of ulna
Head
Of radius {
Neck
Proximal radioulnar joint
Tuberosity
Ulna

C

6.48   **Bones and imaging of elbow region**

A. Anterior view. **B.** Posterior view. **C.** Radiograph of elbow joint, anteroposterior view.

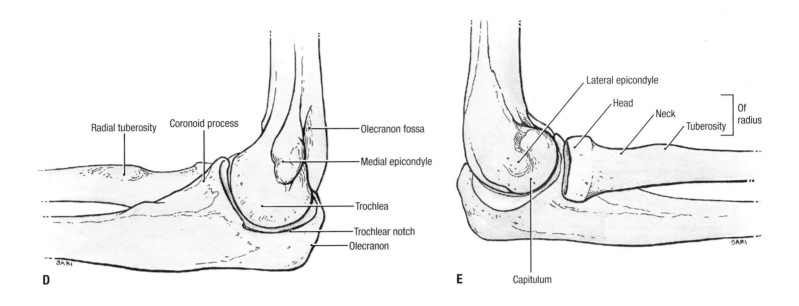

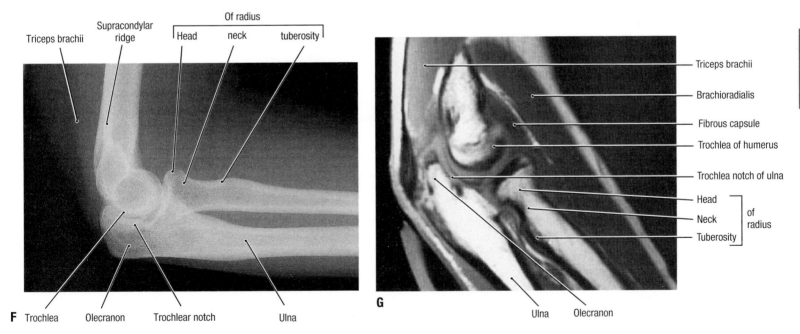

D. Medial view. **E.** Lateral view. **F.** Radiograph of elbow joint, lateral view. **G.** Sagittal MRI of elbow.

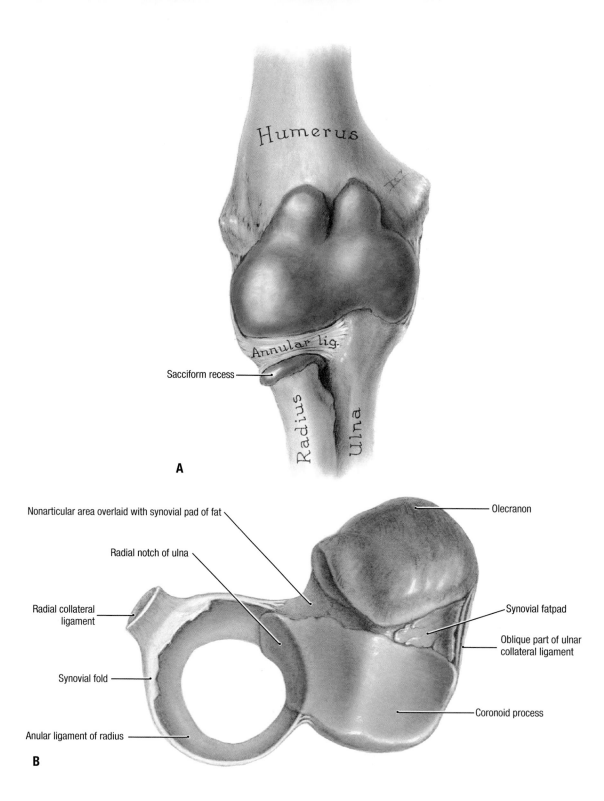

A. Articular cavity of elbow and proximal radioulnar joints, anterior view. The cavity of the elbow was injected with wax. The fibrous capsule was removed, and the synovial capsule remains. **B.** Socket for head of radius and trochlea of humerus, superior view. The anular ligament secures the head of the radius to the radial notch of the ulna,

6.49   Articular cavity of elbow

and with it forms a cup-shaped socket (i.e., wide superiorly, narrow inferiorly). The anular ligament is bound to the humerus by the radial collateral ligament of the elbow. *A common childhood injury is displacement of the head of the radius after traction on a pronated forearm. Part of the anular ligament becomes trapped between the radial head and the capitulum.*

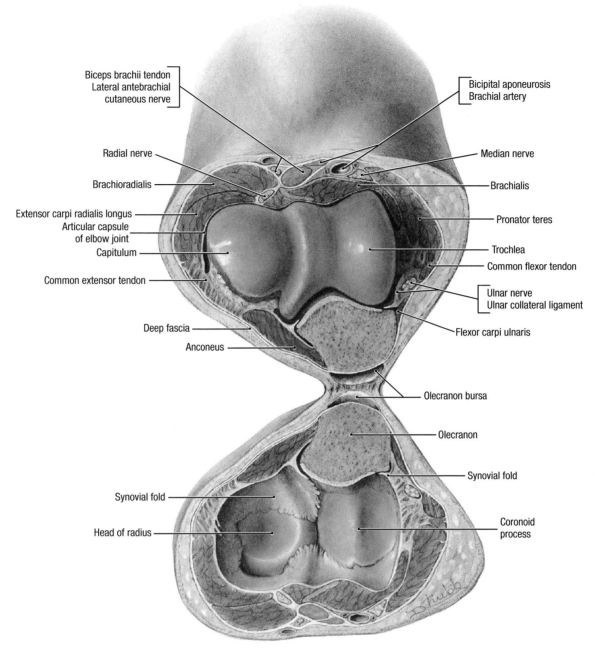

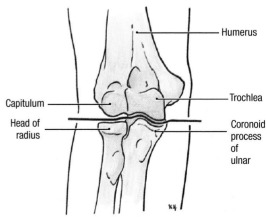

6.50 **Transverse section through elbow joint**

OBSERVE:
1. The radial nerve is in contact with the joint capsule, the ulnar nerve is in contact with the ulnar collateral ligament, and the median nerve is separated from the joint capsule by the brachialis muscle;
2. Synovial folds containing fat overlie the periphery of the head of the radius and the nonarticular indentations on the trochlear notch of the ulna;
3. The olecranon bursa lies between the olecranon process and the skin.

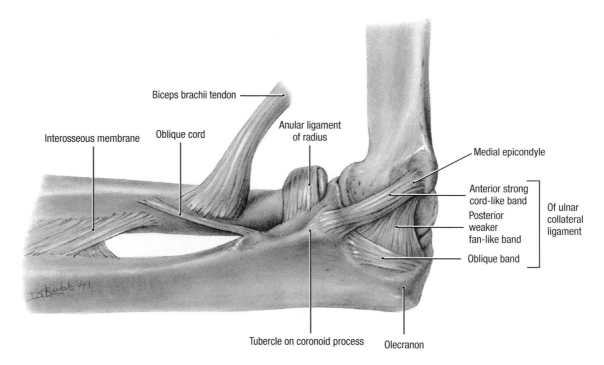

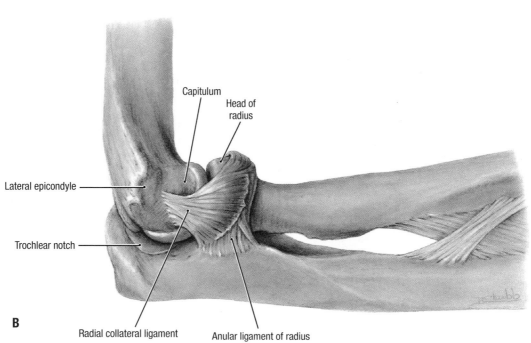

6.51   Collateral ligaments of the elbow

A. Ulnar (medial) collateral ligament, medial view. The anterior band (part) is a strong, round cord that is taut when the elbow joint is extended. The posterior band is a weak fan that is taut in flexion of the joint. The oblique fibers deepen the socket for the trochlea of the humerus. **B.** Radial (lateral) collateral ligament, lateral view. The fan-shaped lateral ligament is attached to the anular ligament of the radius, but the superficial fibers of the lateral ligament continue on to the radius.

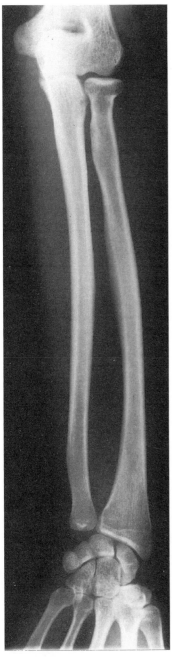

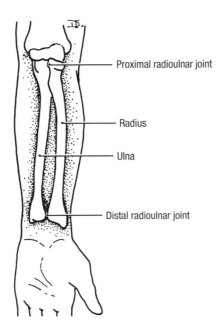

Proximal radioulnar joint

Radius

Ulna

Distal radioulnar joint

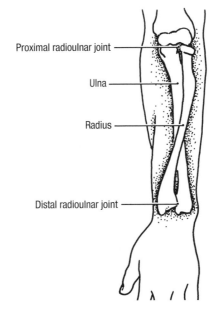

Proximal radioulnar joint

Ulna

Radius

Distal radioulnar joint

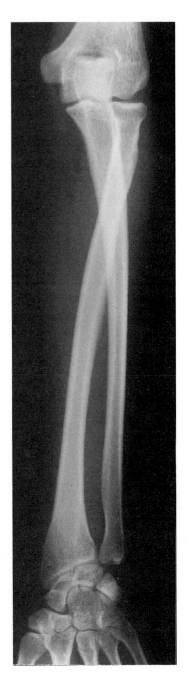

A, Supination

B, Pronation

6.52 **Radioulnar joints**

A. Anterior radiograph of forearm in supination. **B.** Anterior radiograph of forearm in pronation. Note that the radius crosses the ulna when the forearm is pronated.

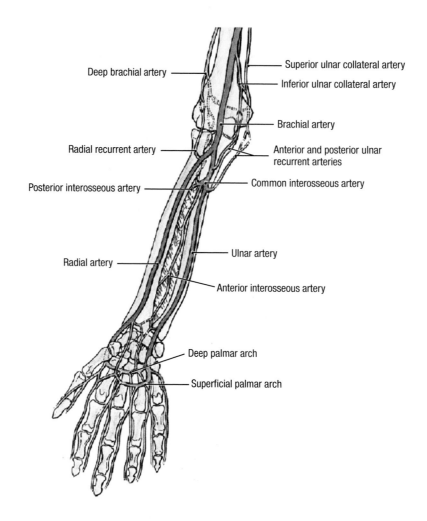

Table 6.5 Arteries of Forearm

Artery	Origin	Course
Radial	Smaller terminal division of brachial in cubital fossa	Runs inferolaterally under cover of brachioradialis and distally lies lateral to flexor carpi radialis tendon; winds around lateral aspect of radius and crosses floor of anatomical snuff box to pierce fascia; ends by forming deep palmar arch with deep branch of ulnar artery
Ulnar	Larger terminal branch of brachial in cubital fossa	Passes inferomedially and then directly inferiorly, deep to pronator teres, palmaris longus, and flexor digitorum superficialis to reach medial side of forearm; passes superficial to flexor retinaculum at wrist and gives a deep palmar branch to deep arch and continues as superficial palmar arch
Radial recurrent	Lateral side of radial, just distal to its origin	Ascends on supinator and then passes between brachioradialis and brachialis
Anterior and posterior ulnar recurrent	Ulnar, just distal to elbow joint	Anterior ulnar recurrent artery passes superiorly and posterior ulnar collateral artery passes posteriorly to anastomose with ulnar collateral and interosseous recurrent arteries
Common interosseous	Ulnar, just distal to bifurcation of brachial	After a short course, terminates by dividing into anterior and posterior interosseous arteries
Anterior and posterior interosseous	Common interosseous artery	Pass to anterior and posterior sides of interosseous membrane

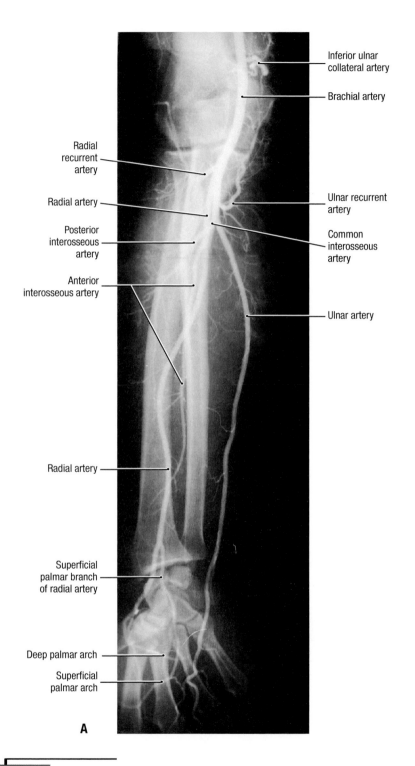

A

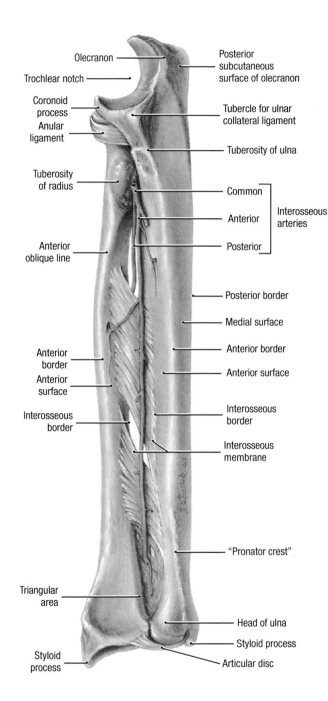

B

6.53   Arteries of the forearm

A. Brachial arteriogram, anteroposterior view. **B.** Radioulnar ligaments and interosseous arteries, anterior view. The ligament of the proximal radioulnar joint is the anular ligament, that of the distal joint is the articular disc, and that of the middle joint is the interosseous membrane. The general direction of the fibers of the membrane is such that a superior thrust to the hand is received by the radius and transmitted to the ulna. The membrane is attached to the interosseous borders of the radius and ulna, but it also spreads onto their surfaces.

6.54 Bones of forearm and hand, showing muscle attachments, anterior view

The proximal attachments of the three palmar interossei are indicated by the letter *P*; those of the four dorsal interossei are indicated by color only. Proximal attachments of the three thenar and two of the hypothenar muscles are omitted.

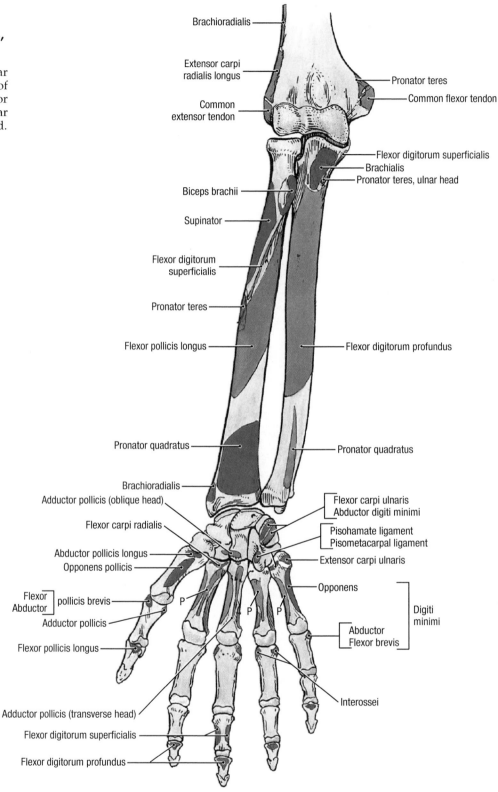

Brachioradialis

Extensor carpi radialis longus

Pronator teres

Common extensor tendon

Common flexor tendon

Flexor digitorum superficialis
Brachialis
Pronator teres, ulnar head

Biceps brachii

Supinator

Flexor digitorum superficialis

Pronator teres

Flexor pollicis longus

Flexor digitorum profundus

Pronator quadratus

Pronator quadratus

Brachioradialis
Adductor pollicis (oblique head)

Flexor carpi ulnaris
Abductor digiti minimi

Flexor carpi radialis

Pisohamate ligament
Pisometacarpal ligament

Abductor pollicis longus
Opponens pollicis

Extensor carpi ulnaris

Opponens

Flexor
Abductor } pollicis brevis

Digiti minimi

Adductor pollicis

Abductor
Flexor brevis

Flexor pollicis longus

Interossei

Adductor pollicis (transverse head)

Flexor digitorum superficialis

Flexor digitorum profundus

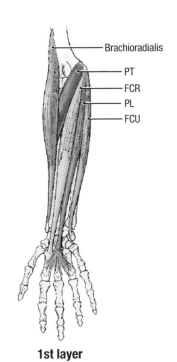
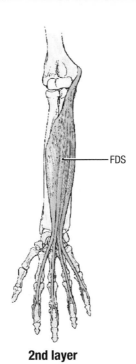
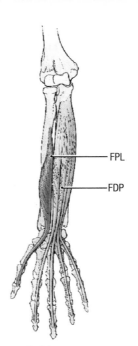
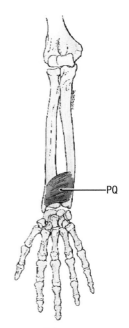

Brachioradialis
PT
FCR
PL
FCU

FDS

FPL
FDP

PQ

1st layer **2nd layer** **3rd layer** **4th layer**

Table 6.6 Muscles on the Anterior Surface of the Forearm

Muscle	Proximal Attachment	Distal Attachment	Innervation	Main Actions
Pronator teres (*PT*)	Medial epicondyle of humerus and coronoid process of ulna	Middle of lateral surface of radius	Median nerve (C6 and **C7**)	Pronates forearm and flexes it
Flexor carpi radialis (*FCR*)	Medial epicondyle of humerus	Base of second metacarpal bone		Flexes hand and abducts it
Palmaris longus (*PL*)	Medial epicondyle of humerus	Distal half of flexor retinaculum and palmar aponeurosis	Median nerve (C7 and **C8**)	Flexes hand and tightens palmar aponeurosis
Flexor carpi ulnaris (*FCU*)	*Humeral head:* medial epicondyle of humerus; *Ulnar head:* olecranon and posterior border of ulna	Pisiform bone, hook of hamate bone, and fifth metacarpal bone	Ulnar nerve (C7 and **C8**)	Flexes hand and adducts it
Flexor digitorum superficialis (*FDS*)	*Humeroulnar head:* medial epicondyle of humerus, ulnar collateral ligament, and coronoid process of ulna; *Radial head:* superior half of anterior border of radius	Bodies of middle phalanges of medial four digits	Median nerve (C7, **C8**, and T1)	Flexes middle phalanges of medial four digits; acting more strongly, it flexes proximal phalanges and hand
Flexor digitorum profundus (*FDP*)	Proximal three quarters of medial and anterior surfaces of ulna and interosseous membrane	Bases of distal phalanges of medial four digits	*Medial part:* ulnar nerve (**C8** and T1); Lateral part: medial nerve (**C8** and T1)	Flexes distal phalanges of medial four digits; assists with flexion of hand
Flexor pollicis longus (*FPL*)	Anterior surface of radius and adjacent interosseous membrane	Base of distal phalanx of thumb	Anterior interosseous nerve from median (**C8** and T1)	Pronates forearm; deep fibers bind radius and ulnar together
Pronator quadratus (*PQ*)	Distal fourth of anterior surface of ulna	Distal fourth of anterior surface of radius		Pronates forearm; deep fibers bind radius and ulna together

6.55   Superficial muscles of forearm and palmar aponeurosis, anterior view

OBSERVE:

1. At the elbow, the brachial artery lies between the biceps tendon and median nerve. It then bifurcates into the radial and ulnar arteries;
2. At the wrist, the radial artery is lateral to the flexor carpi radialis tendon, and the ulnar artery is lateral to flexor carpi ulnaris tendon;
3. In the forearm, the radial artery lies between two muscle groups or two motor territories. The muscles lateral to the artery are supplied by the radial nerve, and those medial to it by the median and ulnar nerves; thus, no motor nerve crosses the radial artery;
4. The lateral group of muscles, represented by the brachioradialis muscle, slightly overlaps the radial artery, which is otherwise superficial;
5. The four superficial muscles (pronator teres, flexor carpi radialis, palmaris longus, and flexor carpi ulnaris) radiate from the medial epicondyle;
6. The palmaris longus muscle, in this specimen, has an anomalous distal belly; this muscle usually has a small belly at the common flexor origin and a long tendon, which is continued into the palm as the palmar aponeurosis. The palmaris longus is absent in approximately 14% of limbs.

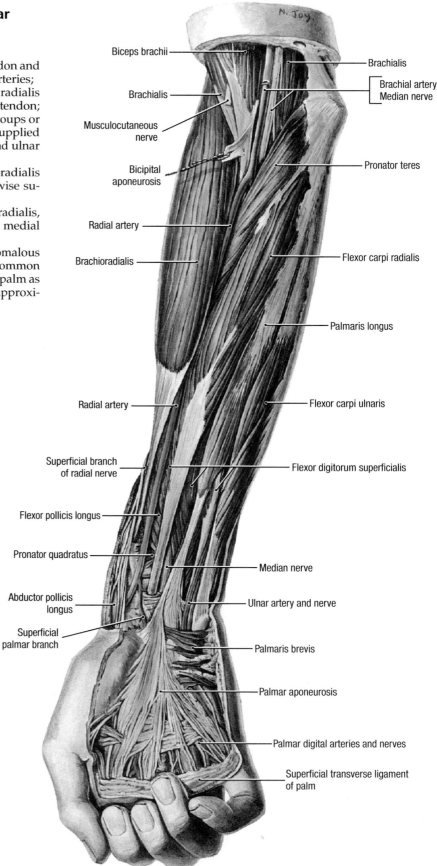

6.56 Flexor digitorum superficialis and related structures, anterior view

OBSERVE:

1. The oblique attachment of the flexor digitorum superficialis muscle;
2. The ulnar artery descends obliquely posterior to the superficialis to meet and accompany the ulnar nerve;
3. The ulnar nerve descends vertically near the medial border of superficialis; it is exposed by splitting the septum between the superficialis and flexor carpi ulnaris muscles;
4. The median nerve descends vertically posterior to superficialis, supplying the muscle as it clings to its posterior surface and appearing distally at its lateral border;
5. The tendons of the superficialis to the 3rd and 4th digits lie superficially side by side, and the tendons to the 5th and 2nd digits lie deeply;
6. The median artery in this specimen persists as an embryologic remnant.

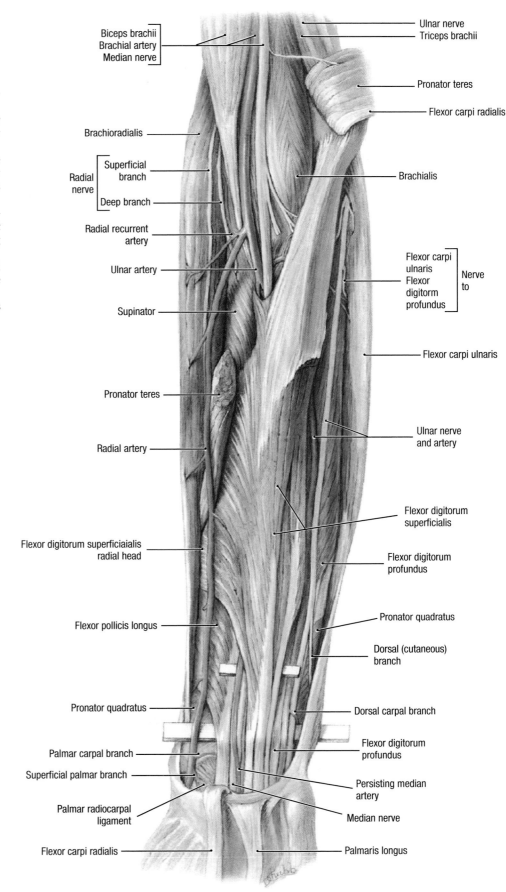

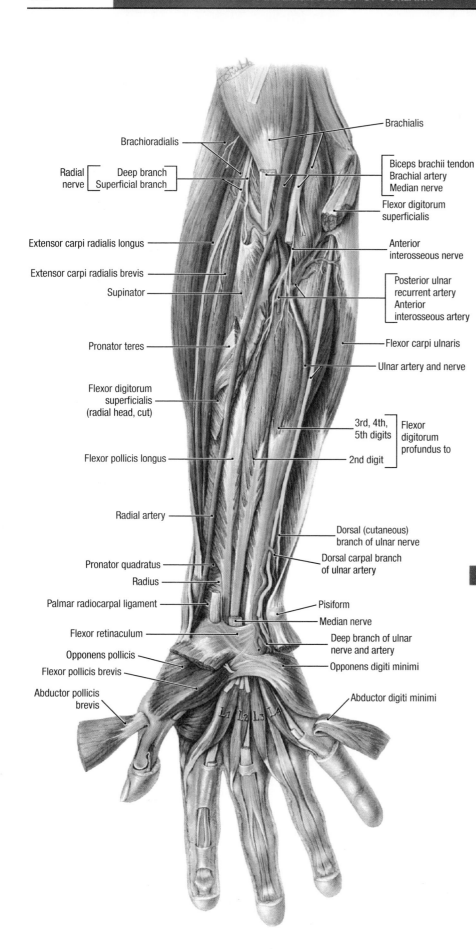

Brachialis

Brachioradialis

Radial nerve { Deep branch / Superficial branch

Biceps brachii tendon
Brachial artery
Median nerve

Flexor digitorum superficialis

Extensor carpi radialis longus

Anterior interosseous nerve

Extensor carpi radialis brevis

Supinator

Posterior ulnar recurrent artery
Anterior interosseous artery

Pronator teres

Flexor carpi ulnaris

Ulnar artery and nerve

Flexor digitorum superficialis (radial head, cut)

3rd, 4th, 5th digits } Flexor digitorum profundus to
2nd digit

Flexor pollicis longus

Radial artery

Dorsal (cutaneous) branch of ulnar nerve

Dorsal carpal branch of ulnar artery

Pronator quadratus

Radius

Pisiform

Palmar radiocarpal ligament

Median nerve

Flexor retinaculum

Deep branch of ulnar nerve and artery

Opponens pollicis

Opponens digiti minimi

Flexor pollicis brevis

Abductor pollicis brevis

Abductor digiti minimi

L1 L2 L3 L4

6.57 Deep flexors of the digits and related structures, anterior view

OBSERVE:

1. The two deep digital flexor muscles, flexor pollicis longus and flexor digitorum profundus arise from the flexor aspects of the radius, interosseous membrane, and ulna between the origin of superficialis proximally and pronator quadratus distally;
2. The median nerve crosses anterior to the ulnar artery at the elbow and posterior to the flexor retinaculum at the wrist.
3. The ulnar nerve is sheltered by the medial epicondyle at the elbow and by the pisiform bone at the wrist;
4. The ulnar nerve enters the forearm posterior to the medial epicondyle, descends on profundus, is joined by the ulnar artery, continues on profundus to the wrist, and there passes anterior to the flexor retinaculum and lateral to the pisiform as it enters the palm. At the elbow, it supplies the flexor carpi ulnaris and the medial half of the profundus muscles; superior to the wrist, it gives off its dorsal branch;
5. The recurrent, common interosseous, and dorsal carpal branches, as well as the muscular branches of the ulnar artery.
6. The four lumbricals (L1–L4) arise from the profundus tendons.

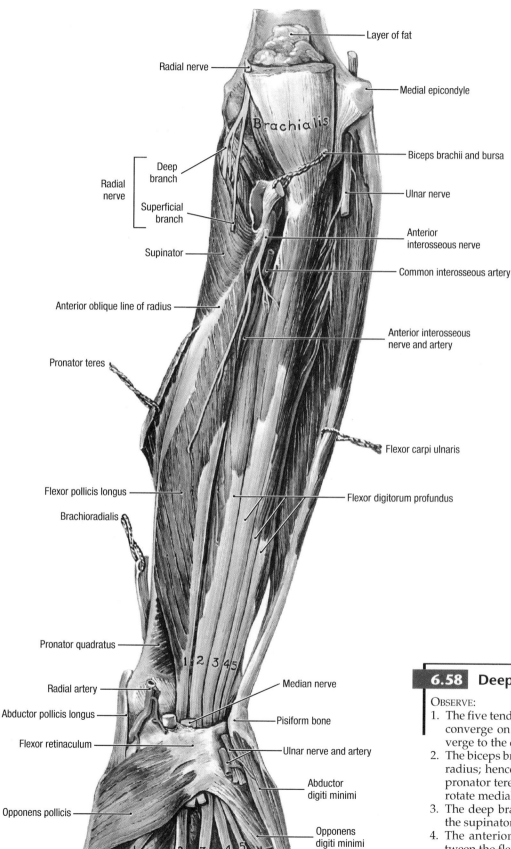

Layer of fat

Radial nerve

Medial epicondyle

Brachialis

Deep branch

Radial nerve

Superficial branch

Biceps brachii and bursa

Ulnar nerve

Anterior interosseous nerve

Supinator

Common interosseous artery

Anterior oblique line of radius

Anterior interosseous nerve and artery

Pronator teres

Flexor carpi ulnaris

Flexor pollicis longus

Flexor digitorum profundus

Brachioradialis

Pronator quadratus

Radial artery

Median nerve

Abductor pollicis longus

Pisiform bone

Flexor retinaculum

Ulnar nerve and artery

Abductor digiti minimi

Opponens pollicis

Opponens digiti minimi

6.58   Deep flexors of the digits, anterior view

OBSERVE:
1. The five tendons (*1–5*) of the deep digital flexors, side by side, converge on the carpal tunnel; having traversed it, they diverge to the distal phalanges of the digits;
2. The biceps brachii muscle attaches to the medial aspect of the radius; hence, it can rotate laterally (supinate), whereas the pronator teres muscle, by attaching to the lateral surface, can rotate medially (pronate);
3. The deep branch of the radial nerve pierces and innervates the supinator muscle;
4. The anterior interosseous nerve and artery disappear between the flexor pollicis longus and flexor digitorum profundus muscles to lie on the interosseous membrane.

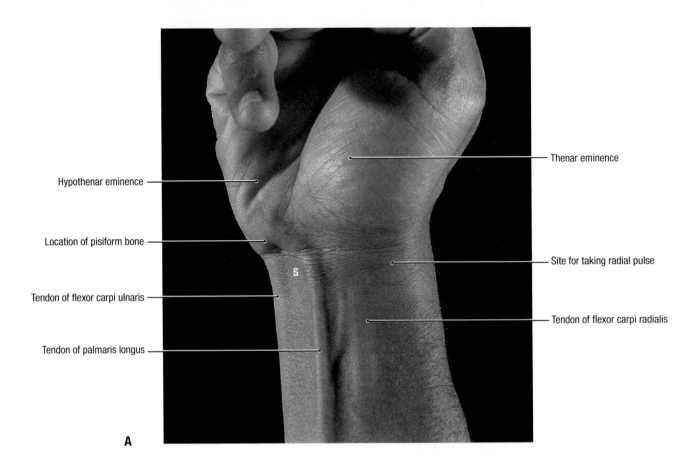

Hypothenar eminence

Location of pisiform bone

Tendon of flexor carpi ulnaris

Tendon of palmaris longus

Thenar eminence

Site for taking radial pulse

Tendon of flexor carpi radialis

A

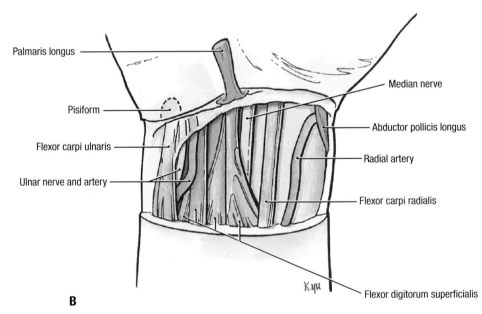

Palmaris longus

Pisiform

Flexor carpi ulnaris

Ulnar nerve and artery

Median nerve

Abductor pollicis longus

Radial artery

Flexor carpi radialis

Flexor digitorum superficialis

B

6.59   Superficial structures at the wrist, anterior views

A. Surface anatomy. (*S,* Location of tendons of flexor digitorum superficialis.) **B.** Wrist structures.

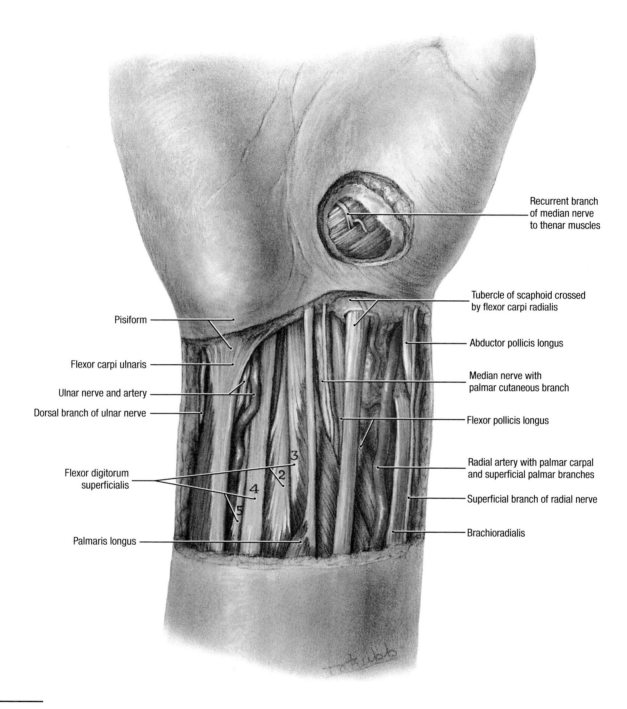

Recurrent branch
of median nerve
to thenar muscles

Tubercle of scaphoid crossed
by flexor carpi radialis

Pisiform

Abductor pollicis longus

Flexor carpi ulnaris

Median nerve with
palmar cutaneous branch

Ulnar nerve and artery

Dorsal branch of ulnar nerve

Flexor pollicis longus

Flexor digitorum
superficialis

Radial artery with palmar carpal
and superficial palmar branches

Superficial branch of radial nerve

Brachioradialis

Palmaris longus

3
2
4
5

6.60   Structures of anterior aspect of wrist

OBSERVE:

1. The distal skin incision follows the transverse skin crease at the wrist, crossing the pisiform, to which the flexor carpi ulnaris muscle is a guide, and the tubercle of the scaphoid muscle, to which the tendon of flexor carpi radialis is a guide;
2. The palmaris longus tendon bisects the crease; deep to its lateral margin is the median nerve;
3. The radial artery disappears deep to the abductor pollicis longus muscle;

4. The ulnar nerve and artery are sheltered by the flexor carpi ulnaris tendon and the expansion this gives to the flexor retinaculum;
5. The flexor digitorum superficialis tendons to the 3rd and 4th digits are somewhat anterior to those of the 2nd and 5th digits;
6. The recurrent branch of the median nerve to the thenar muscles lies within a circle whose center is 2.5 to 4 cm inferior to the tubercle of the scaphoid muscle.

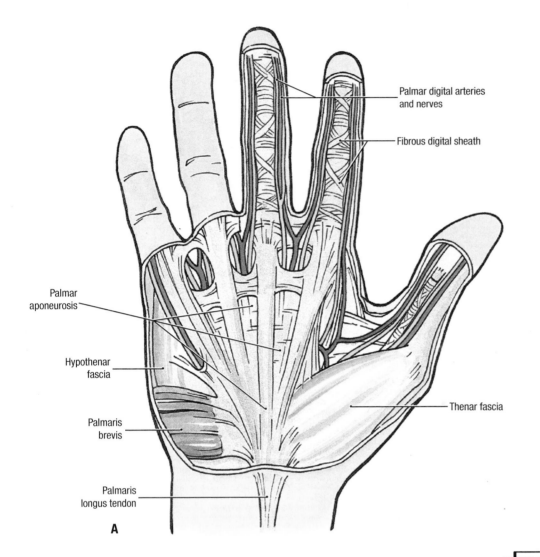

Palmar digital arteries and nerves

Fibrous digital sheath

Palmar aponeurosis

Hypothenar fascia

Palmaris brevis

Palmaris longus tendon

Thenar fascia

A

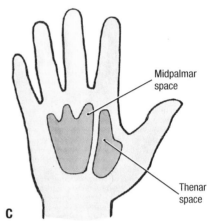

Midpalmar space

Thenar space

C

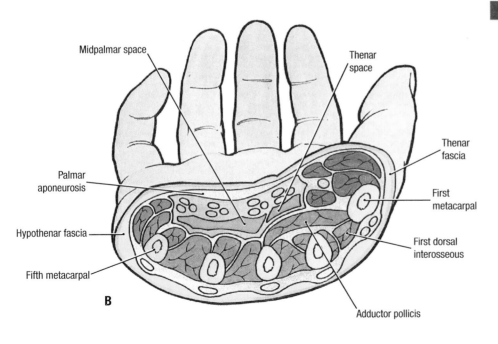

Midpalmar space

Thenar space

Thenar fascia

Palmar aponeurosis

First metacarpal

Hypothenar fascia

First dorsal interosseous

Fifth metacarpal

Adductor pollicis

B

6.61   Fascia of the palm of the hand

A. Palmar aponeurosis, anterior view. **B.** Compartments of hand, transverse section. **C.** Extent of compartments of hand, anterior view.

OBSERVE IN **A**:
1. The palmar fascia is thin over the thenar and hypothenar eminences, but thick centrally, where it forms the palmar aponeurosis, and in the digits, where it forms the fibrous digital sheaths;
2. The distal end of the palmar aponeurosis divides into four digital bands.

OBSERVE IN **B** AND **C**:
3. The three compartments of the palm: (a) thenar (blue), posterior to the thenar fascia; (b) hypothenar (green), posterior to the hypothenar fascia; and between these (c) middle (orange), posterior to the palmar aponeurosis and anterior to the fascia covering the interossei and adductor pollicis muscles, palmar ligaments, and deep transverse metacarpal ligaments;
4. The thenar and midpalmar potential spaces between the flexor tendons and fascia covering the deep palmar muscles.

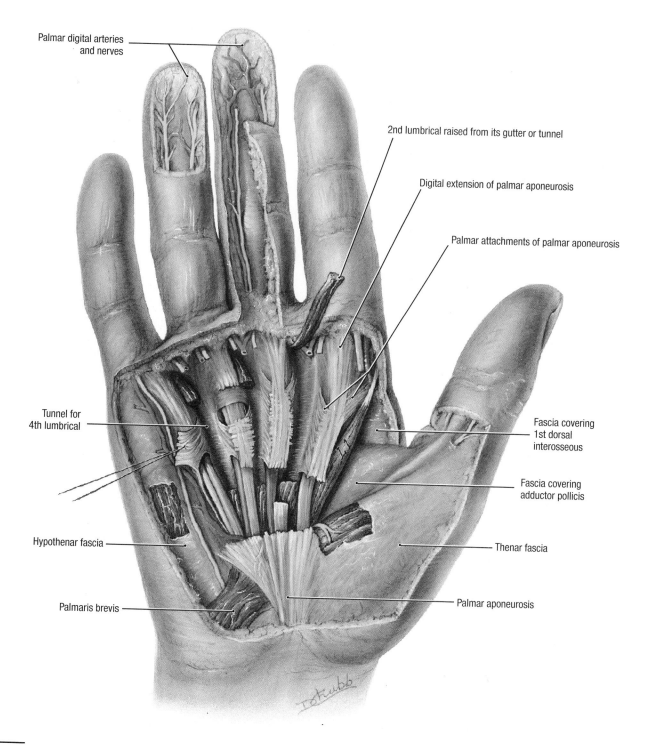

Palmar digital arteries and nerves

2nd lumbrical raised from its gutter or tunnel

Digital extension of palmar aponeurosis

Palmar attachments of palmar aponeurosis

Tunnel for 4th lumbrical

Fascia covering 1st dorsal interosseous

Fascia covering adductor pollicis

Hypothenar fascia

Thenar fascia

Palmaris brevis

Palmar aponeurosis

6.62 **Attachments of palmar aponeurosis, digital vessels, and nerves, anterior view**

OBSERVE:

1. From the palmar aponeurosis, a few longitudinal fibers enter the fingers; the other fibers, forming an extensive fibroareolar septa, pass posteriorly to the palmar ligaments (see Figure 6.69) and, more proximally, to the fascia covering the interossei. Thus, two sets of tunnels exist in the distal half of the palm: (a) tunnels for long flexor tendons, and (b) tunnels for lumbricals, digital vessels, and digital nerves;

2. The absence of fat deep to the skin creases of the fingers;

3. The plane between the fascia covering the 1st dorsal interosseous muscle and that covering the adductor pollicis muscle.

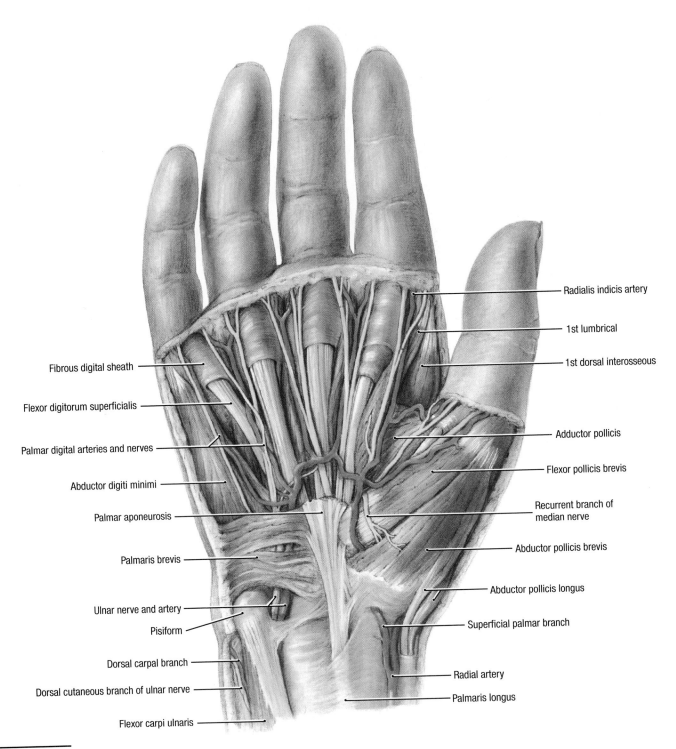

Radialis indicis artery

1st lumbrical

1st dorsal interosseous

Fibrous digital sheath

Flexor digitorum superficialis

Palmar digital arteries and nerves

Adductor pollicis

Flexor pollicis brevis

Abductor digiti minimi

Recurrent branch of
median nerve

Palmar aponeurosis

Abductor pollicis brevis

Palmaris brevis

Abductor pollicis longus

Ulnar nerve and artery

Superficial palmar branch

Pisiform

Dorsal carpal branch

Radial artery

Dorsal cutaneous branch of ulnar nerve

Palmaris longus

Flexor carpi ulnaris

6.63   Superficial dissection of palm, anterior view

The skin, superficial fascia, palmar aponeurosis, and thenar and hypothenar fasciae have been removed.

OBSERVE:

1. The superficial palmar arch is formed by the ulnar artery and completed by the superficial palmar branch of the radial artery. Only the structures removed by dissection and the palmaris brevis cover the arch; it is superficial, as are the digital vessels and nerves and the recurrent branch of the median nerve;
2. The four lumbricals lie posterior to the digital vessels and nerves;
3. The prominent pisiform shelters the ulnar nerve and artery as they pass into the palm;
4. In the digits, a digital artery and nerve lie on the medial and lateral sides of the fibrous digital sheath.

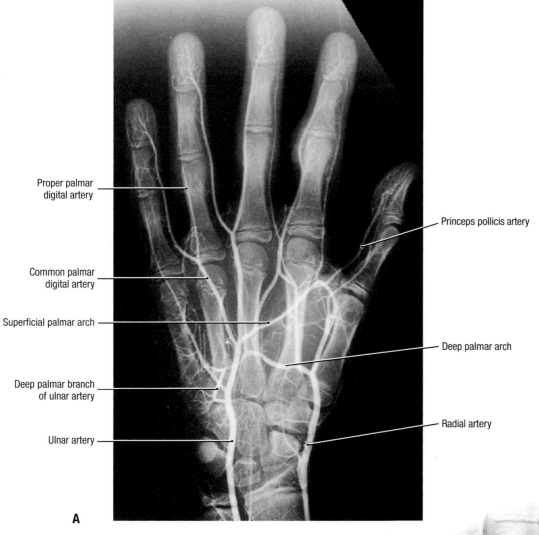

Proper palmar
digital artery

Common palmar
digital artery

Superficial palmar arch

Deep palmar branch
of ulnar artery

Ulnar artery

Princeps pollicis artery

Deep palmar arch

Radial artery

A

6.64   Arterial supply of hand

A. Arteriogram of the hand, anteroposterior view. **B.** Dissection of palmar arterial arches, anterior view. The superficial palmar arch is usually completed by the superficial palmar branch of the radial artery (see Figure 6.64), but in this specimen the dorsalis pollicis artery completes the arch. The deep palmar arch is formed by the radial artery, which enters the palmar surface of the hand and passes between the bases of the 1st and 2nd metacarpals, and between the two heads of the 1st dorsal interosseous and adductor pollicis muscles. The deep branch of the ulnar artery completes the arch.

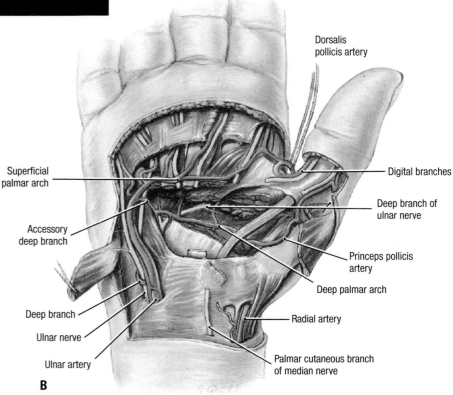

Dorsalis
pollicis artery

Superficial
palmar arch

Accessory
deep branch

Deep branch

Ulnar nerve

Ulnar artery

Digital branches

Deep branch of
ulnar nerve

Princeps pollicis
artery

Deep palmar arch

Radial artery

Palmar cutaneous branch
of median nerve

B

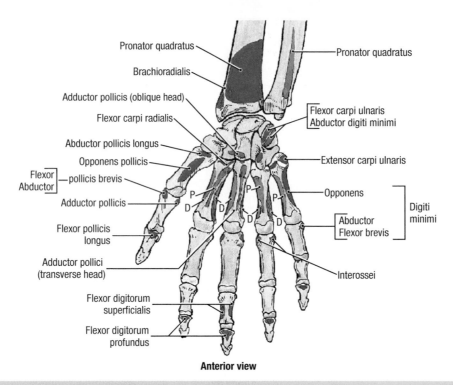

Pronator quadratus
Pronator quadratus
Brachioradialis
Adductor pollicis (oblique head)
Flexor carpi ulnaris
Abductor digiti minimi
Flexor carpi radialis
Abductor pollicis longus
Extensor carpi ulnaris
Opponens pollicis
Flexor
Abductor — pollicis brevis
Opponens
Adductor pollicis
Abductor
Flexor brevis
Digiti minimi
Flexor pollicis longus
Adductor pollici (transverse head)
Interossei
Flexor digitorum superficialis
Flexor digitorum profundus

Anterior view

Table 6.7. Muscles of Hand

Muscle	Proximal Attachment	Distal Attachment	Innervation	Main Actions
Abductor pollicis brevis	Flexor retinaculum and tubercles of scaphoid and trapezium bones	Lateral side of base of proximal phalanx of thumb	Recurrent branch of median nerve (**C8** and T1)	Abducts thumb and helps oppose it
Flexor pollicis brevis	Flexor retinaculum and tubercle of trapezium bone	Lateral side of first metacarpal bone		Flexes thumb
Opponens pollicis				Opposes thumb toward center of palm and rotates it medially
Adductor pollicis	*Oblique head:* bases of second and third metacarpals, capitate, and adjacent carpal bones; *Transverse head:* anterior surface of body of third metacarpal bone	Medial side of base of proximal phalanx of thumb	Deep branch of ulnar nerve (C8 and **T1**)	Adducts thumb toward middle digit
Abductor digiti minimi	Pisiform bone	Medial side of base of proximal phalanx of digit 5	Deep branch of ulnar nerve (C8 and T1)	Abducts digit 5
Flexor digiti minimi brevis	Hook of hamate bone and flexor retinaculum			Flexes proximal phalanx of digit 5
Opponens digiti minimi		Medial border of fifth metacarpal bone		Draws fifth metacarpal bone anteriorly and rotates it, bringing digit 5 into opposition with thumb
Lumbricals 1 and 2	Lateral two tendons of flexor digitorum profundus	Lateral sides of extensor expansions of digitis 2–5	*Lumbricals 1 and 2:* median nerve (C8 and **T1**)	Flex digits at metacarpophalangeal joints and extend interphalangeal joints
Lumbricals 3 and 4	Medial three tendons of flexor digitorum profundus		*Lumbricals 3 and 4:* deep branch of ulnar nerve (C8 and **T1**)	
Dorsal interossei 1–4	Adjacent sides of two metacarpal bones (D)	Extensor expansions and bases of proximal phalanges of digits 2–4	Deep branch of ulnar nerve (C8 and **T1**)	Adduct digits and assist lumbricals
Palmar interossei 1–3	Palmar surfaces of second, fourth, and fifth metacarpal bones (P)	Extensor expansions of digits and bases of proximal phalanges of digits 2, 4, and 5		

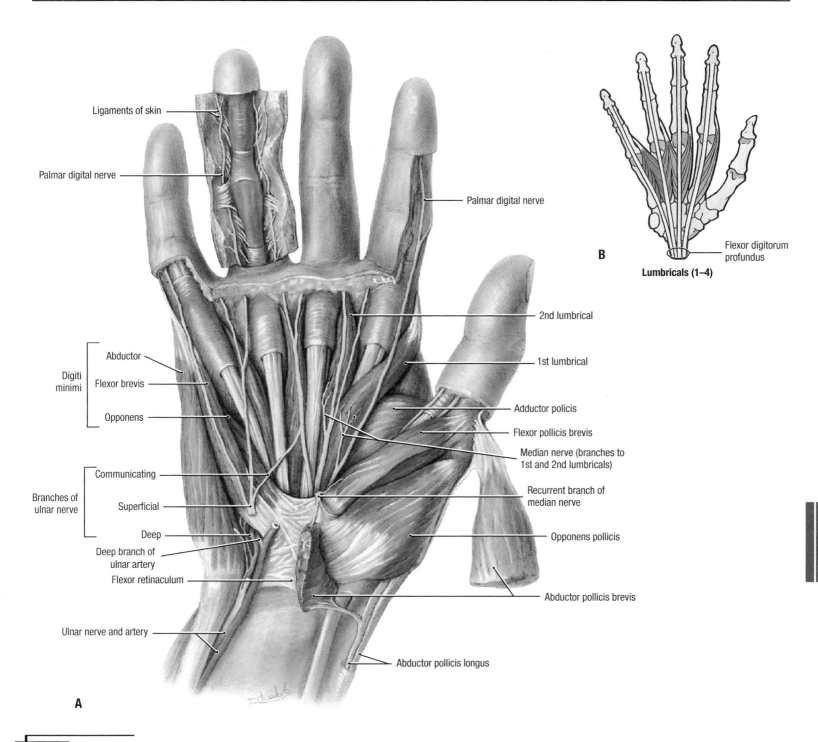

Ligaments of skin

Palmar digital nerve

Palmar digital nerve

B

Flexor digitorum profundus

Lumbricals (1–4)

2nd lumbrical

1st lumbrical

Digiti minimi
- Abductor
- Flexor brevis
- Opponens

Adductor policis

Flexor pollicis brevis

Median nerve (branches to 1st and 2nd lumbricals)

Branches of ulnar nerve
- Communicating
- Superficial
- Deep

Recurrent branch of median nerve

Deep branch of ulnar artery

Opponens pollicis

Flexor retinaculum

Abductor pollicis brevis

Ulnar nerve and artery

Abductor pollicis longus

A

6.65   **Superficial dissection of palm, ulnar and median nerves, anterior views**

A. Thenar and hypothenar eminences, lumbricals, and ulnar and median nerves. **B.** Lumbricals.

OBSERVE:

1. The three thenar (flexor pollicis brevis, abductor pollicis brevis, and opponens pollicis) and three hypothenar (flexor digiti minimi, abductor digiti minimi, and opponens digiti minimi) muscles attach to the flexor retinaculum and the four marginal carpal bones, which are united by the retinaculum;
2. The median nerve is distributed to five muscles (three thenar and two lumbrical) and provides cutaneous branches to three digits;
3. The ulnar nerve supplies all other short (intrinsic) muscles in the hand (three hypothenar, two lumbricals, interossei, and adductor pollicis) and provides cutaneous branches to the medial 1½ digits; the communicating branch joins the ulnar and median nerves;
4. The recurrent branch (motor branch) of the median nerve arises from the lateral side of the nerve at the distal border of the flexor retinaculum muscle and innervates the thenar muscles. *The recurrent branch lies superficially and can easily be severed.*
5. In B, the four lumbricals arise from the lateral sides of the profundus tendons and are inserted into the lateral sides of the dorsal expansions of the corresponding digits; the medial two lumbricals, also arise from the medial sides of adjacent profundus tendons.

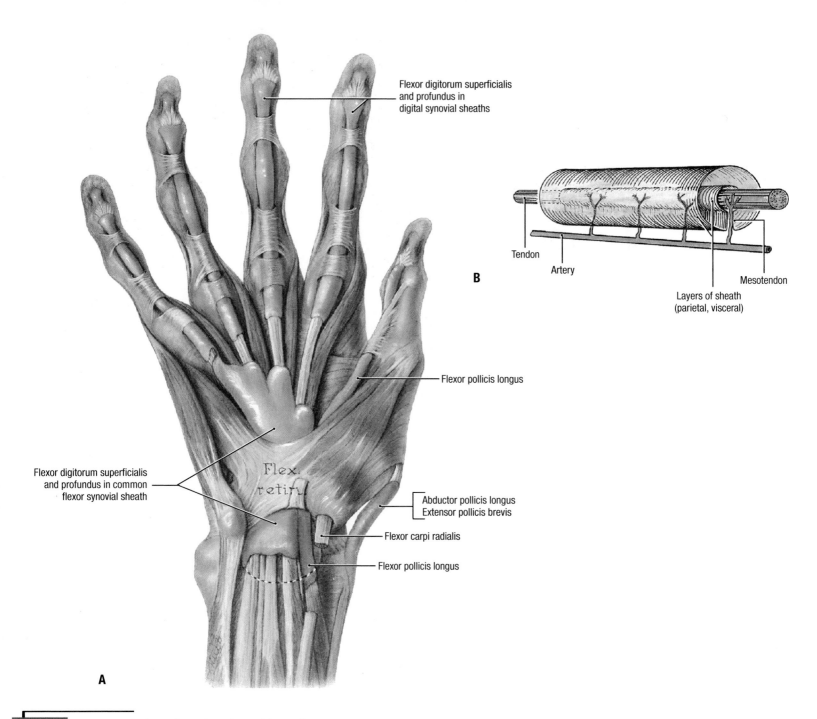

Flexor digitorum superficialis and profundus in digital synovial sheaths

B

Tendon

Artery

Mesotendon

Layers of sheath (parietal, visceral)

Flexor pollicis longus

Flexor digitorum superficialis and profundus in common flexor synovial sheath

Flex. retin.

Abductor pollicis longus
Extensor pollicis brevis

Flexor carpi radialis

Flexor pollicis longus

A

6.66   Synovial sheaths of palm of hand

A. Synovial sheaths of long flexor tendons of the digits, anterior view. **B.** Diagram of distended synovial sheath. A tendon lying within a synovial sheath has, or at one time must have had, a mesotendon conveying vessels to it. The mesotendons of the flexor pollicis longus and flexor digitorum superficialis and profundus remain as vascular folds, called vinculae. (See Fig. 6.70).

OBSERVE IN **A**:

1. There are two sets of synovial sheaths: (a) proximal or carpal, posterior to the flexor retinaculum, and (b) distal or digital, posterior to the fibrous sheaths of the digital flexors;

2. The carpal synovial sheaths, although developmentally separate, unite with one another to form a common flexor sheath, with which the carpal sheath of the thumb tendon usually communicates; this common flexor sheath extends 1 to 2.5 cm proximal to the flexor retinaculum and distally farthest on the thumb and little finger, where it is continuous with the distal sheaths;

3. Each digital sheath extends from the proximal end of the palmar ligament or plate to the base of a distal phalanx;

4. The flexor tendons glide across the prominent anterior border of the inferior articular surface of the radius; hence, the common flexor sheath extends further posteriorly (*broken line*) than anteriorly.

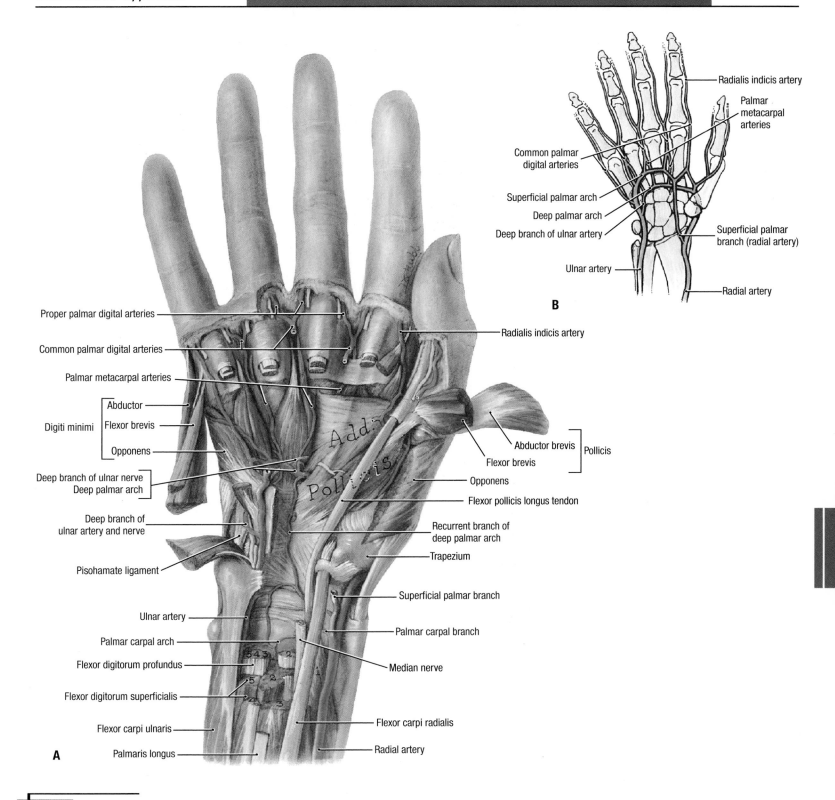

6.67 **Deep dissection of palm, anterior views.**

A. Deep palmar arch and adductor pollicis. **B.** Palmar arterial arches.

OBSERVE:
1. The flexor pollicis longus tendon makes a spiral turn around the flexor carpi radialis muscle;
2. The deep branch of the ulnar artery joins the radial artery to form the deep palmar arch;
3. The transverse and oblique heads of the adductor pollicis muscle

attach to the medial side of the proximal phalanx of the thumb. There is usually a sesamoid bone contained in the tendon of insertion. The radial artery emerges on the palmar surface of the hand between the two heads of the adductor pollicis muscle.
4. In B, the deep palmar arch lies at the level of the bases of the metacarpals; the superficial palmar arch is more distally located.

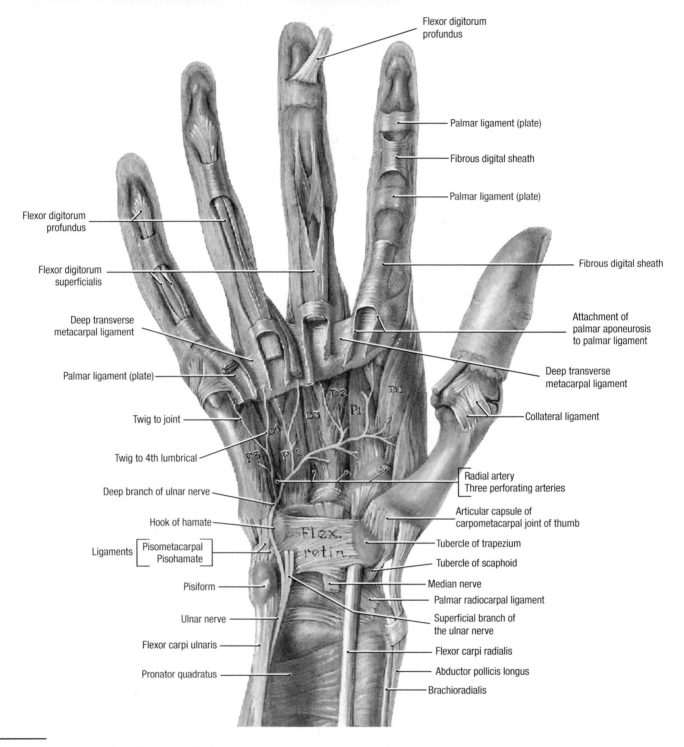

Flexor digitorum profundus

Palmar ligament (plate)

Fibrous digital sheath

Palmar ligament (plate)

Flexor digitorum profundus

Flexor digitorum superficialis

Fibrous digital sheath

Deep transverse metacarpal ligament

Attachment of palmar aponeurosis to palmar ligament

Palmar ligament (plate)

Deep transverse metacarpal ligament

Twig to joint

Collateral ligament

Twig to 4th lumbrical

Deep branch of ulnar nerve

Radial artery
Three perforating arteries

Hook of hamate

Articular capsule of carpometacarpal joint of thumb

Ligaments   Pisometacarpal
            Pisohamate

Tubercle of trapezium

Tubercle of scaphoid

Pisiform

Median nerve

Palmar radiocarpal ligament

Ulnar nerve

Superficial branch of the ulnar nerve

Flexor carpi ulnaris

Flexor carpi radialis

Pronator quadratus

Abductor pollicis longus

Brachioradialis

6.68   Deep dissection of palm and digits with ulnar nerve, anterior view

OBSERVE:
1. The ulnar nerve lies anterior, and the median nerve lies posterior to the flexor retinaculum;
2. The flexor carpi radialis muscle descends vertically anterior to the tubercle of the scaphoid to the 2nd metacarpal;
3. The flexor carpi ulnaris muscle continues beyond the pisiform as the pisohamate and the pisometacarpal ligament;
4. Four dorsal (D1-4) and three palmar interossei (P1-3) muscles;
5. The ulnar nerve crosses the hook of the hamate to be distributed by

its deep branch to the three hypothenar muscles, all seven interossei, medial two lumbricals, adductor pollicis, the superficial branch supplies the palmaris brevis muscle and sensation to the medial 1½ digits;
6. The deep transverse metacarpal ligaments unite the palmar ligaments; the lumbricals pass anterior to the deep transverse metacarpal ligament, and the interossei pass posterior to the ligament.

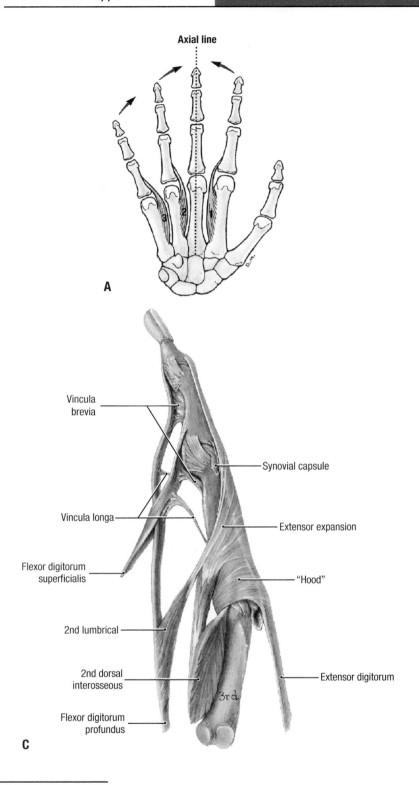

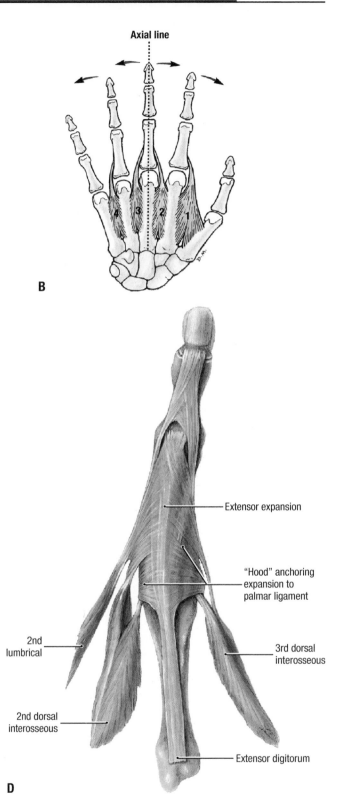

6.69 Interossei

A. Palmar interossei, anterior view. **B.** Dorsal interossei, anterior view. **C.** Extensor expansion of the 3rd (middle) digit, lateral view. **D.** Extensor expansion of 3rd digit, dorsal view.

OBSERVE:

1. Three unipennate palmar and four bipennate dorsal interosseous muscles; the palmar interossei adduct the fingers, and the dorsal interossei abduct the fingers in relation to the axial line, an imaginary line drawn through the long axis of the 3rd digit (A and B);

2. The palmar and dorsal interossei pass posterior to the deep transverse metacarpal ligament and insert into the base of the proximal phalanx and extensor expansion (C and D); the part of the muscle attaching to the base of the proximal phalanx functions in abduction and adduction of the fingers, and the part attaching to the extensor expansion functions in flexion of the metacarpophalangeal joints and extension of the interphalangeal joints.

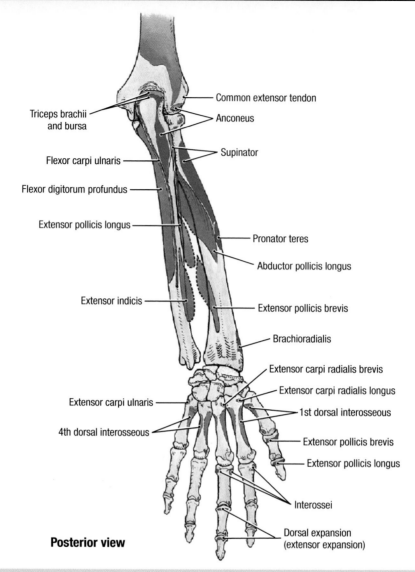

Common extensor tendon
Triceps brachii and bursa
Anconeus
Supinator
Flexor carpi ulnaris
Flexor digitorum profundus
Extensor pollicis longus
Pronator teres
Abductor pollicis longus
Extensor indicis
Extensor pollicis brevis
Brachioradialis
Extensor carpi radialis brevis
Extensor carpi radialis longus
Extensor carpi ulnaris
1st dorsal interosseous
4th dorsal interosseous
Extensor pollicis brevis
Extensor pollicis longus
Interossei
Dorsal expansion (extensor expansion)

Posterior view

Table 6.8. Muscles on the Posterior Surface of the Forearm

Muscle	Proximal Attachment	Distal Attachment	Innervation	Main Actions
Brachioradialis	Proximal two thirds of lateral supracondylar ridge of humerus	Lateral surface of distal end of radius	Radial nerve (C5, **C6**, and C7)	Flexes forearm
Extensor carpi radialis longus	Lateral supracondylar ridge of humerus	Base of second metacarpal bone	Radial nerve (C6 and C7)	Extend and abduct hand at wrist joint
Extensor carpi radialis brevis	Lateral epicondyle of humerus	Base of third metacarpal bone	Deep branch of radial nerve (**C7** and C8)	
Extensor digitorum	Lateral epicondyle of humerus	Extensor expansions of medial four digits		Extends medial four digits at metacarpo-phalangeal joints; extends hand at wrist joint
Extensor digiti minimi	Lateral epicondyle of humerus	Extensor expansion of fifth digit	Posterior interosseous nerve (C7 and C8), a branch of the radial nerve	Extends fifth digit at metacarpophalangeal and interphalangeal joints
Extensor carpi ulnaris	Lateral epicondyle of humerus and posterior border of ulna	Base of fifth metacarpal bone		Extends and adducts hand at wrist joint

Continued

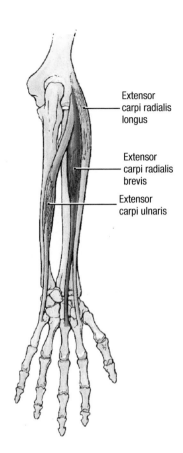

Extensor carpi radialis longus

Extensor carpi radialis brevis

Extensor carpi ulnaris

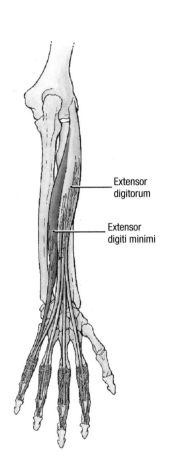

Extensor digitorum

Extensor digiti minimi

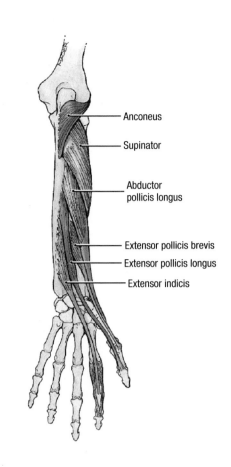

Anconeus

Supinator

Abductor pollicis longus

Extensor pollicis brevis

Extensor pollicis longus

Extensor indicis

Table 6.8. *(Continued)*

Muscle	Proximal Attachment	Distal Attachment	Innervation	Main Actions
Anconeus	Lateral epicondyle humerus	Lateral surface of olecranon and superior part of posterior surface of ulna	Radial nerve (C7, C8, and T1)	Assists triceps in extending elbow joint; stabilizes elbow joint; abducts ulna during pronation
Supinator	Lateral epicondyle of humerus, radial collateral and anular ligaments, supinator fossa, and crest of ulna	Lateral, posterior, and anterior surfaces of proximal third of radius	Deep branch of radial nerve (C5 and **C6**)	Supinates forearm, i.e., rotates radius to turn palm anteriorly
Abductor pollicis longus	Posterior surfaces of ulna, radius, and interosseous membrane	Base of first metacarpal bone		Abducts thumb and extends it at carpometacarpal joint
Extensor pollicis brevis	Posterior surface of radius and interosseous membrane	Base of first metacarpal bone	Posterior interosseous nerve (C7 and **C8**)	Extends proximal phalanx of thumb at carpometacarpal joint
Extensor pollicis longus	Posterior surface of middle third of ulna and interosseous membrane	Base of distal phalanx of thumb		Extends distal phalanx of thumb at metacarpophalangeal and interphalangeal joints
Extensor indicis	Posterior surface of ulna and interosseous membrane	Extensor expansion of second digit		Extends second digit and helps to extend hand

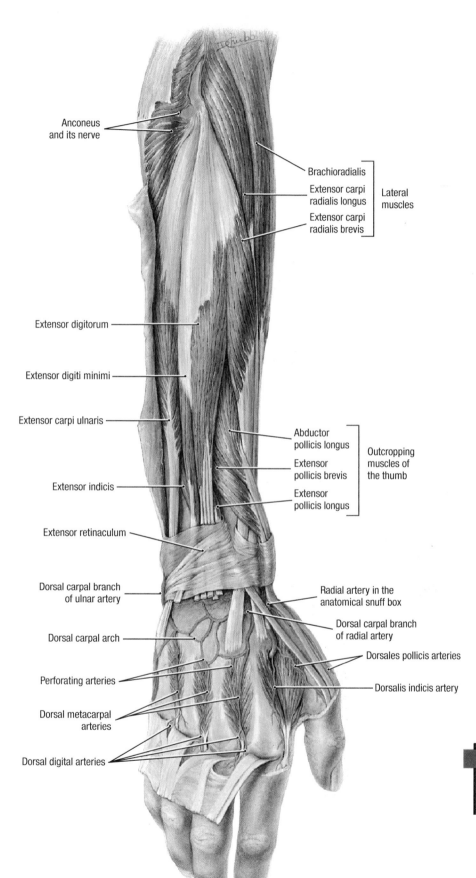

Anconeus
and its nerve

Brachioradialis

Extensor carpi
radialis longus

Extensor carpi
radialis brevis

} Lateral
muscles

Extensor digitorum

Extensor digiti minimi

Extensor carpi ulnaris

Abductor
pollicis longus

Extensor
pollicis brevis

Extensor
pollicis longus

} Outcropping
muscles of
the thumb

Extensor indicis

Extensor retinaculum

Dorsal carpal branch
of ulnar artery

Radial artery in the
anatomical snuff box

Dorsal carpal branch
of radial artery

Dorsal carpal arch

Dorsales pollicis arteries

Perforating arteries

Dorsalis indicis artery

Dorsal metacarpal
arteries

Dorsal digital arteries

6.70   Muscles of extensor region of
forearm, posterior view

OBSERVE:
1. The digital extensors have been reflected without dis-
turbing the arteries because they lie on the skeletal
plane;
2. No muscle is attached to the posterior surface of a
carpal bone;
3. The radial artery disappears between the two heads of
the 1st dorsal interosseous muscle.

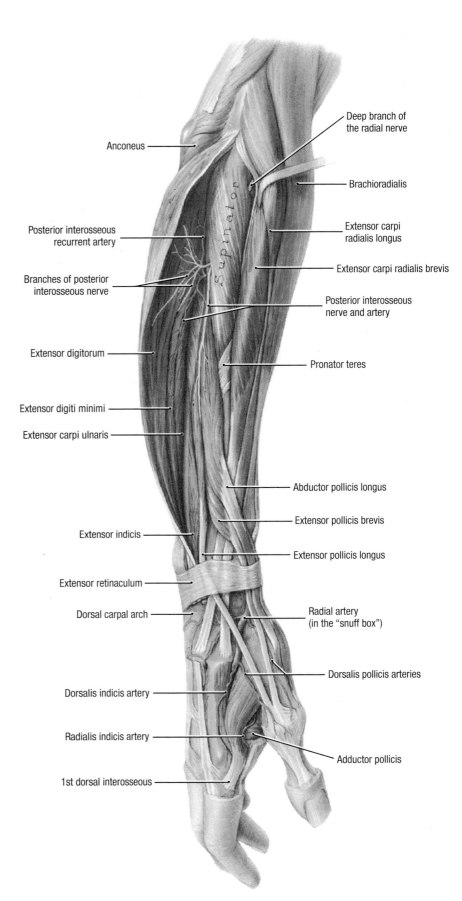

Anconeus

Deep branch of the radial nerve

Brachioradialis

Posterior interosseous recurrent artery

Extensor carpi radialis longus

Branches of posterior interosseous nerve

Extensor carpi radialis brevis

Posterior interosseous nerve and artery

Extensor digitorum

Pronator teres

Extensor digiti minimi

Extensor carpi ulnaris

Abductor pollicis longus

Extensor pollicis brevis

Extensor indicis

Extensor pollicis longus

Extensor retinaculum

Dorsal carpal arch

Radial artery (in the "snuff box")

Dorsalis pollicis arteries

Dorsalis indicis artery

Radialis indicis artery

Adductor pollicis

1st dorsal interosseous

6.71 Deep structures on extensor aspect of forearm, posterolateral view

OBSERVE:
1. Three "outcropping" muscles of the thumb (abductor pollicis longus, extensor pollicis brevis, and extensor pollicis longus) emerge between the extensor carpi radialis brevis and extensor digitorum;
2. The furrow from which the thumb muscles emerge has been opened proximally to the lateral epicondyle, exposing the supinator;
3. The laterally retracted brachioradialis and extensor carpi radialis longus and brevis are innervated by the deep branch of the radial nerve; the other extensor muscles are supplied by the posterior interosseous nerve, which is a continuation of the deep branch of the radial nerve after it pierces supinator and emerges inferior to the head of the radius;
4. The tendons of the three outcropping muscles of the thumb pass to the bases of the three long bones of the thumb: the metacarpal, proximal phalanx, and distal phalanx.

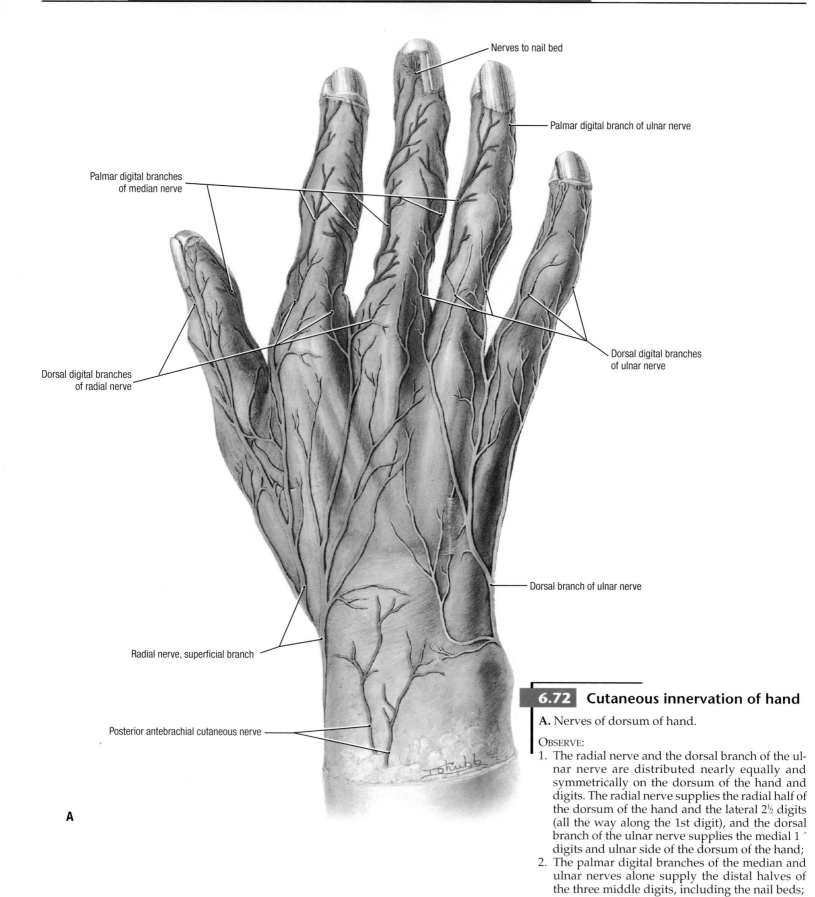

Nerves to nail bed

Palmar digital branch of ulnar nerve

Palmar digital branches
of median nerve

Dorsal digital branches
of ulnar nerve

Dorsal digital branches
of radial nerve

Dorsal branch of ulnar nerve

Radial nerve, superficial branch

Posterior antebrachial cutaneous nerve

A

6.72   Cutaneous innervation of hand

A. Nerves of dorsum of hand.

OBSERVE:
1. The radial nerve and the dorsal branch of the ulnar nerve are distributed nearly equally and symmetrically on the dorsum of the hand and digits. The radial nerve supplies the radial half of the dorsum of the hand and the lateral 2½ digits (all the way along the 1st digit), and the dorsal branch of the ulnar nerve supplies the medial 1 ´ digits and ulnar side of the dorsum of the hand;
2. The palmar digital branches of the median and ulnar nerves alone supply the distal halves of the three middle digits, including the nail beds;
3. Communications between adjacent nerves are numerous.

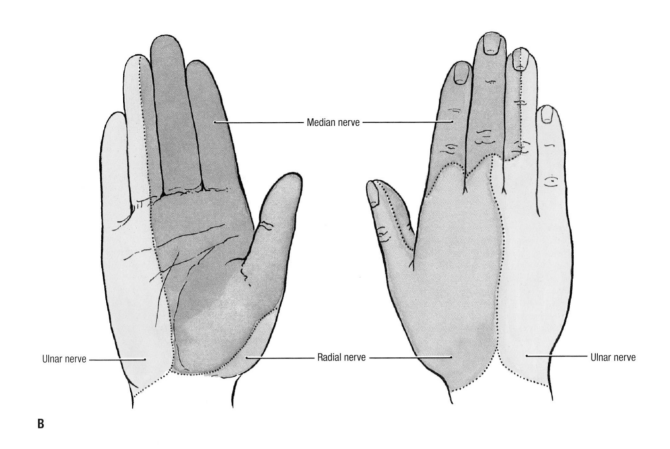

B

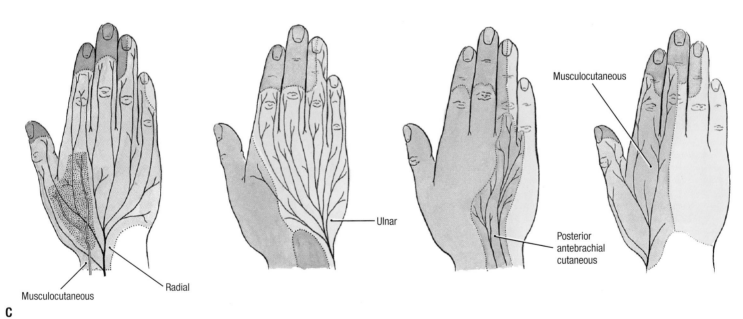

C

B. Distribution of cutaneous nerves to palm and dorsum of hand (left, palmar view; right, dorsal view). **C.** Variations in pattern of cutaneous nerves in dorsum of hand.

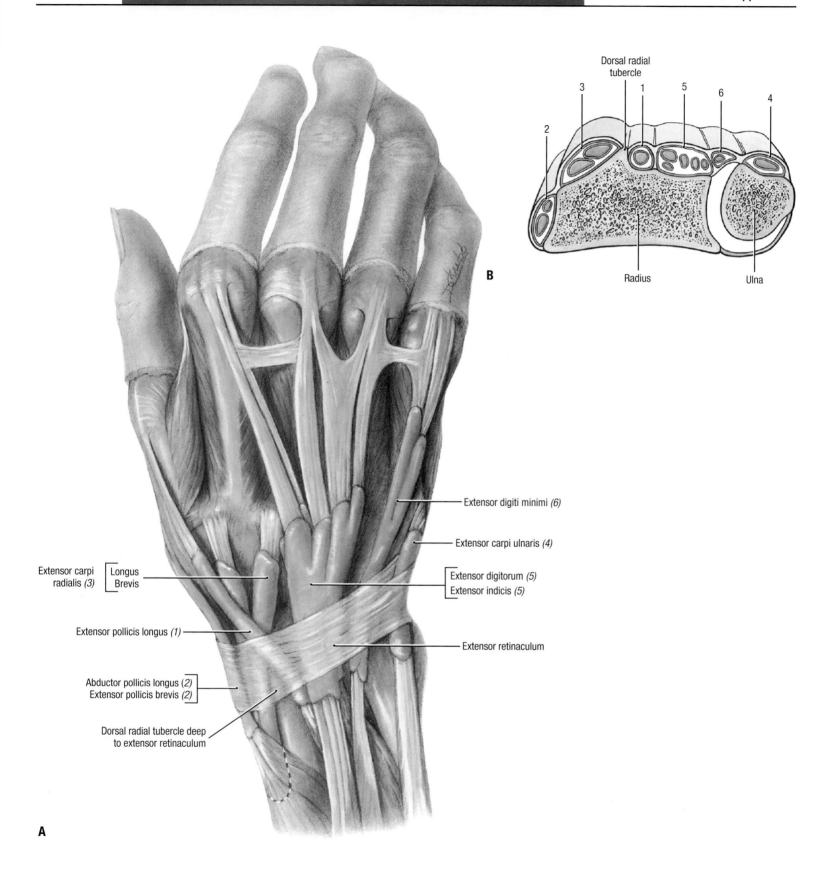

Dorsal radial tubercle

Radius

Ulna

B

Extensor digiti minimi *(6)*

Extensor carpi ulnaris *(4)*

Extensor carpi radialis *(3)*   Longus / Brevis

Extensor digitorum *(5)*
Extensor indicis *(5)*

Extensor pollicis longus *(1)*

Extensor retinaculum

Abductor pollicis longus *(2)*
Extensor pollicis brevis *(2)*

Dorsal radial tubercle deep to extensor retinaculum

A

6.73 Synovial sheaths on dorsum of wrist

A. Synovial sheaths. **B.** Transverse section (numbers refer to structures labeled in **A**).

OBSERVE:

1. Six sheaths occupy the six osseofibrous tunnels deep to the extensor retinaculum. They contain nine tendons: tendons for the thumb in sheaths 1 and 2; tendons for the extensors of the wrist in sheaths 3 and 4; and tendons for the extensors of the wrist and fingers in sheaths 5 and 6;
2. The band of thickened deep fascia and the extensor retinaculum;
3. The tendon of the extensor pollicis longus hooks around the dorsal radial tubercle to pass obliquely across the tendons of the extensor carpi radialis longus and brevis muscles to the thumb.

6.74 Branches of radial artery on dorsum of hand

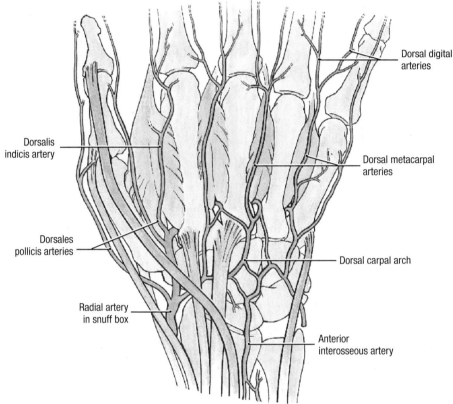

Dorsal digital arteries

Dorsalis indicis artery

Dorsal metacarpal arteries

Dorsales pollicis arteries

Dorsal carpal arch

Radial artery in snuff box

Anterior interosseous artery

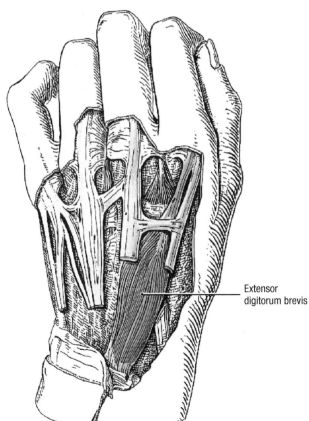

Extensor digitorum brevis

6.75 Extensor digitorum brevis muscle of hand, dorsal view

This muscle is found occasionally on the dorsum of the hand, usually as a single bundle.

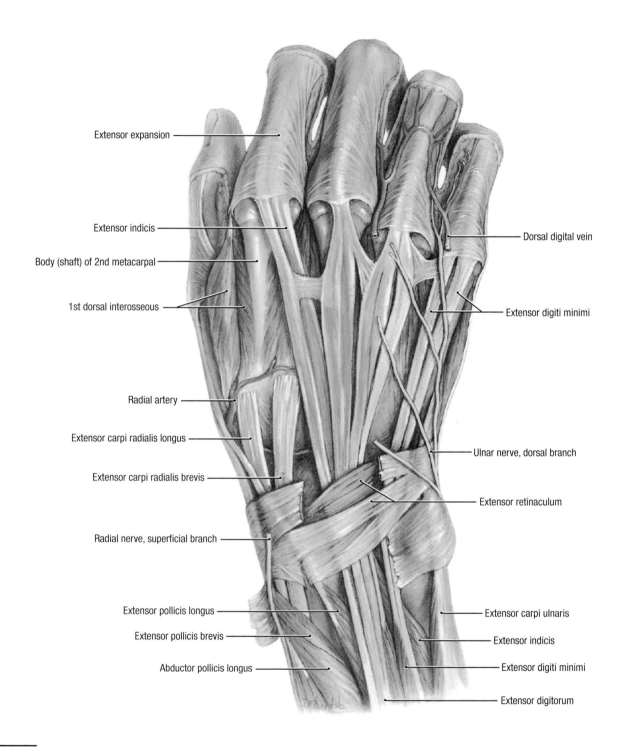

Extensor expansion

Extensor indicis

Body (shaft) of 2nd metacarpal

1st dorsal interosseous

Radial artery

Extensor carpi radialis longus

Extensor carpi radialis brevis

Radial nerve, superficial branch

Extensor pollicis longus

Extensor pollicis brevis

Abductor pollicis longus

Dorsal digital vein

Extensor digiti minimi

Ulnar nerve, dorsal branch

Extensor retinaculum

Extensor carpi ulnaris

Extensor indicis

Extensor digiti minimi

Extensor digitorum

6.76   Tendons on dorsum of hand and extensor retinaculum, dorsal view

OBSERVE:
1. The location of the tendons of the extensor carpi radialis longus and brevis, extensor digitorum, extensor digiti minimi, and extensor carpi ulnaris muscles on the dorsum of the wrist and hand;
2. The deep fascia, here thickened and called the extensor retinaculum, stretches obliquely from one ridge on the radius to another;

medially, it passes distal to the ulna to attach to the pisiform and triquetrum bones, as depicted in Figure 6.81B;
3. Proximal to the knuckles, bands connect the tendons of the digital extensors and thereby restrict the independent action of the fingers;
4. The body (shaft) of the 2nd metacarpal is not covered with an extensor tendon.

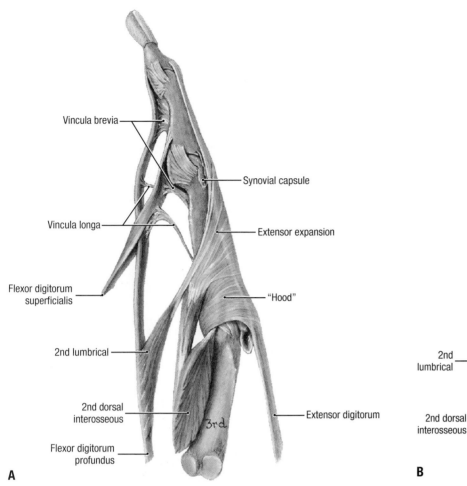

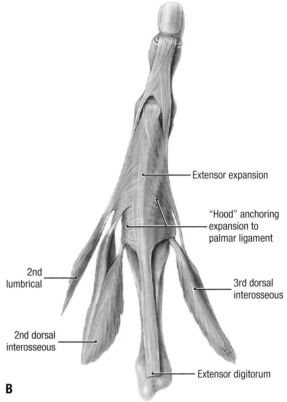

A

B

6.77   Extensor (dorsal) expansion of 3rd digit

A. Lateral view. **B.** Dorsal view.

OBSERVE:

1. The interossei are partly inserted into the bases of the proximal phalanges and partly into the extensor expansion;
2. The 2nd lumbrical inserts into the radial side of the expansion;

3. The hood covering the head of the metacarpal is attached to the palmar ligament; preventing "bowstringing" of the extensor tendon and expansion;
4. The expansion extends to the bases of the middle and distal phalanges.

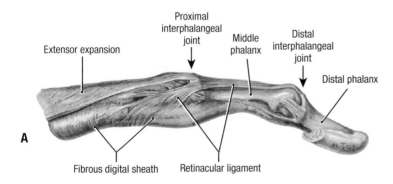

A

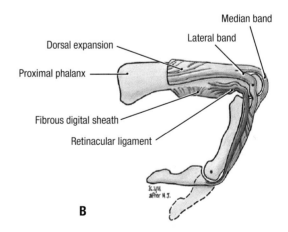

B

6.78   Retinacular ligament, lateral views

A. Extended digit. **B.** Flexed digit.

OBSERVE:

1. The retinacular ligament is a delicate, fibrous band that runs from the proximal phalanx and fibrous digital sheath obliquely across

the middle phalanx and two interphalangeal joints to join the dorsal expansion, and so to the distal phalanx;
2. On flexion of the distal interphalangeal joint, the retinacular ligament becomes taut and pulls the proximal joint into flexion;
3. On extension of the proximal joint, the distal joint is pulled by the retinacular ligament into nearly complete extension.

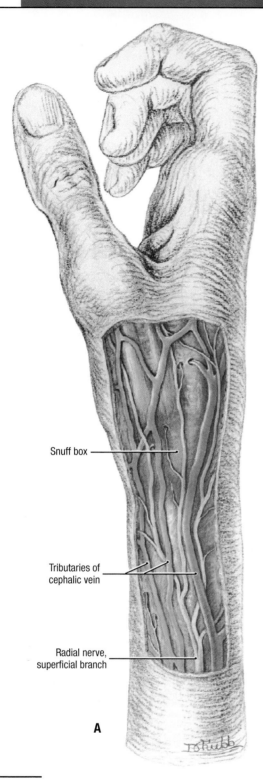

Snuff box

Tributaries of
cephalic vein

Radial nerve,
superficial branch

A

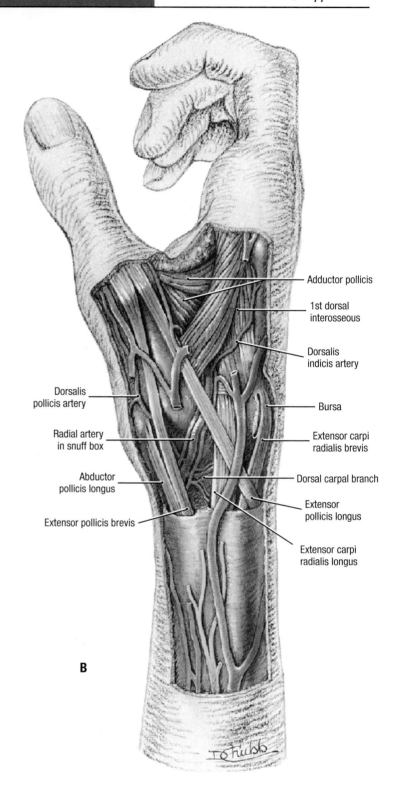

Adductor pollicis

1st dorsal
interosseous

Dorsalis
indicis artery

Dorsalis
pollicis artery

Bursa

Radial artery
in snuff box

Extensor carpi
radialis brevis

Abductor
pollicis longus

Dorsal carpal branch

Extensor
pollicis longus

Extensor pollicis brevis

Extensor carpi
radialis longus

B

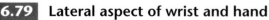

6.79   Lateral aspect of wrist and hand

A. Anatomical snuff box-I. **B.** Anatomical snuff box-II.

OBSERVE IN **A**:
1. The depression at the base of the thumb, the "anatomical snuff box," retains its name from an archaic habit;
2. Superficial veins, including the cephalic vein and/or its tributaries, and cutaneous nerves crossing the snuff box;
3. Perforating veins and articular nerves pierce the deep fascia.

OBSERVE IN **B**:
1. Three long tendons of the thumb form the boundaries of the snuff box;
2. The radial artery and its venae comitantes cross the floor of the snuff box and disappear between the two heads of the 1st dorsal interosseous;
3. The adductor pollicis and 1st dorsal interosseous, proximal to the web between the pollex and index digits, are supplied by the ulnar nerve.

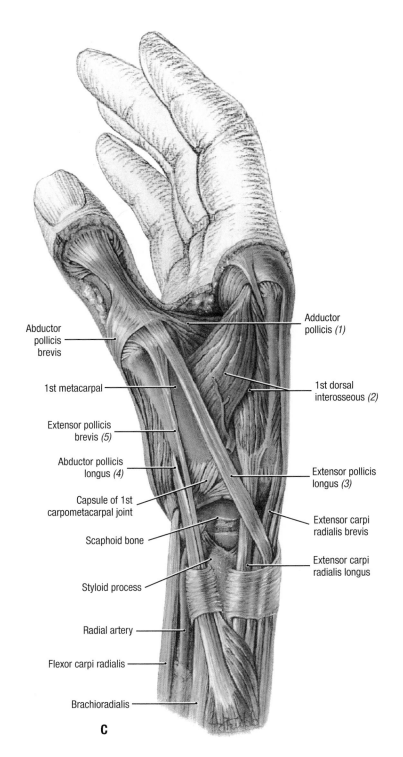

Abductor pollicis brevis

1st metacarpal

Extensor pollicis brevis (5)

Abductor pollicis longus (4)

Capsule of 1st carpometacarpal joint

Scaphoid bone

Styloid process

Radial artery

Flexor carpi radialis

Brachioradialis

Adductor pollicis (1)

1st dorsal interosseous (2)

Extensor pollicis longus (3)

Extensor carpi radialis brevis

Extensor carpi radialis longus

C

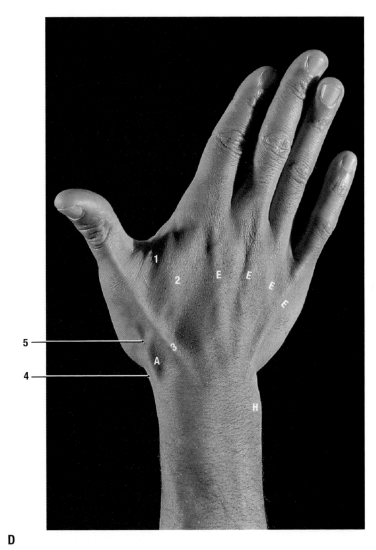

D

C. Anatomical snuff box-III. **D.** Surface anatomy of wrist and hand. *H,* Head of ulna; *E,* Tendons of extensor digitorum longus; *A,* Anatomical snuff box. (Numbers refer to structures labeled in **C**.)

OBSERVE IN **C**:

1. The scaphoid bone, the wrist joint proximal to the scaphoid, and the midcarpal distal to it;
2. The capsule of the 1st carpometacarpal joint;
3. The abductor pollicis brevis and adductor pollicis muscles are partly inserted into the dorsal (extensor) expansion.

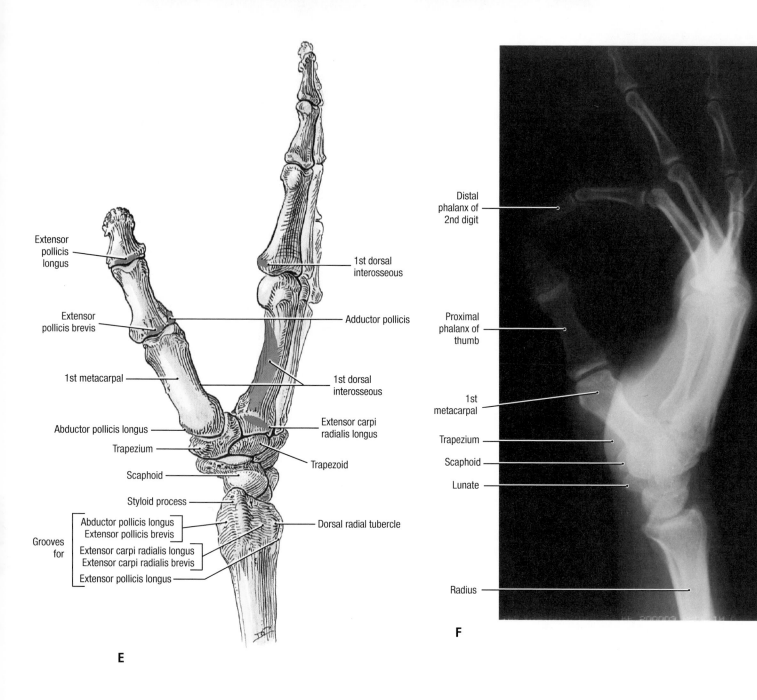

Extensor
pollicis
longus

Extensor
pollicis brevis

1st metacarpal

Abductor pollicis longus

Trapezium

Scaphoid

Styloid process

Grooves
for

> Abductor pollicis longus
> Extensor pollicis brevis

> Extensor carpi radialis longus
> Extensor carpi radialis brevis

> Extensor pollicis longus

1st dorsal
interosseous

Adductor pollicis

1st dorsal
interosseous

Extensor carpi
radialis longus

Trapezoid

Dorsal radial tubercle

E

Distal
phalanx of
2nd digit

Proximal
phalanx of
thumb

1st
metacarpal

Trapezium

Scaphoid

Lunate

Radius

F

E. Bony hand showing muscle attachments. **F.** Radiograph, lateral view.

OBSERVE IN **E**:
1. The attachments of muscles to bone (red and dark blue);
2. Articular surfaces (pale blue);

3. The anatomical snuff box is limited proximally by the styloid process of the radius and distally by the base of the 1st metacarpal;
4. The two lateral marginal bones of the carpus (scaphoid and trapezium) form the floor of the snuff box.

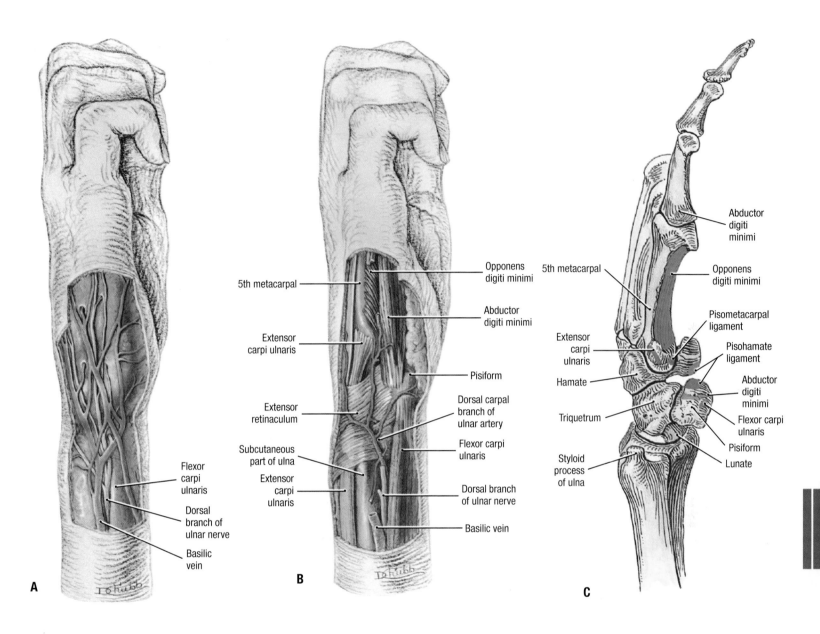

A. Superficial dissection. B. Deep dissection. C. Bony hand showing muscle attachments.

6.80 Medial aspect of wrist and hand

OBSERVE IN A:
1. The superficial veins and their perforating branches;
2. The dorsal branch of the ulnar nerve, a cutaneous nerve, appears from deep to the flexor carpi ulnaris.

OBSERVE IN B:
1. A vertical incision is made along the medial subcutaneous surface of the ulna and along the medial border of the hand; it passes between two motor territories (flexor carpi ulnaris, abductor digiti minimi, and opponens digiti minimi, supplied by the ulnar nerve; and extensor carpi ulnaris by the posterior interosseous nerve);
2. Superficial veins, nerves, and arteries are divided, but no motor nerves are touched.

OBSERVE IN C:
1. The attachments of muscles to bone;
2. The extensor carpi ulnaris is inserted directly into the base of the 5th metacarpal;
3. The flexor carpi ulnaris is inserted indirectly through the pisiform bone and pisometacarpal ligament to the base of the 5th metacarpal.

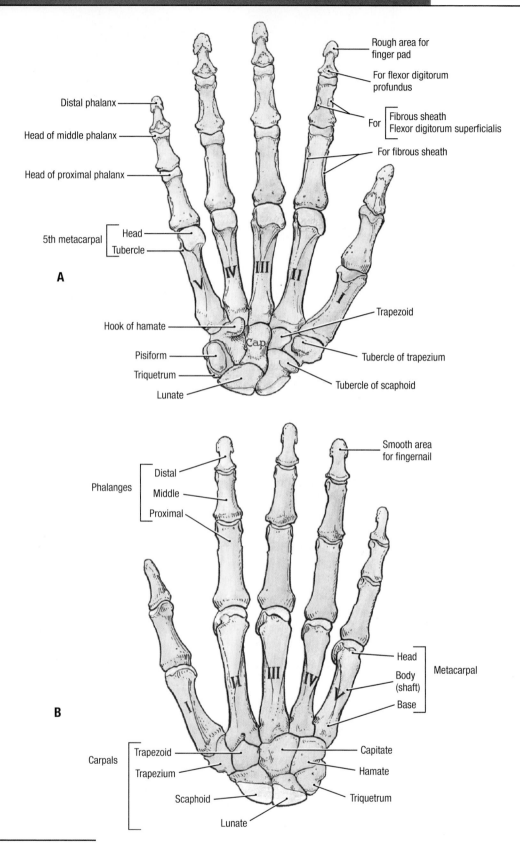

Rough area for
finger pad

For flexor digitorum
profundus

For [Fibrous sheath
Flexor digitorum superficialis

For fibrous sheath

Distal phalanx

Head of middle phalanx

Head of proximal phalanx

5th metacarpal [Head
Tubercle

A

V IV III II I

Hook of hamate

Cap

Trapezoid

Pisiform

Triquetrum

Lunate

Tubercle of trapezium

Tubercle of scaphoid

Smooth area
for fingernail

Phalanges [Distal
Middle
Proximal

B

I II III IV V

Head
Body
(shaft)   Metacarpal
Base

Carpals

Trapezoid
Trapezium

Scaphoid

Lunate

Capitate

Hamate

Triquetrum

6.81   **Bones of hand**

A. Palmar view. **B.** Dorsal view
The eight carpal bones form two rows: in the distal row, the hamate, capitate, trapezoid, and trapezium; the trapezium forming a saddle-shaped joint with the 1st metacarpal; in the proximal row, the scaphoid, lunate, and pisiform; the pisiform superimposed on the triquetrum.

6.82 Imaging of bones of wrist and hand

A. Radiograph, anteroposterior view. **B.** Three-dimensional computer-generated image of wrist and hand. (Letters correspond to structures labeled in **A.**) **C.** Coronal MRI of wrist. *A,* Articular disc; *J,* Distal radioulnar joint. (Letters correspond to structures labeled in **A.**)

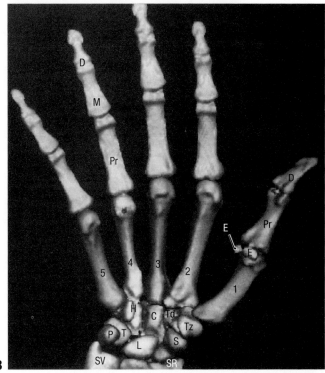

B

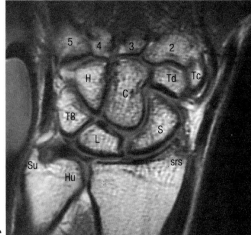

C

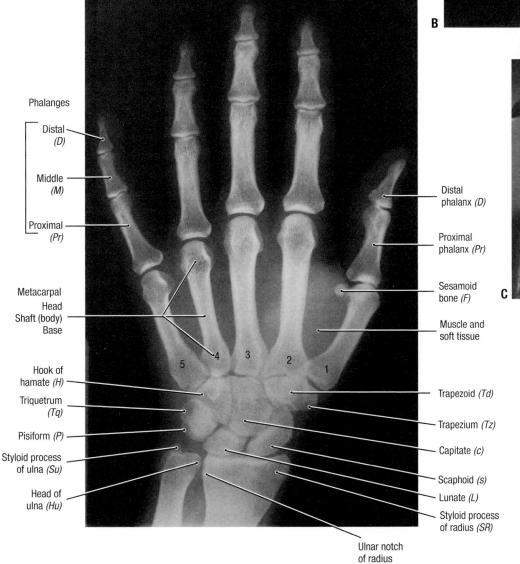

Phalanges

Distal *(D)*

Middle *(M)*

Proximal *(Pr)*

Metacarpal
Head
Shaft (body)
Base

Hook of
hamate *(H)*

Triquetrum
(Tq)

Pisiform *(P)*

Styloid process
of ulna *(Su)*

Head of
ulna *(Hu)*

Distal
phalanx *(D)*

Proximal
phalanx *(Pr)*

Sesamoid
bone *(F)*

Muscle and
soft tissue

Trapezoid *(Td)*

Trapezium *(Tz)*

Capitate *(c)*

Scaphoid *(s)*

Lunate *(L)*

Styloid process
of radius *(SR)*

Ulnar notch
of radius

A

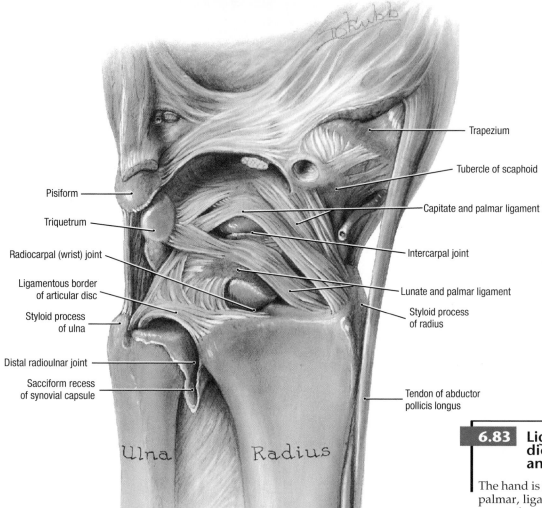

Trapezium

Tubercle of scaphoid

Pisiform

Triquetrum

Capitate and palmar ligament

Radiocarpal (wrist) joint

Intercarpal joint

Ligamentous border
of articular disc

Styloid process
of ulna

Lunate and palmar ligament

Styloid process
of radius

Distal radioulnar joint

Sacciform recess
of synovial capsule

Tendon of abductor
pollicis longus

Ulna   Radius

6.83 **Ligaments of distal radioulnar, radiocarpal, and intercarpal joints,
anterior view**

The hand is forcibly extended. Observe the anterior, or
palmar, ligaments, passing from the radius to the two
rows of carpal bones; they are strong, and directed
such that the hand follows the radius during supination. The dorsal ligaments take the same direction;
hence, the hand is also "obedient" during pronation.

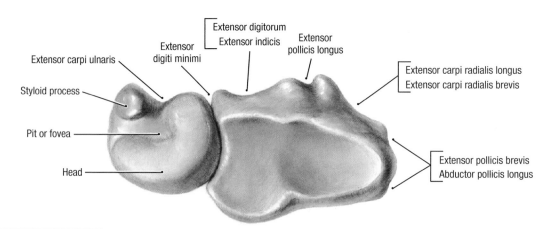

Extensor digitorum
Extensor indicis

Extensor
digiti minimi

Extensor
pollicis longus

Extensor carpi ulnaris

Extensor carpi radialis longus
Extensor carpi radialis brevis

Styloid process

Pit or fovea

Head

Extensor pollicis brevis
Abductor pollicis longus

6.84 **Distal ends of radius and ulna, inferior view**

OBSERVE:
1. The four features of the distal end of the ulna: head, fovea, styloid process, and groove for the tendon of ex-
    tensor carpi ulnaris;
2. The grooves for the tendons at the posterior aspect of the wrist; Figure 6.74 shows these tendons in their
    synovial sheaths.

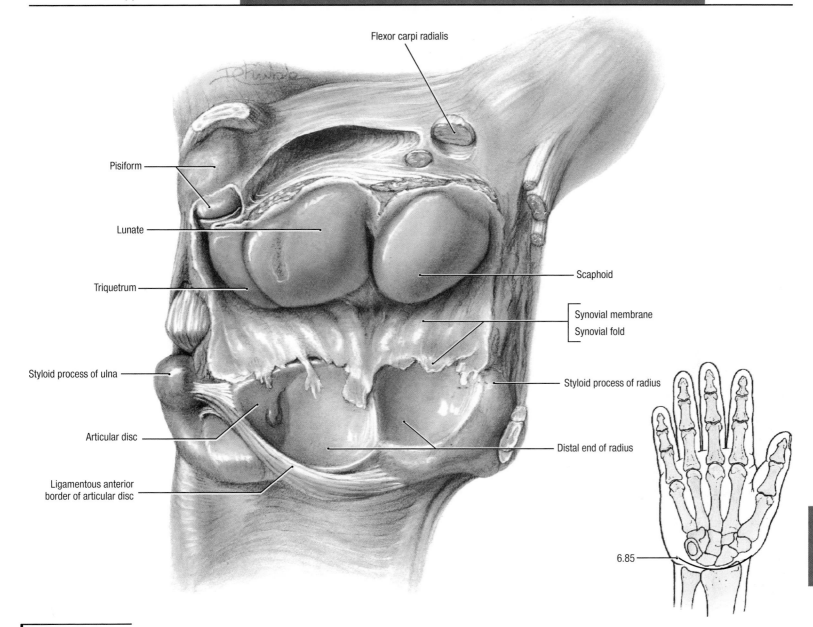

Flexor carpi radialis

Pisiform

Lunate

Triquetrum

Scaphoid

Synovial membrane
Synovial fold

Styloid process of ulna

Styloid process of radius

Articular disc

Distal end of radius

Ligamentous anterior
border of articular disc

6.85

6.85 **Surfaces of radiocarpal, or wrist, joint
opened anteriorly**

OBSERVE:
1. The proximal articular surfaces of the scaphoid and lunate are
nearly equal;

2. The lunate articulates with the radius and articular disc; only
during adduction of the wrist does the triquetrum come into
articulation with the disc;
3. *The perforation in the disc and the associated roughened surface of the
lunate are a common occurrence;*
4. The pisiform joint communicates with the radiocarpal joint.

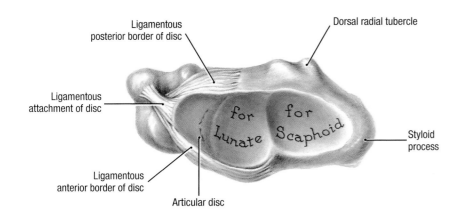

Ligamentous
posterior border of disc

Dorsal radial tubercle

Ligamentous
attachment of disc

for
Lunate

for
Scaphoid

Styloid
process

Ligamentous
anterior border of disc

Articular disc

6.86 **Articular disc of distal radioulnar
joint, inferior view**

This disc unites the distal ends of the radius and ulna;
it is fibrocartilaginous, smooth, and stiff at the triangular area compressed between the head of the ulna and
the lunate bone, but ligamentous and pliable elsewhere. The cartilaginous part is commonly fissured, as
here, but the ligamentous parts are not.

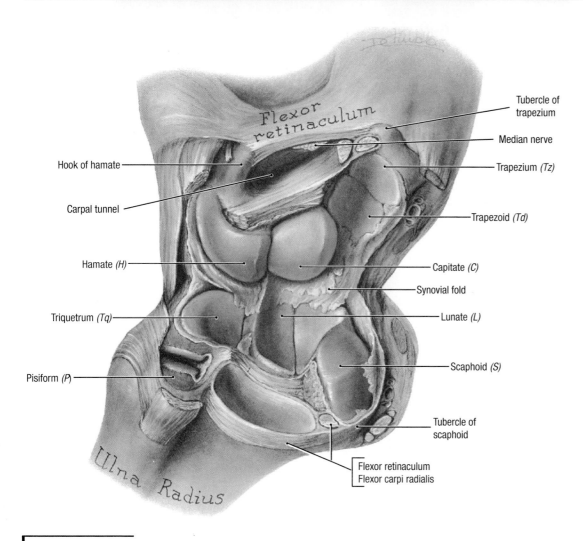

Flexor retinaculum

Hook of hamate

Carpal tunnel

Hamate (H)

Triquetrum (Tq)

Pisiform (P)

Ulna   Radius

Tubercle of trapezium

Median nerve

Trapezium (Tz)

Trapezoid (Td)

Capitate (C)

Synovial fold

Lunate (L)

Scaphoid (S)

Tubercle of scaphoid

Flexor retinaculum
Flexor carpi radialis

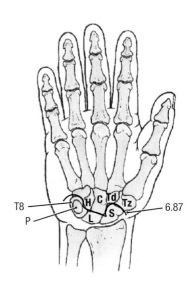

T8
P
H C Td Tz
L S
6.87

6.87   Surfaces of midcarpal (transverse carpal) joint, opened anteriorly

Letters in parentheses correlate to Figure 6.88.

OBSERVE:
1. The flexor retinaculum has been divided;
2. The sinuous surfaces of the opposed bones: the trapezium and trapezoid together present a concave, oval surface to the scaphoid, and the capitate and hamate together present a convex surface to the scaphoid, lunate, and triquetrum. The triquetrum is slightly broken by the linear facet on the apex of the hamate for its counterpart on the lunate; the proximal part of the flexor retinaculum, which stretches from the movable pisiform to the scaphoid, is relatively weak; the distal part, which stretches from the hook of the hamate to the tubercle of the trapezium, is strong.

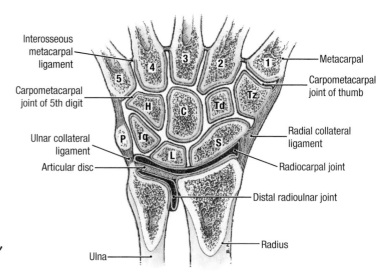

Interosseous
metacarpal
ligament

Carpometacarpal
joint of 5th digit

Ulnar collateral
ligament

Articular disc

Ulna

Metacarpal

Carpometacarpal
joint of thumb

Radial collateral
ligament

Radiocarpal joint

Distal radioulnar joint

Radius

6.88   Coronal section of wrist and hand, anterior view

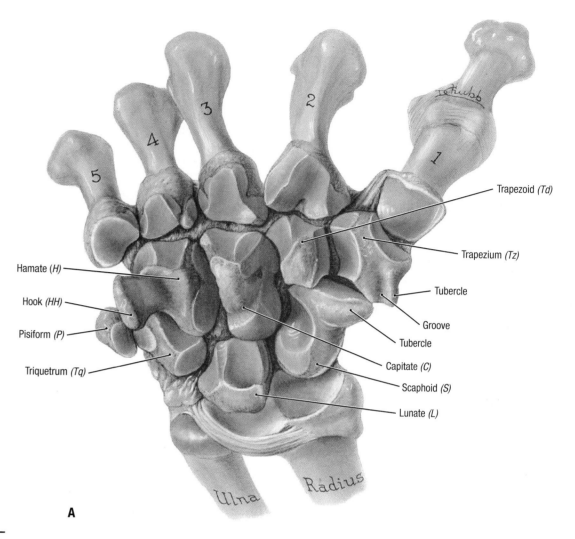

Hamate *(H)*

Hook *(HH)*

Pisiform *(P)*

Triquetrum *(Tq)*

Trapezoid *(Td)*

Trapezium *(Tz)*

Tubercle

Groove

Tubercle

Capitate *(C)*

Scaphoid *(S)*

Lunate *(L)*

Ulna　Radius

A

6.89　Carpal bones and bases of metacarpals, anterior views

The dorsal ligaments remain as a binding, allowing for the study of articular facets.

A. Open intercarpal and carpometacarpal joints. **B.** Diagram of the articular surfaces of the carpometacarpal joints (letters refer to structures labeled in **A**).

OBSERVE:

1. The radius supports two proximal carpals (scaphoid and lunate); these, in turn, support three distal carpals (trapezium, trapezoid, and capitate) and articulate with the apex of the hamate. The four distal carpals support the five metacarpals; the triquetrum is unsupported;
2. The flexor retinaculum attaches to the marginal projections (pisiform, hook of hamate, tubercle of scaphoid, and tubercle of trapezium);
3. The triquetrum has an isolated facet for the pisiform muscle;
4. The capitate articulates with three metacarpals (2nd, 3rd, and 4th);
5. The 2nd metacarpal articulates with three carpals (trapezium, trapezoid, and capitate);
6. The 2nd and 3rd carpometacarpal joints are practically immobile; the 1st is saddle-shaped, and the 4th and 5th are hinge-shaped.

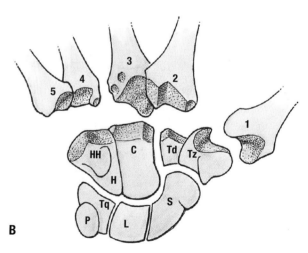

B

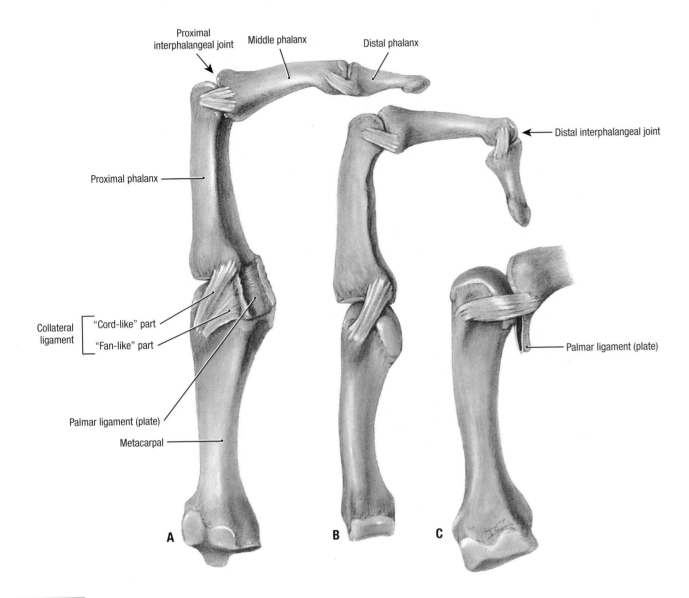

Proximal interphalangeal joint

Middle phalanx

Distal phalanx

Distal interphalangeal joint

Proximal phalanx

Collateral ligament

"Cord-like" part

"Fan-like" part

Palmar ligament (plate)

Palmar ligament (plate)

Metacarpal

A   B   C

6.90   Collateral ligaments of metacarpophalangeal and interphalangeal joints, lateral views

A. Extended metacarpophalangeal and distal interphalangeal joints. **B.** Flexed distal interphalangeal joint. **C.** Flexed metacarpophalangeal joint.

OBSERVE:

1. A fibrocartilaginous plate, the palmar ligament, hangs from the base of the proximal phalanx, is fixed to the head of the metacarpal by the weaker, fan-like part of the collateral ligament (**A**), and moves like a visor across the metacarpal head (**C**);

2. The extremely strong, cord-like parts of the collateral ligaments of this joint (**A** and **B**) are eccentrically attached to the metacarpal heads; they are slack during extension and taut during flexion (**C**), so the fingers cannot be spread (abducted) unless the hand is open;

3. The interphalangeal joints have corresponding ligaments, but the distal ends of the proximal and middle phalanges, because they are flattened anteroposteriorly and have two small condyles, permit neither adduction nor abduction.

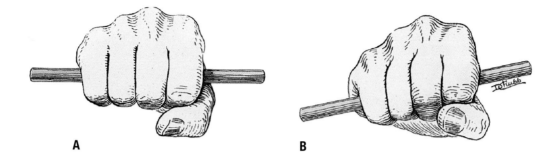

A   **B**

6.91   Grasping hand

A. Loosely held. **B.** Firmly gripped. The 2nd and 3rd carpometacarpal joints are rigid and stable, but the 4th and 5th are hinge joints that permit flexion and extension. This is apparent on inspection of the skeleton and on grasping a cylindrical structure; it is a forward movement, or flexion, of the 4th and 5th metacarpals that gives tenacity to the grip on a rod.

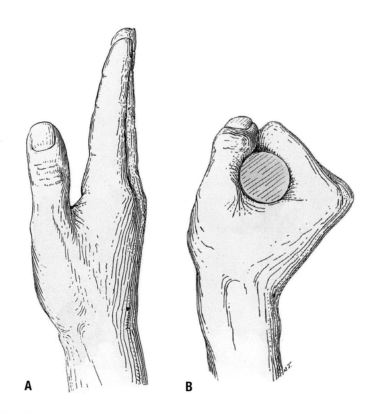

A   **B**

6.92   Wrist extension of the grasping hand

A. The extended hand. **B.** Grasping an object. When grasping an object, the metacarpophalangeal and interphalangeal joints are flexed, but the radiocarpal and transverse carpal joints are extended. The grasping hand requires an extended wrist; without this extension, the grip is feeble and insecure. The extensor carpi radialis longus and brevis and extensor carpi ulnaris muscles, as synergists, are essential to the digital flexors for strength when grasping.

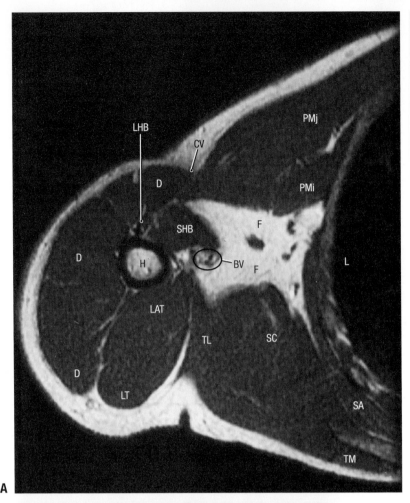

BB	Biceps brachii
BC	Brachialis
BR	Brachioradialis
BS	Basilic vein
BV	Brachial vessels and nerves
CV	Cephalic vein
D	Deltoid
F	Fat in axilla
H	Humerus
L	Lung
LAT	Lateral head of triceps brachii
LHB	Long head of biceps brachii
LI	Lateral intermuscular septum
LT	Long head of triceps brachii
MI	Medial intermuscular septum
MT	Medial head of triceps brachii
PMi	Pectoralis minor
PMj	Pectoralis major
SA	Serratus anterior
SC	Subscapularis
SHB	Short head of biceps brachii
T	Deltoid tuberosity
TL	Teres major and latissimus dorsi
Tm	Teres minor

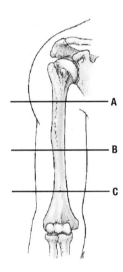

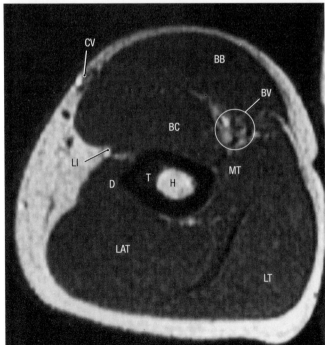

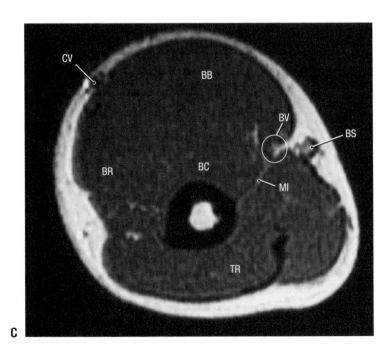

6.93   Axial (transverse) MRIs of arm

A. Proximal. **B.** Middle. **C.** Distal.

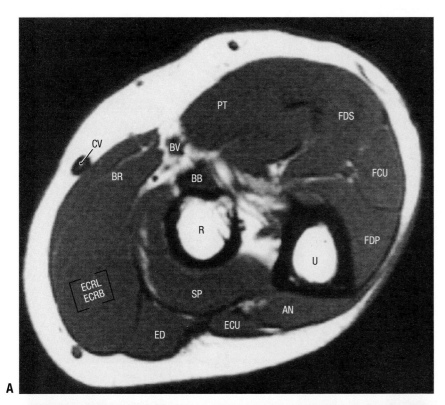

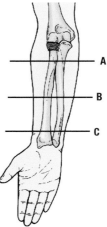

AN	Anconeus
APL	Abductor pollicis longus
AV	Anterior interosseous vessels and nerve
BB	Biceps brachii
BR	Brachioradialis
BV	Brachial vessels
CV	Cephalic vein
ECRB	Extensor carpi radialis brevis
ECRL	Extensor carpi radialis longus
ECU	Extensor carpi ulnaris
ED	Extensor digitorum
EPB	Extensor pollicis brevis
EPL	Extensor pollicis longus
FCR	Flexor carpi radialis
FCU	Flexor carpi ulnaris
FDP	Flexor digitorum profundus
FDS	Flexor digitorum superficialis
FPL	Flexor pollicis longus
INT	Interosseous membrane
PQ	Pronator quadratus
PT	Pronator teres
R	Radius
RV	Radial vessels
SP	Supinator
U	Ulna
UV	Ulnar vessels and nerve

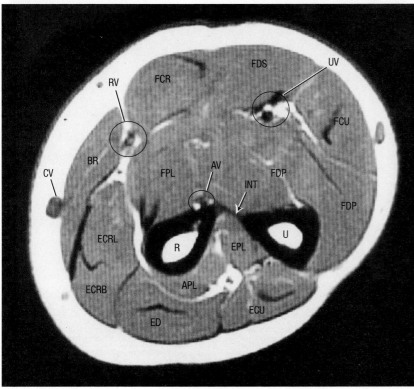

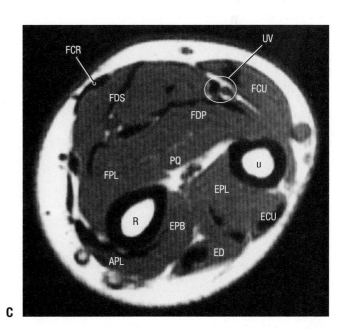

6.94 **Axial (transverse) MRIs of forearm**

A. Proximal. **B.** Middle. **C.** Distal.

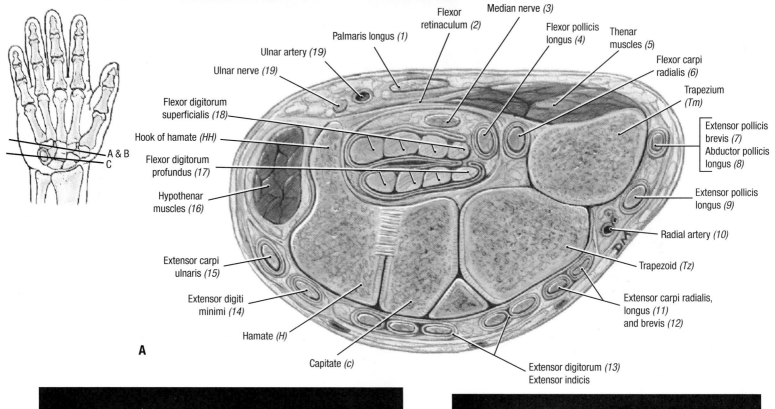

A. Section through distal carpal tunnel.

Palmaris longus (1)
Flexor retinaculum (2)
Median nerve (3)
Flexor pollicis longus (4)
Thenar muscles (5)
Flexor carpi radialis (6)
Trapezium (Tm)
Extensor pollicis brevis (7)
Abductor pollicis longus (8)
Extensor pollicis longus (9)
Radial artery (10)
Trapezoid (Tz)
Extensor carpi radialis, longus (11) and brevis (12)
Extensor digitorum (13)
Extensor indicis
Capitate (c)
Hamate (H)
Extensor digiti minimi (14)
Extensor carpi ulnaris (15)
Hypothenar muscles (16)
Flexor digitorum profundus (17)
Hook of hamate (HH)
Flexor digitorum superficialis (18)
Ulnar nerve (19)
Ulnar artery (19)

A

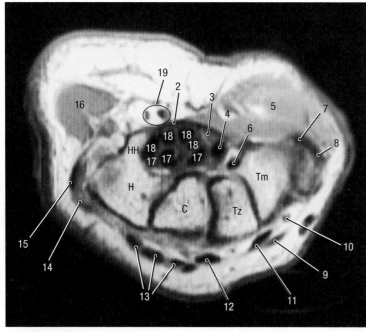

B

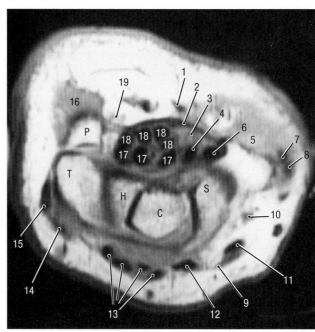

C

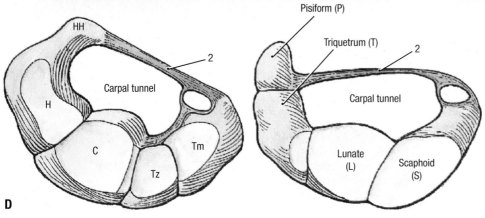

Pisiform (P)
Triquetrum (T)
Carpal tunnel
Lunate (L)
Scaphoid (S)
Carpal tunnel
HH
H
C
Tm
Tz

D

6.95 Axial (transverse) section and MRIs through carpal tunnel

A. Section through distal carpal tunnel.
B. MRI of distal carpal tunnel **C.** MRI of proximal carpal tunnel. **D.** Distal row of carpal bones (*top*) and proximal row of carpal bones (*bottom*). Numbers in MRIs refer to structures in **A.** Letters on bones in MRIs refer to bones labeled on **A** and **D.**

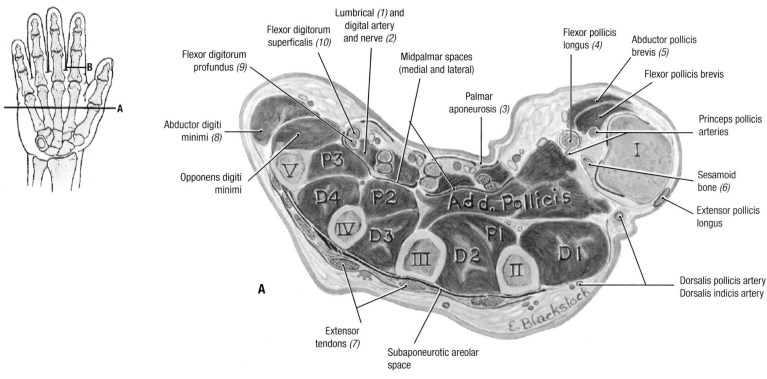

Lumbrical (1) and digital artery and nerve (2)

Flexor digitorum superficalis (10)

Flexor digitorum profundus (9)

Midpalmar spaces (medial and lateral)

Palmar aponeurosis (3)

Flexor pollicis longus (4)

Abductor pollicis brevis (5)

Flexor pollicis brevis

Abductor digiti minimi (8)

Opponens digiti minimi

Princeps pollicis arteries

Sesamoid bone (6)

Extensor pollicis longus

Dorsalis pollicis artery
Dorsalis indicis artery

Extensor tendons (7)

Subaponeurotic areolar space

A

Add. Pollicis

E. Blackstock

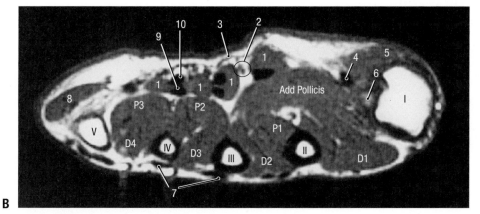

B

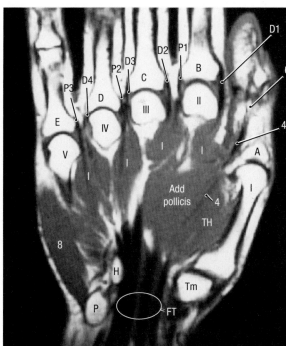

C

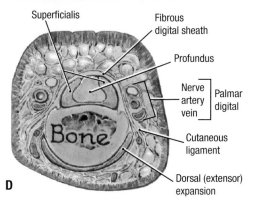

Superficialis

Fibrous digital sheath

Profundus

Nerve
artery
vein } Palmar digital

Cutaneous ligament

Dorsal (extensor) expansion

Bone

D

6.96　Sections and MRIs through head

A. Transverse section through adductor pollicis. *D1–D4*, Dorsal interossei; *P1–P3*, Palmar interossei; *I–V*, Metacarpals; *Add. pollicis,* Adductor pollicis. **B.** Axial (transverse) MRI through adductor pollicis. **C.** Coronal MRI of wrist and hand. Numbers and letters in MRIs refer to structures in **A.** *FT*, Long flexor tendons in carpal tunnel; *TH*, Thenar muscles; *P,* Pisiform; *H* Hook of hamate; *Tm,* Trapezium; *I,* Interossei, *A–E*, Proximal phalanges. **D.** Transverse section of proximal phalanx.

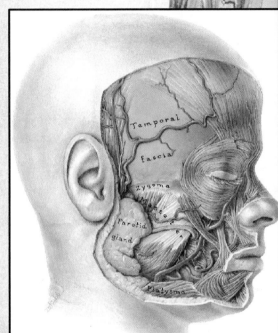

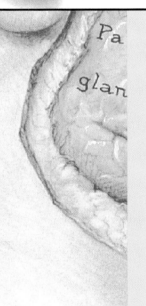

CHAPTER 7

Head

7.1   **Skull, anterior views**

A. Bony skull. **B.** Diagram of skull. Orbital cavity, see Fig 7.42.

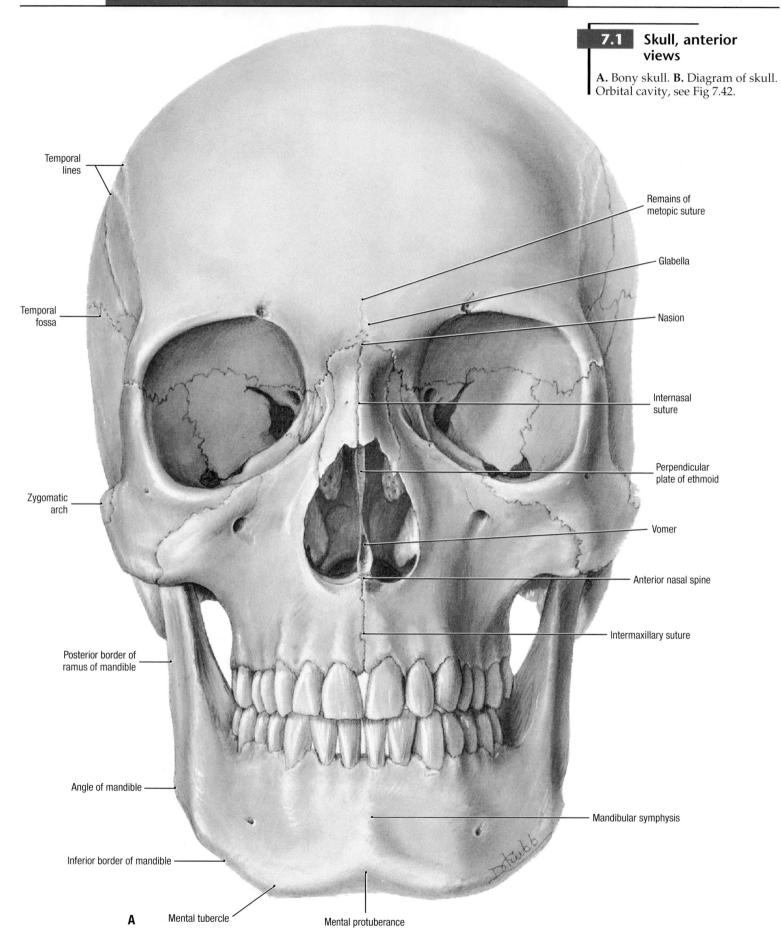

Temporal lines

Temporal fossa

Zygomatic arch

Posterior border of ramus of mandible

Angle of mandible

Inferior border of mandible

A   Mental tubercle

Mental protuberance

Remains of metopic suture

Glabella

Nasion

Internasal suture

Perpendicular plate of ethmoid

Vomer

Anterior nasal spine

Intermaxillary suture

Mandibular symphysis

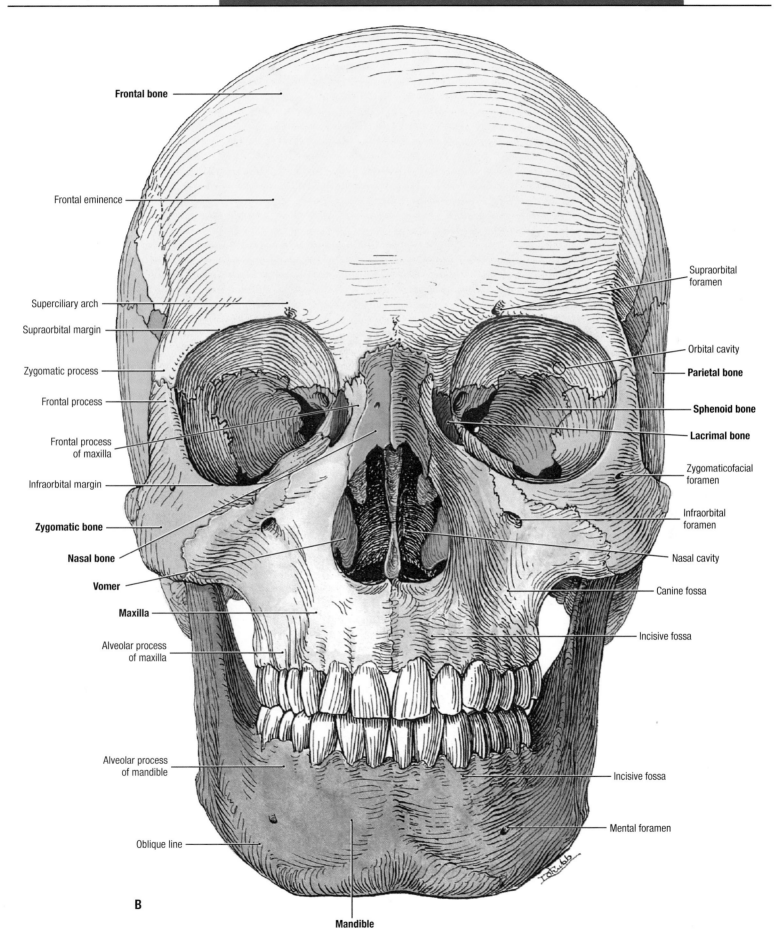

Frontal bone

Frontal eminence

Superciliary arch

Supraorbital margin

Zygomatic process

Frontal process

Frontal process of maxilla

Infraorbital margin

Zygomatic bone

Nasal bone

Vomer

Maxilla

Alveolar process of maxilla

Alveolar process of mandible

Oblique line

Supraorbital foramen

Orbital cavity

Parietal bone

Sphenoid bone

Lacrimal bone

Zygomaticofacial foramen

Infraorbital foramen

Nasal cavity

Canine fossa

Incisive fossa

Incisive fossa

Mental foramen

B

Mandible

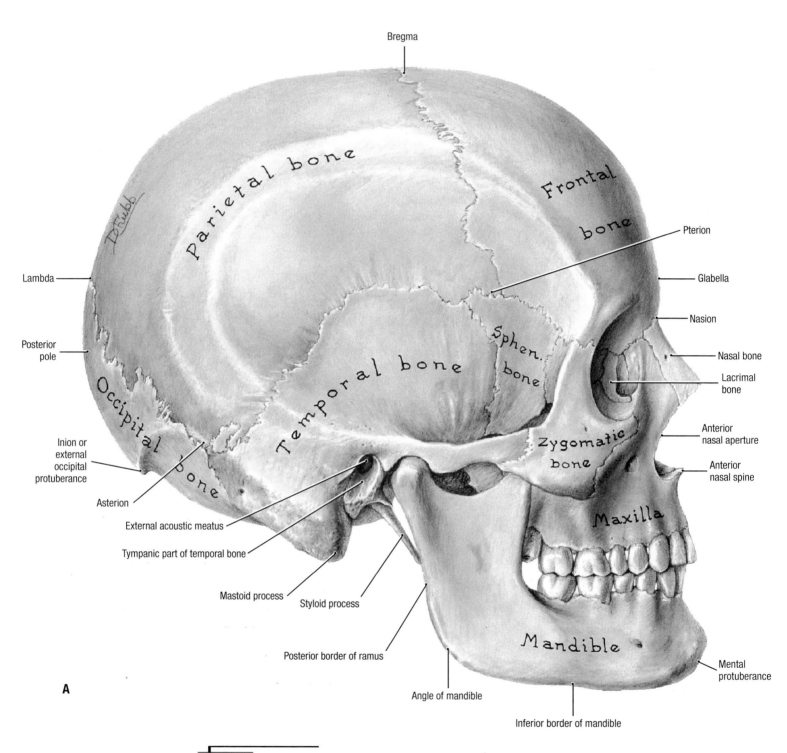

A

7.2   Skull, lateral views

A. Bony skull. **B.** Diagram of skull.

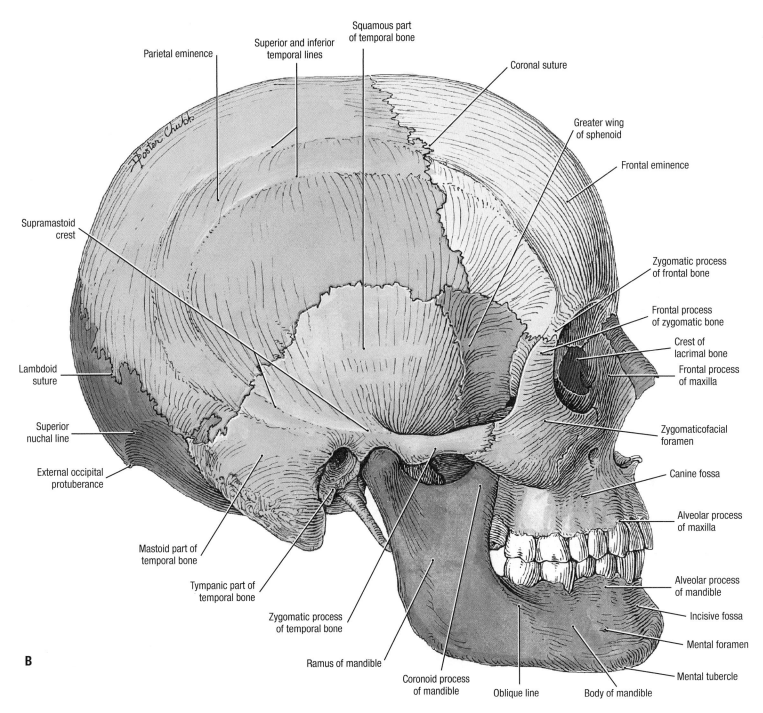

B. Diagram.

Parietal eminence

Superior and inferior temporal lines

Squamous part of temporal bone

Coronal suture

Greater wing of sphenoid

Frontal eminence

Zygomatic process of frontal bone

Frontal process of zygomatic bone

Crest of lacrimal bone

Frontal process of maxilla

Zygomaticofacial foramen

Canine fossa

Alveolar process of maxilla

Alveolar process of mandible

Incisive fossa

Mental foramen

Mental tubercle

Supramastoid crest

Lambdoid suture

Superior nuchal line

External occipital protuberance

Mastoid part of temporal bone

Tympanic part of temporal bone

Zygomatic process of temporal bone

Ramus of mandible

Coronoid process of mandible

Oblique line

Body of mandible

B

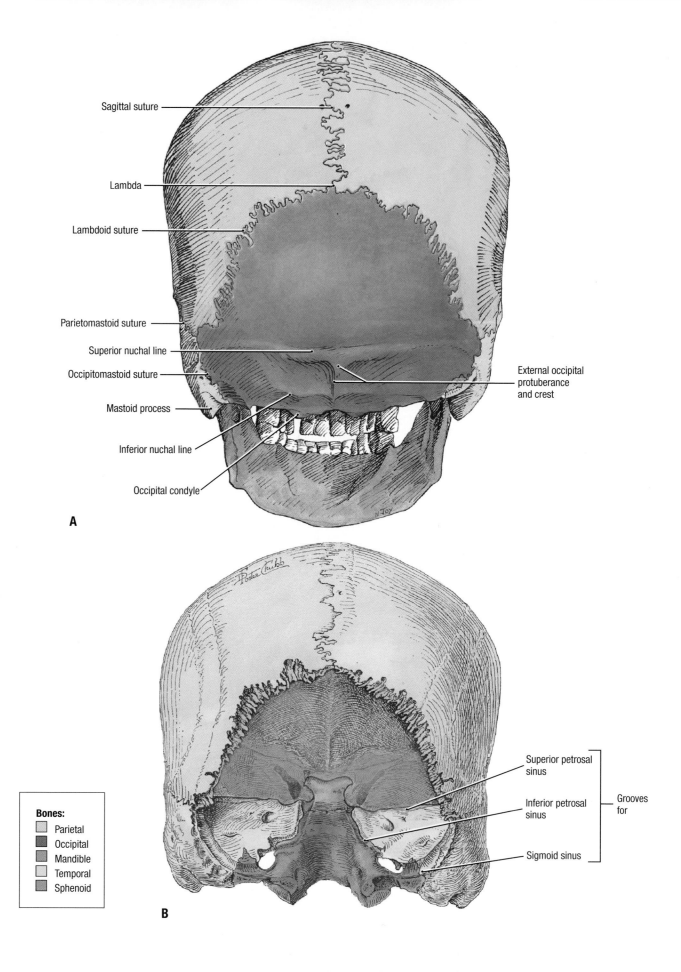

Sagittal suture

Lambda

Lambdoid suture

Parietomastoid suture

Superior nuchal line

Occipitomastoid suture

Mastoid process

Inferior nuchal line

Occipital condyle

External occipital protuberance and crest

A

Superior petrosal sinus

Inferior petrosal sinus

Sigmoid sinus

Grooves for

Bones:
- Parietal
- Occipital
- Mandible
- Temporal
- Sphenoid

B

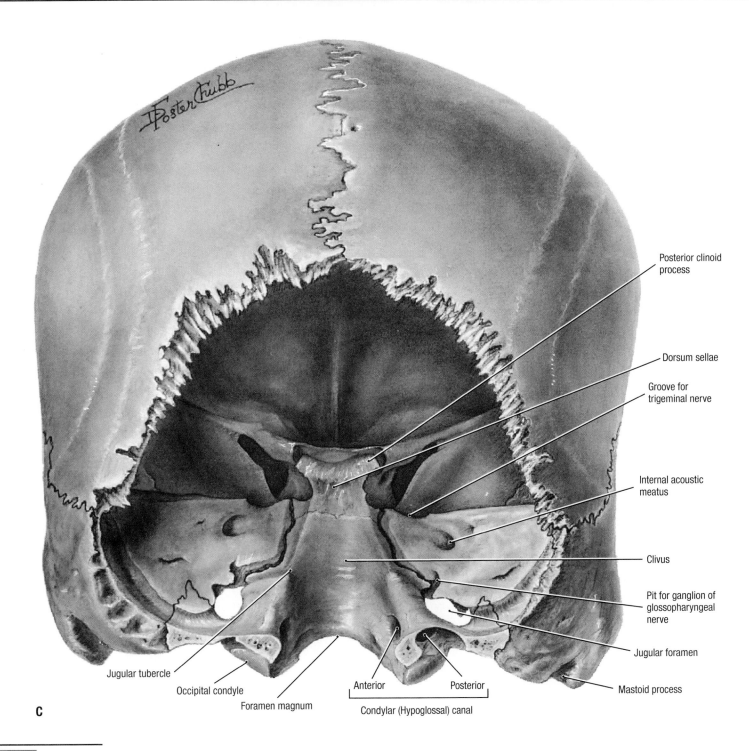

Poster Crubb

Posterior clinoid process

Dorsum sellae

Groove for trigeminal nerve

Internal acoustic meatus

Clivus

Pit for ganglion of glossopharyngeal nerve

Jugular foramen

Mastoid process

Jugular tubercle

Occipital condyle

Foramen magnum

Anterior   Posterior

Condylar (Hypoglossal) canal

C

7.3   **Skull posterior and posterior cranial fossa, posterior views**

A. Skull posterior. **B.** Bones and sinuses of posterior cranial fossa. The squamous part of the occipital bone is removed. **C.** Bony features of posterior cranial fossa.

OBSERVE IN **A**:
1. The surface of the skull is convex and includes parts of the parietal, occipital, and temporal (mastoid part) bones; near the center is the lambda, at the junction of the sagittal and lambdoid sutures;
2. The superior nuchal line curves laterally from the midline external occipital protuberance to the mastoid process.

OBSERVE IN **B** AND **C**:
3. The dorsum sellae is a plate of bone that rises from the body of the sphenoid; at its superior angles are the posterior clinoid processes;
4. The clivus is the sloping surface between the dorsum sellae and foramen magnum; it is formed by the basilar part of the occipital bone (basiocciput) and body of the sphenoid;
5. The grooves for the sigmoid sinus and inferior petrosal sinus lead inferiorly to the jugular foramen.

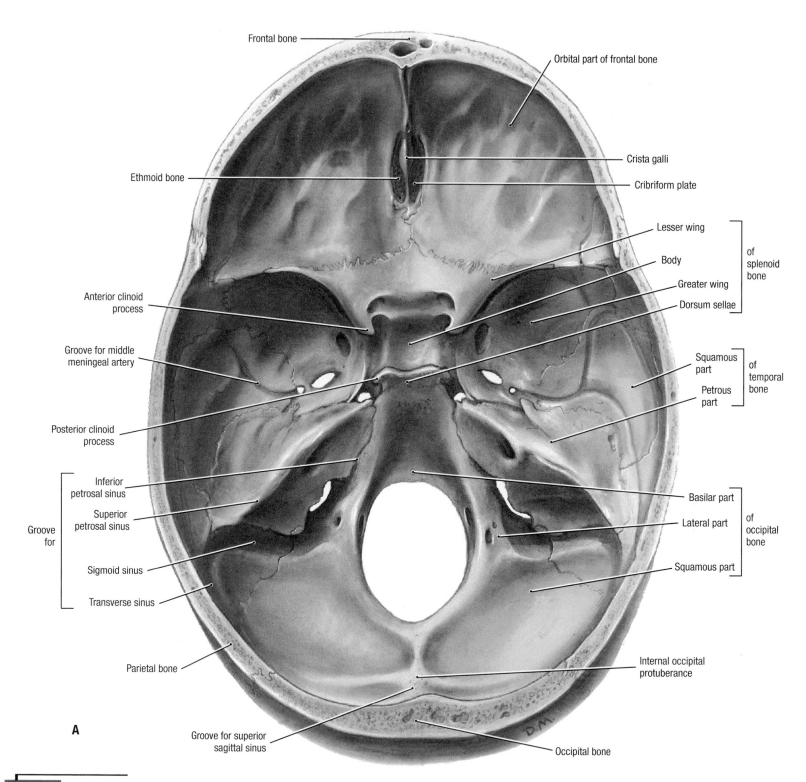

Frontal bone

Orbital part of frontal bone

Crista galli

Ethmoid bone

Cribriform plate

Lesser wing

Body

of splenoid bone

Greater wing

Anterior clinoid process

Dorsum sellae

Groove for middle meningeal artery

Squamous part

of temporal bone

Petrous part

Posterior clinoid process

Inferior petrosal sinus

Basilar part

Lateral part

of occipital bone

Superior petrosal sinus

Groove for

Sigmoid sinus

Squamous part

Transverse sinus

Internal occipital protuberance

Parietal bone

A

Groove for superior sagittal sinus

Occipital bone

7.4   Interior of base of skull, superior views

A. Bony skull. **B.** Diagram.

OBSERVE IN **A:**

1. Three bones contribute to the anterior cranial fossa: the orbital part of the frontal bone, cribriform plate of the ethmoid, and lesser wing of the sphenoid;

2. The four developmental parts of the occipital bone are the basilar, right and left lateral, and squamous;

3. The anterior clinoid processes on the lesser wing of the sphenoid and the posterior clinoid processes project from the dorsum sellae for the attachment of the tentorium cerebelli.

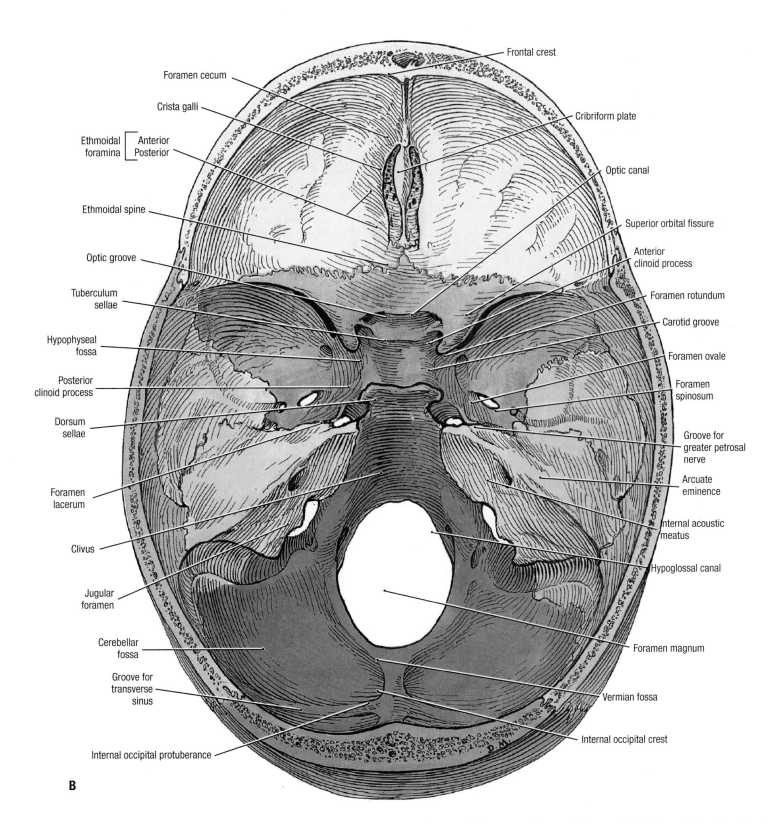

Frontal crest

Foramen cecum

Crista galli

Cribriform plate

Ethmoidal foramina — Anterior / Posterior

Optic canal

Ethmoidal spine

Superior orbital fissure

Optic groove

Anterior clinoid process

Tuberculum sellae

Foramen rotundum

Carotid groove

Hypophyseal fossa

Foramen ovale

Posterior clinoid process

Foramen spinosum

Dorsum sellae

Groove for greater petrosal nerve

Arcuate eminence

Foramen lacerum

Internal acoustic meatus

Clivus

Hypoglossal canal

Jugular foramen

Cerebellar fossa

Foramen magnum

Groove for transverse sinus

Vermian fossa

Internal occipital crest

Internal occipital protuberance

B

OBSERVE IN **B** THE FOLLOWING FEATURES IN THE MEDIAN PLANE:

4. In the anterior cranial fossa: the frontal crest and crista galli for attachment of the falx cerebri; between them is the foramen cecum, which usually transmits a vein connecting the superior sagittal sinus with the veins of the frontal sinus and root of the nose;

5. In the middle cranial fossa: the tuberculum sellae, hypophyseal fossa, and dorsum sellae, which constitute the sella turcica (Turkish saddle);

6. In the posterior cranial fossa: the clivus, foramen magnum, vermian fossa (for vermis of the cerebellum), internal occipital crest for attachment of the falx cerebelli, and the internal occipital protuberance, from which the grooves for the transverse sinuses curve laterally.

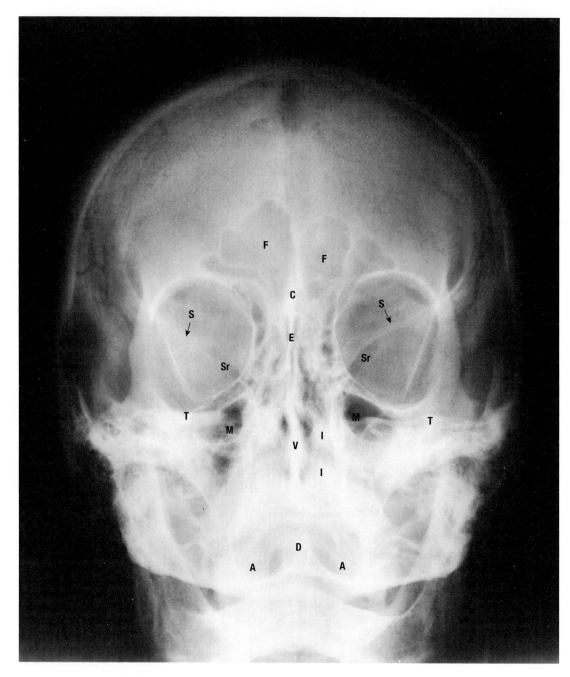

A, Anteroposterior view

7.5   Radiograph of skull

A. Anteroposterior radiograph. **B.** Lateral radiograph.

OBSERVE IN **A:**
1. The superior orbital fissure (*Sr*), lesser wing of sphenoid (*S*), and superior surface of the petrous part of the temporal bone (*T*);
2. The nasal septum is formed by the perpendicular plate of the ethmoid (*E*) and the vomer (*V*); note the inferior and middle conchae (*I*) of the lateral wall of the nose;
3. The crista galli (*C*), frontal sinus (*F*), and maxillary sinus (*M*);
4. Superimposed on the facial skeleton is the dens (*D*) and lateral masses of the atlas (*A*).

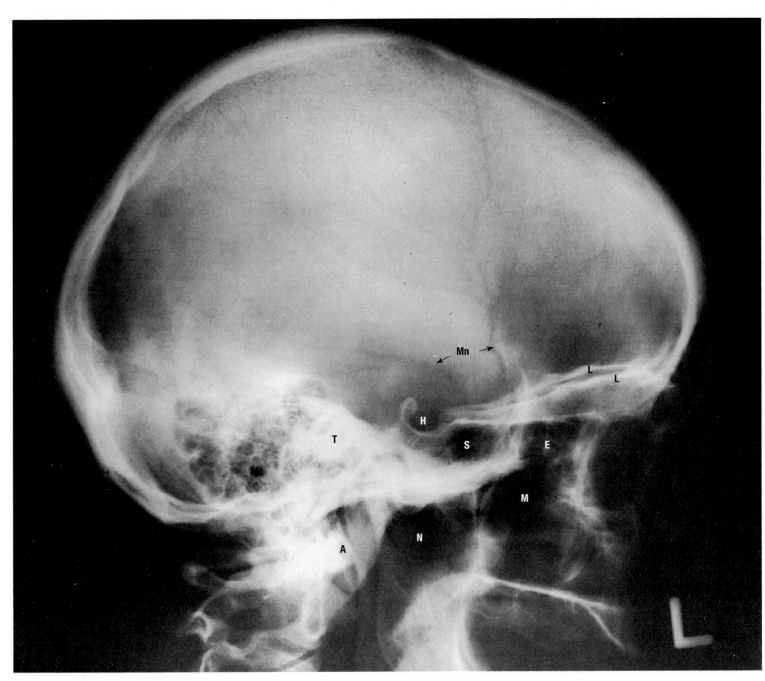

B, Lateral view

OBSERVE IN **B:**
  5. The paranasal sinuses: frontal (*F*), ethmoidal (*E*), sphenoidal (*S*), and maxillary (*M*);
  6. The hypophyseal fossa (*H*) for the pituitary gland;
  7. The great density of the petrous part of the temporal bone (*T*) and the mastoid cells (*Mc*);
  8. The right and left orbital plates of the frontal bone are not superimposed; thus, the floor of the anterior cranial fossa appears as two lines (*L*);
  9. The grooves for the branches of the middle meningeal vessels (*Mn*);
  10. The arch of the atlas (*A*) and the nasopharynx (*N*).

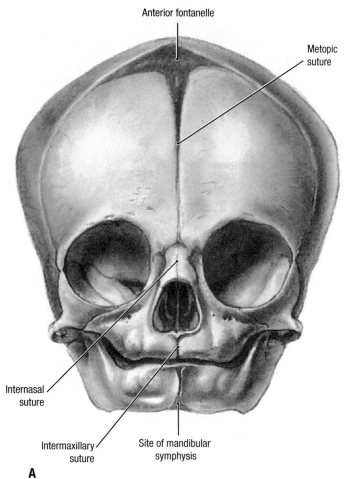

A

Anterior fontanelle

Metopic suture

Internasal suture

Intermaxillary suture

Site of mandibular symphysis

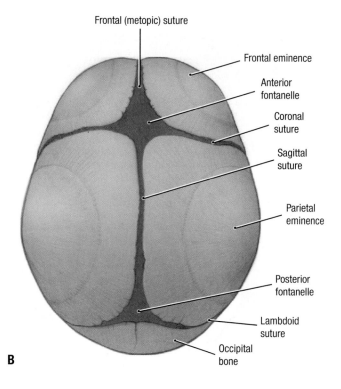

B

Frontal (metopic) suture

Frontal eminence

Anterior fontanelle

Coronal suture

Sagittal suture

Parietal eminence

Posterior fontanelle

Lambdoid suture

Occipital bone

Parietal eminence

Anterior fontanelle

Posterior fontanelle

Frontal eminence

Anterolateral fontanelle

Maxilla

Mandible

Posterolateral fontanelle

Tympanic membrane in external acoustic meatus

C

7.6   Skull at birth

A. Anterior view. **B.** Superior view. **C.** Lateral view.

OBSERVE:

1. The teeth have not erupted;
2. The maxilla and mandible are small, and the angle of the mandible is obtuse; thus, the ramus and body of the mandible are nearly in line, and the inferior border of the mandible is level with the foramen magnum;
3. The orbital cavities are large, but the face is small, forming 1/8 of the whole skull; in the adult, it forms 1/3;
4. The mandibular symphysis (symphysis menti), which closes during the 2nd year, and the metopic suture, which closes during the 6th year, are still open;
5. The eminence of the parietal bone, like that of the frontal bone, is conical. Ossification, which starts at the eminences, has not yet reached the four angles of the parietal bone; accordingly, these regions are membranous, and the membrane is blended with the pericranium externally and the dura mater internally to form the fontanelles. The fontanelles are usually closed by the 2nd year;
6. There is no mastoid process until the 2nd year;
7. The external acoustic meatus is short;
8. The tympanic membrane is close to the surface of the skull.

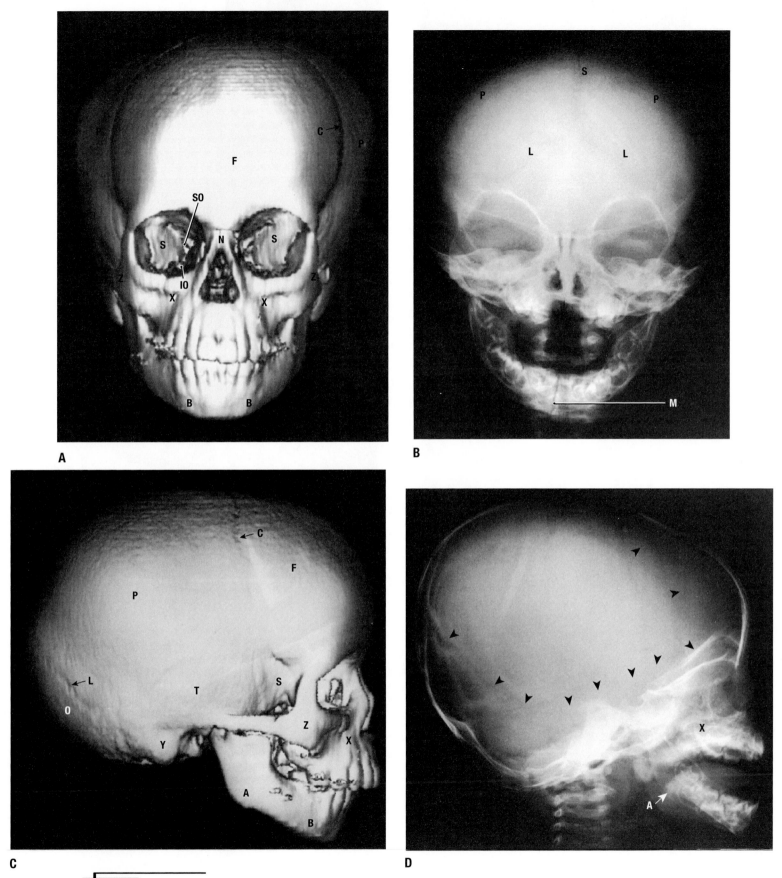

7.7 Images of child's skull

A. and **C.** Three-dimensional computer-generated images of 3-year-old child's skull, anterior (**A**) and lateral (**C**) views. **B** and **D.** Radiographs of 6½-month-old child, posterioanterior (**B**) and lateral (**D**) views. *A*, Angle of mandible; *X*, Maxilla; *M*, Symphysis menti; *S*, Sagittal suture; *L*, Lambdoid suture; *P*, Parietal eminence; *B*, Body of mandible; *C*, Coronal suture; *F*, Frontal bone; *T*, Temporal bone; *S*, Sphenoid; *Z*, Zygomatic bone; *Y*, Mastoid process; *O*, Occipital bone; *N*, Nasal bone; *SO*, Superior orbital fissure; *IO*, Inferior orbital fissure; *arrowheads*, Membranous outline of the parietal bone.

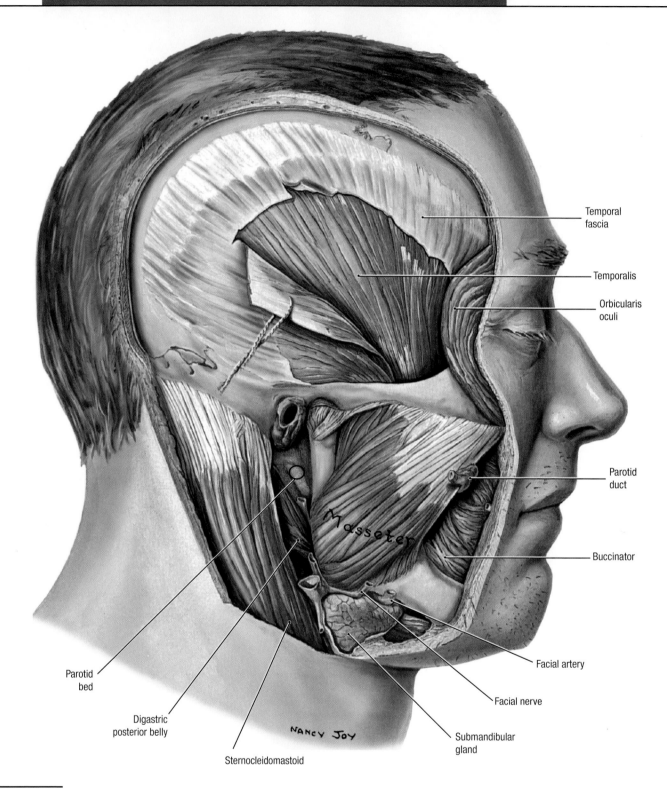

Temporal fascia

Temporalis

Orbicularis oculi

Parotid duct

Masseter

Buccinator

Facial artery

Facial nerve

Submandibular gland

Parotid bed

Digastric posterior belly

NANCY JOY

Sternocleidomastoid

7.8   Great muscles of skull, lateral view

OBSERVE:

1. The temporalis and masseter muscles are supplied by the trigeminal nerve, and both close the jaw. The temporalis arises, in part, from the overlying fascia;
2. The orbicularis oculi and buccinator muscles are supplied by the facial nerve; one closes the eye and the other prevents food from collecting between the cheeks and teeth;
3. The sternocleidomastoid muscle is the chief flexor of the head and neck; it forms the posterior boundary of the parotid region;
4. The facial artery passes deep to the submandibular gland, and the facial vein passes superficial to it.

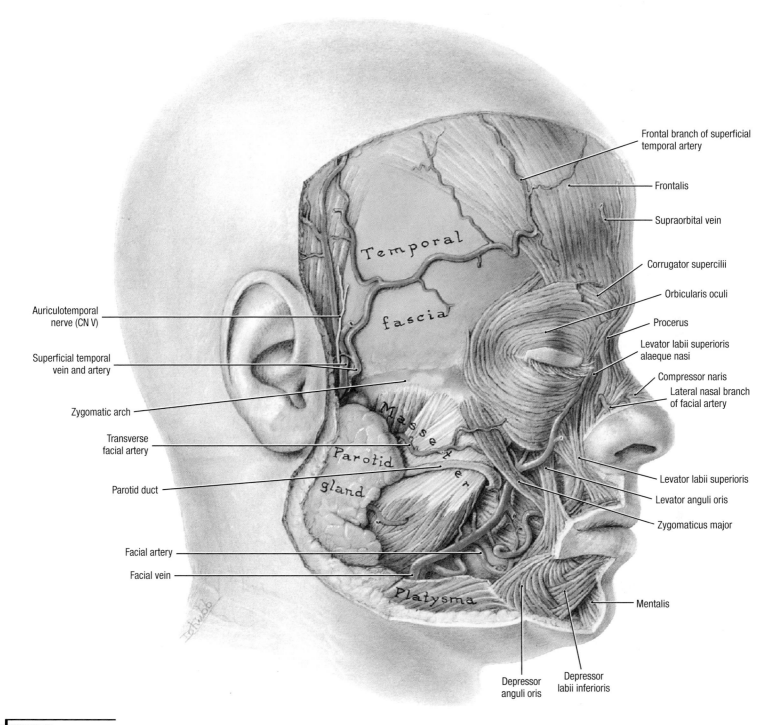

Frontal branch of superficial temporal artery

Frontalis

Supraorbital vein

Corrugator supercilii

Orbicularis oculi

Procerus

Levator labii superioris alaeque nasi

Compressor naris

Lateral nasal branch of facial artery

Levator labii superioris

Levator anguli oris

Zygomaticus major

Mentalis

Auriculotemporal nerve (CN V)

Superficial temporal vein and artery

Zygomatic arch

Transverse facial artery

Parotid duct

Facial artery

Facial vein

Temporal fascia

Masseter

Parotid gland

Platysma

Depressor anguli oris

Depressor labii inferioris

7.9   Muscles of facial expression and arteries of face, lateral view

OBSERVE:
1. The muscles of facial expression are the superficial sphincters and dilators of the orifices of the head; all are supplied by the facial nerve (CN VII);
2. There are muscles of facial expression around the eyes, ears, nose, and mouth, blending into the upper lip, lower lip, chin, and cheek;
3. The facial artery crosses the base of the mandible at the anterior border of the masseter muscle, passing within 1 cm of the angle of the mouth and lying anterior to the facial vein, which takes a straight and more superficial course;

4. The auriculotemporal nerve ascends with the superficial temporal vessels;
5. *The pulse can be taken at the facial artery, where it winds around the inferior border of the mandible; it can also be felt at the superficial temporal artery, where the vessel passes anterior to the ear and crosses the zygomatic arch;*
6. The masseter and temporalis (covered by temporal fascia) are muscles of mastication that are innervated by the trigeminal nerve.

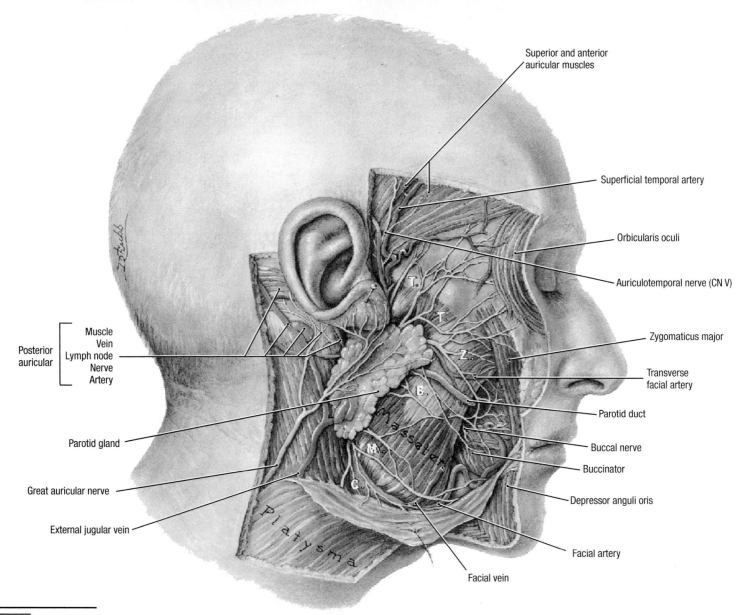

Superior and anterior auricular muscles

Superficial temporal artery

Orbicularis oculi

Auriculotemporal nerve (CN V)

Zygomaticus major

Transverse facial artery

Parotid duct

Buccal nerve

Buccinator

Depressor anguli oris

Facial artery

Facial vein

Posterior auricular {
Muscle
Vein
Lymph node
Nerve
Artery
}

Parotid gland

Great auricular nerve

External jugular vein

7.10 Relationships of the branches of the facial nerve and vessels to parotid gland and duct, lateral view

OBSERVE:

1. The parotid gland and duct cross the masseter muscle one finger-breadth inferior to the zygomatic arch and turn medially to pierce the buccinator; *Infection of the parotid gland (e.g., mumps) causes inflammation (parotiditis) of the gland. Because the capsule of the parotid gland is tightly bound around the gland, swelling of the gland is limited, which can result in pain.*

2. The facial nerve (CN VII) supplies motor innervation to the mus-

cles of facial expression; its branches pass through the parotid gland and radiate over the face to anastomose with each other and the branches of the trigeminal nerve. The facial nerve is divided into temporal (*T*), zygomatic (*Z*), buccal (*B*), mandibular (*M*), cervical (*C*), and posterior auricular branches. *During parotidectomy (surgical excision of the gland), the identification, dissection, and preservation of the facial nerve is critical.*

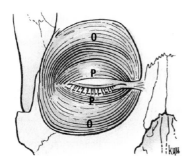

7.11 Orbicularis oculi, anterior view

Palpebral (*P*) and orbital (*O*) parts of the orbicularis oculi muscle. The palpebral part gently closes and the orbital part tightly closes the eyelids. The lacrimal portion (not shown) passes posterior to the lacrimal sac, and helps spread lacrimal secretions.

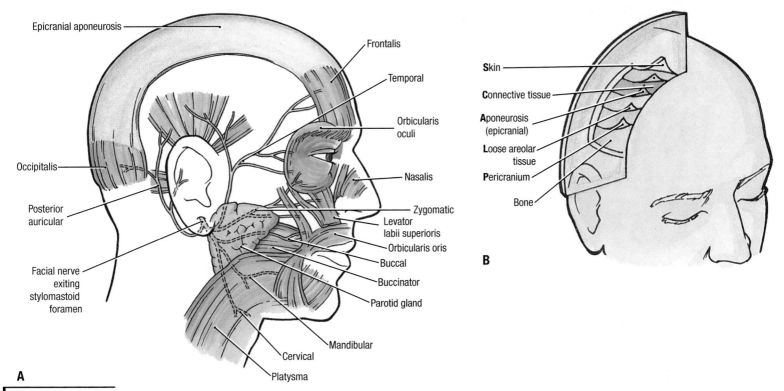

A. Lateral view. **B.** Anterolateral view.

OBSERVE:
1. One of the most common causes of facial paralysis is inflammation of the facial nerve in the area of the stylomastoid foramen. Patients with Bell's palsy cannot close their lips and eyelids, nor chew effectively and empty the gutter between the teeth and cheek on the affected side, and have a drooping of the mouth on the affected side, resulting in dribbling of food and saliva from the corner of the mouth. The cornea on the affected side is not lubricated with lacrimal fluid and can become ulcerated.
2. In **B,** the layers of the scalp: the skin is bound tightly to the epicranial aponeurosis, which is attached to the skull laterally, the occipitalis posteriorly, and the frontalis anteriorly; *thus blood from a torn vessel can spread widely over the skull deep to the aponeurosis and leak out anteriorly, appearing as bruising in the area of the eyelids.*

Table 7.1. Main Muscles of Facial Expression

Muscle[a]	Origin	Insertion	Action(s)
Frontalis	Epicranial aponeurosis	Skin of forehead	Elevates eyebrows and forehead
Orbicularis oculi	Medial orbital margin, medial palpebral ligament, and lacrimal bone	Skin around margin of orbit; tarsal plate	Closes eyelids
Nasalis	Superior part of canine ridge of maxilla	Nasal cartilages	Draws ala (side) of nose toward nasal septum
Orbicularis oris	Some fibers arise near median plane of maxilla superiorly and mandible inferiorly; other fibers arise from deep surface of skin	Mucous membrane of lips	Compresses and protrudes lips (e.g., purses them during whistling an sucking)
Levator labii superioris	Frontal process of maxilla and infraorbital region	Skin of upper lip and alar cartilage of nose	Elevates lip, dilates nostril, and raises angle of mouth
Platysma	Superficial fascia of deltoid and pectoral regions	Mandible, skin of cheek, angle of mouth, and orbicularis oris	Depresses mandible and tenses skin of lower face and neck
Mentalis	Incisive fossa of mandible	Skin of chin	Protrudes lower lip
Buccinator	Mandible, pterygomandibular raphe, and alveolar processes of maxilla and mandible	Angle of mouth	Presses cheek against molar teeth, thereby aiding chewing; expels air from oral cavity as occurs when playing a wind instrument

[a] All these muscles are supplied by the facial nerve (CN VII).

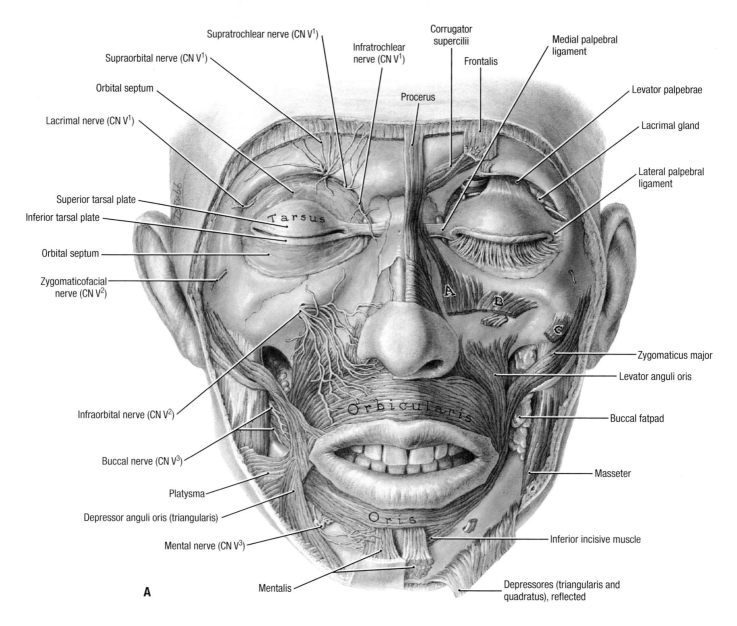

A. Face, anterior view.

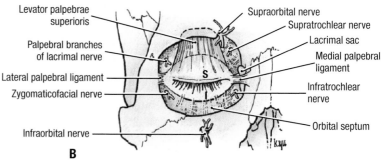

B. Orbital septum and eyelid, anterior view.

7.13 Cutaneous branches of trigeminal nerve, muscles of facial expression, and eyelid

A. Face, anterior view. **B.** Orbital septum and eyelid, anterior view.

OBSERVE:

1. The cutaneous branches of the ophthalmic (CN V1), maxillary (CN V2), and mandibular (CN V3) nerves;
2. Three sectional muscles: *A*, levator labii superioris alaeque nasi: *B*, levator labii superioris; and *C*, zygomaticus minor;
3. The buccal pad of fat fills the space between the buccinator medially and the ramus of the jaw and masseter laterally;
4. The medial palpebral ligament crosses anterior to the lacrimal gland and attaches the superior and inferior tarsal plates to the frontal process of the maxilla;
5. Diagram B shows the superior (*S*) and inferior (*I*) tarsal plates and their attachments. Their ciliary margins are free, but the peripheral margins are attached to the orbital septum;

6. The angles of the tarsal plates are anchored by medial and lateral palpebral ligaments;
7. The orbital septum is attached to the orbital margin, and medially passes posterior to the lacrimal sac to the crest of the lacrimal bone;
8. The fan-shaped aponeurosis of levator palpebrae superioris is attached to the anterior surface and superior edge of the superior tarsal plate.

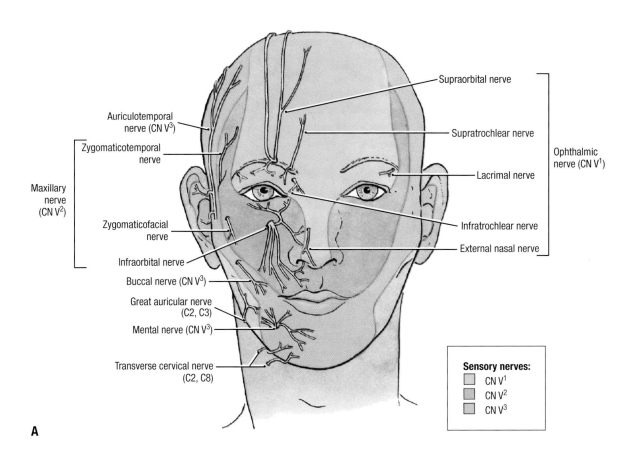

A

Sensory nerves:
- CN V^1
- CN V^2
- CN V^3

7.14 Sensory nerves of face and scalp

A. Anterior view. **B.** Superior view.

OBSERVE IN **A**:
1. The ophthalmic nerve supplies the area of the embryonic frontonasal prominence; the maxillary nerve (CN V2) supplies the maxillary prominence; and the mandibular nerve (CN V3) supplies the mandibular prominence. These nerves supply the whole thickness of the prominences, from skin to mucous surface, as far as the median plane (i.e., falx cerebri, nasal septum, and septum of tongue);
2. Branches of the supraorbital and auriculotemporal nerves extend posteriorly in the scalp;
3. The buccal nerve supplies the skin and mucous membrane of the cheek, reaching the angle of the mouth;
4. *Trigeminal neuralgia (tic douloureux) is a sensory disorder of the sensory division of the trigeminal nerve that is characterized by sudden attacks of excruciating facial pain. The cause is unknown, but may involve an anomalous blood vessel that compresses the nerve. The pain is often in the distribution of the mandibular division.*

OBSERVE IN **B**:
5. The arteries supplying the scalp anastomose freely; the supraorbital and supratrochlear arteries are derived from the internal carotid artery through the ophthalmic artery, and the superficial temporal, posterior auricular, and occipital arteries are branches of the external carotid artery;
6. *Hemorrhage from a scalp injury is often profuse because of the vascularity of the scalp and lack of constriction of the arterial vessels on injury. Because scalp arteries supply little blood to the bones of the calvaria (skull cap), loss of the scalp does not produce necrosis of the cranial bones;*

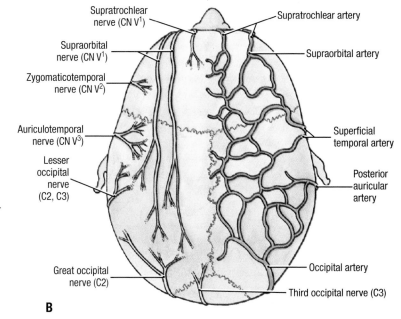

B

7. The nerves innervating the scalp appear in sequence: CN V1, CN V2, CN V3, lesser occiptal nerve (ventral primary rami of C2 and C3), and great and third occipital nerves (dorsal primary rami of C2 and C3); C1 has no cutaneous branch.

7.15 Surface anatomy of cranium, lateral view

The middle meningeal artery (*red*) and venous sinus (*blue*) were located on the external surface of the skull by drilling a series of holes from the interior of the skull along the grooves in which these structures lie.

OBSERVE:

1. The pterion is located two fingersbreadth superior to the zygomatic arch and one thumb breadth posterior to the frontal process of the zygomatic bone (approximately 4 cm superior to the midpoint of the zygomatic arch); the anterior branch of the middle meningeal artery crosses the pterion;

2. The supramastoid crest is located approximately at the level of the floor of the middle cranial fossa. A hole drilled inferior to the crest and superior to the suprameatal spine enters the mastoid (tympanic) antrum, whereas one drilled superior to the crest enters the middle cranial fossa;

3. The transverse (*T*) and sigmoid (*S*) sinuses.

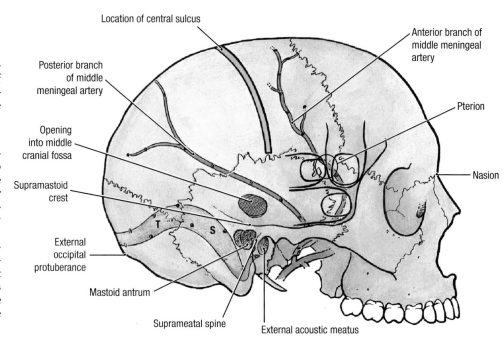

7.16 Diploic veins, lateral view

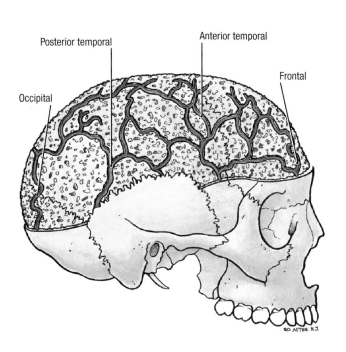

The outer layer of the compact bone of the skull has been filed away, exposing the channels for the diploic veins in the cancellous bone of the diploe.

OBSERVE:

1. The four (paired) diploic veins: the frontal opens into the supraorbital vein at the supraorbital notch; the anterior temporal opens into the sphenoparietal sinus; and the posterior temporal and occipital both open into the transverse sinus, although they may open into surface veins;

2. *Connections between intracranial and extracranial venous channels allow infection to travel freely among the scalp, skull, meninges, and brain;*

3. There are no accompanying diploic arteries.

7.17 Middle meningeal artery, sagittal section of skull

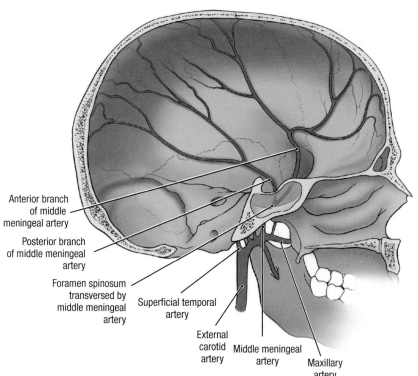

OBSERVE:

1. The middle meningeal artery passes anterolaterally in a groove in the petrous temporal bone and then divides into anterior and posterior branches;

2. *The anterior branch courses anterosuperiorly to reach the pterion, a site at which the artery is frequently torn, resulting in an extradural (epidural) hematoma;*

3. The posterior branch courses posteriorly over the squamous temporal and parietal bones.

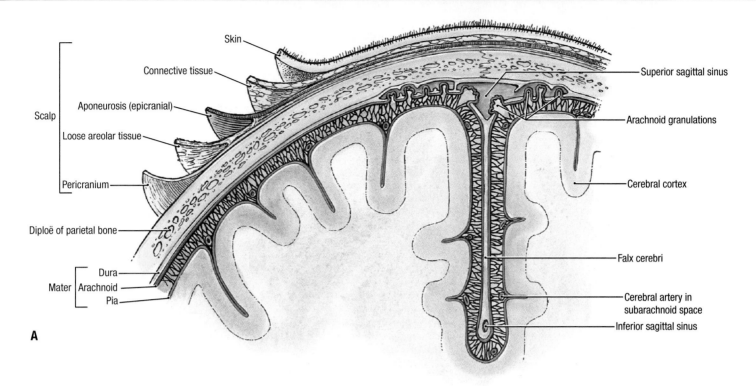

A

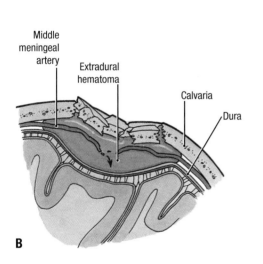

B

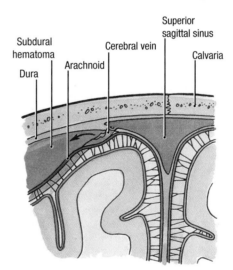

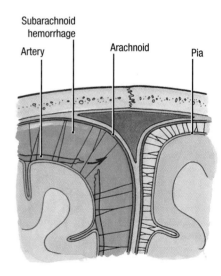

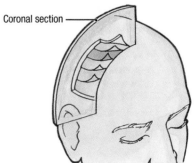

Coronal section

7.18

A. Scalp, skull, and meninges, coronal section. **B.** Intracranial hemorrhage, coronal sections.

OBSERVE IN **A:**

1. The layers of the meninges: the outer, tough dura mater encloses the venous sinuses; the arachnoid mater is in contact with the dura and bridges sulci on the cortical surface; and the most internal, delicate vascular membrane is the pia mater;

2. The three meningeal spaces: the extradural (epidural) space between the cranial bones and dura is a potential space (becomes a real space if blood accumulates in it); the potential subdural space is between the dura and arachnoid; and the subarachnoid space is between the arachnoid and pia, and contains cerebrospinal fluid;

OBSERVE IN **B:**

3. *Extradural (epidural) hematomas (left) result from bleeding from a torn middle meningeal artery; subdural hematomas (middle) commonly result* *from tearing of a cerebral vein as it enters the superior sagittal sinus; and subarachnoid hemorrhage (right) is caused by bleeding into the subarachnoid space, e.g., from rupture of an aneurysm.*

ANTERIOR

Outer layer of dura
Inner layer of dura
Arachnoid
Superior sagittal
sinus, opened

Branches
of middle
Anterior   meningeal
artery and
Posterior   vein

Opened to
show arachnoid   Lacuna
granulations   lateralis

Closed

POSTERIOR

7.19 External surface of dura mater and arachnoid granulations, superior view

The calvaria (skull cap) is removed. In the median plane, the thick roof of the superior sagittal sinus is partly pinned aside and, laterally, the thin roofs of two lacunae laterales are reflected.

OBSERVE:

1. On the right of the specimen, an angular flap of dura is turned anteriorly; the subdural space is thereby opened, and the convolutions of the cerebral cortex are visible through the arachnoid mater;
2. The middle meningeal artery lies in a venous channel (middle meningeal vein), which enlarges superiorly into the lacuna lateralis; a channel or channels drain the lacuna lateralis into the superior sagittal sinus;
3. Arachnoid granulations in the lacunae are responsible for absorption of cerebrospinal fluid from the subarachnoid space into the venous system.

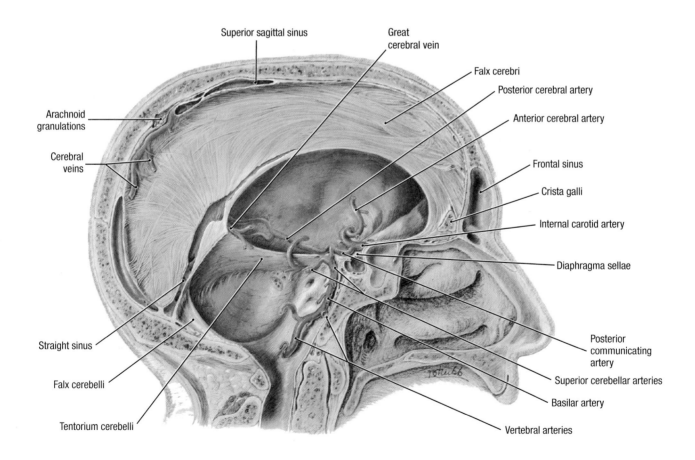

Superior sagittal sinus
Great
cerebral vein
Falx cerebri
Posterior cerebral artery
Anterior cerebral artery
Arachnoid
granulations
Frontal sinus
Cerebral
veins
Crista galli
Internal carotid artery
Diaphragma sellae
Posterior
communicating
artery
Straight sinus
Superior cerebellar arteries
Falx cerebelli
Basilar artery
Tentorium cerebelli
Vertebral arteries

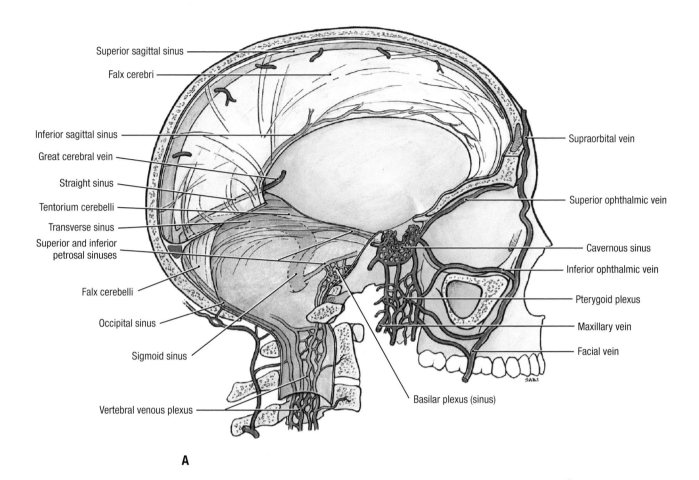

Superior sagittal sinus

Falx cerebri

Inferior sagittal sinus

Great cerebral vein

Straight sinus

Tentorium cerebelli

Transverse sinus

Superior and inferior petrosal sinuses

Falx cerebelli

Occipital sinus

Sigmoid sinus

Vertebral venous plexus

Supraorbital vein

Superior ophthalmic vein

Cavernous sinus

Inferior ophthalmic vein

Pterygoid plexus

Maxillary vein

Facial vein

Basilar plexus (sinus)

A

7.21 Venous sinuses of dura mater

A. Sagittal section of head. **B.** Anteroposterior venogram of sinuses. *C*, confluence of sinuses; *T*, transverse sinus; *S*, sigmoid sinus; *I*, internal jugular vein. **C.** Lateral venogram of sinuses.

OBSERVE:

1. The superior sagittal sinus is at the superior border of the falx cerebri, and the inferior sagittal sinus is in its free border. The great cerebral vein joins the inferior sagittal sinus to form the straight sinus, which runs obliquely in the junction between the falx cerebri and tentorium cerebelli. The occipital sinus is in the attached border of the falx cerebelli;

2. The superior sagittal sinus usually becomes the right transverse sinus, right sigmoid sinus, and right internal jugular vein; the straight sinus similarly drains into the left transverse sinus, which then continues into the left sigmoid sinus and left internal jugular vein;

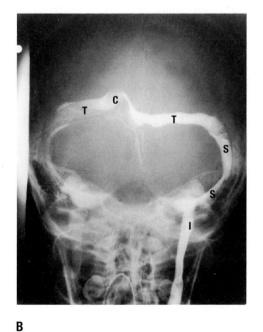

B

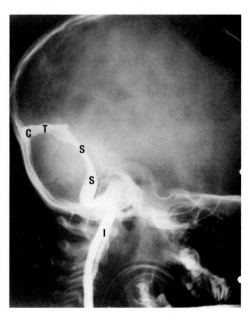

C

3. The cavernous sinus communicates with the veins of the face through the ophthalmic veins and pterygoid plexus of veins, and empties through the superior and inferior petrosal sinuses;

4. The basilar plexus (sinus) connects the inferior petrosal sinuses of the opposite sides and, like the occipital sinus, communicates inferiorly with the vertebral venous plexus.

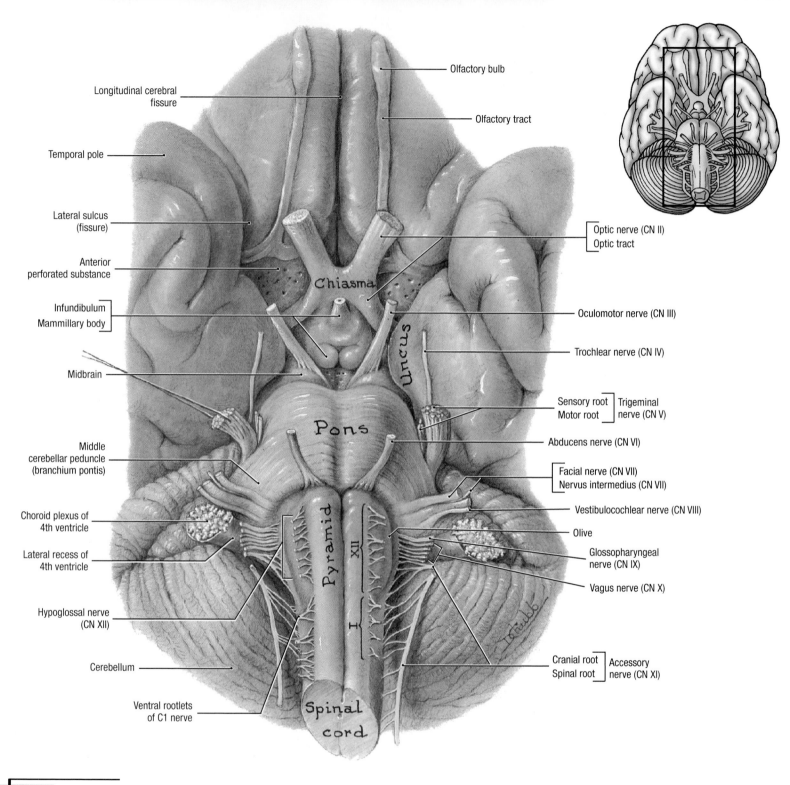

Olfactory bulb

Longitudinal cerebral fissure

Olfactory tract

Temporal pole

Optic nerve (CN II)
Optic tract

Lateral sulcus (fissure)

Anterior perforated substance

Chiasma

Infundibulum
Mammillary body

Oculomotor nerve (CN III)

Uncus

Trochlear nerve (CN IV)

Midbrain

Pons

Sensory root ⎤ Trigeminal
Motor root ⎦ nerve (CN V)

Abducens nerve (CN VI)

Middle cerebellar peduncle (branchium pontis)

Facial nerve (CN VII)
Nervus intermedius (CN VII)

Vestibulocochlear nerve (CN VIII)

Choroid plexus of 4th ventricle

Pyramid

Olive

Lateral recess of 4th ventricle

XII

Glossopharyngeal nerve (CN IX)

I

Vagus nerve (CN X)

Hypoglossal nerve (CN XII)

Cerebellum

Cranial root ⎤ Accessory
Spinal root ⎦ nerve (CN XI)

Ventral rootlets of C1 nerve

Spinal cord

7.22   Base of brain and superficial origins of cranial nerves

OBSERVE:
1. The locations of the 12 pairs of cranial nerves;
2. The olfactory nerves that end in the olfactory bulbs are not shown;
3. The rootlets of the hypoglossal nerve (CN XII) arise between the pyramid and the olive and are in line with the ventral rootlets of the 1st cervical nerve.

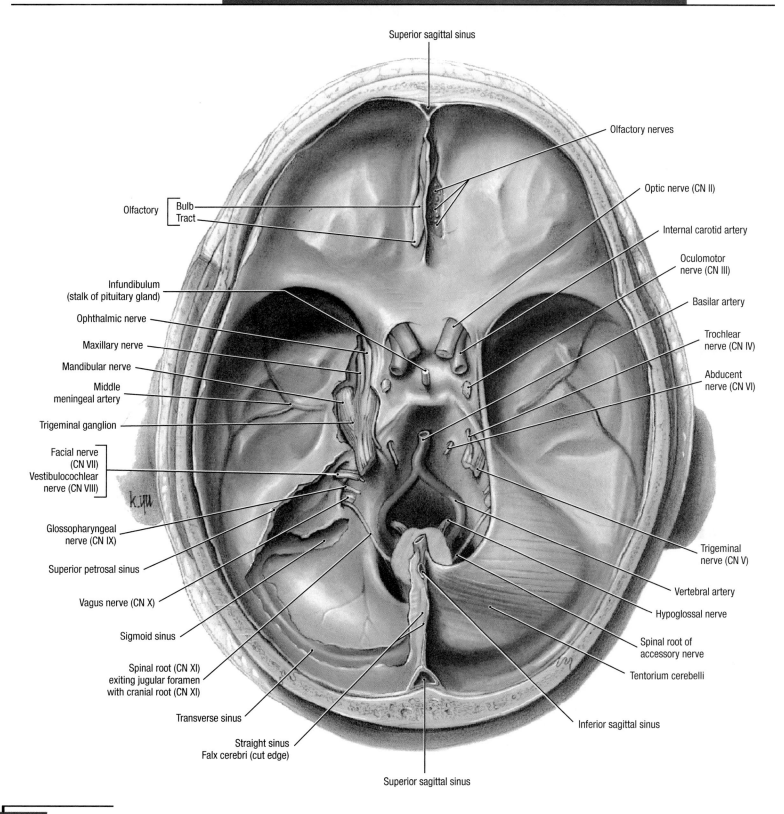

Superior sagittal sinus

Olfactory nerves

Optic nerve (CN II)

Olfactory { Bulb / Tract

Internal carotid artery

Infundibulum (stalk of pituitary gland)

Oculomotor nerve (CN III)

Ophthalmic nerve

Basilar artery

Maxillary nerve

Trochlear nerve (CN IV)

Mandibular nerve

Middle meningeal artery

Abducent nerve (CN VI)

Trigeminal ganglion

Facial nerve (CN VII)
Vestibulocochlear nerve (CN VIII)

k.yu

Glossopharyngeal nerve (CN IX)

Trigeminal nerve (CN V)

Superior petrosal sinus

Vagus nerve (CN X)

Vertebral artery

Hypoglossal nerve

Sigmoid sinus

Spinal root of accessory nerve

Spinal root (CN XI) exiting jugular foramen with cranial root (CN XI)

Tentorium cerebelli

Transverse sinus

Inferior sagittal sinus

Straight sinus
Falx cerebri (cut edge)

Superior sagittal sinus

7.23   **Nerves and vessels of the interior of base of skull, superior view**

OBSERVE:
1. On the left of the specimen, the dura mater is cut away to expose the trigeminal nerve, its three branches, and the sigmoid sinus; the tentorium cerebelli is removed to reveal the transverse and superior petrosal sinuses;

2. The frontal lobes are located in the anterior cranial fossa, the temporal lobes in the middle cranial fossa, and the brainstem and cerebellum in the posterior cranial fossa;
3. The location of the 12 cranial nerves and the internal carotid, vertebral, basilar, and middle meningeal arteries.

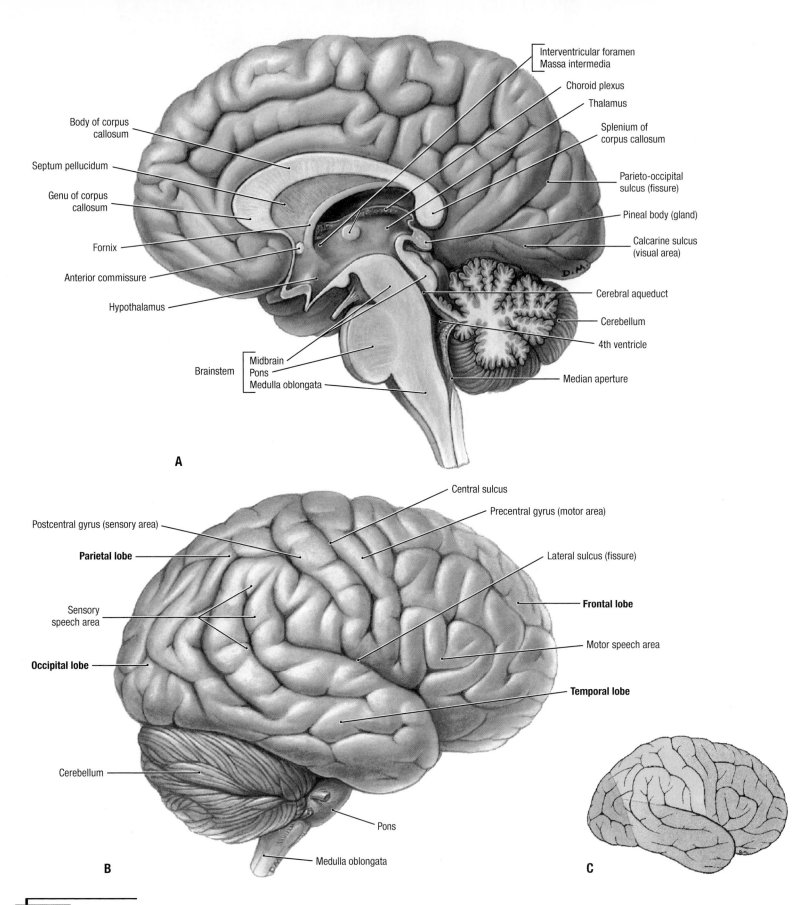

Body of corpus callosum

Septum pellucidum

Genu of corpus callosum

Fornix

Anterior commissure

Hypothalamus

Brainstem
{ Midbrain
Pons
Medulla oblongata

Interventricular foramen
Massa intermedia

Choroid plexus

Thalamus

Splenium of corpus callosum

Parieto-occipital sulcus (fissure)

Pineal body (gland)

Calcarine sulcus (visual area)

Cerebral aqueduct

Cerebellum

4th ventricle

Median aperture

A

Postcentral gyrus (sensory area)

Parietal lobe

Sensory speech area

Occipital lobe

Cerebellum

Central sulcus

Precentral gyrus (motor area)

Lateral sulcus (fissure)

Frontal lobe

Motor speech area

Temporal lobe

Pons

Medulla oblongata

B

C

7.24 Brain

A. Median section. **B.** Lateral view. **C.** Lobes of cerebral hemisphere, lateral view. The cerebrum can be divided into lobes in relation to the overlying cranial bones: frontal (*purple*), parietal (*orange*), occipital (*green*), and temporal (*blue*). Observe the cerebral cortex, consisting of gyri (folds) and sulci (grooves), the parts of the brainstem (medulla oblongata, pons, and midbrain), and the cerebellum.

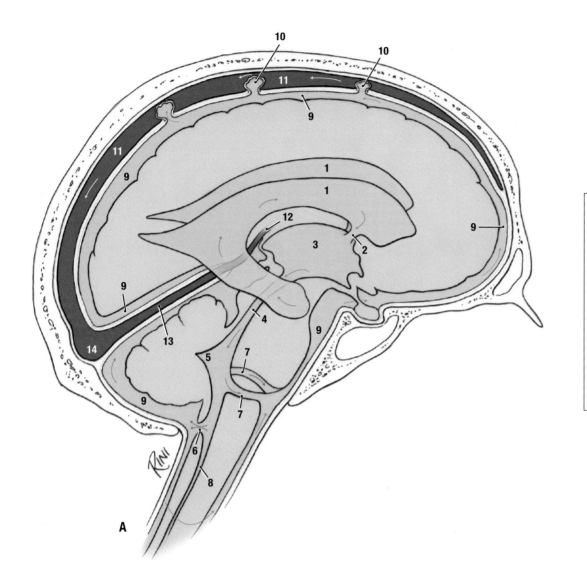

1.	Right and left lateral ventricles
2.	Interventricular foramen
3.	Third ventricle
4.	Cerebral aqueduct
5.	Fourth ventricle
6.	Median aperture
7.	Lateral apertures
8.	Central canal
9.	Subarachnoid space
10.	Arachnoid granulations
11.	Superior sagittal sinus
12.	Great cerebral vein
13.	Straight sinus
14.	Confluence of sinuses

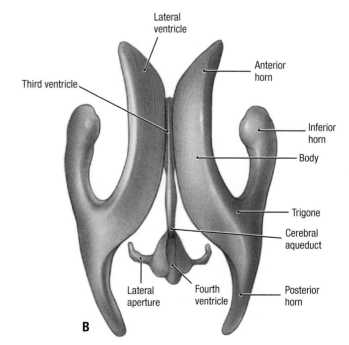

7.25   Ventricular system

A. Circulation of cerebrospinal fluid, lateral view. **B.** Ventricles, superior view.

OBSERVE:

1. The ventricular system consists of two lateral ventricles located in the cerebral hemispheres, a third ventricle located between the right and left halves of the diencephalon, and a fourth ventricle located in the posterior parts of the pons and medulla;
2. Cerebrospinal fluid (CSF) secreted by choroid plexus in the ventricles drains via the interventricular foramen from the lateral to third ventricle, via the cerebral aqueduct from the third to the fourth ventricle, and via median and lateral apertures into the subarachnoid space; CSF is absorbed by arachnoid granulations into the venous sinuses (especially superior sagittal sinus).

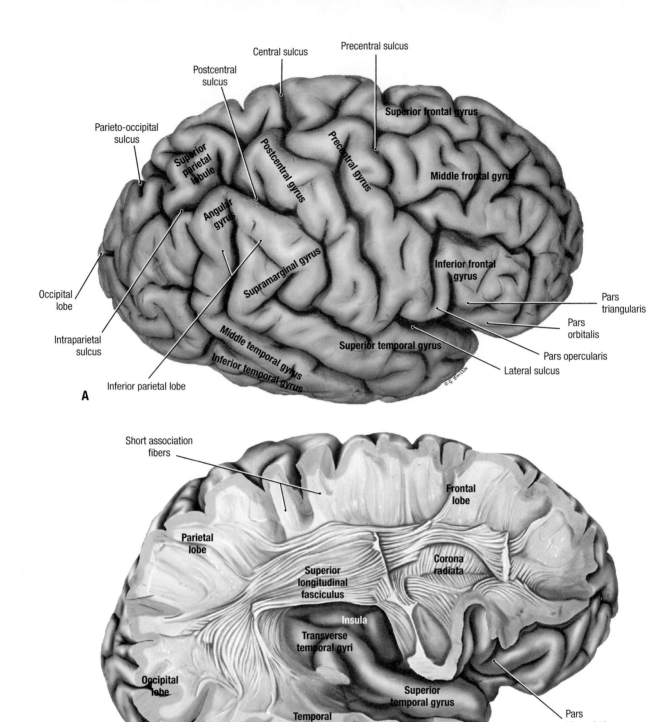

A. Sulci and gyri of the lateral surface of the cerebral hemisphere.

Labels in A (clockwise):
Postcentral sulcus · Central sulcus · Precentral sulcus · Superior frontal gyrus · Middle frontal gyrus · Inferior frontal gyrus · Pars triangularis · Pars orbitalis · Pars opercularis · Lateral sulcus · Superior temporal gyrus · Inferior temporal gyrus · Middle temporal gyrus · Inferior parietal lobe · Intraparietal sulcus · Occipital lobe · Parieto-occipital sulcus · Superior parietal lobule · Postcentral gyrus · Precentral gyrus · Angular gyrus · Supramarginal gyrus

Labels in B:
Short association fibers · Frontal lobe · Parietal lobe · Corona radiata · Superior longitudinal fasciculus · Insula · Transverse temporal gyri · Occipital lobe · Temporal lobe · Superior temporal gyrus · Pars triangularis

7.26 Serial dissections of lateral aspect of cerebral hemisphere, lateral views

The dissections begin from the lateral surface of the cerebral hemisphere (A) and proceed sequentially medially (**B** to **F**).
A. Sulci and gyri of the lateral surface of the cerebral hemisphere. Each gyrus is a fold of cerebral cortex with a core of white matter. The furrows are called sulci. The pattern of sulci and gyri formed shortly before birth is recognizable in some adult brains, as shown in this specimen. Usually the expanding cortex acquires secondary foldings, which make identification of this basic pattern more difficult. **B.** Superior longitudinal fasciculus, transverse temporal gyri, and insula. The cortex and short association fiber bundles around the lateral fissure have been removed.

OBSERVE IN **B**:
1. The superior longitudinal fasciculus, a long association fiber bundle, interconnects the cortices of the frontal, parietal, and occipital lobes; the inferior part, called the arcuate fasciculus, links the frontal and temporal lobes;
2. The transverse temporal gyrus is located on the inferior wall of the lateral sulcus;
3. The insula, an island of cortex, is situated in the floor of the lateral sulcus.

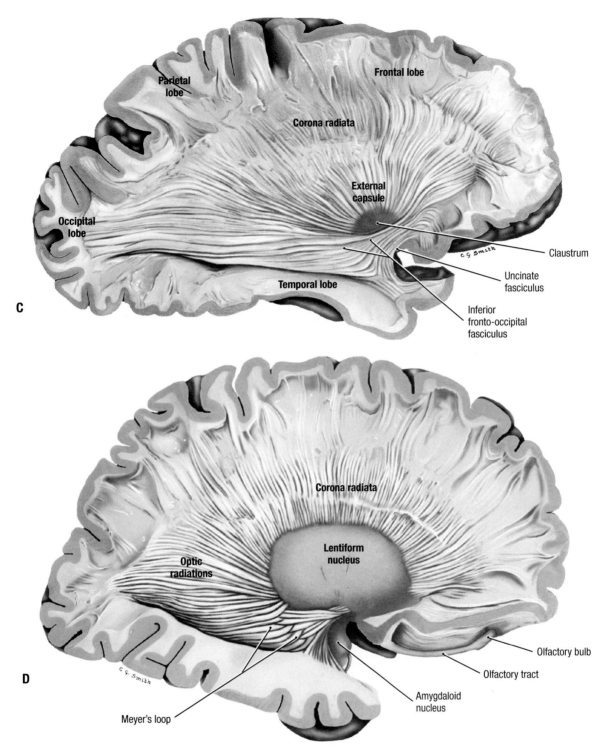

C. Uncinate and inferior fronto-occipital fasciculi and external capsule. **D.** Lentiform nucleus and corona radiata. The inferior longitudinal and uncinate fasciculi, claustrum, and external capsule have been removed. **E.** Caudate and amygdaloid nuclei and internal capsule. The lateral wall of the lateral ventricle, the marginal part of the internal capsule, the anterior commissure, and the superior part of the lentiform nucleus have been removed. **F.** Lateral ventricle, hippocampus and diencephalon. The inferior part of the lentiform nucleus, internal capsule, and caudate nucleus have been removed.

OBSERVE IN **C:**
4. The uncinate fasciculus connects the frontal and temporal lobes, and the inferior frontooccipital fasciculus connects the frontal, temporal, and occipital lobes;
5. The external capsule consists of projection fibers that pass between the claustrum laterally and the lentiform nucleus medially.

OBSERVE IN **D:**
6. The corona radiata is a crown-like ridge of projection fibers that connects the higher and lower levels of the central nervous system;
7. The fibers of the optic radiations convey impulses from the right half of the retina of each eye; the fibers extending closest to the temporal pole (Meyer's loop) carry impulses from the lower portion of each retina; the anterior commissure connecting the right and left temporal lobes.

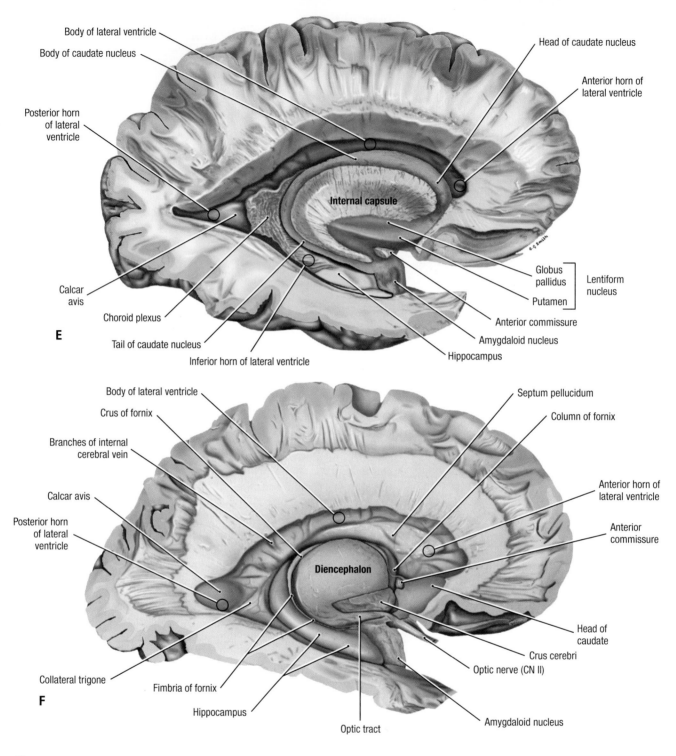

Body of lateral ventricle

Body of caudate nucleus

Head of caudate nucleus

Anterior horn of lateral ventricle

Posterior horn of lateral ventricle

Internal capsule

Globus pallidus ⎤
　　　　　　　⎬ Lentiform nucleus
Putamen ⎦

Calcar avis

Choroid plexus

Tail of caudate nucleus

Inferior horn of lateral ventricle

Anterior commissure

Amygdaloid nucleus

Hippocampus

E

Body of lateral ventricle

Crus of fornix

Septum pellucidum

Column of fornix

Branches of internal cerebral vein

Calcar avis

Anterior horn of lateral ventricle

Posterior horn of lateral ventricle

Diencephalon

Anterior commissure

Head of caudate

Crus cerebri

Optic nerve (CN II)

Collateral trigone

Fimbria of fornix

Hippocampus

Optic tract

Amygdaloid nucleus

F

OBSERVE IN **E:**

8. The internal capsule lies medial, posterior, and inferior to the lentiform nucleus; the lentiform nucleus consists of the putamen laterally and globus pallidus medially; at the tip of the inferior horn of the lateral ventricle, the caudate nucleus connects to the amygdaloid nucleus.

9. The caudate nucleus, a C-shaped mass of gray matter, extends posteriorly, medial to the fibers of the internal capsule; here, it forms a part of the wall of the anterior horn, the body and roof of the inferior horn of the lateral ventricle;

OBSERVE IN **F:**

10. The hippocampus lies in the inferior horn of the lateral ventricle;

11. The fornix forms medial to the hippocampus (fimbria of fornix), courses along the medial border of the hippocampus to reach the midline, turns anteriorly along the inferior margin of the septum pellucidum, and enters the diencephalon just anterior to the interventicular foramen to terminate in the mammillary bodies;

12. The calcar avis is an elevation in the posterior horn of the lateral ventricle, produced by the calcarine sulcus on the medial surface of the brain.

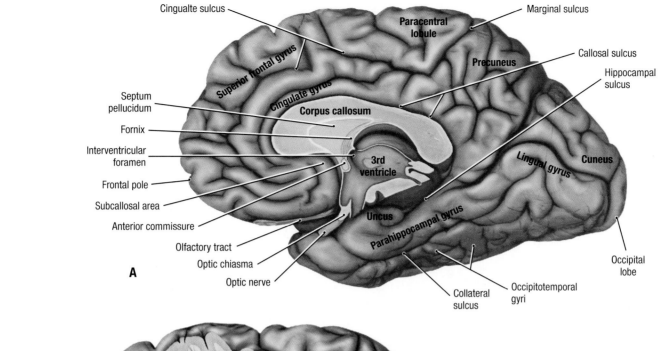

A

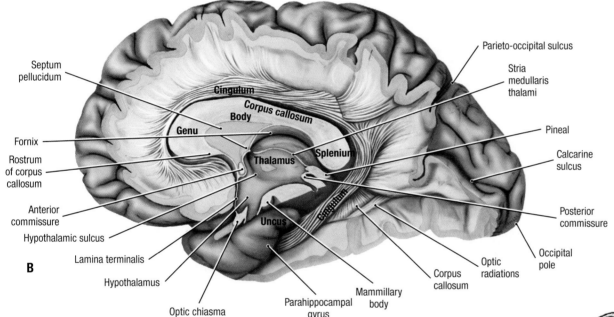

B

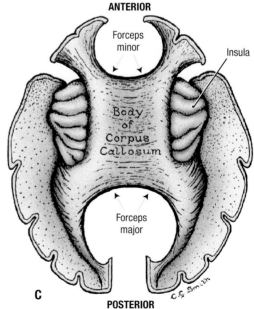

ANTERIOR

Forceps minor

Insula

Body of Corpus Callosum

Forceps major

C

POSTERIOR

7.27 Serial dissections of medial aspect of cerebral hemisphere

The dissections begin from the medial surface of the cerebral hemisphere (**A**) and proceed sequentially laterally (**B, D,** and **E**).
A. Sulci and gyri of medial surface of cerebral hemisphere, medial veiw. **B.** Cingulum, medial view. The cortex and short-association fibers were removed from the medial aspect of the hemisphere **C.** Corpus callosum, superior view. The body of the corpus callosum connects the two cerebral hemispheres; the forceps minor (at genu of corpus callosum) connects the frontal lobes, and the forceps minor (at splenium) connects the occipital lobes.

OBSERVE IN **A:**

1. The corpus callosum consisting of the rostrum, genu, body, and splenium;
3. The cingulate and parahippocampal gyri from the limbic lobe;
4. The paracentral lobule uniting the precentral and postcentral gyri around the end of the central sulcus.

OBSERVE IN **B:**

5. The cingulum is a long-association fiber bundle that lies in the core of the cingulate and parahippocampal gyri;
6. The wall of the third ventricle is formed by the thalamus and hypothalmus.

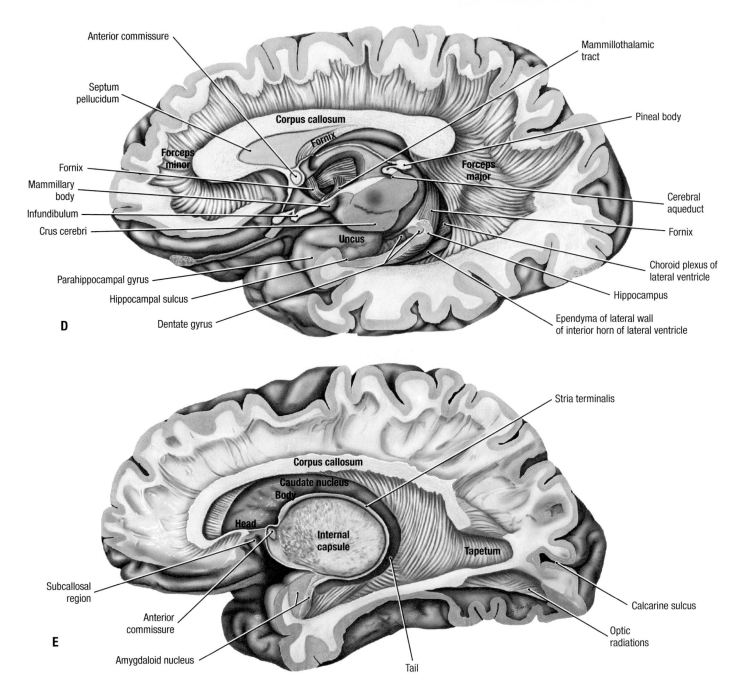

D. Fornix, mamillothalamic tract, and forceps major and minor, medial view. The cingulum and a portion of the wall of the third ventricle have been removed. **E.** Caudate nucleus and internal capsule, medial view. The diencephalon was removed, along with the ependyma of the lateral ventricle, except where it covers the caudate and amygdaloid nuclei.

OBSERVE IN **D:**

7. The forceps major and minor are the anterior and posterior portions of the corpus callosum, respectively;
8. The fornix begins at the hippocampus and terminates in the mammillary body; the fornix passes anterior to the interventricular foramen posterior to the anterior commissure;
9. The mamillothalamic tract emerges from the mammillary body and terminates in the anterior nucleus of the thalamus.

OBSERVE IN **E:**

10. The head, body, and tail of the caudate nucleus; the continuity of the caudate nucleus with the amygdaloid nucleus;
11. The amygdaloid nucleus extends anterior to the inferior horn of the lateral ventricle to form part of the uncus;
12. The tapetum, fibers of the corpus callsum, lines the wall of the posterior and inferior horns of the lateral ventricle;
13. The stria terminalis conveys impulses from the amygdaloid nucleus to the hypothalamus;

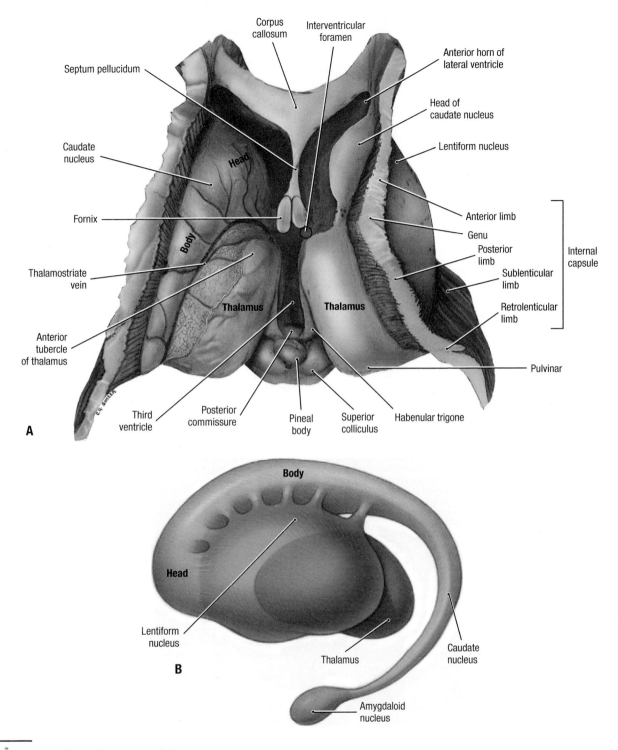

Corpus callosum

Interventricular foramen

Septum pellucidum

Anterior horn of lateral ventricle

Head of caudate nucleus

Caudate nucleus

Head

Lentiform nucleus

Fornix

Body

Anterior limb

Genu

Posterior limb

Internal capsule

Sublenticular limb

Thalamostriate vein

Retrolenticular limb

Thalamus

Thalamus

Anterior tubercle of thalamus

Pulvinar

A

Third ventricle

Posterior commissure

Pineal body

Superior colliculus

Habenular trigone

Body

Head

Lentiform nucleus

Thalamus

Caudate nucleus

B

Amygdaloid nucleus

7.28 Caudate and lentiform nuclei

A. Relationship to the lateral ventricles and internal capsule, posterosuperior view. The dorsal surface of the diencephalon has been exposed by dissecting away the two cerebral hemispheres, except the anterior part of the corpus callosum, the inferior part of the septum pellucidum, the internal capsule, and the caudate and lentiform nuclei. On the right side of the specimen, the thalamus, caudate, and lentiform nuclei have been cut horizontally at the level of the interventricular foramen. **B.** Schematic illustration of nuclei, lateral view.

OBSERVE IN **A**:
1. The interventricular foramen lies between the anterior tubercle (anterior nucleus) of the thalamus and fornix;
2. The pulvinar is the posterior portion of the thalamus that projects posteriorly;
3. The head of the caudate nucleus, corpus callosum, and septum pellucidum forms the walls of the anterior horn of the lateral ventricle;
4. The parts of the internal capsule: anterior, posterior, retrolenticular sublenticular limbs, and genu.

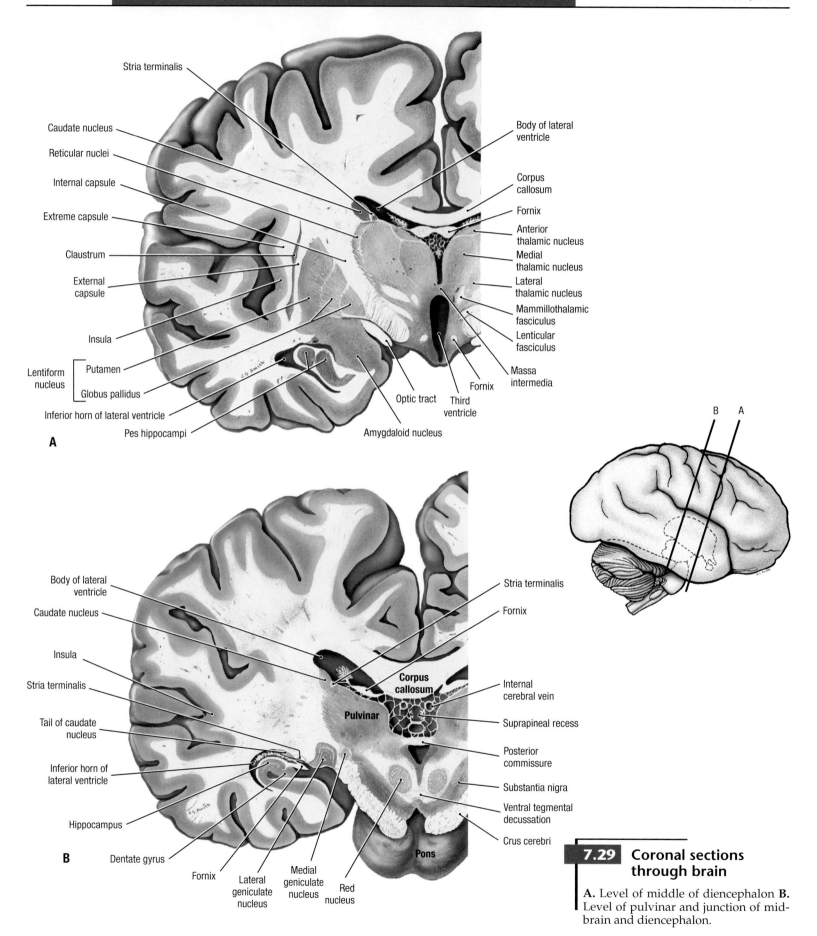

A.

Stria terminalis

Caudate nucleus

Reticular nuclei

Internal capsule

Extreme capsule

Claustrum

External capsule

Insula

Lentiform nucleus { Putamen — Globus pallidus }

Inferior horn of lateral ventricle

Pes hippocampi

Body of lateral ventricle

Corpus callosum

Fornix

Anterior thalamic nucleus

Medial thalamic nucleus

Lateral thalamic nucleus

Mammillothalamic fasciculus

Lenticular fasciculus

Massa intermedia

Fornix

Third ventricle

Optic tract

Amygdaloid nucleus

B.

Body of lateral ventricle

Caudate nucleus

Insula

Stria terminalis

Tail of caudate nucleus

Inferior horn of lateral ventricle

Hippocampus

Dentate gyrus

Fornix

Lateral geniculate nucleus

Medial geniculate nucleus

Red nucleus

Stria terminalis

Fornix

Corpus callosum

Pulvinar

Internal cerebral vein

Suprapineal recess

Posterior commissure

Substantia nigra

Ventral tegmental decussation

Crus cerebri

Pons

B   A

7.29   Coronal sections through brain

A. Level of middle of diencephalon **B.** Level of pulvinar and junction of midbrain and diencephalon.

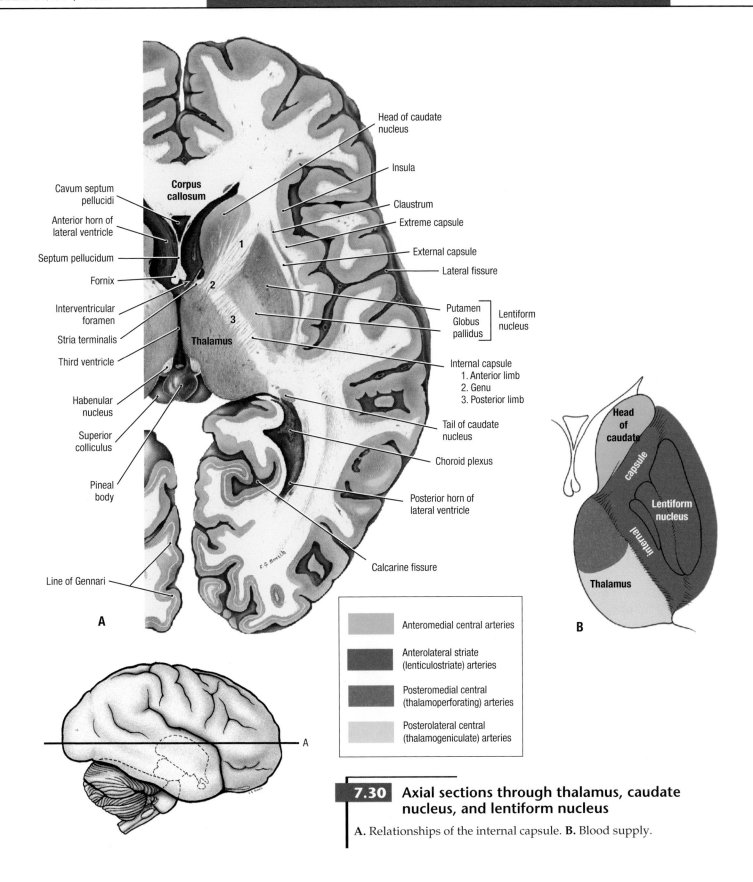

7.30 **Axial sections through thalamus, caudate nucleus, and lentiform nucleus**

A. Relationships of the internal capsule. **B.** Blood supply.

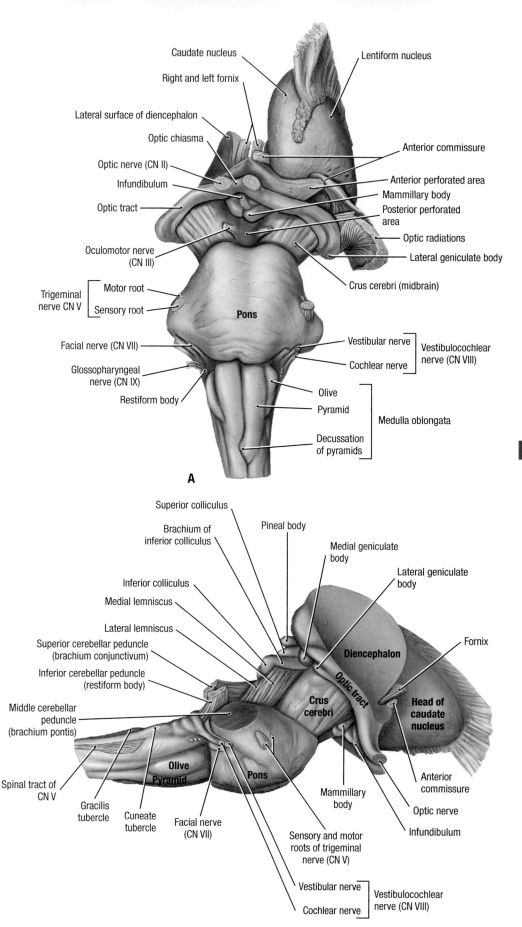

Caudate nucleus

Lentiform nucleus

Right and left fornix

Lateral surface of diencephalon

Optic chiasma

Anterior commissure

Optic nerve (CN II)

Anterior perforated area

Infundibulum

Mammillary body

Optic tract

Posterior perforated area

Optic radiations

Oculomotor nerve (CN III)

Lateral geniculate body

Crus cerebri (midbrain)

Trigeminal nerve CN V — Motor root / Sensory root

Pons

Facial nerve (CN VII)

Vestibular nerve

Cochlear nerve

Vestibulocochlear nerve (CN VIII)

Glossopharyngeal nerve (CN IX)

Restiform body

Olive

Pyramid

Medulla oblongata

Decussation of pyramids

A

Superior colliculus

Brachium of inferior colliculus

Pineal body

Medial geniculate body

Lateral geniculate body

Inferior colliculus

Medial lemniscus

Lateral lemniscus

Superior cerebellar peduncle (brachium conjunctivum)

Inferior cerebellar peduncle (restiform body)

Middle cerebellar peduncle (brachium pontis)

Spinal tract of CN V

Gracilis tubercle

Cuneate tubercle

Facial nerve (CN VII)

Sensory and motor roots of trigeminal nerve (CN V)

Vestibular nerve

Cochlear nerve

Vestibulocochlear nerve (CN VIII)

Diencephalon

Fornix

Optic tract

Crus cerebri

Head of caudate nucleus

Olive

Pyramid

Pons

Anterior commissure

Mammillary body

Optic nerve

Infundibulum

B

7.31   Brainstem

The brainstem has been exposed by removing the cerebellum, all of the right cerebral hemisphere, and the major portion of the left hemisphere.

A. Ventral aspect. **B.** Lateral aspect. **C.** Posterior aspect.

OBSERVE IN **A:**
1. The brainstem consists of the medulla oblongata, pons, and midbrain;
2. The pyramid is on the ventral surface of the medulla; the decussation of the pyramids is formed by the decussating (crossing) lateral corticospinal tract;
3. The trigeminal nerve (CN V) consists of sensory and motor tract;
4. The crus cerebri of the midbrain; the oculomotor nerve emerges from the interpeduncular fossa.

OBSERVE IN **B:**
5. The vestibulocochlear nerve (CN VIII) has two parts: the vestibular and cochlear parts;
6. The spinal tract of the trigeminal nerve is exposed where it comes to the surface of the medulla to form the tuberculum cinereum;
7. The three cerebellar peduncles: superior, middle, and inferior;
8. The medial and lateral lemnisci on the lateral aspect of the midbrain.

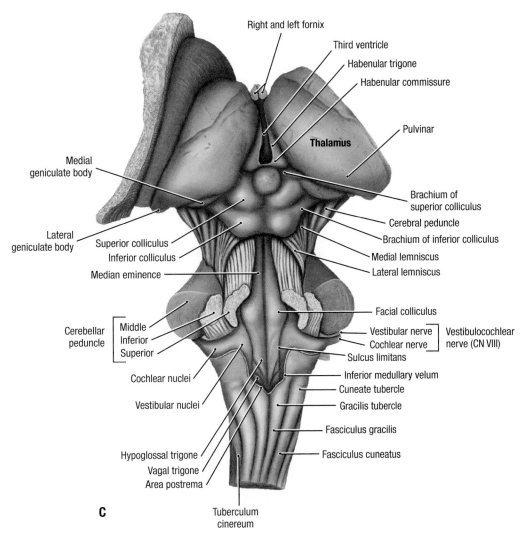

Right and left fornix

Third ventricle

Habenular trigone

Habenular commissure

Pulvinar

Thalamus

Medial geniculate body

Brachium of superior colliculus

Cerebral peduncle

Brachium of inferior colliculus

Lateral geniculate body

Superior colliculus

Inferior colliculus

Median eminence

Medial lemniscus

Lateral lemniscus

Facial colliculus

Cerebellar peduncle

Middle
Inferior
Superior

Vestibular nerve
Cochlear nerve

Vestibulocochlear nerve (CN VIII)

Sulcus limitans

Cochlear nuclei

Inferior medullary velum

Cuneate tubercle

Vestibular nuclei

Gracilis tubercle

Fasciculus gracilis

Hypoglossal trigone

Fasciculus cuneatus

Vagal trigone

Area postrema

C

Tuberculum cinereum

OBSERVE IN **C**:
  9. Ridges are formed by the fasciculus gracilis and cuneatus;
 10. The gracilis and cuneate tubercles are the site of the nucleus cuneatus and nucleus gracilis;
 11. The diamond-shaped floor of the fourth ventricle; lateral to the sulcus limitans are the vestibular and cochlear nuclei and medially are the hypoglossal and vagal trigones and the facial colliculus;
 12. The superior and inferior colliculi form the dorsal surface of the midbrain;

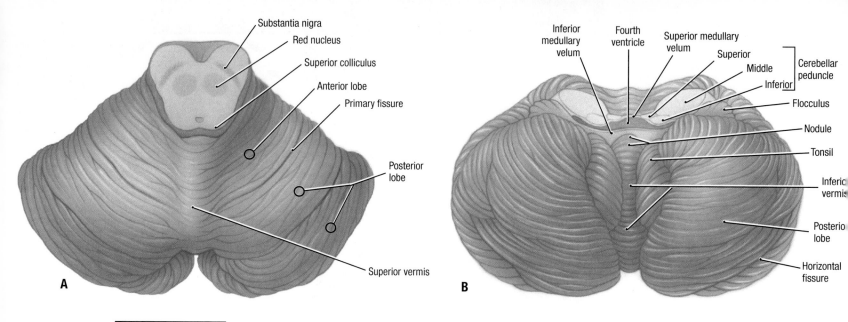

A. Superior view.
- Substantia nigra
- Red nucleus
- Superior colliculus
- Anterior lobe
- Primary fissure
- Posterior lobe
- Superior vermis

B. Inferior view.
- Inferior medullary velum
- Fourth ventricle
- Superior medullary velum
- Superior
- Middle
- Inferior
- Cerebellar peduncle
- Flocculus
- Nodule
- Tonsil
- Inferior vermis
- Posterior lobe
- Horizontal fissure

7.32   **Cerebellum**

A. Superior view. **B.** Inferior view.

OBSERVE:
1. In **A**, the right and left cerebellar hemispheres are united by the superior vermis; the anterior and posterior lobes are separated by the primary fissure;
2. In **B**, the flocculonodular lobe, the oldest part of the cerebellum, consists of the flocculus and nodule; *the cerebellar tonsils, on herniation through the foramen magun, compress the medulla.*

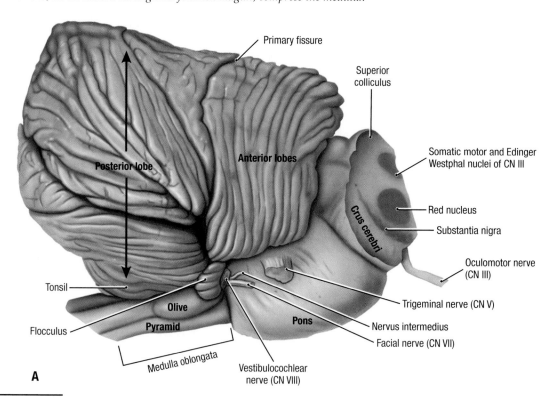

- Primary fissure
- Superior colliculus
- Posterior lobe
- Anterior lobes
- Somatic motor and Edinger Westphal nuclei of CN III
- Crus cerebri
- Red nucleus
- Substantia nigra
- Oculomotor nerve (CN III)
- Trigeminal nerve (CN V)
- Tonsil
- Olive
- Pyramid
- Pons
- Nervus intermedius
- Flocculus
- Facial nerve (CN VII)
- Medulla oblongata
- Vestibulocochlear nerve (CN VIII)

A

7.33   **Serial dissections of the cerebellum, lateral views**

The dissection begin from the lateral surface of the cerebellar hemispheres (**A**) and proceed sequentially medially (**B** to **D**).

A. Cerebellum and brainstem. Note the anterior and posterior lobes separated by the primary fissure, the flocculus, and the relationship of the cerebellar tonsil to the medulla. **B.** Middle cerebellar peduncle. The fibers of the middle cerebellar peduncle were exposed by peeling away the lateral portion of the lobules of the cerebellar hemisphere.

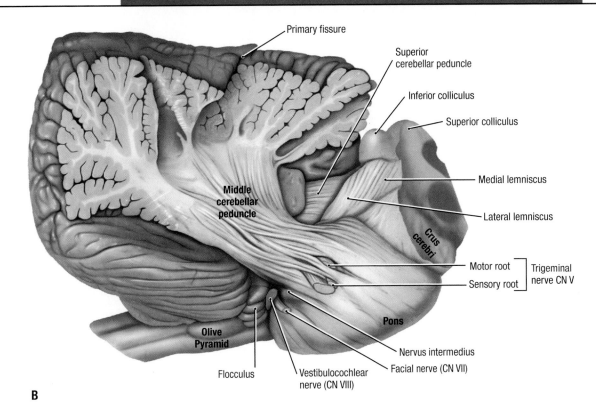

B

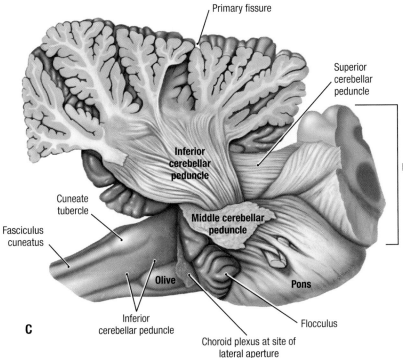

C

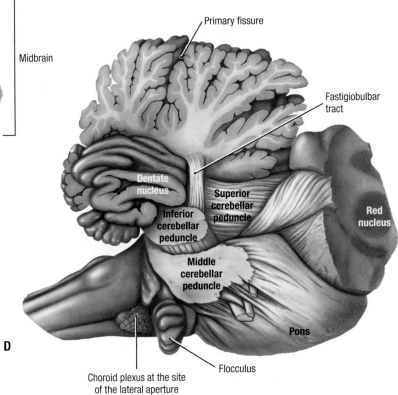

D

C. Inferior cerebellar peduncle. The fibers of the middle cerebellar peduncle were cut dorsal to the trigeminal nerve and peeled away to expose the fibers of the inferior cerebellar peduncle. **D.** Superior cerebellar peduncle and dentate nucleus. The fibers of the inferior cerebellar peduncle were cut just dorsal to the perviously sectioned middle peduncle and peeled away until the gray matter of the dentate nucleus could be seen. The dentate nucleus was then completely uncovered, and its deep longitudinal furrows were revealed. In carrying out this dissection, all of the lobules of the hemisphere were removed.

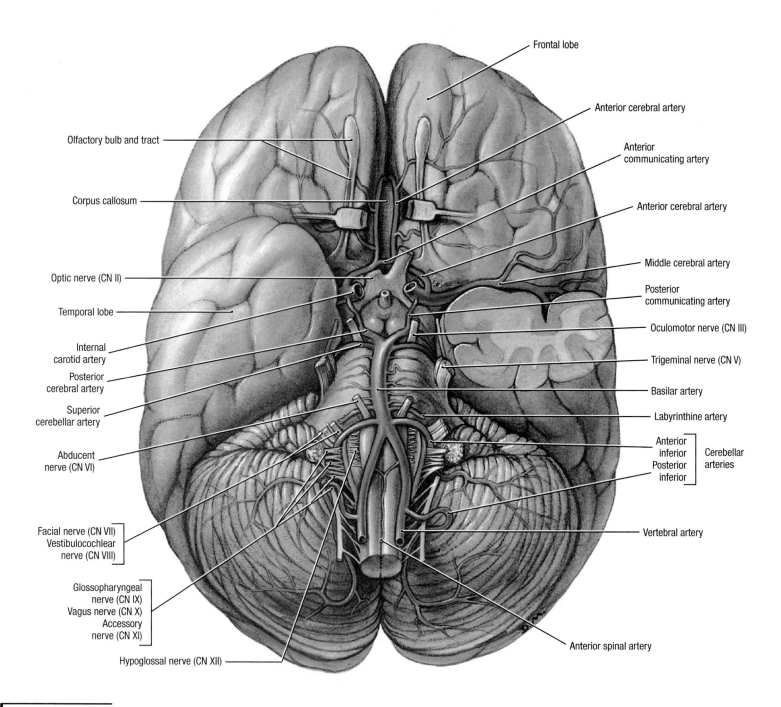

Frontal lobe

Anterior cerebral artery

Anterior communicating artery

Anterior cerebral artery

Middle cerebral artery

Posterior communicating artery

Oculomotor nerve (CN III)

Trigeminal nerve (CN V)

Basilar artery

Labyrinthine artery

Anterior inferior

Posterior inferior
} Cerebellar arteries

Vertebral artery

Anterior spinal artery

Olfactory bulb and tract

Corpus callosum

Optic nerve (CN II)

Temporal lobe

Internal carotid artery

Posterior cerebral artery

Superior cerebellar artery

Abducent nerve (CN VI)

Facial nerve (CN VII)
Vestibulocochlear nerve (CN VIII)

Glossopharyngeal nerve (CN IX)
Vagus nerve (CN X)
Accessory nerve (CN XI)

Hypoglossal nerve (CN XII)

7.34   Base of brain and cerebral arterial circle, ventral view

The left temporal pole is removed to enable visualization of the middle cerebral artery in the lateral fissure. The frontal lobes are separated to expose the anterior cerebral arteries and corpus callosum.

OBSERVE:
1. Three arterial stems ascend to supply the brain: the right and left internal carotids and the basilar artery, which results from the union of the two vertebral arteries. These three stems form an arterial cir-

cle (the circle of Willis) at the base of the brain. The cerebral arterial circle is formed by the posterior cerebral, posterior communicating, internal carotid, anterior cerebral, and anterior communicating arteries. Variations in the size of the vessels that form the circle are common;
2. The cerebellum is mainly supplied by branches from the vertebral and basilar arteries.

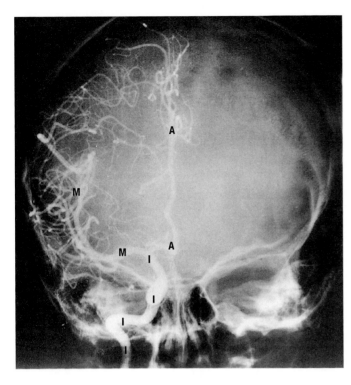

A

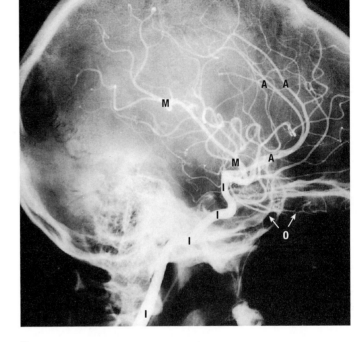

B

7.35   Arteriograms

A. Carotid arteriogram, posteroanterior view. **B.** Carotid arteriogram, lateral view. **C.** Vertebral arteriogram, lateral view.

OBSERVE IN **A** AND **B**:
1. The four letter *I*'s indicate the parts of the internal carotid artery: cervical, before entering the skull; petrous, within the temporal bone; cavernous, within that venous sinus; and cerebral, within the cranial subarachnoid space;
2. The anterior cerebral artery and its branches (*A*); the middle cerebral artery and its branches (*M*); and the ophthalmic artery (*O*).

OBSERVE IN **C**:
3. The vertebral artery curves to lie in contact with the posterior arch of the atlas before its passage through the dura mater (*1*);
4. The vertebral artery enters the skull through the foramen magnum within the subarachnoid space (*2*);
5. The posterior inferior cerebellar artery (*3*);
6. The anterior inferior cerebellar artery (*4*);
7. The basilar artery, formed by the union of the right and left vertebral arteries (*5*);
8. The superior cerebellar artery (*6*);
9. The posterior cerebral artery, with branches going to the occipital and temporal lobes (*7*);
10. The posterior communicating arteries (*8*).

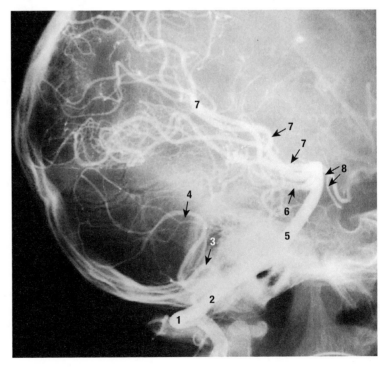

C

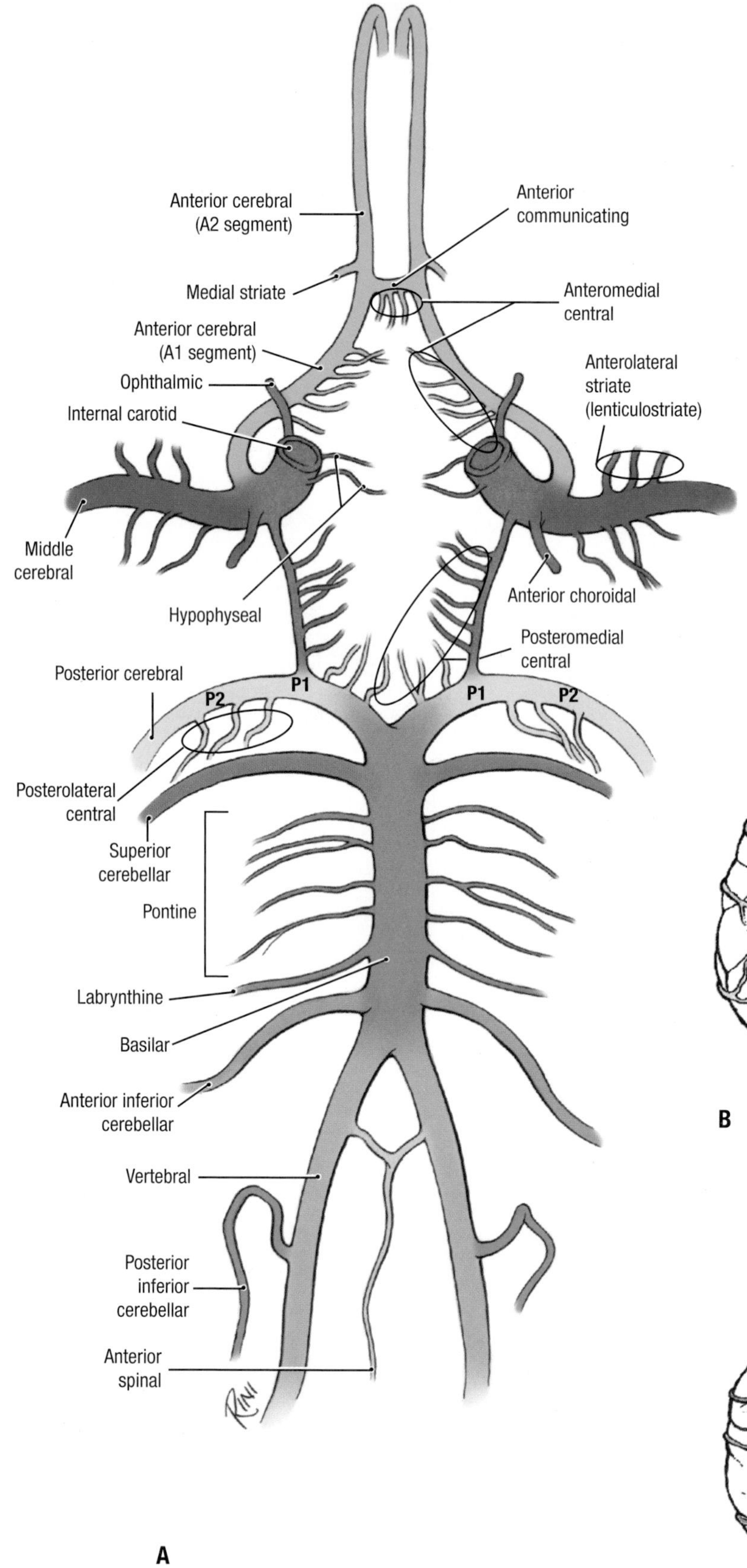

Anterior cerebral
(A2 segment)

Anterior
communicating

Medial striate

Anteromedial
central

Anterior cerebral
(A1 segment)

Ophthalmic

Anterolateral
striate
(lenticulostriate)

Internal carotid

Middle
cerebral

Hypophyseal

Anterior choroidal

Posteromedial
central

Posterior cerebral

P1   P1   P2

P2

Posterolateral
central

Superior
cerebellar

Pontine

Labrynthine

Basilar

Anterior inferior
cerebellar

Vertebral

Posterior
inferior
cerebellar

Anterior
spinal

A

7.36 Blood supply of cerebral hemispheres

A. Cerebral arterial circle (of Willis), ventral view. **B.** Cerebral hemisphere, lateral view. **C.** Cerebral hemisphere, medial view. Blood is supplied to the cerebral hemispheres by the anterior and middle cerebral arteries from the internal carotids and the posterior cerebral arteries from the basilar. In these schematic diagrams, the general areas of supply are shown for the three cerebral arteries: anterior (*green*), middle (*purple*), and posterior (*yellow*).

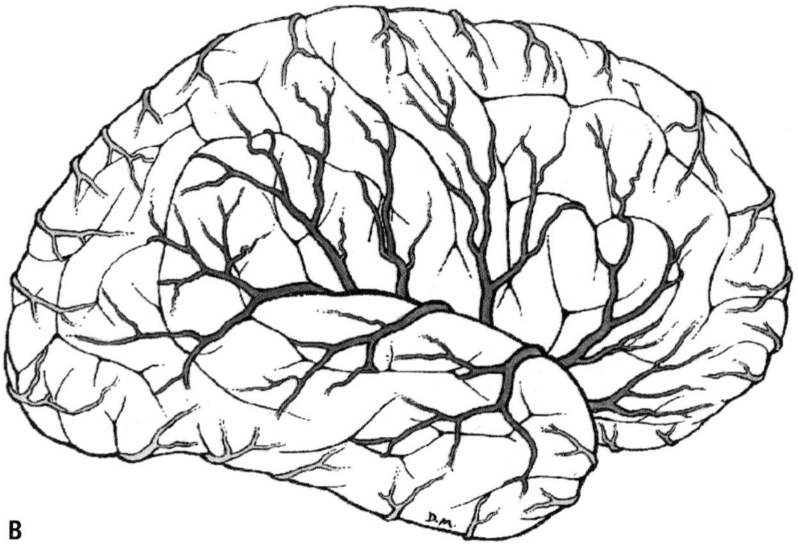

B

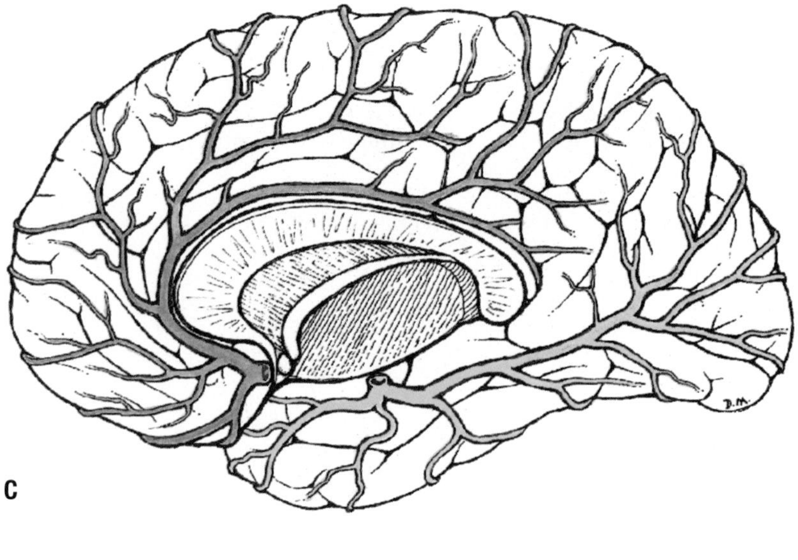

C

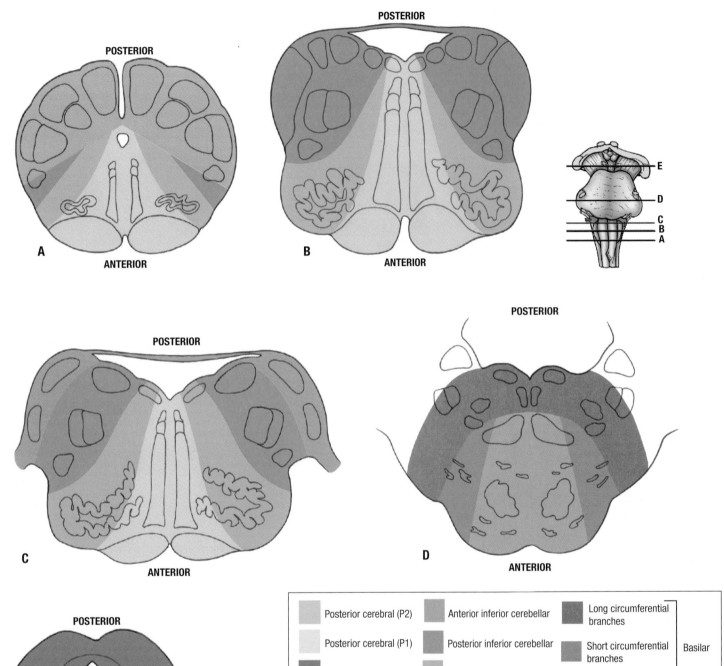

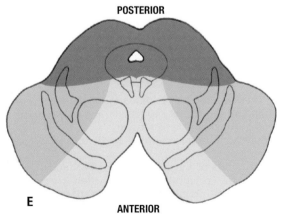

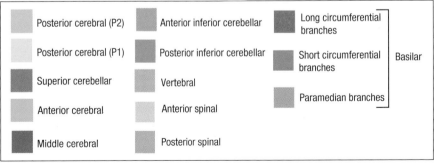

Posterior cerebral (P2)

Posterior cerebral (P1)

Superior cerebellar

Anterior cerebral

Middle cerebral

Anterior inferior cerebellar

Posterior inferior cerebellar

Vertebral

Anterior spinal

Posterior spinal

Long circumferential branches

Short circumferential branches

Paramedian branches

Basilar

7.37   **Blood supply to brainstem, horizontal sections**

A. Lower medulla. **B.** Middle medulla. **C.** Upper medulla. **D.** Pons. **E.** Midbrain.

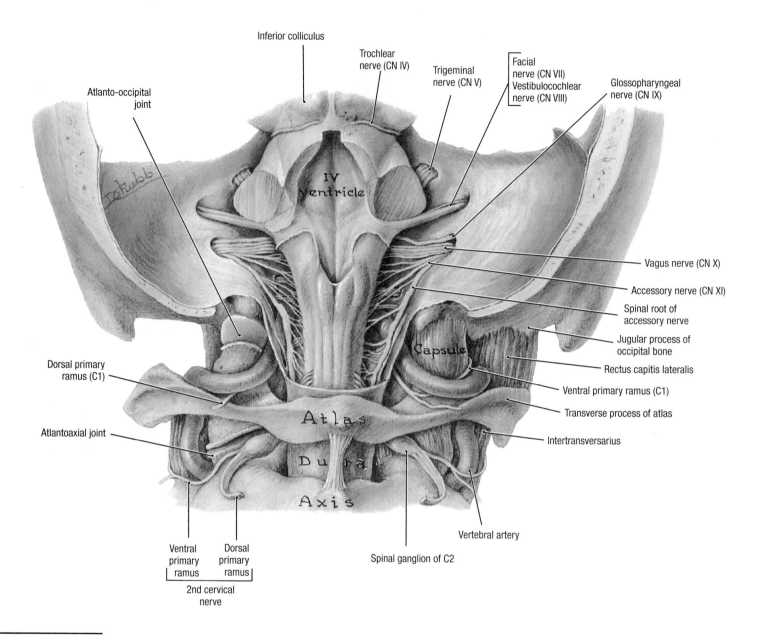

7.38   **Posterior exposure of cranial nerves, posterior view**

OBSERVE:

1. The trochlear nerves (CN IV) arise from the dorsal aspect of the midbrain just inferior to the inferior colliculi; the trigeminal nerves (CN V) ascend to enter the mouths of the trigeminal caves; the facial (CN VII) and vestibulocochlear (CN VIII) nerves course superiorly to the internal acoustic meatus; the glossopharyngeal nerves (CN IX) pierce the dura mater separately and pass with the vagus (CN X) and accessory (CN XI) nerves through the jugular foramina; and the rootlets of the accessory nerves of opposite sides leave the medulla and spinal cord asymmetrically;

2. The abducens nerves (CN VI) are not shown; the hypoglossal nerves (CN XII) lie anterior to the spinal roots of nerves XI and just superior to the vertebral arteries;

3. The transverse process of the atlas is joined to the jugular process of the occipital bone by the rectus capitis lateralis muscle, which morphologically is an intertransverse muscle;

4. The vertebral arteries are raised from their "beds" on the posterior arch of the atlas;

5. The dorsal primary ramus of the 1st cervical nerve (suboccipital nerve) passes between the vertebral artery and posterior arch of the atlas; its ventral primary ramus curves around the atlanto-occipital joint;

6. The 2nd cervical nerve has a large spinal ganglion, large dorsal primary ramus (greater occipital nerve), and smaller ventral primary ramus.

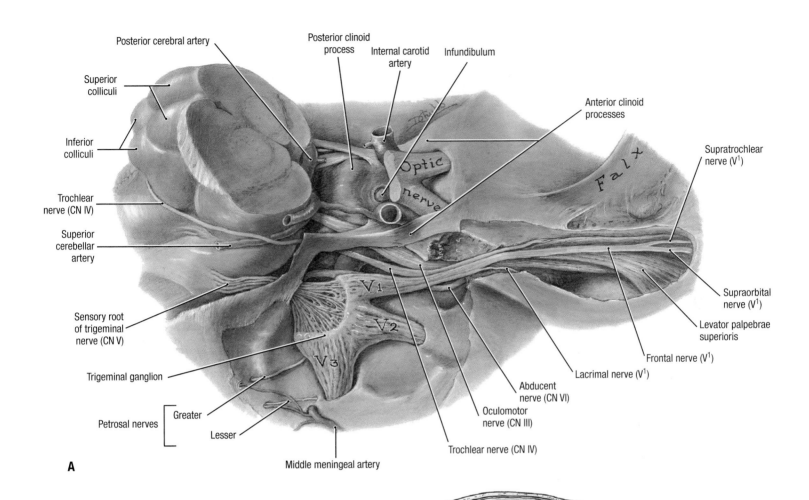

A. Superficial dissection.

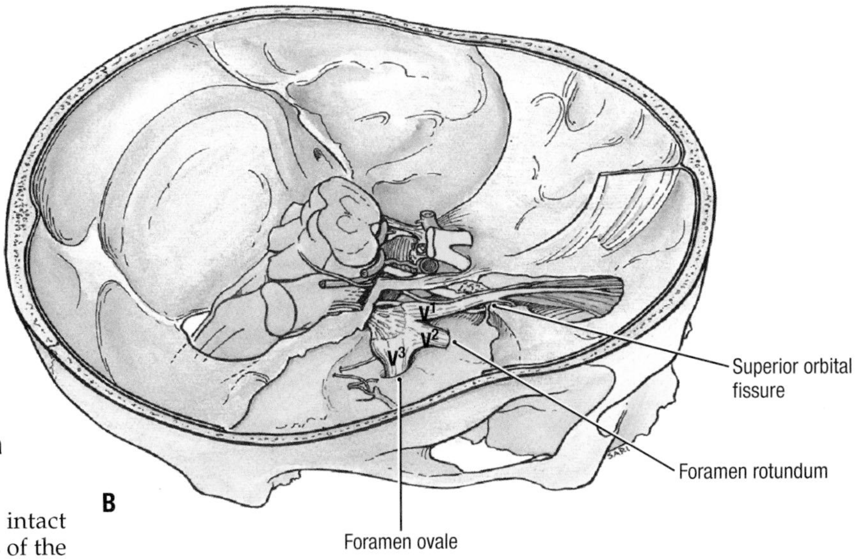

Labels (figure A), clockwise:
Posterior cerebral artery · Posterior clinoid process · Internal carotid artery · Infundibulum · Anterior clinoid processes · Supratrochlear nerve (V¹) · Supraorbital nerve (V¹) · Levator palpebrae superioris · Frontal nerve (V¹) · Lacrimal nerve (V¹) · Abducent nerve (CN VI) · Oculomotor nerve (CN III) · Trochlear nerve (CN IV) · Middle meningeal artery · Petrosal nerves (Greater, Lesser) · Trigeminal ganglion · Sensory root of trigeminal nerve (CN V) · Superior cerebellar artery · Trochlear nerve (CN IV) · Inferior colliculi · Superior colliculi

Labels (figure B):
Superior orbital fissure · Foramen rotundum · Foramen ovale

7.39 Nerves and vessels of middle cranial fossa superolateral views.

A. Superficial dissection. **B.** Superficial dissection in situ in intact skull. The tentorium cerebelli is cut away to reveal the courses of the trochlear and trigeminal nerves in the posterior cranial fossa. The dura is largely removed from the middle cranial fossa. The roof of the orbit is partly removed.

OBSERVE:

1. The trigeminal (semilunar) ganglion and its three divisions: the mandibular, maxillary, and ophthalmic nerves;
2. The mandibular nerve (CN V3) passes inferiorly through the foramen ovale into the infratemporal fossa;
3. The maxillary nerve (CN V2) passes anteriorly through the foramen rotundum into the pterygopalatine fossa;
4. The ophthalmic nerve (CN V1) ascends slightly, close to the trochlear nerve (CN IV), and divides into frontal and lacrimal branches; the trochlear, frontal, and lacrimal nerves run anteriorly through the superior orbital fissure just deep to the roof of the orbital cavity (removed).

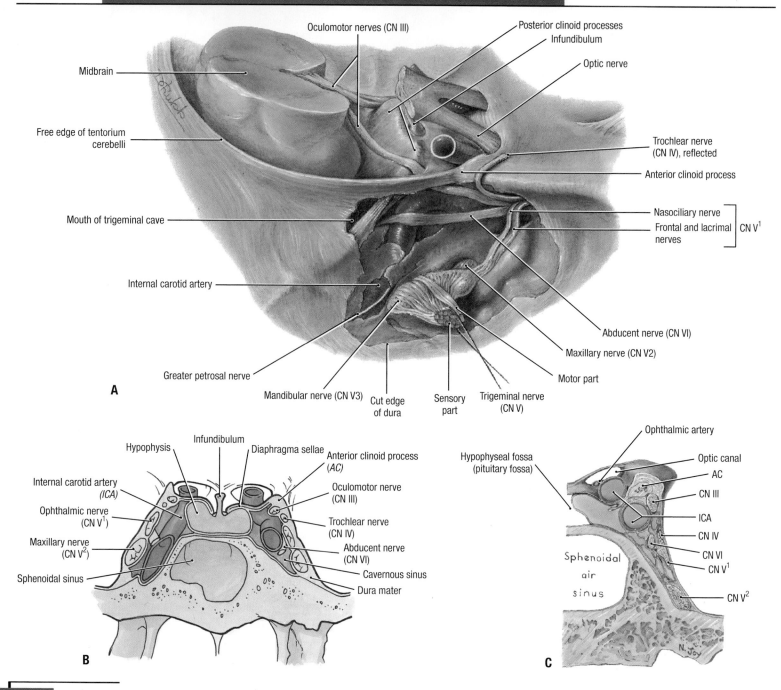

Oculomotor nerves (CN III)

Posterior clinoid processes
Infundibulum

Optic nerve

Midbrain

Free edge of tentorium
cerebelli

Trochlear nerve
(CN IV), reflected

Anterior clinoid process

Mouth of trigeminal cave

Nasociliary nerve
Frontal and lacrimal
nerves } CN V¹

Internal carotid artery

Abducent nerve (CN VI)

Maxillary nerve (CN V2)

Greater petrosal nerve

Motor part

A

Mandibular nerve (CN V3)   Cut edge
of dura

Sensory
part

Trigeminal nerve
(CN V)

Hypophysis
Infundibulum
Diaphragma sellae
Anterior clinoid process
(*AC*)

Internal carotid artery
(*ICA*)

Oculomotor nerve
(CN III)

Ophthalmic nerve
(CN V¹)

Trochlear nerve
(CN IV)

Maxillary nerve
(CN V²)

Abducent nerve
(CN VI)

Cavernous sinus

Sphenoidal sinus

Dura mater

B

Ophthalmic artery

Hypophyseal fossa
(pituitary fossa)

Optic canal

AC

CN III

ICA

CN IV

CN VI

CN V¹

Sphenoidal
air
sinus

CN V²

C

7.40   Nerves and vessels of middle cranial fossa—II

A. Deep dissection, superolateral view. **B** and **C.** Coronal sections through the cavernous sinus, posterior views. The trigeminal nerve is divided, withdrawn from the mouth of the trigeminal cave, and turned anteriorly. The trochlear nerve is reflected anteriorly.

OBSERVE IN **A:**
1. The "bed" of the trigeminal ganglion is partly formed by the greater petrosal nerve and internal carotid artery, with the dura intervening;
2. The motor part of nerve CN V (the nerve to the muscles of mastication) crosses the ganglion diagonally to join CN V3;
3. CN V1 gives off the nasociliary nerve and passes with cranial nerves III, IV, and VI through the superior orbital fissure;
4. The anterior clinoid process is located between the optic nerve and internal carotid artery medially, and the oculomotor nerve inferiorly;
5. The abducent nerve (CN VI) makes a right angle turn at the apex

of the petrous bone and then, as it runs horizontally, lies lateral to the internal carotid artery;
6. The course of the internal carotid artery is sinuous.

OBSERVE IN **B** AND **C:**
7. The cavernous venous sinuses are situated lateral to the sphenoidal air sinus and hypophyseal fossa;
8. Cranial nerves III, IV, V1, and V2 are in a sheath in the lateral wall of the sinus;
9. The internal carotid artery, surrounded by the internal carotid plexus (not shown), and the abducent nerve (CN VI) run through the cavernous sinus; they are vulnerable in thrombosis of the sinus;
10. The internal carotid artery, having made an acute bend, is cut twice; this artery and the oculomotor nerve lie adjacent to the anterior clinoid process.

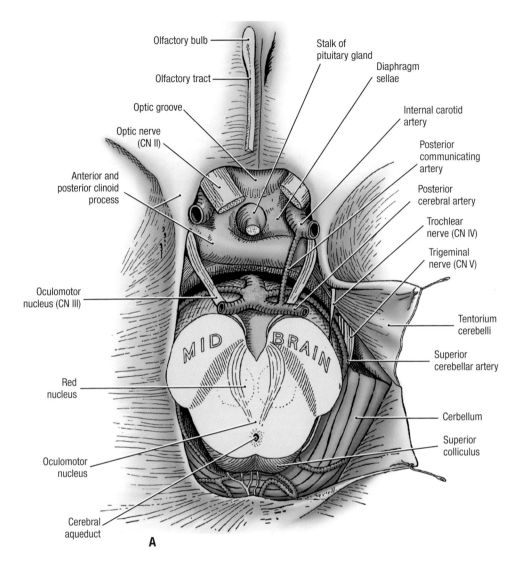

A

7.41   Middle and posterior cranial fossae

A. Midline structures, superior view. The forebrain has been removed by cutting through the midbrain. On the right side of the specimen, the tentorium cerebelli is divided and reflected. **B.** Internal carotid artery, coronal section through carotid canal, posterior view. Follow the course of the internal carotid artery in the carotid canal and cavernous sinus. The artery takes an inverted, L-shaped course from the inferior surface of the petrous bone to its apex. There, at the superior end of foramen lacerum, it enters the cranial cavity and takes an S-shaped course. Note its relationships to the optic, oculomotor, trochlear, and abducent nerves.

OBSERVE IN **A**:

1. There is a circular opening in the diaphragma sellae for the infundibulum stalk of the pituitary gland;
2. The oculomotor nerve (CN III) passes between the posterior cerebral and superior cerebellar arteries, and then passes laterally around the posterior clinoid process;
3. On the right of the specimen, the trochlear nerve (CN IV) passes around the midbrain under the free edge of the tentorium cerebelli; the trigeminal nerve (CN V) enters the mouth of the trigeminal cave.

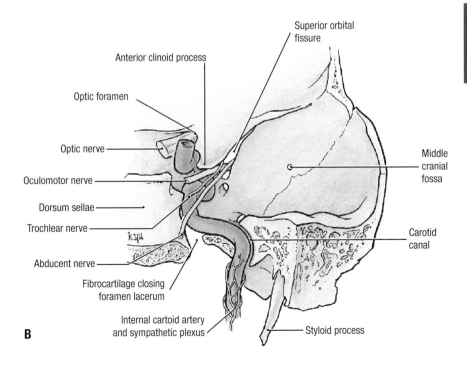

B

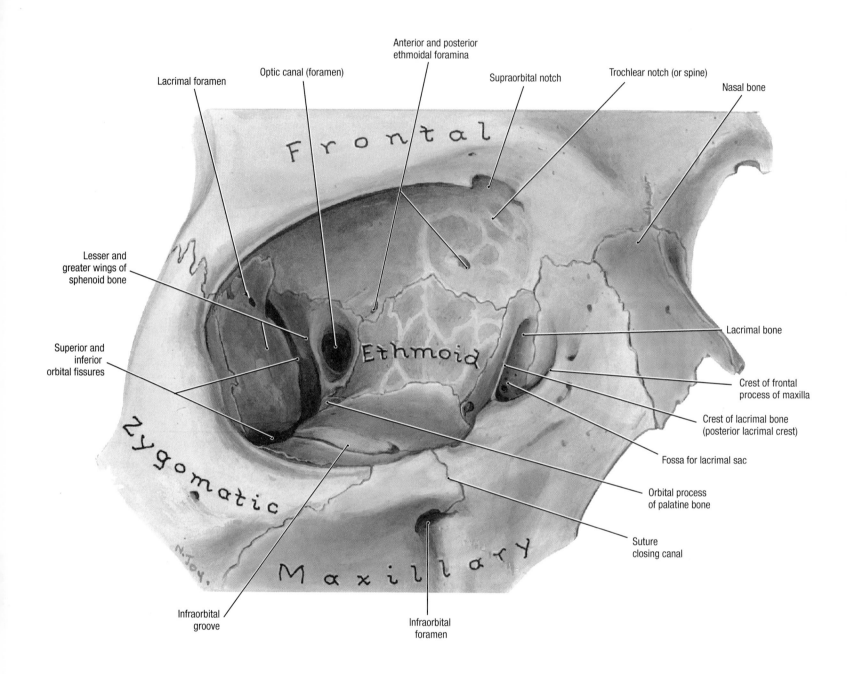

7.42 Orbital cavity, anterior view

OBSERVE:
1. The quadrangular orbital margin is formed by the frontal, maxillary, and zygomatic bones;
2. The fossa for the lacrimal sac is located between the crest of the lacrimal bone (posterior lacrimal crest) and crest of the frontal process of the maxilla;
3. The optic canal is situated at the apex of the pear-shaped orbital cavity;
4. The superior wall, or roof, is formed by the orbital plate of the frontal bone;
5. The inferior wall, or floor, is formed by the orbital plate of the maxilla and the zygomatic bone; it is crossed by the infraorbital groove,

the anterior end of which is converted into the infraorbital canal, which ends at the infraorbital foramen;
6. The thick lateral wall is formed by the frontal process of the zygomatic bone and the greater wing of the sphenoid;
7. The superior and inferior orbital fissures together form a V-shaped fissure;
8. The thin medial wall is formed by the lacrimal bone and orbital plate of the ethmoid bone;
9. The lacrimal foramen for the anastomosis between the middle meningeal and lacrimal arteries is located just beyond the superolateral end of the superior orbital fissure.

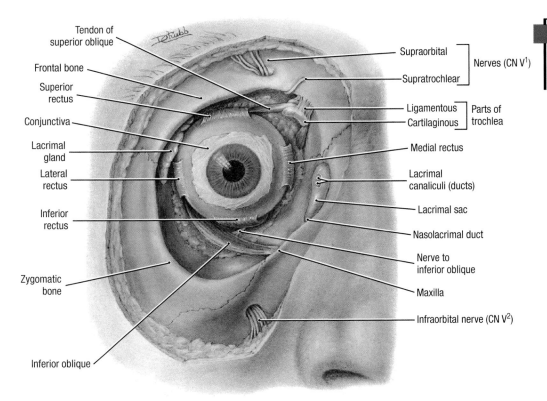

Tendon of superior oblique
Frontal bone
Superior rectus
Conjunctiva
Lacrimal gland
Lateral rectus
Inferior rectus
Zygomatic bone
Inferior oblique

Supraorbital } *Nerves (CN V¹)*
Supratrochlear
Ligamentous } Parts of
Cartilaginous } *trochlea*
Medial rectus
Lacrimal canaliculi (ducts)
Lacrimal sac
Nasolacrimal duct
Nerve to inferior oblique
Maxilla
Infraorbital nerve (CN V²)

7.43   **Dissection of orbital cavity, anterior view**

The eyelids, orbital septum, levator palpebrae superioris, and some fat are removed.

OBSERVE:

1. The aponeurotic insertions of the four recti;
2. The tendon of the superior oblique muscle lies in a cartilaginous pulley or trochlea that is fixed by ligamentous fibers just posterior to the superomedial angle of the orbital margin;
3. The nerve to the inferior oblique muscle enters its posterior border;
4. The lacrimal gland is placed between the bony orbital wall laterally and the eyeball and lateral rectus muscle medially.

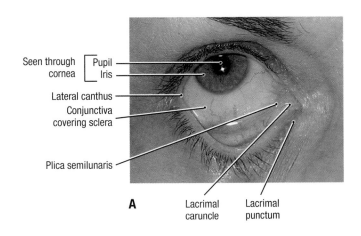

Seen through cornea [*Pupil* / *Iris*]
Lateral canthus
Conjunctiva covering sclera
Plica semilunaris
A
Lacrimal caruncle   *Lacrimal punctum*

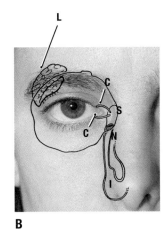

B

7.44   **Surface anatomy of eye and lacrimal apparatus, anterior views**

A. Surface features. **B.** Lacrimal apparatus. Tears are secreted by the lacrimal gland (*L*), located in the superolateral angle of the bony orbit. Tears, after passing over the eyeball, drain into the lacrimal sac (*S*) through puncta in the superior and inferior lids, which lead to the lacrimal canaliculi (*C*). The lacrimal sac drains into the nasolacrimal duct (*N*), which empties into the inferior meatus (*I*) of the nose.

OBSERVE IN **A**:
1. The tough, white, fibrous outer coat of the eyeball is the sclera; the inferior lid has been everted to show the reflection of conjunctiva from the anterior surface of the eyeball to the inner surface of the lid;

2. Through the central, transparent cornea is the pigmented iris with its aperture, the pupil;
3. The superior and inferior lids meet at angles called the medial and lateral canthi;
4. An arrow points to the inferior lacrimal punctum;
5. Near the medial angle is a vertical fold of conjunctiva called the plica semilunaris;
6. In the medial angle is a mound of modified skin, called the lacrimal caruncle;

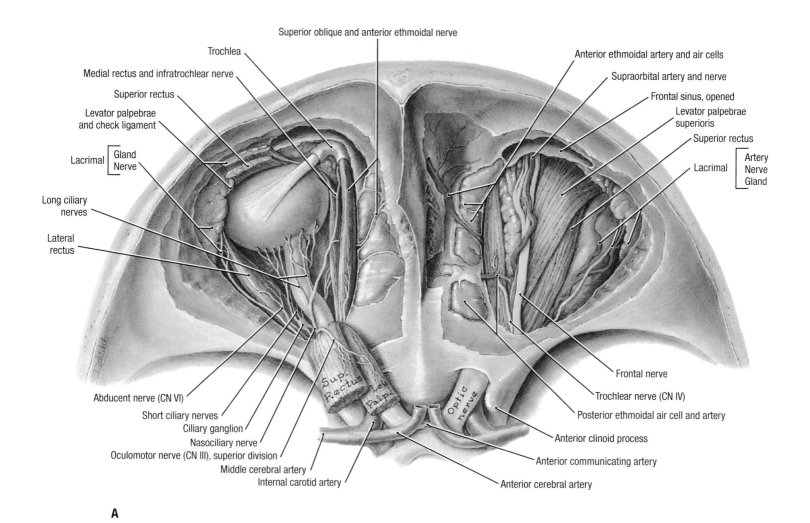

Superior oblique and anterior ethmoidal nerve

Trochlea

Medial rectus and infratrochlear nerve

Superior rectus

Levator palpebrae and check ligament

Lacrimal [Gland / Nerve]

Long ciliary nerves

Lateral rectus

Anterior ethmoidal artery and air cells

Supraorbital artery and nerve

Frontal sinus, opened

Levator palpebrae superioris

Superior rectus

Lacrimal [Artery / Nerve / Gland]

Frontal nerve

Trochlear nerve (CN IV)

Posterior ethmoidal air cell and artery

Anterior clinoid process

Anterior communicating artery

Anterior cerebral artery

Internal carotid artery

Middle cerebral artery

Oculomotor nerve (CN III), superior division

Nasociliary nerve

Ciliary ganglion

Short ciliary nerves

Abducent nerve (CN VI)

A

7.45 Orbital cavity, superior views

A. Superficial dissection. **B.** Deep dissection.

OBSERVE ON THE RIGHT OF FIGURE **A:**
1. The orbital plate of the frontal bone is removed;
2. The levator palpebrae superioris muscle overlies the superior rectus muscle;
3. The trochlear, frontal, and lacrimal nerves lie just deep to the roof of the orbital cavity;
4. The supraorbital, lacrimal, and anterior and posterior ethmoidal branches of the ophthalmic artery.

OBSERVE ON THE LEFT OF FIGURE **A:**
5. The levator palpebrae and superior rectus muscles are reflected;
6. The superior division of the oculomotor nerve (CN III) supplies the superior rectus and levator palpebrae muscles;
7. The entire course of the superior oblique muscle and the trochlear nerve (CN IV) that supplies it;

8. The lateral rectus muscle and the abducent nerve (CN VI) that supplies it;
9. The lacrimal nerve runs superior to the lateral rectus muscle giving branches to the conjunctiva and skin of the superior eyelid; it receives a communicating branch of the zygomaticotemporal nerve carrying secretory motor fibers from the facial nerve to the lacrimal gland;
10. The ciliary ganglion is placed between the lateral rectus muscle and the optic nerve (CN II) and gives off many short ciliary nerves;
11. The nasociliary nerve gives off two long ciliary nerves that anastomose with each other and the short ciliary nerves.

OBSERVE ON THE RIGHT OF FIGURE **B:**
12. The four recti muscles (superior, medial, inferior, lateral) are supplied on their ocular surfaces, and the two oblique muscles (superior, inferior) are supplied near their borders; the superior rectus and inferior obliques are not shown.

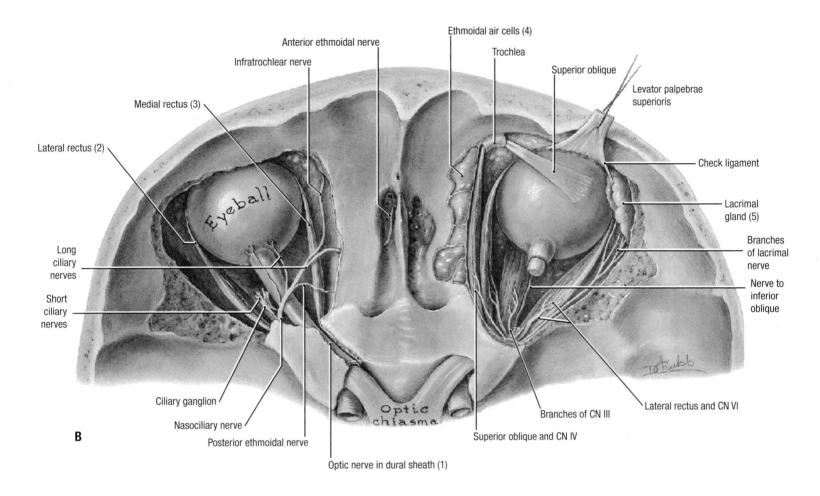

Eyeball (labeled on left orbit)

B

Labels (clockwise from top):
- Anterior ethmoidal nerve
- Infratrochlear nerve
- Medial rectus (3)
- Lateral rectus (2)
- Long ciliary nerves
- Short ciliary nerves
- Ciliary ganglion
- Nasociliary nerve
- Posterior ethmoidal nerve
- Optic nerve in dural sheath (1)
- Optic chiasma
- Superior oblique and CN IV
- Branches of CN III
- Lateral rectus and CN VI
- Nerve to inferior oblique
- Branches of lacrimal nerve
- Lacrimal gland (5)
- Check ligament
- Levator palpebrae superioris
- Superior oblique
- Trochlea
- Ethmoidal air cells (4)

OBSERVE ON THE LEFT OF FIGURE **B**:

13. The eyeball occupies the anterior half of the orbital cavity;

14. The ciliary ganglion lies posteriorly between the lateral rectus muscle and sheath of the optic nerve. It receives a twig (sensory and sympathetic) from the nasociliary nerve and a twig (motor to sphincter pupillae and ciliary muscle) from the nerve to the inferior oblique muscle, and gives off short ciliary nerves (cut short);

15. The nasociliary nerve sends a twig to the ciliary ganglion, crosses the optic nerve, gives off two long ciliary nerves (sensory to the eyeball and cornea) and the posterior ethmoidal nerve (to the sphenoidal sinus and posterior ethmoidal cells), and divides into the anterior ethmoidal and infratrochlear nerves.

C. Transverse magnetic resonance image (MRI) of orbital cavity. (Numbers refer to structures labeled in **B**.)

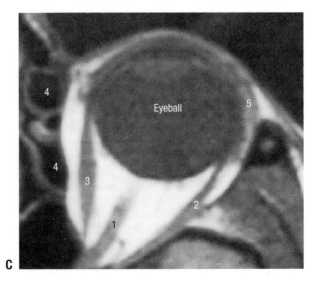

C

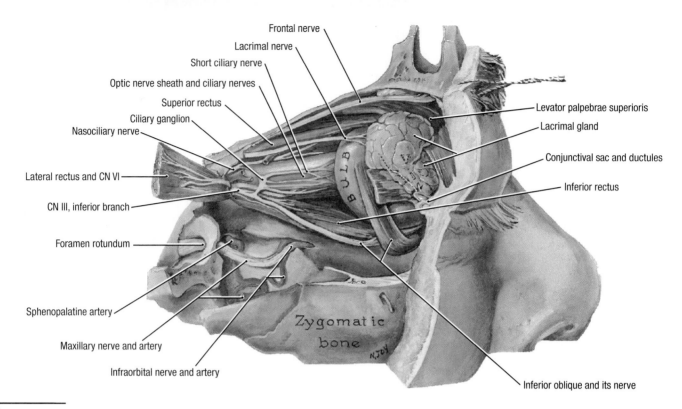

Frontal nerve

Lacrimal nerve

Short ciliary nerve

Optic nerve sheath and ciliary nerves

Superior rectus

Ciliary ganglion

Nasociliary nerve

Lateral rectus and CN VI

CN III, inferior branch

Foramen rotundum

Sphenopalatine artery

Maxillary nerve and artery

Infraorbital nerve and artery

Levator palpebrae superioris

Lacrimal gland

Conjunctival sac and ductules

Inferior rectus

Inferior oblique and its nerve

BULB

Zygomatic bone

7.46   Dissection of orbit, lateral view

OBSERVE:
1. The ciliary ganglion receives sensory fibers from the nasociliary branches of V1, sympathetic fibers from the internal carotid plexus traveling around the ophthalmic artery, and parasympathetic fibers (which synapse in the ganglion) from the inferior branch of the oculomotor nerve;

2. Eight to ten short ciliary nerves go to the eyeball;
3. *Interruption of a cervical sympathetic trunk results in paralysis of the superior tarsal muscle supplied by sympathetic fibers, causing ptosis. This is part of Horner's syndrome, which also includes a constricted pupil, sinking of the eye, and redness, dryness, and increased temperature on the affected side of the face.*

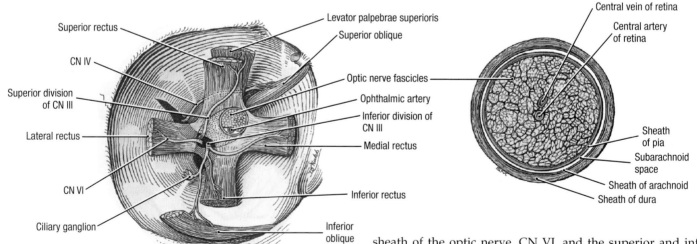

Superior rectus

CN IV

Superior division of CN III

Lateral rectus

CN VI

Ciliary ganglion

Levator palpebrae superioris

Superior oblique

Optic nerve fascicles

Ophthalmic artery

Inferior division of CN III

Medial rectus

Inferior rectus

Inferior oblique

Central vein of retina

Central artery of retina

Sheath of pia

Subarachnoid space

Sheath of arachnoid

Sheath of dura

7.47   Nerves of orbit, anterior view

OBSERVE:
1. The optic nerve lies within its pial, arachnoid, and dural sheaths;
2. The four recti arise from a tendinous ring that encircles the dural sheath of the optic nerve, CN VI, and the superior and inferior branches of CN III; the nasociliary nerve (not shown) also passes through this cuff, but CN IV clings to the bony roof of the cavity;
3. Cranial nerves IV and VI supply one muscle each, and CN III supplies the remaining five orbital muscles; two through its superior branch, and three through its inferior branch;
4. The oculomotor nerve (CN III) through the ciliary ganglion supplies parasympathetic fibers to the ciliary muscle and sphincter iridis.

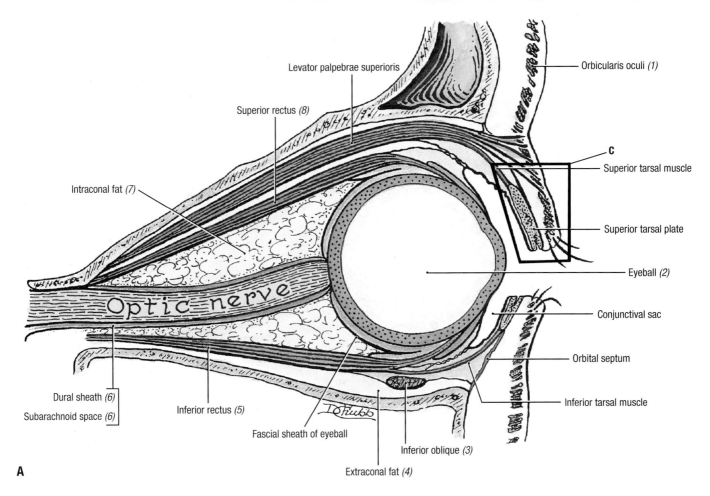

Levator palpebrae superioris

Superior rectus (8)

Intraconal fat (7)

C

Superior tarsal muscle

Superior tarsal plate

Eyeball (2)

Conjunctival sac

Orbital septum

Inferior tarsal muscle

Dural sheath (6)

Subarachnoid space (6)

Inferior rectus (5)

Fascial sheath of eyeball

Inferior oblique (3)

Extraconal fat (4)

A

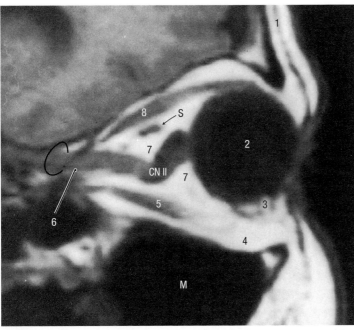

B

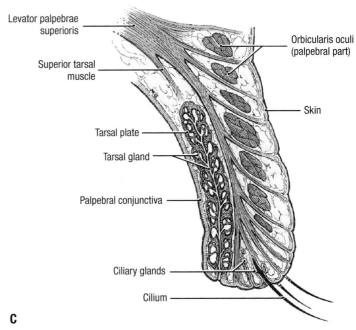

Levator palpebrae superioris

Superior tarsal muscle

Orbicularis oculi (palpebral part)

Skin

Tarsal plate

Tarsal gland

Palpebral conjunctiva

Ciliary glands

Cilium

C

7.48   Orbital contents and upper eyelid, sagittal sections

A. Orbital contents. (The boxed area is enlarged in **C**.) **B.** Sagittal MRI through optic nerve. (Numbers refer to structures labeled in **A.** *S*, superior ophthalmic vein; *M*, maxillary sinus; *circled,* optic foramen.) **C.** Upper eyelid. The lid has a superficial, ciliary part and a deeper, tarsal part. The ciliary part is covered with skin, contains the fibers of the palpebral part of orbicularis oculi, and bears the eyelashes. The tarsal part is lined with conjunctiva; embedded in the tarsal plate, which forms its skeleton, are modified sebaceous glands that open on the margin of the eyelid.

7.49 Eyeball and muscle attachments

A. Attachments of the four recti, anterior view. **B.** Insertions of the two obliques, posterior view.

OBSERVE:

1. The conjunctiva is loose and wrinkled over the sclera, but adherent to the cornea;
2. The four recti are spread out to show the insertions of their aponeuroses into the anterior half of the eyeball, 6 to 8 mm posterior to the sclerocorneal junction;
3. The two obliques are inserted by aponeuroses into the posterolateral quadrant of the eyeball; when in situ, the inferior rectus passes superior to the inferior oblique muscle.

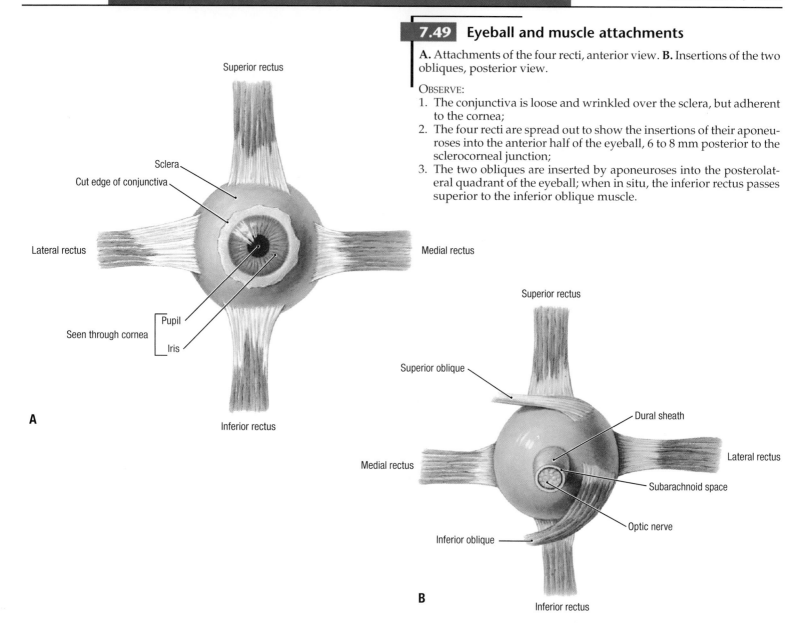

Table 7.2. Muscles of the Orbit

Muscle	Origin	Insertion	Innervation
Levator palpebrae superioris	Lesser wing of sphenoid bone and superior and anterior to optic canal	Tarsal plate and skin of upper eyelid	Oculomotor nerve; deep layer (superior tarsal muscle) is supplied by sympathetic fibers
Superior rectus			
Inferior rectus			
Lateral rectus	Common tendinous ring	Sclera just posterior to cornea	Oculomotor nerve
Medial rectus	Body of sphenoid bone		Abducent nerve
Superior oblique		Its tendon passes through a fibrous ring or trochlea and changes its direction and inserts into sclera deep to superior rectus muscle	Oculomotor nerve Trochlear nerve
Inferior oblique	Anterior part of floor of orbit	Sclera deep to lateral rectus muscle	Oculomotor nerve

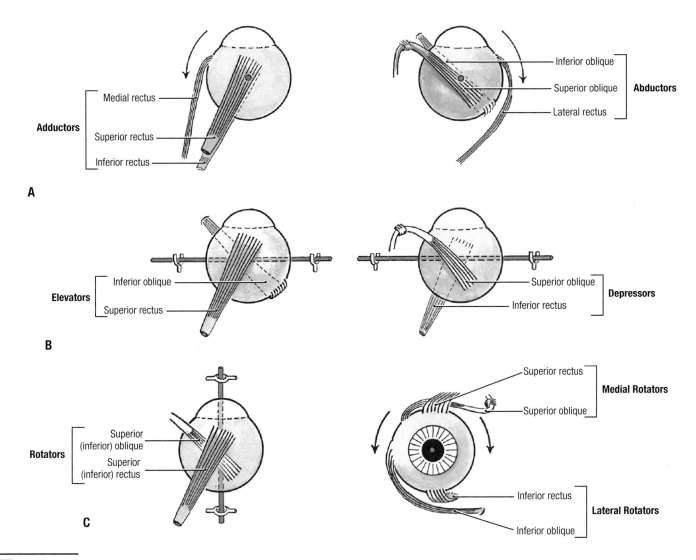

7.50　**Movement of eyeball around the vertical, horizontal, and anteroposterior axes**

A. Vertical axis, superior views. **B.** Horizontal axis, superior views. **C.** Anteroposterior axis, superior and anterior views. The right eyeball is represented for each movement. Of the six ocular muscles, the medial rectus and lateral rectus move the eyeball on one axis only; each of the four other muscles moves it on all three axes. The two obliques also protract (protrude) the eyeball, whereas the four recti retract it. *For clinical testing, each muscle is examined in its position of greatest efficiency.*

Table 7.3. Actions of Muscles of Orbit

	Actions			Clinical Testing
Muscle	*Vertical Axis*	*Horizontal Axis*	*Anteroposterior Axis*	*(The patient is asked to look …)*
Superior Rectus	Elevates	Adducts	Rotates medially	Upward and outward
Inferior Rectus	Depresses	Adducts	Rotates laterally	Downward and outward
Superior Oblique	Depresses	Abducts	Rotates Medially	Downward and inward
Inferior Oblique	Elevates	Abducts	Rotates laterally	Upward and inward
Medial Rectus	N/A	Adducts	N/A	Inward
Lateral Rectus	N/A	Abducts	N/A	Outward

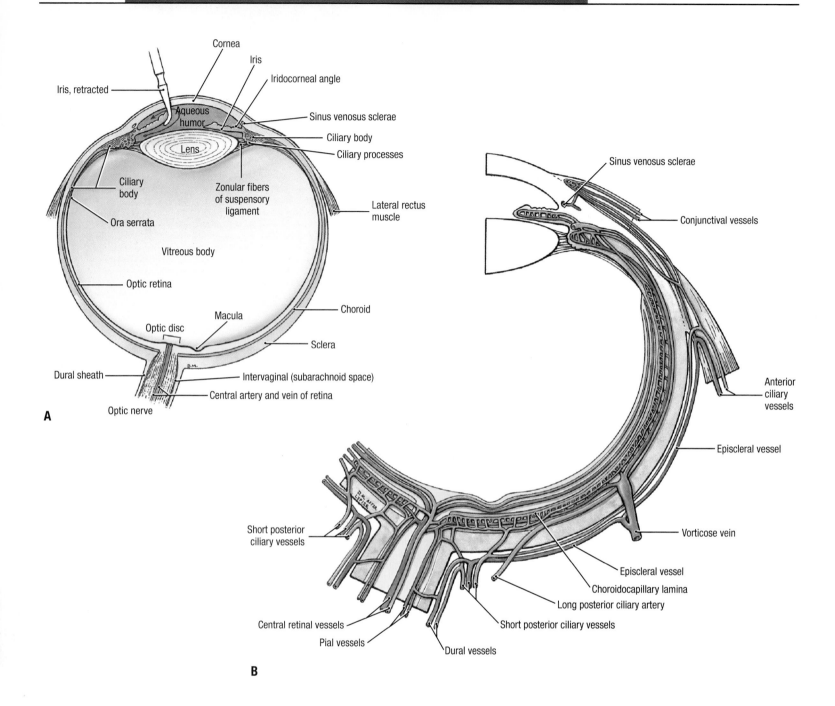

A

Cornea
Iris
Iridocorneal angle
Iris, retracted
Aqueous humor
Sinus venosus sclerae
Ciliary body
Ciliary processes
Lens
Ciliary body
Zonular fibers of suspensory ligament
Ora serrata
Lateral rectus muscle
Vitreous body
Optic retina
Choroid
Macula
Optic disc
Sclera
Dural sheath
Intervaginal (subarachnoid space)
Central artery and vein of retina
Optic nerve

B

Sinus venosus sclerae
Conjunctival vessels
Anterior ciliary vessels
Episcleral vessel
Vorticose vein
Episcleral vessel
Choroidocapillary lamina
Long posterior ciliary artery
Short posterior ciliary vessels
Short posterior ciliary vessels
Central retinal vessels
Pial vessels
Dural vessels

7.51 Right eyeball, horizontal sections

Parts of eyeball. **B.** Blood supply to eyeball.

OBSERVE:

1. The eyeball, or bulbus oculi, has three layers: a) the external, fibrous layer is the sclera and cornea; b) the middle, vascular layer is the choroid, ciliary body, and iris; and c) the internal, neural layer or retina consists of a pigment cell layer and a neural layer;

2. The four refractive media are: a) the cornea; b) the aqueous humor, which fills two chambers—an anterior in front of the iris and a posterior behind the iris; c) the lens; and d) the vitreous humor, a transparent gel that occupies the vitreous body between the lens and retina;

3. The central artery of the retina, a branch of the ophthalmic artery, is an end artery. Of the eight or so posterior ciliary arteries, six sup-

ply the choroid, which, in turn, nourishes the outer, nonvascular layer of the retina. Two long posterior ciliary arteries, one on each side of the eyeball, run between the sclera and choroid to anastomose with the anterior ciliary arteries, which are derived from muscular branches;

4. The aqueous humor is produced by the ciliary processes and provides nutrients for the avascular cornea and lens; the aqueous humor drains into the venous sinus of the sclera, called the sinus venosus sclerae (canal of Schlemm). *When drainage of the aqueous humor is reduced significantly, pressure builds up in the chambers of the eye (glaucoma);*

5. The four to five vorticose veins drain into the posterior ciliary and ophthalmic veins.

7.52 Right ocular fundus, ophthalmoscopic view

OBSERVE:

1. The oval optic disc has retinal vessels radiating from its center; composed of nerve fibers, the disc is called the "blind spot";
2. Retinal veins are wider than the arteries;
3. The central retinal artery (a branch of the ophthalmic artery) enters the optic nerve posterior to the eyeball and divides into superior and inferior branches; each then divides into medial (nasal) and lateral (temporal) branches;
4. The round, dark area lateral to the disc is the macula; branches of vessels extend into this area, but do not reach its center, the fovea centralis;
5. The fovea centralis is a depressed spot that is the area of most acute vision; it is avascular and nourished by the choroidal circulation.

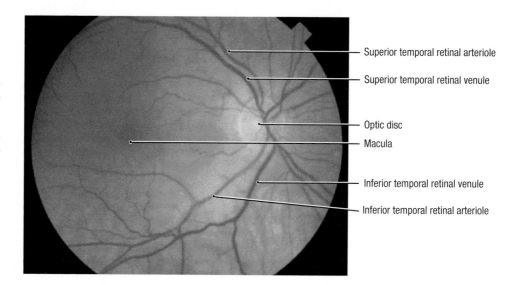

- Superior temporal retinal arteriole
- Superior temporal retinal venule
- Optic disc
- Macula
- Inferior temporal retinal venule
- Inferior temporal retinal arteriole

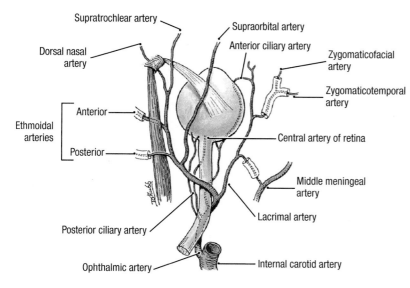

Supratrochlear artery
Supraorbital artery
Dorsal nasal artery
Anterior ciliary artery
Zygomaticofacial artery
Zygomaticotemporal artery
Ethmoidal arteries
  Anterior
  Posterior
Central artery of retina
Middle meningeal artery
Lacrimal artery
Posterior ciliary artery
Ophthalmic artery
Internal carotid artery

A

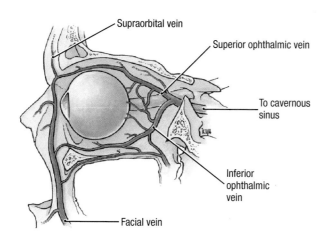

Supraorbital vein
Superior ophthalmic vein
To cavernous sinus
Inferior ophthalmic vein
Facial vein

B

7.53 Ophthalmic vessels

A. Ophthalmic artery, superior view. **B.** Ophthalmic veins, lateral view.

OBSERVE IN **A**:

1. The ophthalmic artery, a branch of the internal carotid artery, enters the orbit through the optic canal within the dural sheath of the optic nerve; it supplies the contents of the orbit;
2. Of its branches, the central artery of the retina is an end artery. *Because these vessels are end arteries, their obstruction by an embolus results in total, unilateral blindness;*
3. Six branches pass beyond the orbit; the a) supratrochlear and b) supraorbital arteries to the forehead; c) dorsal nasal to the face; d) lacrimal to the eyelid and, through its zygomatic branches, to the cheek and temporal region; and e) and f) anterior and posterior ethmoidal arteries to the nasal cavity. These six arteries, which extend beyond the orbit, anastomose freely with branches of the external carotid artery.

OBSERVE IN **B**:

4. The superior and inferior ophthalmic veins empty into the cavernous sinus posteriorly and communicate with the facial and supraorbital veins anteriorly;
5. The superior ophthalmic vein travels with the ophthalmic artery and its branches;
6. The inferior ophthalmic vein runs in the floor of the orbit and enters the cavernous sinus; it may join the superior ophthalmic vein before entering the sinus. *Because the central vein of the retina enters the cavernous sinus, thrombophlebitis of this sinus or vein may result in passage of thrombi to the central retinal veins and produce clotting in the small retinal veins. This results in slow painless loss of vision.*

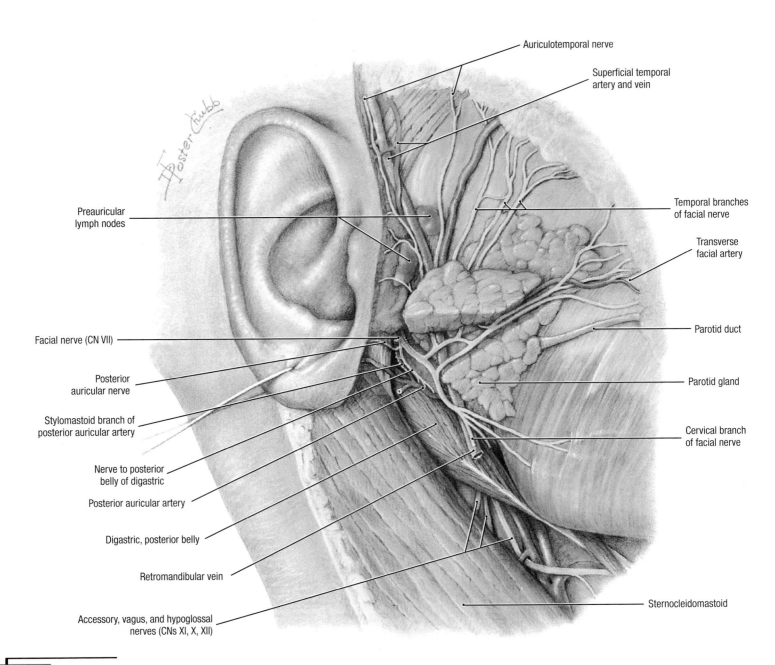

Auriculotemporal nerve

Superficial temporal artery and vein

Temporal branches of facial nerve

Transverse facial artery

Parotid duct

Parotid gland

Cervical branch of facial nerve

Sternocleidomastoid

Preauricular lymph nodes

Facial nerve (CN VII)

Posterior auricular nerve

Stylomastoid branch of posterior auricular artery

Nerve to posterior belly of digastric

Posterior auricular artery

Digastric, posterior belly

Retromandibular vein

Accessory, vagus, and hypoglossal nerves (CNs XI, X, XII)

7.54 Parotid region—I, lateral view

(See Fig. 7.10 for a more superficial dissection.)

OBSERVE:
1. The facial nerve (CN VII) descends from the stylomastoid foramen approximately 1 cm before curving anteriorly to penetrate the parotid gland;
2. The nerve to the posterior belly of the digastric muscle arises from the facial nerve;

3. The posterior auricular artery gives off a branch, the stylomastoid artery, which accompanies the facial nerve through the stylomastoid foramen;
4. The cervical branch of the facial nerve and the retromandibular vein cross superficial to the posterior belly of the digastric muscle;
5. The preauricular lymph nodes are located anterior to the ear.

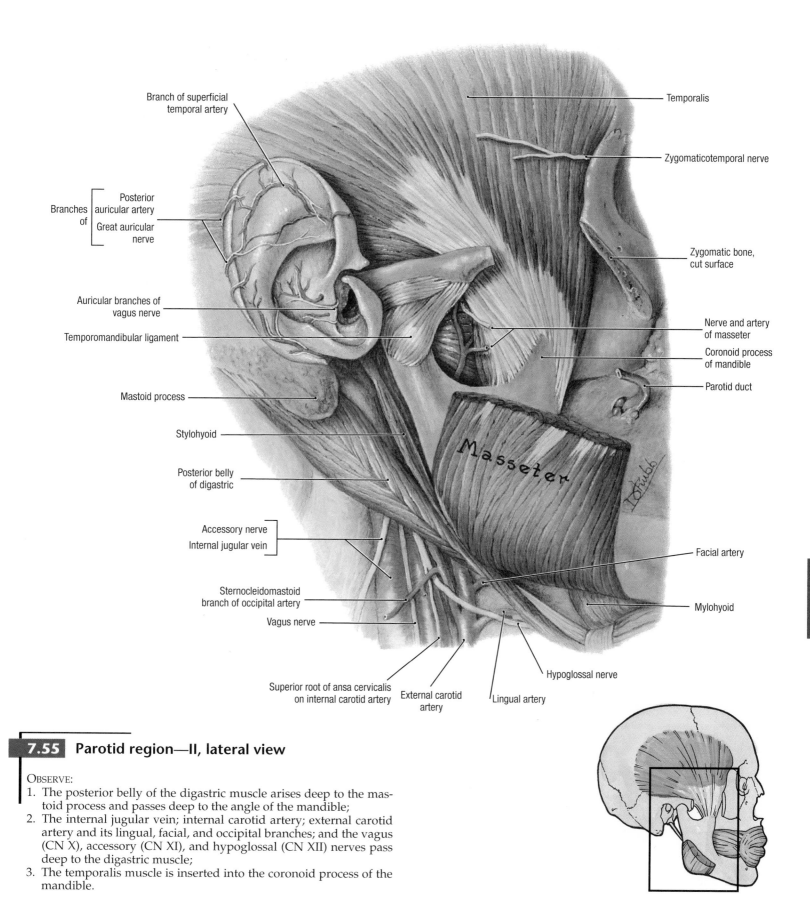

Branch of superficial temporal artery

Branches of { Posterior auricular artery / Great auricular nerve

Auricular branches of vagus nerve

Temporomandibular ligament

Mastoid process

Stylohyoid

Posterior belly of digastric

Accessory nerve
Internal jugular vein

Sternocleidomastoid branch of occipital artery

Vagus nerve

Superior root of ansa cervicalis on internal carotid artery

External carotid artery

Lingual artery

Hypoglossal nerve

Masseter

Temporalis

Zygomaticotemporal nerve

Zygomatic bone, cut surface

Nerve and artery of masseter

Coronoid process of mandible

Parotid duct

Facial artery

Mylohyoid

7.55 Parotid region—II, lateral view

OBSERVE:
1. The posterior belly of the digastric muscle arises deep to the mastoid process and passes deep to the angle of the mandible;
2. The internal jugular vein; internal carotid artery; external carotid artery and its lingual, facial, and occipital branches; and the vagus (CN X), accessory (CN XI), and hypoglossal (CN XII) nerves pass deep to the digastric muscle;
3. The temporalis muscle is inserted into the coronoid process of the mandible.

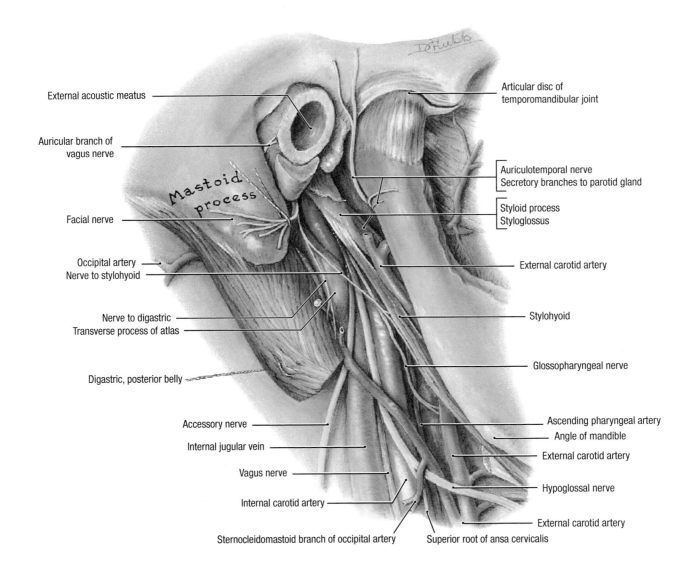

External acoustic meatus

Auricular branch of vagus nerve

Mastoid process

Facial nerve

Occipital artery
Nerve to stylohyoid

Nerve to digastric
Transverse process of atlas

Digastric, posterior belly

Accessory nerve

Internal jugular vein

Vagus nerve

Internal carotid artery

Sternocleidomastoid branch of occipital artery

Articular disc of temporomandibular joint

Auriculotemporal nerve
Secretory branches to parotid gland

Styloid process
Styloglossus

External carotid artery

Stylohyoid

Glossopharyngeal nerve

Ascending pharyngeal artery

Angle of mandible

External carotid artery

Hypoglossal nerve

External carotid artery

Superior root of ansa cervicalis

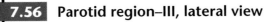

7.56   Parotid region–III, lateral view

The facial nerve, posterior belly of the digastric muscle, and its nerve are retracted; the external carotid artery, stylohyoid muscle, and nerve to stylohyoid remain in situ.

OBSERVE:
1. The tip of the transverse process of the atlas lies about midway between the tip of the mastoid process and the angle of the mandible;
2. The internal jugular vein, internal carotid artery, and glossopharyngeal (CN IX), vagus (CN X), accessory (CN XI), and hypoglossal (CN XII) nerves cross anterior to the transverse process of the atlas and deep to the styloid process;
3. The internal and external carotid arteries are separated by the styloid process;
4. The two nerves that pass anteriorly to the tongue: a) glossopharyngeal (CN IX) nerve, superior to the level of the angle of the mandible and passing between the external and internal carotid arteries; and b) hypoglossal (CN XII) nerve, inferior to the angle of the mandible and passing superficial to both carotids and all of the arteries it meets, except the occipital artery and its sternocleidomastoid branch;
5. The auricular branch of the vagus and the auriculotemporal nerve supply the external acoustic meatus and external surface of the tympanic membrane;
6. *Care must be taken during surgical procedures involving the temporomandibular joint to preserve the branches of the facial nerve that overlie the joint and the articular branches of the auriculotemporal nerve that enter the joint.*

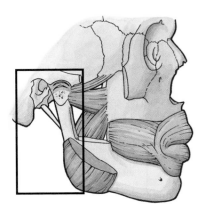

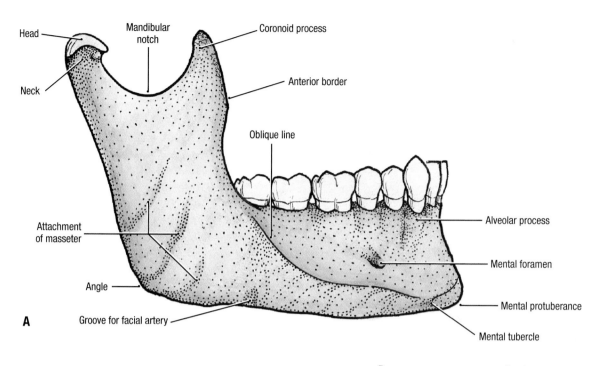

Head
Mandibular notch
Coronoid process
Neck
Anterior border
Oblique line
Alveolar process
Attachment of masseter
Mental foramen
Angle
Mental protuberance
Groove for facial artery
Mental tubercle

A

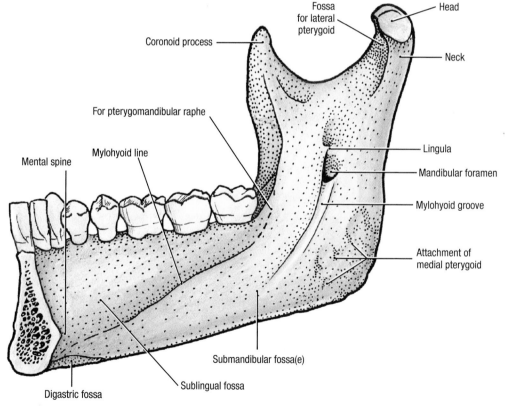

Fossa for lateral pterygoid
Head
Coronoid process
Neck
For pterygomandibular raphe
Mental spine
Mylohyoid line
Lingula
Mandibular foramen
Mylohyoid groove
Attachment of medial pterygoid
Submandibular fossa(e)
Sublingual fossa
Digastric fossa

B

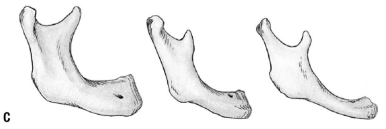

C

7.57　Mandible

A. External surface, lateral view. **B.** Internal surface, medial view. **C.** Mental foramen in edentulous jaws, lateral view. The position of the mental foramen in edentulous jaws varies with the extent of the absorption of the alveolar process. *The pressure of a dental prosthesis on a vulnerable mental nerve in an edentulous jaw can produce pain.*

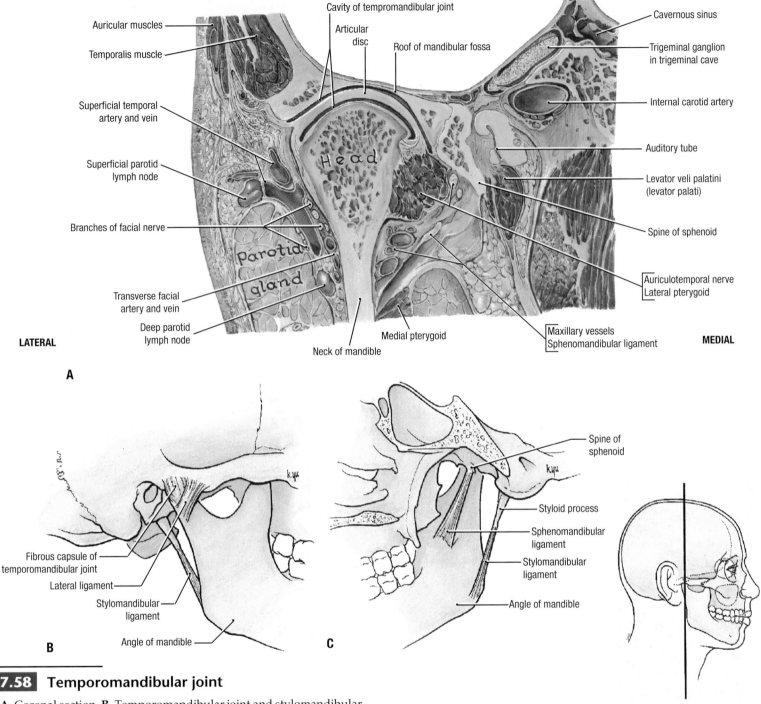

A. Coronal section. B. Temporomandibular joint and stylomandibular ligament, lateral view. The fibrous capsule of the temporomandibular joint attaches to the margins of the articular area of the temporal bone and around the neck of the mandible; the lateral (temporomandibular) ligament strengthens the lateral aspect of the joint. C. Stylomandibular and sphenomandibular ligaments, medial view. The sphenomandibular ligament, which descends from near the spine of the sphenoid to the lingula of the mandible and the stylomandibular ligament, joins the styloid process to the angle of the mandible.

7.58 Temporomandibular joint

OBSERVE IN **A:**
1. The articular disc attaches to the neck of the mandible medially and laterally; part of the lateral pterygoid is inserted into the anterior aspect of the disc;

2. The roof of the mandibular fossa, which separates the head and disc from the middle cranial fossa, is thin centrally and thick elsewhere;
3. The spine of the sphenoid is at the medial end of the mandibular fossa, and the two parts of the auriculotemporal nerve cross lateral to it;
4. The auditory tube has a closed, slit-like opening (lumen); the levator veli palatini (levator palati) lies inferior to it;
5. The trigeminal ganglion in the trigeminal cave is separated from the internal carotid artery by a membrane;
6. The maxillary vessels cross the neck of the mandible on its medial side.

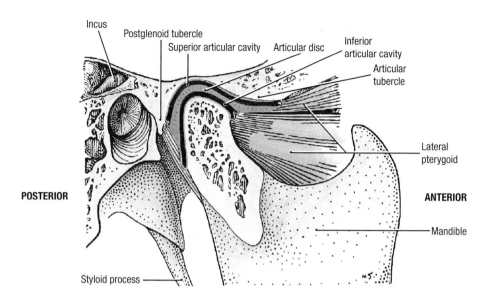

Incus
Postglenoid tubercle
Superior articular cavity
Articular disc
Inferior articular cavity
Articular tubercle
Lateral pterygoid
Mandible
POSTERIOR
ANTERIOR
Styloid process

7.59　Temporomandibular joint, sagittal section

The articular disc divides the articular cavity into superior and inferior compartments. There are two synovial membranes: one lines the fibrous capsule superior to the disc, and the other lines the capsule inferior to the disc. *During yawning or taking large bites, excessive contraction of the lateral pterygoids can cause the head of the mandible to dislocate (pass anterior to the articular tubercle). In this position, the mouth remains wide open, and the person cannot close it.*

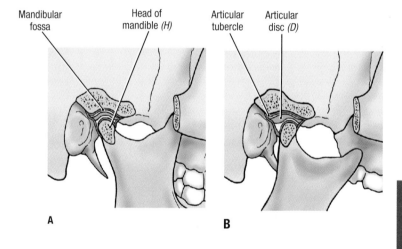

Mandibular fossa
Head of mandible (H)
Articular tubercle
Articular disc (D)

A　　　　　　　　　　　B

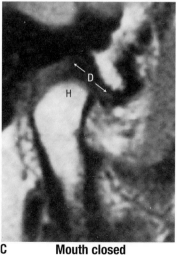
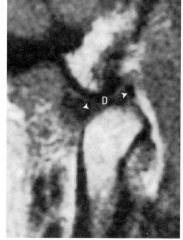

C　**Mouth closed**　　　　D　**Mouth open**

Table 7.4. Movements of the Temporomandibular Joint

Movements	Muscle(s)
Elevation (close mouth)	Temporal, masseter, and medial pterygoid
Depression (open mouth)	Lateral pterygoid and suprahyoid and infrahyoid muscles[a]
Protrusion (protrude chin)	Lateral pterygoid, masseter, and medial pterygoid[b]
Retrusion (retrude chin)	Temporal (posterior oblique and near horizontal fibers) and masseter
Lateral movements (grinding and chewing)	Temporal of same side, pterygoids of opposite side, and masseter

[a]Prime mover normally is gravity—these muscles are mainly active against resistance.
[b]The lateral pterygoid is the prime mover here, with very secondary roles played by masseter and medial pterygoid.

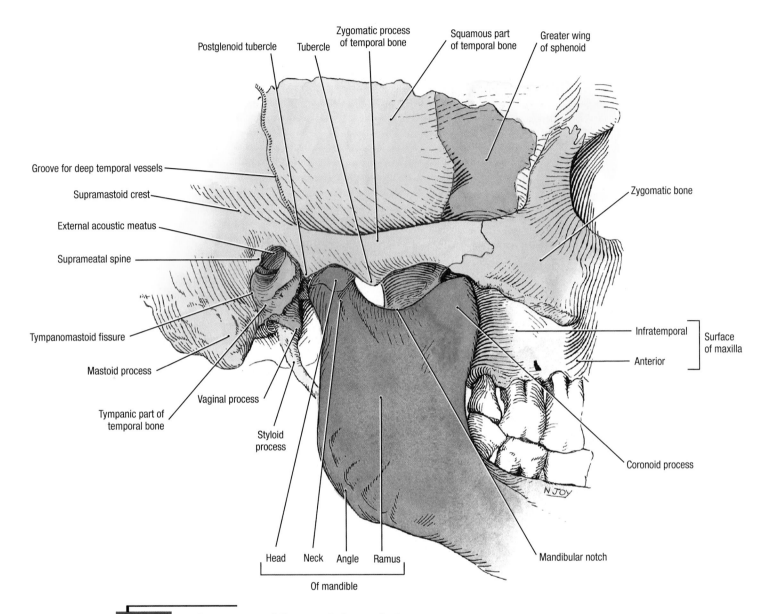

Postglenoid tubercle

Tubercle

Zygomatic process of temporal bone

Squamous part of temporal bone

Greater wing of sphenoid

Groove for deep temporal vessels

Supramastoid crest

External acoustic meatus

Suprameatal spine

Tympanomastoid fissure

Mastoid process

Vaginal process

Tympanic part of temporal bone

Styloid process

Zygomatic bone

Infratemporal
Anterior } Surface of maxilla

Coronoid process

Mandibular notch

Head   Neck   Angle   Ramus

Of mandible

7.60   Infratemporal fossa—I, lateral view

OBSERVE:
1. The lateral wall of the infratemporal fossa is the ramus of the mandible;
2. The zygomatic process of the temporal bone and the zygomatic bone form the zygomatic arch;
3. The zygomatic process of the temporal bone is the boundary between the temporal fossa superiorly and the infratemporal fossa inferiorly.

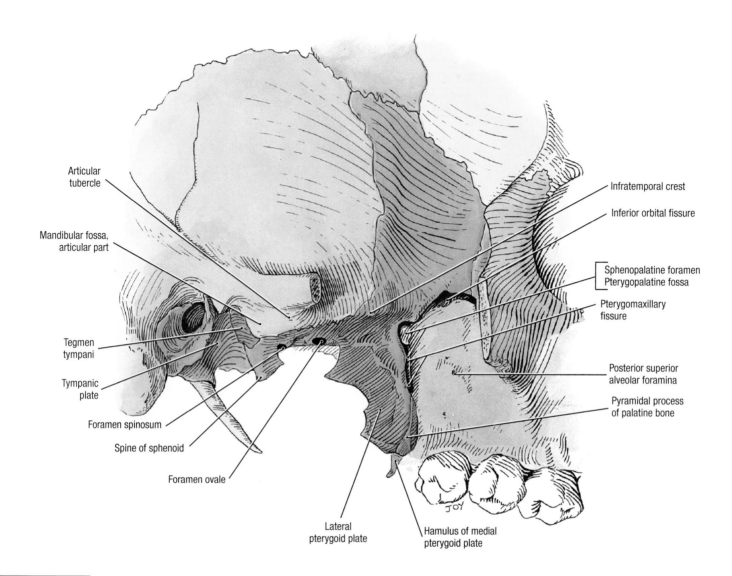

Articular
tubercle

Mandibular fossa,
articular part

Tegmen
tympani

Tympanic
plate

Foramen spinosum

Spine of sphenoid

Foramen ovale

Infratemporal crest

Inferior orbital fissure

Sphenopalatine foramen
Pterygopalatine fossa

Pterygomaxillary
fissure

Posterior superior
alveolar foramina

Pyramidal process
of palatine bone

Lateral
pterygoid plate

Hamulus of medial
pterygoid plate

7.61 Infratemporal fossa—II, lateral view

The mandible and part of the zygomatic arch have been removed.

OBSERVE:
1. The medial wall of the fossa is formed by the lateral pterygoid plate;
2. When followed superiorly, the posterior free border of the lateral pterygoid plate leads to the foramen ovale in the roof of the infratemporal fossa. Posterolateral to the foramen ovale, at the base of the spine of the sphenoid, is the foramen spinosum; the roof of the infratemporal fossa is separated from the temporal fossa by the infratemporal crest;

3. Inferiorly, the anterior border of the lateral pterygoid plate is separated from the maxilla by the pyramidal process of the palatine bone. Superiorly, the border is free and forms the posterior limit of the pterygomaxillary fissure, which is the entrance to the pterygopalatine fossa. On the medial wall of the pterygopalatine fossa is the sphenopalatine foramen, which leads to the nasal cavity;
4. The thin, rounded anterior wall of the infratemporal fossa is formed by the infratemporal surface of the maxilla; the anterior wall is limited superiorly by the inferior orbital fissure and is pierced by two (or more) posterior superior alveolar foramina for the vessels and nerves of the same name.

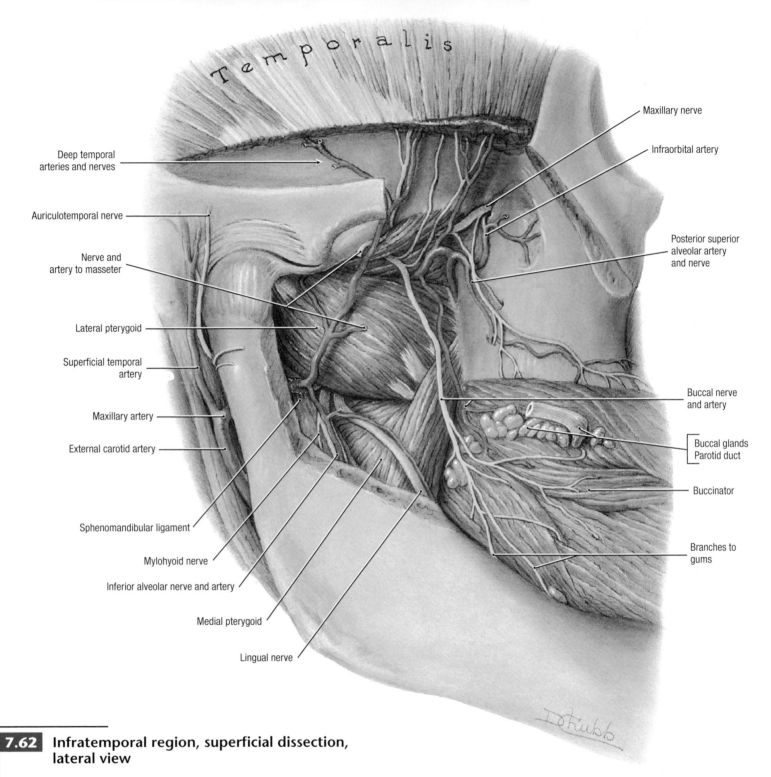

Deep temporal
arteries and nerves

Auriculotemporal nerve

Nerve and
artery to masseter

Lateral pterygoid

Superficial temporal
artery

Maxillary artery

External carotid artery

Sphenomandibular ligament

Mylohyoid nerve

Inferior alveolar nerve and artery

Medial pterygoid

Lingual nerve

Maxillary nerve

Infraorbital artery

Posterior superior
alveolar artery
and nerve

Buccal nerve
and artery

Buccal glands
Parotid duct

Buccinator

Branches to
gums

7.62   **Infratemporal region, superficial dissection,
lateral view**

OBSERVE:
1. The lateral pterygoid, medial pterygoid, and buccinator muscles;
2. The maxillary (CN V2) nerve gives off the posterior superior alve-olar nerve;
3. There are sensory and motor branches of the mandibular (CN V3) nerve;
4. The maxillary artery, the larger of two terminal branches of the ex-ternal carotid, is divided into three parts by the lateral pterygoid muscle: the first part sends branches to accompany the branches of CN V3 (inferior alveolar arteries); the second part supplies blood to the muscles of the region; and the third part sends branches to ac-company the branches of CN V2 (infraorbital and posterior supe-rior alveolar arteries);
5. The buccinator is pierced by the parotid duct, the ducts of the buc-cal (molar) glands, and sensory branches of the buccal nerve;
6. The lateral pterygoid muscle arises by two heads (parts), one head from the roof, and the other head from the medial wall of the in-fratemporal fossa; both heads insert together into the articular disc of the temporomandibular joint and the anterior aspect of the neck of the mandible.

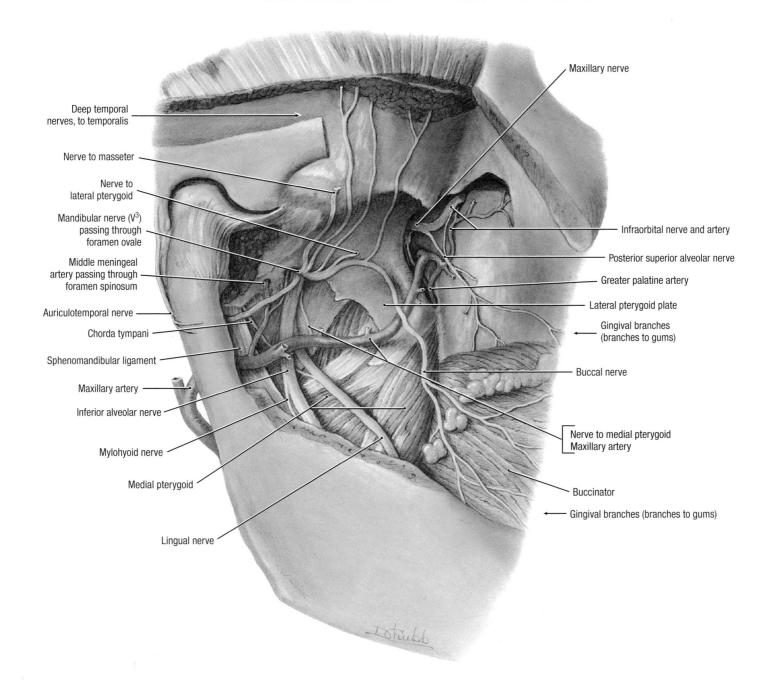

Deep temporal nerves, to temporalis

Nerve to masseter

Nerve to lateral pterygoid

Mandibular nerve (V³) passing through foramen ovale

Middle meningeal artery passing through foramen spinosum

Auriculotemporal nerve

Chorda tympani

Sphenomandibular ligament

Maxillary artery

Inferior alveolar nerve

Mylohyoid nerve

Medial pterygoid

Lingual nerve

Maxillary nerve

Infraorbital nerve and artery

Posterior superior alveolar nerve

Greater palatine artery

Lateral pterygoid plate

Gingival branches (branches to gums)

Buccal nerve

Nerve to medial pterygoid
Maxillary artery

Buccinator

Gingival branches (branches to gums)

7.63 **Infratemporal region, deeper dissection, lateral view**

The lateral pterygoid muscle and most of the branches of the maxillary artery have been removed.

OBSERVE:
1. The medial pterygoid muscle arises from the medial surface of the lateral pterygoid plate; it has a small, superficial head that arises from the pyramidal process of the palatine bone;
2. The maxillary artery and the auriculotemporal nerve pass between the sphenomandibular ligament and neck of the mandible;
3. The mandibular (CN V3) nerve enters the infratemporal fossa through the foramen ovale, which also transmits the accessory meningeal artery (not shown);
4. The middle meningeal artery and vein (not shown) pass through the foramen spinosum;

5. The inferior alveolar and lingual nerves descend on the medial pterygoid muscle. The inferior alveolar gives off the mylohyoid nerve to the mylohyoid muscle and anterior belly of the digastric muscle, and the lingual receives the chorda tympani, which carries secretory parasympathetic fibers and fibers of taste;
6. The nerves to the four muscles of mastication: the masseter, temporalis, and lateral and medial pterygoids. The buccal branch of the mandibular nerve is sensory, and the buccal branch of the facial nerve is the motor supply to the buccinator muscle;
7. The maxillary (CN V2) nerve becomes the infraorbital nerve that enters the infraorbital groove at the inferior orbital fissure.

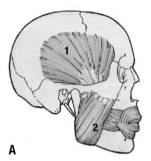
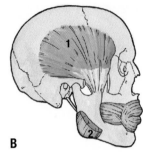
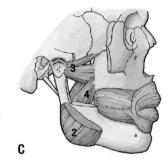

A   B   C

Table 7.5. Muscles Acting on Temporomandibular Joint

Muscle	Origin	Insertion	Innervation	Main Actions
Temporalis (*1*)	Floor of temporal fossa and deep surface of temporal fascia	Tip and medial surface of coronoid process and anterior border of ramus of mandible	Deep temporal branches of mandibular nerve (CN V^3)	Elevates mandible, closing jaws; its posterior fibers retrude mandible after protrusion
Masseter (*2*)	Inferior border and medial surface of zygomatic arch	Lateral surface of ramus of mandible and its coronoid process	Mandibular nerve through masseteric nerve that enters its deep surface	Elevates and protrudes mandible, thus closing jaws; deep fibers retrude it
Lateral pterygoid (*3*)	*Superior head:* infratemporal surface and infratemporal crest of greater wing of sphenoid bone *Inferior head:* lateral surface of lateral pterygoid plate	Neck of mandible, articular disc, and capsule of temporomandibular joint	Mandibular nerve (CN V^3) through lateral pterygoid nerve from anterior trunk, which enters its deep surface	Acting together, they protrude mandible and depress chin; acting alone and alternately, they produce side-to-side movements of mandible
Medial pterygoid (*4*)	*Deep head:* medial surface of lateral pterygoid plate and pyramidal process of palatine bone *Superficial head:* tuberosity of maxilla	Medial surface of ramus of mandible, inferior to mandibular foramen	Mandibular nerve (CN V^3) through medial pterygoid nerve	Helps elevate mandible, closing jaws; acting together, they help protrude mandible; acting alone, it protrudes side of jaw; acting alternately, they produce a grinding motion

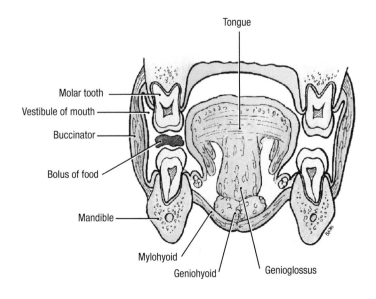

7.64   **Coronal section through mouth and buccinator, posterior view**

The tongue and buccinator retain food between the molar teeth during the act of chewing. The buccinator is innervated by the buccal branch of the facial nerve (CN VII), and the muscle of the tongue is innervated by the hypoglossal nerve (CN XII).

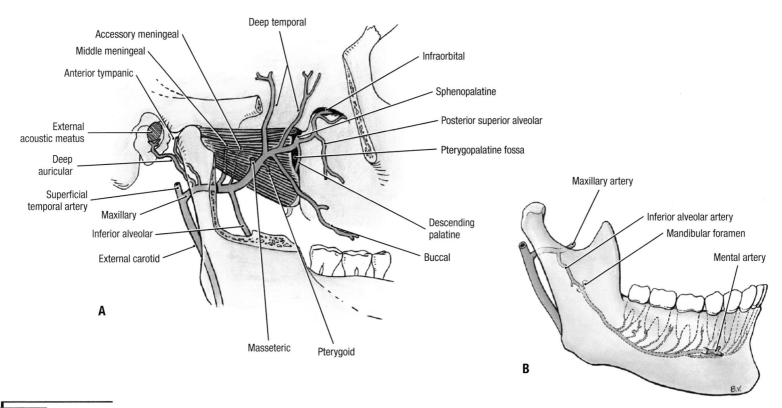

7.65 Branches of maxillary artery, lateral views

A. Infratemporal region. **B.** Mandible.

OBSERVE:
1. The maxillary artery arises at the neck of the mandible and is divided into three parts by the lateral pterygoid; it can pass medial or lateral to the lateral pterygoid;
2. The branches of the first part pass through foramina or canals; the deep auricular to the external acoustic meatus, the anterior tympanic to the tympanic cavity, the middle and accessory meningeal to the cranial cavity, and the inferior alveolar to the mandible and teeth;
3. The branches of the second part supply muscles through the masseteric, deep temporal, pterygoid, and buccal branches;
4. The branches of the third part (posterior superior alveolar, infraorbital, descending palatine, and sphenopalatine arteries) arise just before and within the pterygopalatine fossa. The descending palatine artery divides into the greater and lesser palatine arteries; the sphenopalatine artery divides into the posterior nasal septal and posterior lateral nasal arteries;

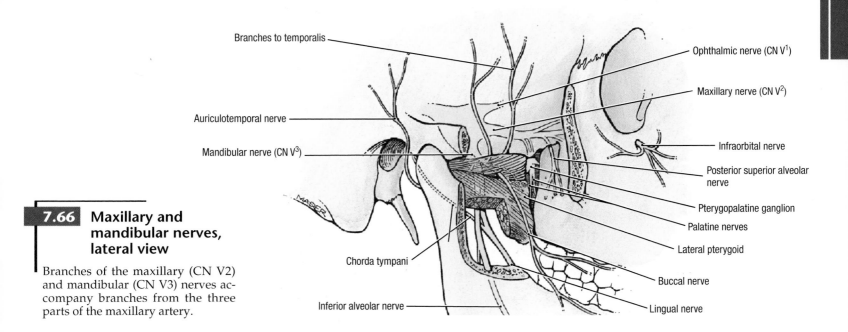

7.66 Maxillary and mandibular nerves, lateral view

Branches of the maxillary (CN V2) and mandibular (CN V3) nerves accompany branches from the three parts of the maxillary artery.

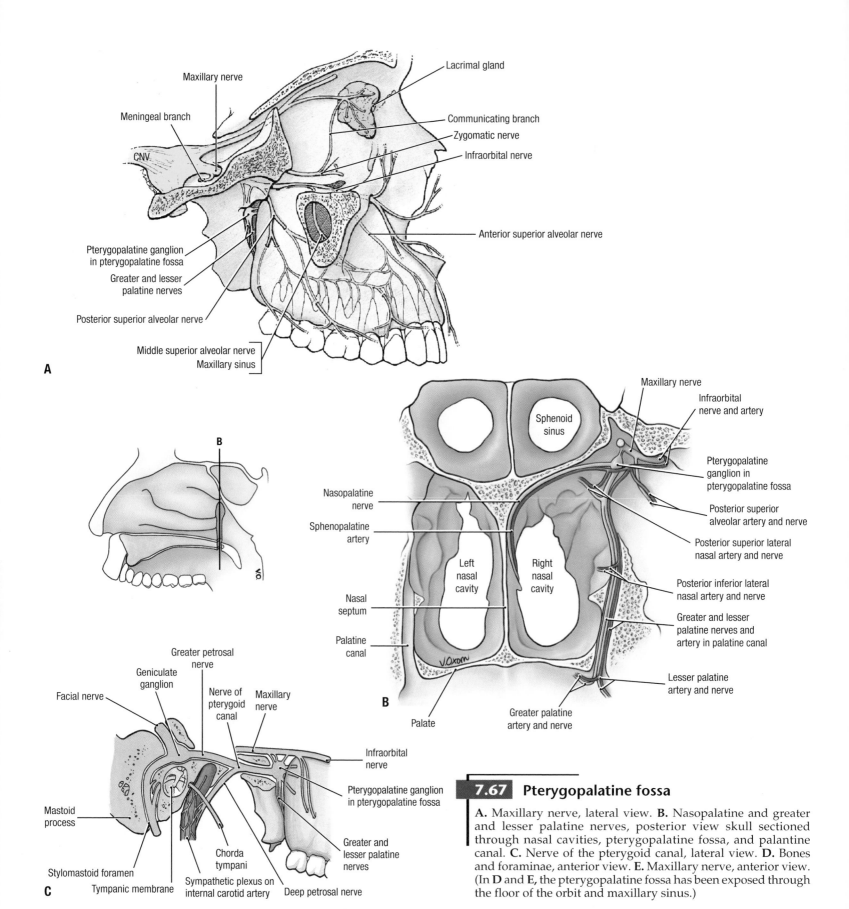

A. Maxillary nerve, lateral view.

Maxillary nerve

Meningeal branch

CNV

Pterygopalatine ganglion in pterygopalatine fossa

Greater and lesser palatine nerves

Posterior superior alveolar nerve

Middle superior alveolar nerve
Maxillary sinus

Lacrimal gland

Communicating branch

Zygomatic nerve

Infraorbital nerve

Anterior superior alveolar nerve

B

Maxillary nerve

Infraorbital nerve and artery

Sphenoid sinus

Nasopalatine nerve

Sphenopalatine artery

Left nasal cavity

Right nasal cavity

Nasal septum

Palatine canal

Palate

Greater palatine artery and nerve

Pterygopalatine ganglion in pterygopalatine fossa

Posterior superior alveolar artery and nerve

Posterior superior lateral nasal artery and nerve

Posterior inferior lateral nasal artery and nerve

Greater and lesser palatine nerves and artery in palatine canal

Lesser palatine artery and nerve

Greater petrosal nerve

Geniculate ganglion

Facial nerve

Nerve of pterygoid canal

Maxillary nerve

Mastoid process

Stylomastoid foramen

Tympanic membrane

Chorda tympani

Sympathetic plexus on internal carotid artery

Deep petrosal nerve

Infraorbital nerve

Pterygopalatine ganglion in pterygopalatine fossa

Greater and lesser palatine nerves

C

7.67 Pterygopalatine fossa

A. Maxillary nerve, lateral view. **B.** Nasopalatine and greater and lesser palatine nerves, posterior view skull sectioned through nasal cavities, pterygopalatine fossa, and palantine canal. **C.** Nerve of the pterygoid canal, lateral view. **D.** Bones and foraminae, anterior view. **E.** Maxillary nerve, anterior view. (In **D** and **E**, the pterygopalatine fossa has been exposed through the floor of the orbit and maxillary sinus.)

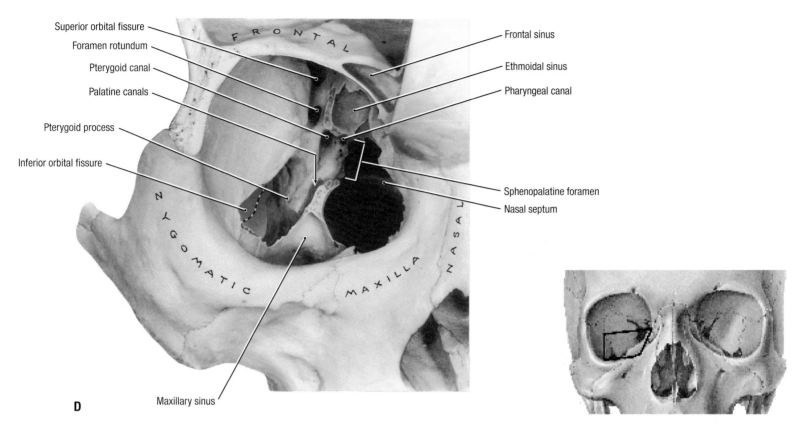

Superior orbital fissure
Foramen rotundum
Pterygoid canal
Palatine canals
Pterygoid process
Inferior orbital fissure
Frontal sinus
Ethmoidal sinus
Pharyngeal canal
Sphenopalatine foramen
Nasal septum
Maxillary sinus

D

OBSERVE IN **E:**

1. The maxillary nerve (CN V2) enters the pterygopalatine fossa through the foramen rotundum;

2. Within the pterygopalatine fossa the maxillary nerve gives off the zygomatic nerve, which divides into the zygomaticofacial and zygomaticotemporal nerves, the pterygopalatine nerves that suspend the pterygopalatine ganglion;

3. The maxillary nerve leaves the pterygopalatine fossa through the inferior orbital fissure, after which it becomes the infraorbital nerve;

4. Sensory fibers of the maxillary nerve pass through the pterygopalatine ganglion without synapsing to supply the nose, palate, tonsil, teeth, and gingivae;

5. The greater petrosal nerve brings parasympathetic fibers to the pterygopalatine ganglion through the nerve of pterygoid canal; the postsynaptic fibers are distributed, with the zygomatic branch of CN V2, as secretomotor fibers to the lacrimal gland.

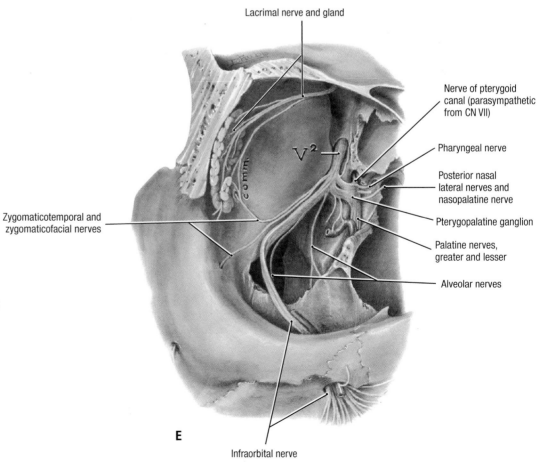

Lacrimal nerve and gland
Nerve of pterygoid canal (parasympathetic from CN VII)
Pharyngeal nerve
Posterior nasal lateral nerves and nasopalatine nerve
Pterygopalatine ganglion
Palatine nerves, greater and lesser
Alveolar nerves
Zygomaticotemporal and zygomaticofacial nerves
Infraorbital nerve

E

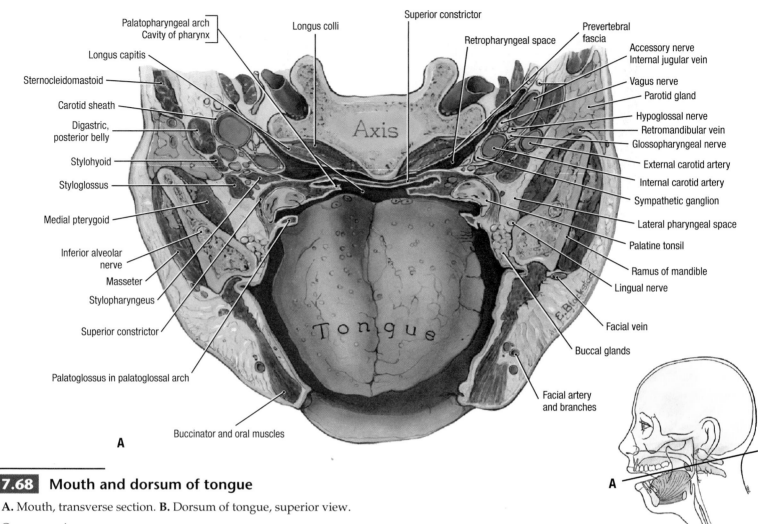

A

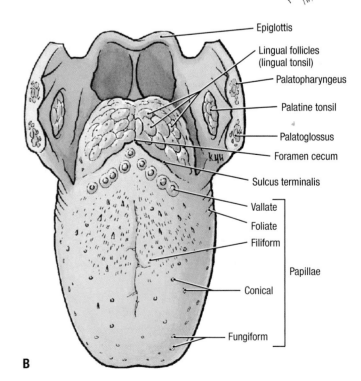

A

7.68 **Mouth and dorsum of tongue**

A. Mouth, transverse section. **B.** Dorsum of tongue, superior view.

OBSERVE IN **A:**

1. The masseter muscle is inserted into the lateral surface of the ramus of the mandible, and the medial pterygoid muscle is inserted into the medial surface; the lingual nerve lies in contact with it;
2. The pharynx is flattened anteroposteriorly, and the palatine tonsil lies in its wall; the tonsil bed is formed by the superior constrictor and palatopharyngeus muscles;
3. The retropharyngeal space (opened up in this specimen) allows the pharynx to contract and relax during swallowing; the retropharyngeal space is closed laterally at the carotid sheath and limited posteriorly by the prevertebral fascia;
4. The three styloid muscles are the stylohyoid, innervated by CN VII styloglossus by CN XII, and stylopharyngeus by CN IX.

OBSERVE IN **B:**

5. The foramen cecum is the patent upper end of the primitive thyroglossal duct; the arms of the V-shaped sulcus terminalis, which diverge from the foramen demarcate the posterior one third of the tongue from the anterior two thirds.

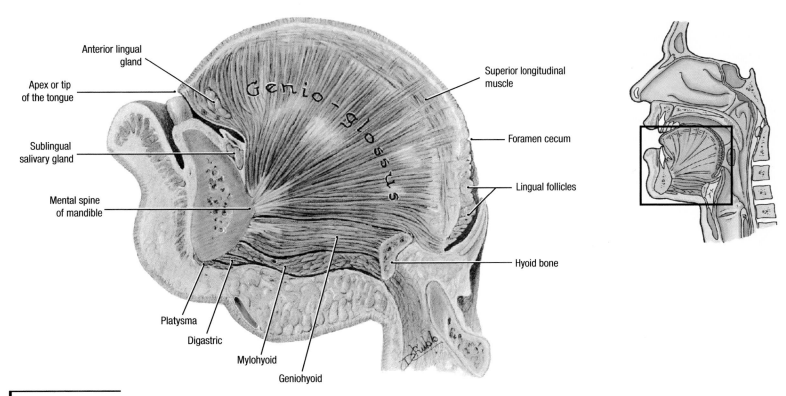

Anterior lingual gland
Apex or tip of the tongue
Sublingual salivary gland
Mental spine of mandible
Platysma
Digastric
Mylohyoid
Geniohyoid

Genio-glossus

Superior longitudinal muscle
Foramen cecum
Lingual follicles
Hyoid bone

7.69 **Tongue and floor of mouth, medial section**

OBSERVE:

1. The tongue is composed mainly of muscles; the extrinsic muscles alter the position of the tongue, and intrinsic muscles alter its shape. In this illustration, the extrinsic muscles are represented by the genioglossus muscle, and the intrinsic by the superior longitudinal muscle;

2. The anterior lingual gland is covered with a layer of muscle; the several ducts of this mixed mucoserous gland open inferior to the tongue, but are not in view.

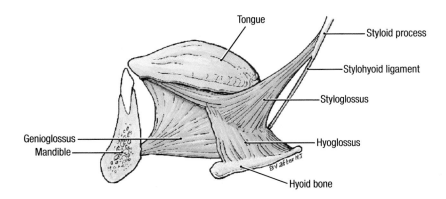

Tongue
Styloid process
Stylohyoid ligament
Styloglossus
Hyoglossus
Genioglossus
Mandible
Hyoid bone

Table 7.6. Extrinsic Muscles of Tongue

Muscle[a]	Origin	Insertion	Innervation	Actions
Genioglossus	Superior part of mental spine of mandible			Depresses tongue; its posterior part protrudes tongue
Hyoglossus	Body and greater horn of hyoid bone	Dorsum of tongue and body of hyoid bone	Hypoglossal nerve (CN XII)	Depresses and retracts tongue
Styloglossus	Styloid process and stylohyoid ligament	Side and inferior aspect of tongue		Retracts tongue and draws it up to create a trough for swallowing

[a]Palatoglossus, see Table 7.7.

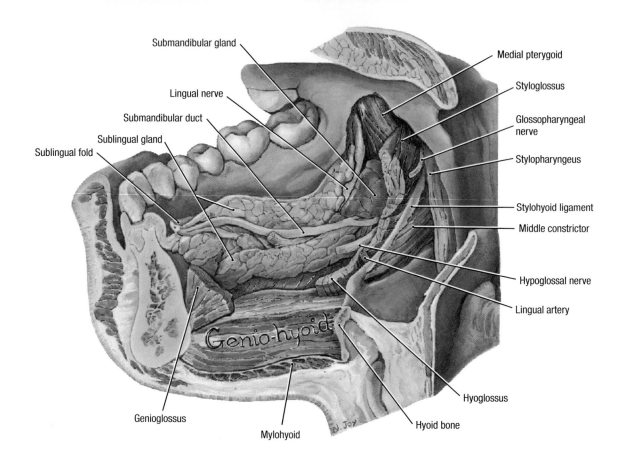

Submandibular gland
Lingual nerve
Submandibular duct
Sublingual gland
Sublingual fold
Genioglossus
Mylohyoid
Geniohyoid
Medial pterygoid
Styloglossus
Glossopharyngeal nerve
Stylopharyngeus
Stylohyoid ligament
Middle constrictor
Hypoglossal nerve
Lingual artery
Hyoglossus
Hyoid bone

7.70 Sublingual and submandibular glands, medial view

The tongue has been excised. The geniohyoid muscle inferiorly, the middle constrictor posteriorly, and the cut edge of the mucous membrane superiorly are undisturbed. The genioglossus muscle anteriorly, hyoglossus inferiorly, and styloglossus posteriorly are divided.

OBSERVE:
1. The lingual nerve appears between the medial pterygoid muscle and ramus of the mandible, and hooks around the submandibular duct;
2. The hypoglossal nerve is separated from the lingual artery by the hyoglossus muscle;

3. The deep part of the submandibular gland lies in the angle between the lingual nerve and submandibular duct, which separates it from the sublingual gland;
4. The orifice of the submandibular duct is seen at the anterior end of the sublingual fold;
5. The submandibular duct adheres to the medial side of the sublingual gland and here receives a large accessory duct from the inferior part of the sublingual gland.

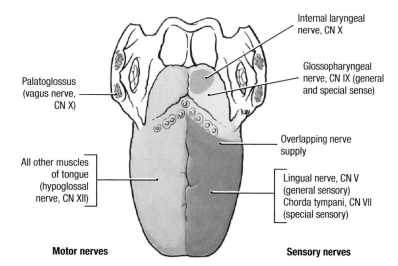

Internal laryngeal nerve, CN X
Glossopharyngeal nerve, CN IX (general and special sense)
Palatoglossus (vagus nerve, CN X)
All other muscles of tongue (hypoglossal nerve, CN XII)
Overlapping nerve supply
Lingual nerve, CN V (general sensory)
Chorda tympani, CN VII (special sensory)

Motor nerves   **Sensory nerves**

7.71 Innervation of tongue, superior view

OBSERVE:
1. All of the muscles of the tongue, except the palatoglossus, are supplied by the hypoglossal nerve (CN XII);
2. For general sensation, the anterior two thirds of the tongue is supplied by the lingual nerve, and the posterior one third by the glossopharyngeal nerve; the internal laryngeal nerve, a branch of the vagus nerve (CN X), supplies a small area of the tongue anterior to the epiglottis;
3. For taste sensation, the anterior two thirds of the tongue is supplied by the corda tympani, and the posterior one third by the glossopharyngeal nerve.

7.72 Muscles and vessels of mandible and base of skull, medial view

OBSERVE:

1. The mylohyoid muscle has a thick, free, posterior edge;
2. The medial pterygoid muscle is oriented in the same direction on the medial side of the ramus of the mandible as the masseter muscle on the lateral side;
3. The tensor veli palatini muscle in this specimen sends some fibers to the hamulus;
4. The lingual nerve is joined superior to the medial pterygoid muscle by the chorda tympani;
5. The otic ganglion lies medial to the mandibular nerve (CN V3) and between the foramen ovale superiorly and the medial pterygoid muscle inferiorly; the tensor veli palatini muscle usually covers the ganglion. The otic ganglion receives sensory fibers from the auriculotemporal branch of CN V3, sympathetic fibers from the plexus on the middle meningeal artery, and the site of synapse of parasympathetic fibers from the lesser petrosal branch of CN IX; it connects with CN VII and allows the motor fibers to the tensors to pass through it.

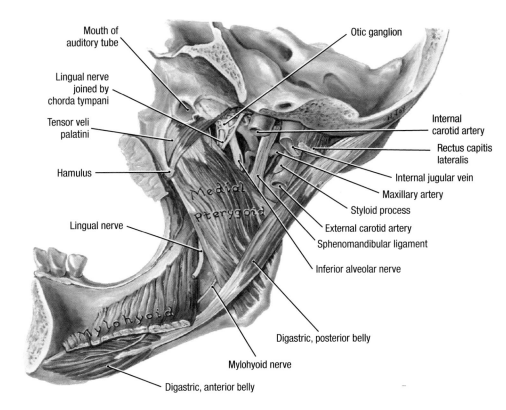

7.73 Muscles of floor of mouth, superior view

OBSERVE:

1. The paired, horizontal geniohyoid muscles lie between the mental spine and body of the hyoid bone; their lateral borders are in contact with mylohyoid muscle;
2. The mylohyoid muscle arises from the mylohyoid line of the mandible; it has a thick, free posterior border that thins as it is traced anteriorly and ends in a delicate, free anterior border as it nears the origin of the geniohyoid and genioglossus muscles.

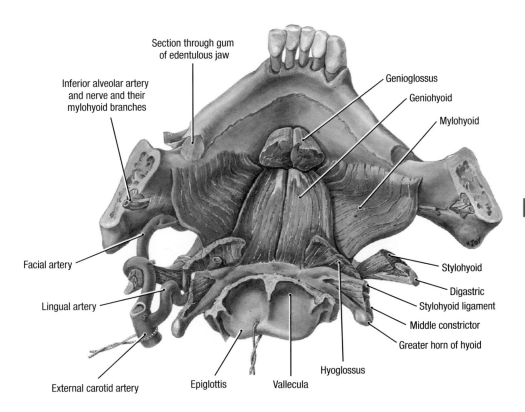

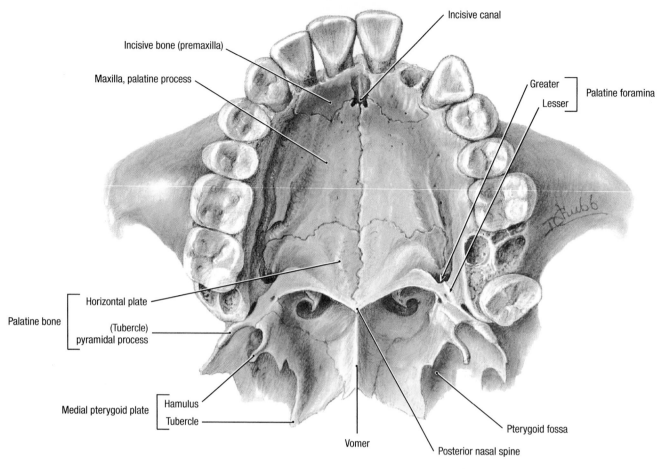

Incisive canal

Incisive bone (premaxilla)

Maxilla, palatine process

Greater

Lesser

Palatine foramina

Horizontal plate

(Tubercle) pyramidal process

Palatine bone

Hamulus

Medial pterygoid plate

Tubercle

Pterygoid fossa

Vomer

Posterior nasal spine

A

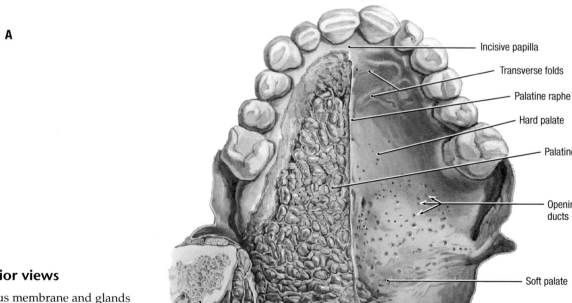

Incisive papilla

Transverse folds

Palatine raphe

Hard palate

Palatine glands

Openings of ducts

Soft palate

Palatoglossal arch

Palatine tonsil

Mandible

Parotid gland

Palatoglossus

Uvula

Palatopharyngeal arch

B

7.74   Palate—I, inferior views

A. Bones of palate. **B.** Mucous membrane and glands of palate.

OBSERVE:

1. The orifices of the ducts of the palatine glands; the palate ends posteriorly in the midline in the uvula and on each side in the palatopharyngeal arch;
2. The palate has bony (hard palate), aponeurotic, and muscular (soft palate) parts;
3. The tensor veli palatini muscle hooks around the hamulus to join the palatine aponeurosis.

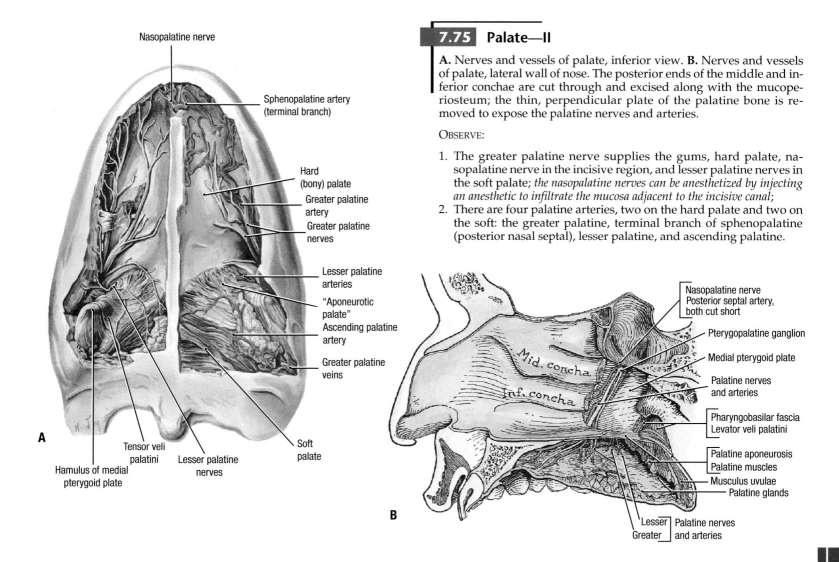

A. Nerves and vessels of palate, inferior view. **B.** Nerves and vessels of palate, lateral wall of nose. The posterior ends of the middle and inferior conchae are cut through and excised along with the mucoperiosteum; the thin, perpendicular plate of the palatine bone is removed to expose the palatine nerves and arteries.

OBSERVE:

1. The greater palatine nerve supplies the gums, hard palate, nasopalatine nerve in the incisive region, and lesser palatine nerves in the soft palate; *the nasopalatine nerves can be anesthetized by injecting an anesthetic to infiltrate the mucosa adjacent to the incisive canal;*
2. There are four palatine arteries, two on the hard palate and two on the soft: the greater palatine, terminal branch of sphenopalatine (posterior nasal septal), lesser palatine, and ascending palatine.

7.75   Palate—II

(Figure A labels: Nasopalatine nerve; Sphenopalatine artery (terminal branch); Hard (bony) palate; Greater palatine artery; Greater palatine nerves; Lesser palatine arteries; "Aponeurotic palate"; Ascending palatine artery; Greater palatine veins; Soft palate; Lesser palatine nerves; Tensor veli palatini; Hamulus of medial pterygoid plate; A)

(Figure B labels: Nasopalatine nerve, Posterior septal artery, both cut short; Pterygopalatine ganglion; Medial pterygoid plate; Palatine nerves and arteries; Pharyngobasilar fascia; Levator veli palatini; Palatine aponeurosis; Palatine muscles; Musculus uvulae; Palatine glands; Lesser / Greater Palatine nerves and arteries; Mid. concha; Inf. concha; B)

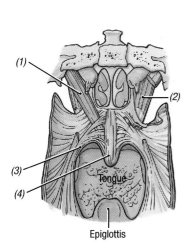

(Labels: (1), (2), (3), (4), Tongue, Epiglottis)

Table 7.7. Muscle of Soft Palate

Muscle	Superior Attachment	Inferior Attachment	Innervation	Main Action(s)
Levator veli (1)	Cartilage of auditory tube and petrous part of temporal bone	Palatine aponeurosis	Pharyngeal branch of vagus nerve through pharyngeal plexus	Elevates soft palate during swallowing and yawning
Tensor veli palatini (2)	Scaphoid fossa of medial pterygoid plate, spine of sphenoid bone, and cartilage of auditory tube		Medial pterygoid nerve (a branch of mandibular nerve) through otic ganglion	Tenses soft palate and opens mouth of auditory tube during swallowing and yawning
Palatoglossus (Fig. 8.43A)	Palatine aponeurosis	Side of tongue	Cranial part of CN XI through pharyngeal branch of vagus nerve (CN X) through	Elevates posterior part of tongue and draws soft palate onto tongue
Palatopharyngeus (3)	Hard palate and palatine aponeurosis	Lateral wall of pharynx		Tenses soft palate and pulls walls of pharynx superiorly, anteriorly, and medially during swallowing
Musculus uvulae (4)	Posterior nasal spine and palatine aponeurosis	Mucosa of uvula		Shortens uvula and pulls it superiorly

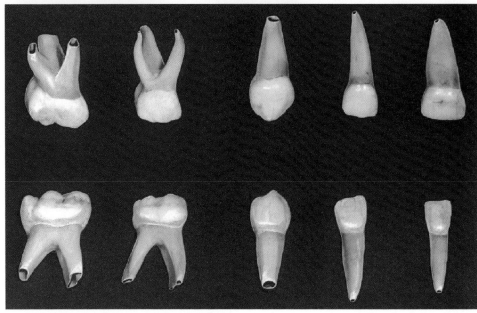

A   2nd molar   1st molar   Canine   Lateral incisor   Central incisor

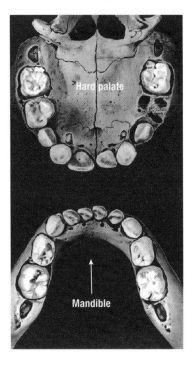

B

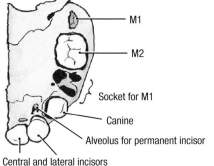

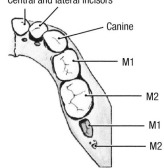

7.76 Primary teeth

A. Teeth removed. **B.** Teeth in situ, younger than 2 years of age.

OBSERVE IN **A:**
1. Our first set of teeth consist of 20 primary, or deciduous, teeth, five in each half of the mandible and five in each maxilla. They are named: central incisor, lateral incisor, canine, 1st molar (*M1*), and 2nd molar (*M2*);
2. The first primary teeth to erupt through the gums are the lower central incisors, at approximately 6 months; the last to erupt are the 2nd upper molars, at approximately the end of 2 years. The three roots of the upper molars and two roots of the lower molars are spread to grasp the developing permanent premolars;
3. Primary teeth differ from permanent teeth in that the primary teeth are smaller and whiter; the molars also have more bulbous crowns and more divergent roots.

OBSERVE IN **B:**
4. The canines have not fully erupted, and the 2nd molars have just started to erupt.
5. The 2nd molars have much larger crowns than the 1st molars;
6. The socket for the three-pronged root of the 1st upper molar is seen;
7. Permanent teeth are colored orange; the crowns of the unerupted 1st and 2nd permanent molars are partly visible.

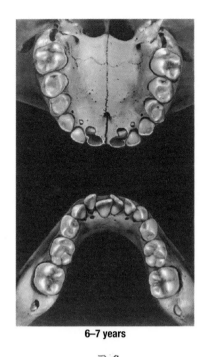
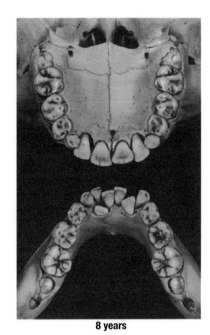
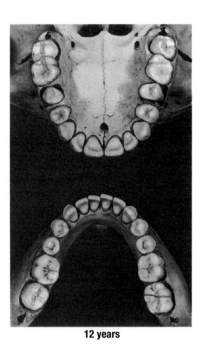

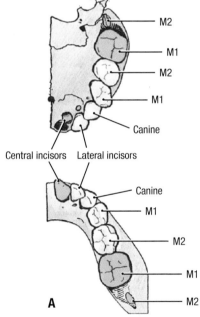
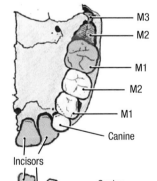
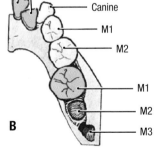
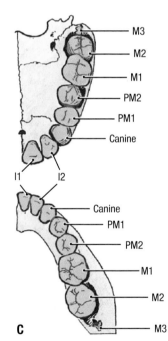

6–7 years   **8 years**   **12 years**

A   **B**   **C**

7.77 Eruption of permanent teeth

Between 6 and 12 years, the primary teeth are shed and succeeded by permanent teeth (orange). **A.** Age 6 to 7 years. The 1st molars (6-year molars) have fully erupted; the primary central incisors have been shed; the lower central incisors nearly have fully erupted; and the upper central incisors are moving downward into the empty sockets. **B.** Age 8 years. All of the permanent incisors have erupted; the upper and lower central and the upper lateral are fully erupted, and the lower lateral are partially erupted. The alveolus has not yet closed around the upper lateral incisors; in this specimen, the root of the left lower lateral primary incisor has not been resorbed, so the tooth has not been shed. **C.** Age 12 years. The 20 primary teeth have been replaced by 20 permanent teeth, and the 1st molars and 2nd molars (12-year molars) have erupted; the canines, 2nd premolars, and 2nd molars (especially those in the upper jaw) have not erupted fully, nor have their bony sockets closed around them. By age 12, 28 permanent teeth are in evidence; the last four teeth, the 3rd molars, may erupt any time after this, or never (*I*, incisor, *PM*, premolar, *M*, molar teeth).

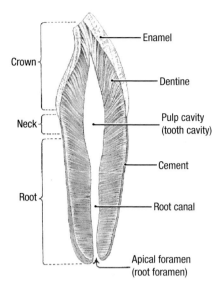

Crown

Neck

Root

Enamel

Dentine

Pulp cavity (tooth cavity)

Cement

Root canal

Apical foramen (root foramen)

Incisor tooth

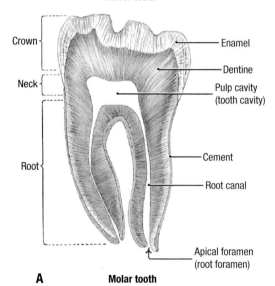

Crown

Neck

Root

Enamel

Dentine

Pulp cavity (tooth cavity)

Cement

Root canal

Apical foramen (root foramen)

A   **Molar tooth**

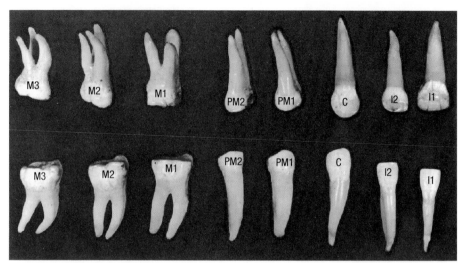

B

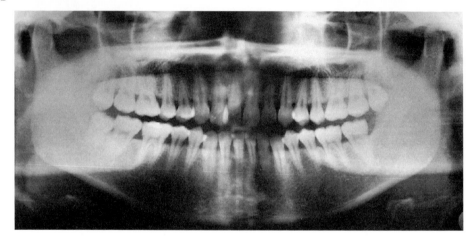

C

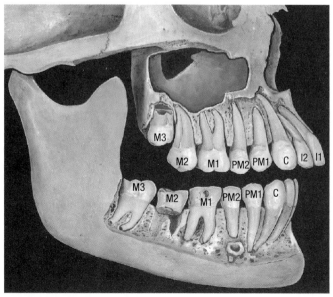

D

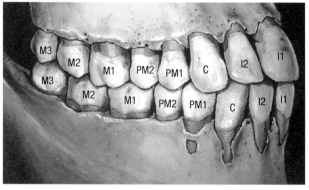

E

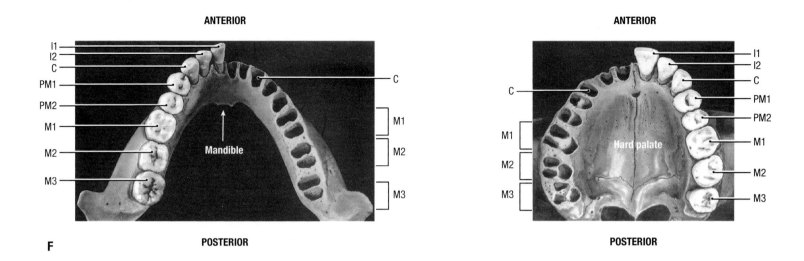

ANTERIOR

I1
I2
C
PM1
PM2
M1
M2
M3

C

M1
M2
M3

Mandible

F   POSTERIOR

ANTERIOR

I1
I2
C
PM1
PM2
M1
M2
M3

C

M1
M2
M3

Hard palate

POSTERIOR

7.78 Permanent teeth

The second set of teeth consist of 32 permanent teeth; eight are on each side of each dental arch on the top and bottom: two incisors, one canine, two premolars, and three molars. **A.** Longitudinal sections of incisor and molar teeth. **B.** Roots, teeth removed. The mandibular (lower) teeth include the incisor (*I*), canine (*C*), and premolar (*PM1* and *PM2*), or bicuspid, teeth; each has one root. Molars (*M1*, *M2*, and *M3*) have two roots: mesial (anterior) and distal (posterior); the mesial roots generally have two root canals. The maxillary (upper) teeth include the incisor and canine teeth; each has one root. Premolars have one or two roots; the 1st premolar usually has two, and the 2nd usually has one, although sometimes, as here, both premolars have two roots; each of the three molars has three roots. **C.** Pantomographic radiograph of mandible and maxilla. Left lower M3 is not present. **D.**

Teeth in situ with roots exposed, lateral view. The roots of the 2nd lower molar have been removed. Note the upper canine ("eye tooth") is the longest tooth with the longest root. The roots of the three upper molars almost penetrate the maxillary sinus; the upper and lower 3rd molars are not yet fully developed. **E.** Teeth in occlusion, lateral view. The maxillary and mandibular teeth are in centric occlusion, with the upper dental arch overlapping the lower dental arch. All teeth, except the lower central incisor and 3rd upper molar, bite on two opposing teeth; **F.** Permanent teeth and their sockets. An incisor tooth has a cutting edge; a canine tooth, or cuspid, has one cusp on its crown; a premolar tooth, or bicuspid, has two or three cusps; and a molar tooth has from three to five cusps.

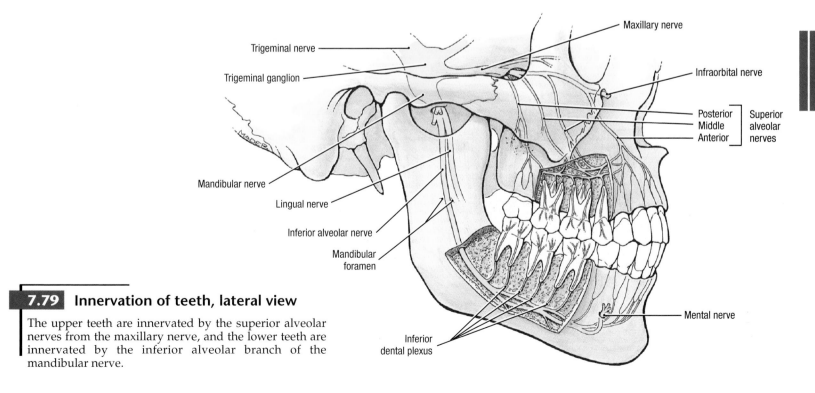

Trigeminal nerve

Trigeminal ganglion

Maxillary nerve

Infraorbital nerve

Posterior
Middle
Anterior
Superior alveolar nerves

Mandibular nerve

Lingual nerve

Inferior alveolar nerve

Mandibular foramen

Mental nerve

Inferior dental plexus

7.79 Innervation of teeth, lateral view

The upper teeth are innervated by the superior alveolar nerves from the maxillary nerve, and the lower teeth are innervated by the inferior alveolar branch of the mandibular nerve.

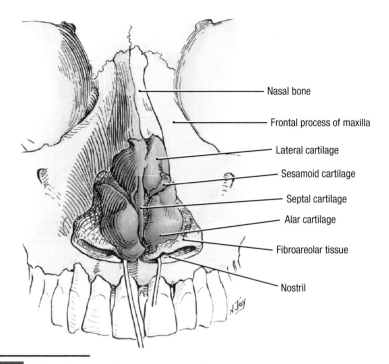

A

- Nasal bone
- Frontal process of maxilla
- Lateral cartilage
- Sesamoid cartilage
- Septal cartilage
- Alar cartilage
- Fibroareolar tissue
- Nostril

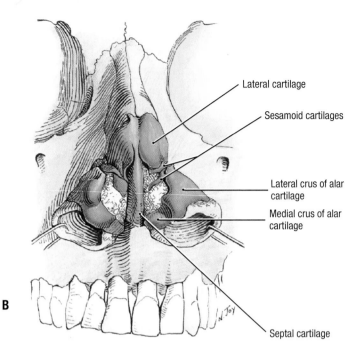

B

- Lateral cartilage
- Sesamoid cartilages
- Lateral crus of alar cartilage
- Medial crus of alar cartilage
- Septal cartilage

7.80 Cartilages of nose, anterior views

A. Alar cartilages pulled inferiorly. **B.** Alar cartilages separated and retracted laterally.

OBSERVE:
1. The lateral nasal cartilages (in this specimen fixed by suture to the nasal bones) are continuous with the septal cartilage;

2. The alar nasal cartilages are free, movable, and U-shaped;
3. The sesamoid cartilages are between the lateral and alar cartilages;
4. The distal part of the nose is formed of fibroareolar tissue; the nasal cartilages are hyaline cartilage; and the cartilage of the auricle is elastic cartilage.

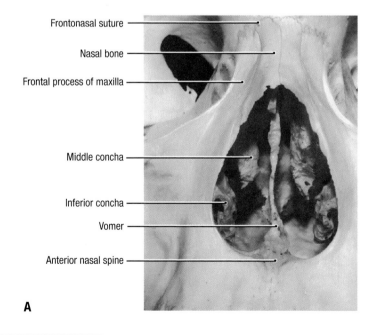

A

- Frontonasal suture
- Nasal bone
- Frontal process of maxilla
- Middle concha
- Inferior concha
- Vomer
- Anterior nasal spine

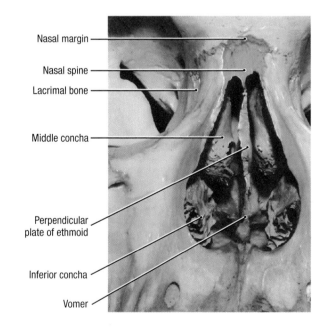

B

- Nasal margin
- Nasal spine
- Lacrimal bone
- Middle concha
- Perpendicular plate of ethmoid
- Inferior concha
- Vomer

7.81 Bones of nose, anterior views

A. Anterior nasal aperture. The margin of the anterior nasal aperture is sharp and formed by the maxillae and nasal bones.
B. Nasal bones removed. The areas on the frontal processes of the

maxillae (*yellow*) and the frontal bone (*blue*) that articulate with the nasal bones can be seen.

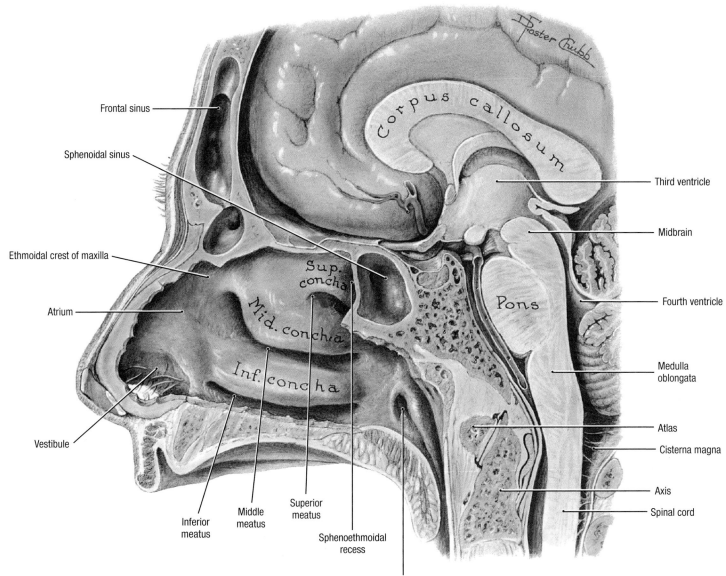

Frontal sinus

Sphenoidal sinus

Ethmoidal crest of maxilla

Atrium

Vestibule

Inferior meatus

Middle meatus

Superior meatus

Sphenoethmoidal recess

Pharyngeal orifice of auditory tube

Sup. concha

Mid. concha

Inf. concha

Corpus callosum

Pons

Third ventricle

Midbrain

Fourth ventricle

Medulla oblongata

Atlas

Cisterna magna

Axis

Spinal cord

7.82 **Lateral wall of nasal cavity**

OBSERVE:
1. The vestibule is superior to the nostril and anterior to the inferior meatus; hairs grow from its skin-lined surface;
2. The atrium is superior to the vestibule and anterior to the middle meatus;
3. The inferior and middle conchae curve inferiorly and medially from the lateral wall, dividing it into three nearly equal parts and covering the inferior and middle meatuses, respectively. The middle concha, with an angled inferior border, ends inferior to the sphenoidal sinus; the inferior concha, with a slightly curved inferior border, ends inferior to the middle concha, just anterior to the orifice of the auditory tube;

4. The superior concha is small and anterior to the sphenoidal sinus;
5. The floor of the nose is inclined slightly inferiorly and posteriorly at the level of the atlas;
6. The roof is composed of an anterior sloping part corresponding to the bridge of the nose; an intermediate horizontal part; a perpendicular part anterior to the sphenoidal sinus; and a curved part, inferior to the sinus, that is continuous with the roof of the nasopharynx;
7. The pons and 4th ventricle of the brain are at the level of the sphenoidal sinus.

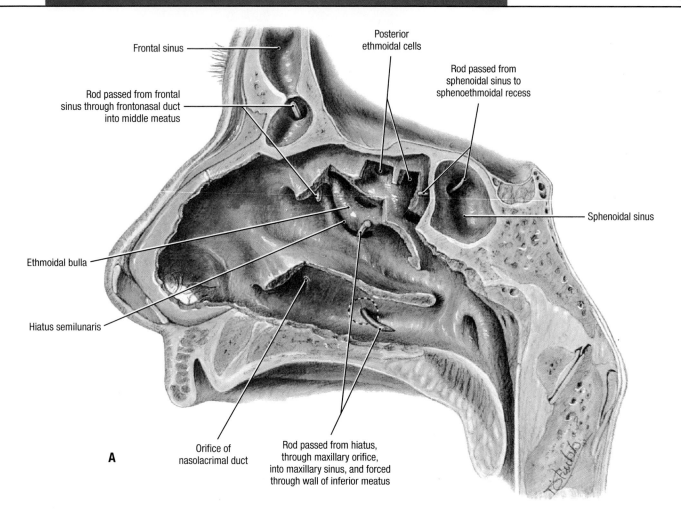

Frontal sinus

Posterior ethmoidal cells

Rod passed from sphenoidal sinus to sphenoethmoidal recess

Rod passed from frontal sinus through frontonasal duct into middle meatus

Sphenoidal sinus

Ethmoidal bulla

Hiatus semilunaris

Orifice of nasolacrimal duct

Rod passed from hiatus, through maxillary orifice, into maxillary sinus, and forced through wall of inferior meatus

A

7.83 Openings on lateral wall of nasal cavity—I, medial view

A. Dissection. Parts of the superior, middle, and inferior conchae are cut away. **B.** Bones. (Frontal, *light yellow*; nasal, *green*; maxilla, *purple*; lacrimal, *blue*; ethmoid, *bright yellow*; palatine, *red*; sphenoid, *gray*.) Note one arrow passing from the frontal sinus through the frontonasal duct into the middle meatus, and another arrow traversing the nasolacrimal canal. Accessory maxillary ostio can occur in the membrane that closes the maxillary hiatus.

OBSERVE IN **A**:
1. The sphenoidal sinus is in the body of the sphenoid bone; its orifice opens into the sphenoethmoidal recess;
2. The orifices of the posterior ethmoidal cells open into the superior meatus;
3. In this specimen, a cell opens onto the superior surface of the ethmoidal bulla;
4. The orifice of the nasolacrimal duct is inferior to the inferior concha;

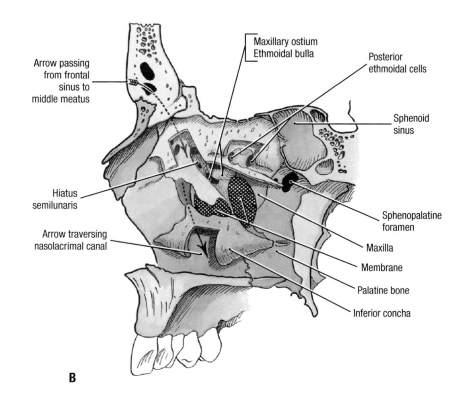

Arrow passing from frontal sinus to middle meatus

Maxillary ostium
Ethmoidal bulla

Posterior ethmoidal cells

Sphenoid sinus

Hiatus semilunaris

Arrow traversing nasolacrimal canal

Sphenopalatine foramen

Maxilla

Membrane

Palatine bone

Inferior concha

B

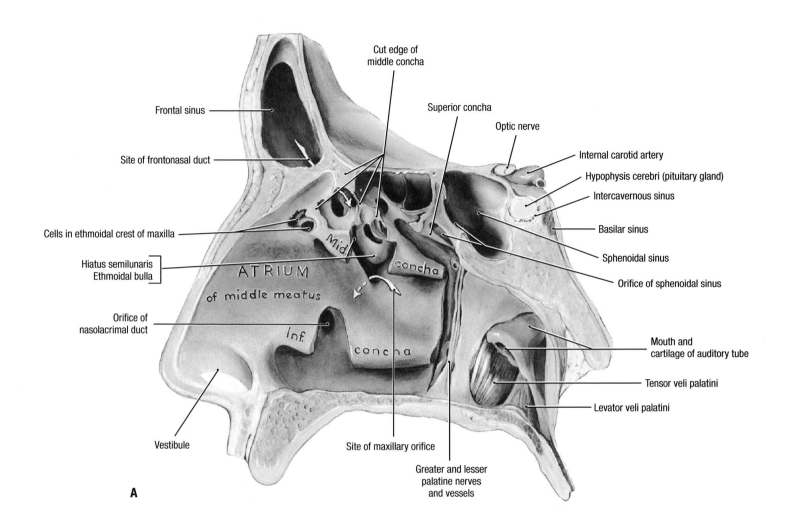

Frontal sinus

Cut edge of middle concha

Superior concha

Site of frontonasal duct

Optic nerve

Internal carotid artery

Hypophysis cerebri (pituitary gland)

Intercavernous sinus

Cells in ethmoidal crest of maxilla

Basilar sinus

Hiatus semilunaris
Ethmoidal bulla

Sphenoidal sinus

Orifice of sphenoidal sinus

Orifice of nasolacrimal duct

Mouth and cartilage of auditory tube

Tensor veli palatini

Levator veli palatini

Vestibule

Site of maxillary orifice

Mouth and cartilage of auditory tube

Greater and lesser palatine nerves and vessels

A

ATRIUM of middle meatus

Mid. concha

Inf. concha

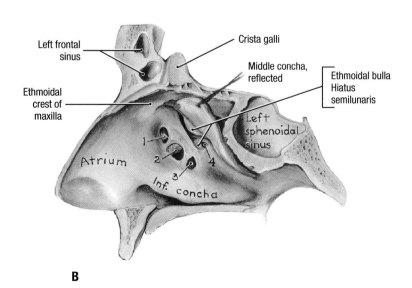

Left frontal sinus

Crista galli

Middle concha, reflected

Ethmoidal crest of maxilla

Ethmoidal bulla
Hiatus semilunaris

Left sphenoidal sinus

Atrium

Inf. concha

B

7.84 Openings on lateral wall of nasal cavity— II, medial view

A. Paranasal air sinuses and hypophysis cerebri. **B.** Accessory maxillary orifices.

OBSERVE IN **A:**
1. The frontal sinus, with its outlet (*arrow*) at its most inferior point, the frontonasal duct, leads into the middle meatus medial to the hiatus semilunaris;
2. Anteriorly, the hiatus semilunaris ends blindly as an anterior ethmoidal cell, and posteriorly as the maxillary orifice (*arrow*);
3. The sphenoidal sinus is of average size, with a large orifice.

OBSERVE IN **B:**
4. In addition to the primary, or normal, ostium (not shown), there are four secondary, or acquired, ostia; these result from the breaking down of the membrane shown in cross-hatching in Figure 7.83B;
5. The septum is between the right and left sphenoidal sinus; in this specimen, it occupies the median plane, whereas it is usually deflected to one side.

ANTERIOR   POSTERIOR

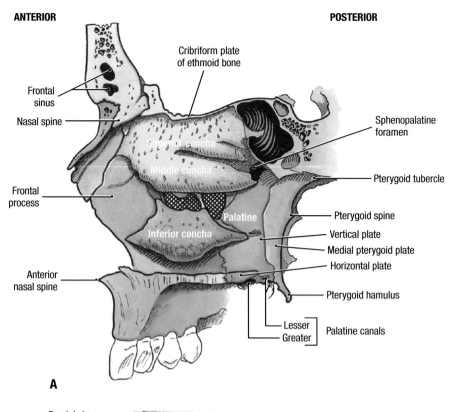

Frontal sinus

Cribriform plate of ethmoid bone

Nasal spine

Superior concha

Middle concha

Sphenopalatine foramen

Frontal process

Palatine

Inferior concha

Pterygoid tubercle

Anterior nasal spine

Vertical plate

Pterygoid spine

Medial pterygoid plate

Horizontal plate

Pterygoid hamulus

Lesser
Greater } Palatine canals

A

7.85 Lateral wall of nose, medial view of median section

7.85 Lateral wall of nose, medial view of median section

A. Bones. (Frontal, *peach*; nasal, *green*; maxilla, *purple*; lacrimal, *blue*; ethmoid, *bright yellow*; palatine, *red*; sphenoid, *gray*.) The superior and middle conchae are parts of the ethmoid bone, whereas the inferior concha is itself a bone. The fragile, perpendicular plate of the palatine bone has a notch at its superior border; when in articulation with the body of the sphenoid bone, it forms the sphenopalatine foramen. **B.** Arteries. The lateral wall of the nose is supplied by the anterior and posterior ethmoidal branches of the ophthalmic artery, which enter the nasal cavity through the cribriform plate. The sphenopalatine artery arises from the maxillary artery and the ascending palatine artery and lateral nasal branches of the facial artery. **C.** Innervation. The lateral wall of the nose is supplied by posterolateral nasal branches of the maxillary nerve (CN V2), the greater palatine nerve, and the anterior ethmoidal nerve. The olfactory neuroepithelium is in the superior part of the lateral and septal walls of the nasal cavity. The central processes of the bipolar olfactory neurosensory cells of this epithelium form approximately 20 bundles on each side, which together form the olfactory nerves. The olfactory nerves pass through the cribriform plate to enter the olfactory bulbs. *An extension of the cranial meninges surrounds the olfactory nerve as it leaves the cribriform plate. Tearing of the meninges results in leakage of cerebrospinal fluid (CSF) into the nose, a condition called CSF rhinorrhea.*

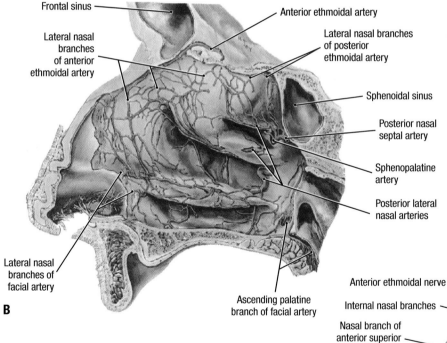

Frontal sinus

Anterior ethmoidal artery

Lateral nasal branches of anterior ethmoidal artery

Lateral nasal branches of posterior ethmoidal artery

Sphenoidal sinus

Posterior nasal septal artery

Sphenopalatine artery

Posterior lateral nasal arteries

Lateral nasal branches of facial artery

Ascending palatine branch of facial artery

B

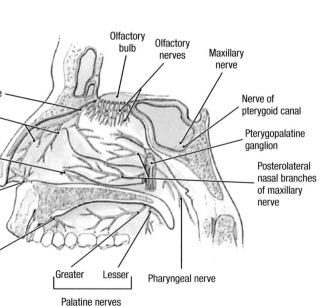

Olfactory bulb

Olfactory nerves

Maxillary nerve

Anterior ethmoidal nerve

Internal nasal branches

Nasal branch of anterior superior alveolar nerve

Nerve of pterygoid canal

Pterygopalatine ganglion

Internal nasal branch of infraorbital nerve

Posterolateral nasal branches of maxillary nerve

Nasopalatine nerve

Greater   Lesser   Pharyngeal nerve

Palatine nerves

C

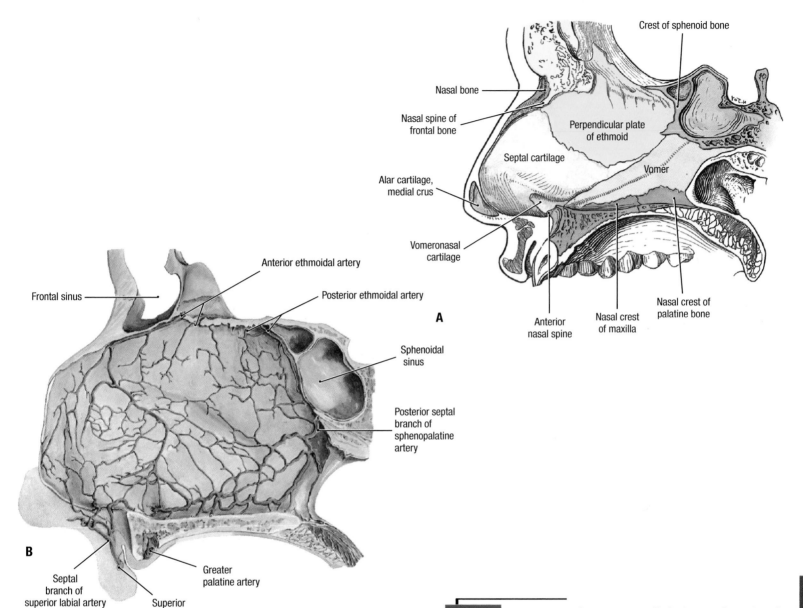

A

Crest of sphenoid bone

Nasal bone

Nasal spine of frontal bone

Perpendicular plate of ethmoid

Septal cartilage

Vomer

Alar cartilage, medial crus

Vomeronasal cartilage

Anterior nasal spine

Nasal crest of maxilla

Nasal crest of palatine bone

B

Frontal sinus

Anterior ethmoidal artery

Posterior ethmoidal artery

Sphenoidal sinus

Posterior septal branch of sphenopalatine artery

Septal branch of superior labial artery

Superior labial branch of facial artery

Greater palatine artery

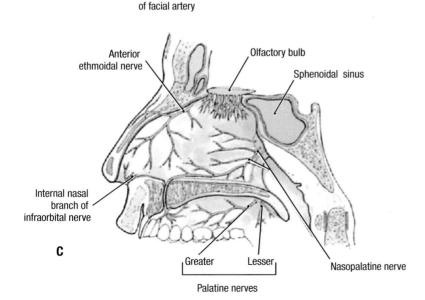

C

Anterior ethmoidal nerve

Olfactory bulb

Sphenoidal sinus

Internal nasal branch of infraorbital nerve

Greater   Lesser

Palatine nerves

Nasopalatine nerve

7.86 Septum of nose, medial view of sagittal section

A. Bones. (Nasal, *green*; frontal, *light yellow*; sphenoid, *dark gray*; ethmoid, *yellow*; palatine, *red*; maxilla, *purple*; vomer, *peach*; septal and alar cartilage, *light gray*) The septum of the nose has hard and soft parts. The skeleton of the hard septum consists of three parts, the perpendicular plate of the ethmoid, septal cartilage, and the vomer. Around the circumference of these, the adjacent bones (frontal, nasal, maxillary, palatine, and sphenoid) make minor contributions to the hard septum. The soft (mobile) septum is composed of the medial crura of the alar cartilages and the skin and soft tissues between the tip of the nose and the nasal spine of the frontal bone. **B. Arteries.** *Epistaxis (nosebleed) is a relatively common condition because of the rich blood supply to the nasal mucosa. In most cases, the cause is trauma, and the bleeding is located in the anterior third of the nose. Epistaxis is also associated with infections and hypertension.* **C. Innervation.** The nasopalatine nerve from the pterygopalatine ganglion (see Fig. 7.85C) supplies the posteroinferior two thirds of the septum, and the anterior ethmoidal nerve (branch of V1) supplies the anterior portion.

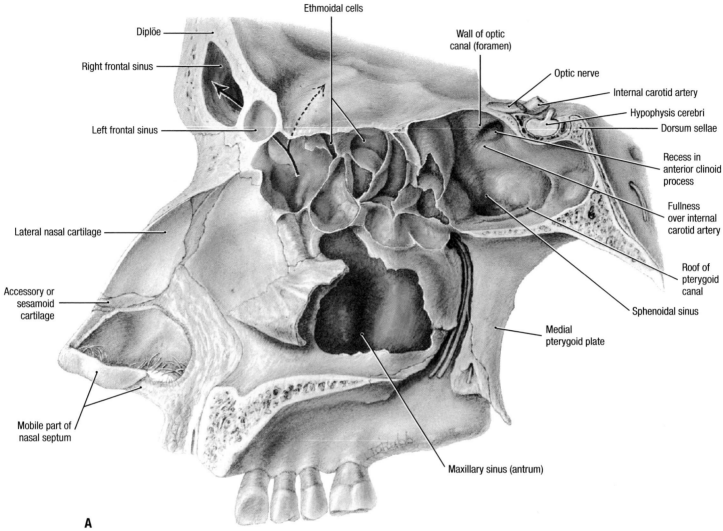

A. Opened sinuses, medial view.

A

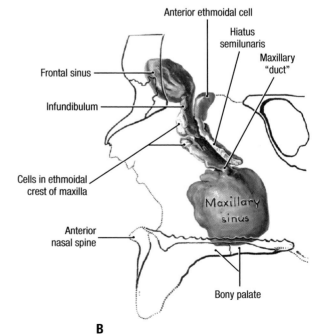

B

7.87 Paranasal sinuses

A. Opened sinuses, medial view. **B.** Cast of frontal and maxillary sinuses, medial view.

OBSERVE IN **A**:

1. The ethmoidal cells (*blue*), collectively called a sinus, have the thin, orbital plate of the frontal bone for a "roof";
2. An anterior ethmoidal cell (*pink*) invades the diploî of the frontal bone to become a frontal sinus (*arrow*); it is ethmoidal in origin, but frontal in location;
3. The sphenoidal sinus (*yellow*) in this specimen is extensive, extending (a) posteriorly, inferior to the hypophysis cerebri to the dorsum sellae; (b) laterally, inferior to the optic nerve; and (c) inferiorly, to the pterygoid process, consisting of the medial and lateral pterygoid plates;
4. The maxillary sinus (*purple*) is pyramidal.

OBSERVE IN **B**:

5. The frontal sinus lies superior to the orbital cavity, with its opening at its most inferior point; the maxillary sinus lies inferior to the orbital cavity, and its opening is level with its most superior point.

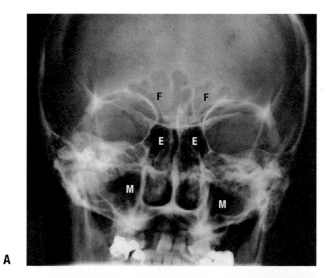

A

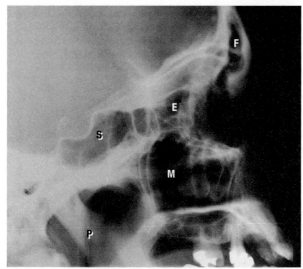

B

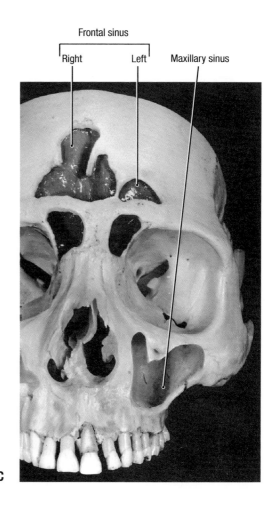

Frontal sinus

Right   Left   Maxillary sinus

C

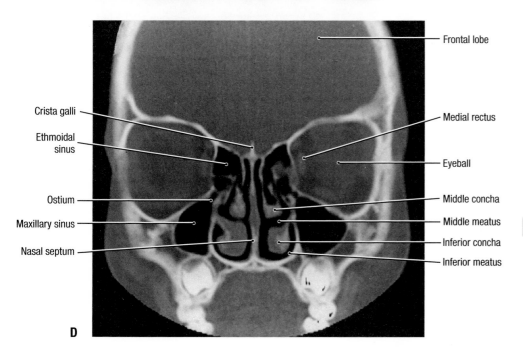

Frontal lobe

Crista galli

Ethmoidal sinus

Medial rectus

Eyeball

Ostium

Maxillary sinus

Nasal septum

Middle concha

Middle meatus

Inferior concha

Inferior meatus

D

7.88 **Imaging of paranasal sinuses**

A. Radiograph, posteroanterior view. **B.** Radiograph, lateral view. *F,* frontal sinus; *E,* ethmoidal sinus; *S,* sphenoidal sinus; M, maxillary sinus; *P,* pharynx. **C.** Opened frontal and maxillary sinuses, anterior view. **D.** Computed tomographic (CT) scan, coronal plane.

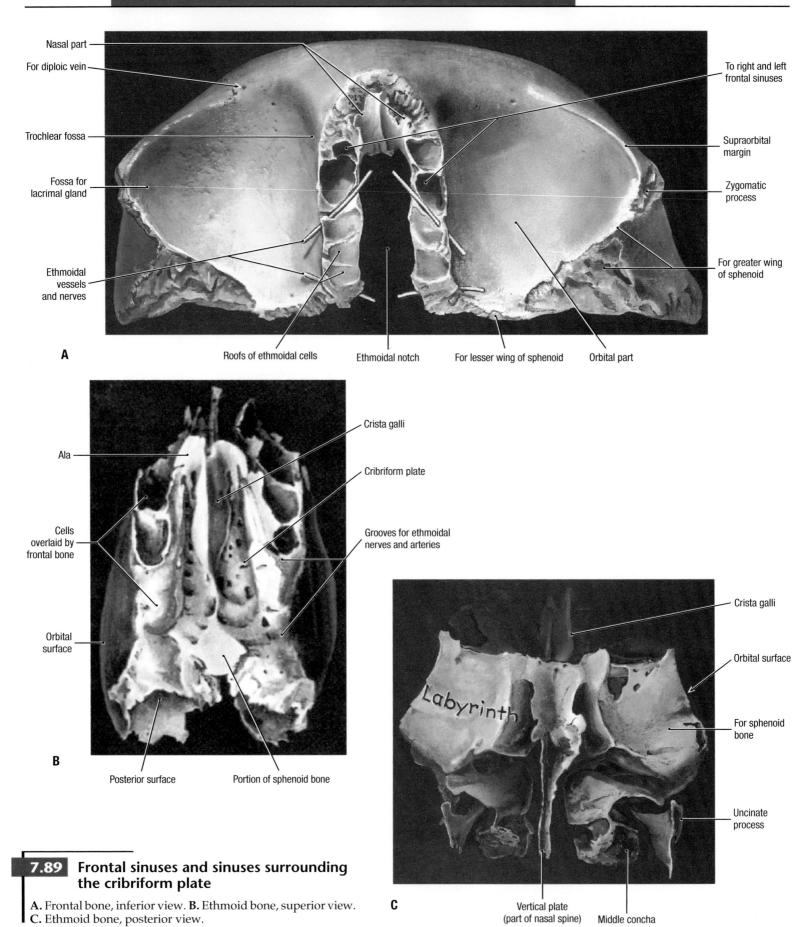

Nasal part

For diploic vein

Trochlear fossa

Fossa for lacrimal gland

Ethmoidal vessels and nerves

To right and left frontal sinuses

Supraorbital margin

Zygomatic process

For greater wing of sphenoid

A

Roofs of ethmoidal cells   Ethmoidal notch   For lesser wing of sphenoid   Orbital part

Ala

Cells overlaid by frontal bone

Orbital surface

B

Crista galli

Cribriform plate

Grooves for ethmoidal nerves and arteries

Posterior surface   Portion of sphenoid bone

Crista galli

Orbital surface

For sphenoid bone

Labyrinth

Uncinate process

C

Vertical plate (part of nasal spine)   Middle concha

7.89 Frontal sinuses and sinuses surrounding the cribriform plate

A. Frontal bone, inferior view. **B.** Ethmoid bone, superior view.
C. Ethmoid bone, posterior view.

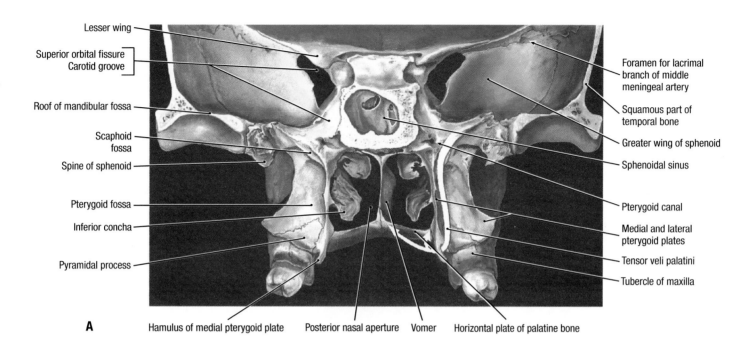

Lesser wing

Superior orbital fissure
Carotid groove

Roof of mandibular fossa

Scaphoid fossa

Spine of sphenoid

Pterygoid fossa

Inferior concha

Pyramidal process

Foramen for lacrimal branch of middle meningeal artery

Squamous part of temporal bone

Greater wing of sphenoid

Sphenoidal sinus

Pterygoid canal

Medial and lateral pterygoid plates

Tensor veli palatini

Tubercle of maxilla

A   Hamulus of medial pterygoid plate   Posterior nasal aperture   Vomer   Horizontal plate of palatine bone

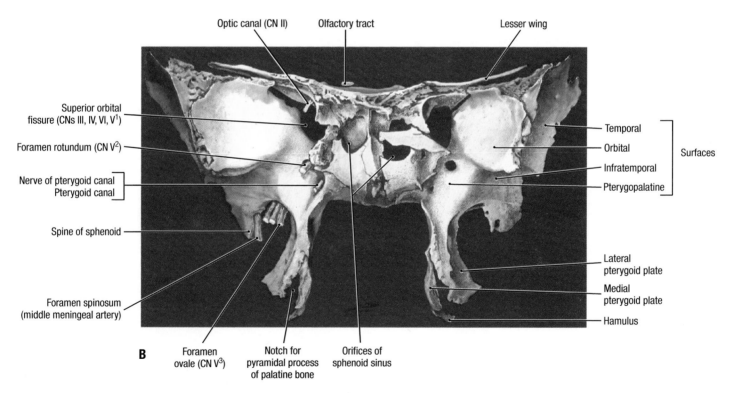

Optic canal (CN II)   Olfactory tract   Lesser wing

Superior orbital fissure (CNs III, IV, VI, V¹)

Foramen rotundum (CN V²)

Nerve of pterygoid canal
Pterygoid canal

Spine of sphenoid

Foramen spinosum (middle meningeal artery)

Temporal

Orbital

Infratemporal

Pterygopalatine

Surfaces

Lateral pterygoid plate

Medial pterygoid plate

Hamulus

B   Foramen ovale (CN V³)   Notch for pyramidal process of palatine bone   Orifices of sphenoid sinus

7.90   Sphenoidal sinus and sphenoid bone

A. Skull, coronal section. **B.** Sphenoid bone, anterior view.

OBSERVE IN **A**:
1. The two posterior nasal apertures are separated by the vomer; superior to these apertures is the sphenoidal sinus (*yellow*);
2. The tensor veli palatini (*white arrow*) attaches to the spine of the sphenoid, scaphoid fossa, and cartilage of the auditory tube, and

passes inferiorly to hook around the hamulus of the medial pterygoid plate before passing into the palatine aponeurosis.

OBSERVE IN **B**:
3. The relationships of the first six cranial nerves (*yellow*) to the sphenoid bone;
4. The maxillary nerve in the foramen rotundum and the nerve of the pterygoid canal in the pterygoid canal can be seen emerging from the sphenoid bone to enter the pterygopalatine fossa.

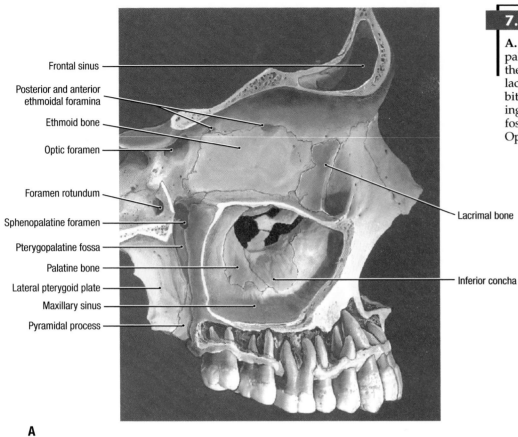

Frontal sinus

Posterior and anterior ethmoidal foramina

Ethmoid bone

Optic foramen

Foramen rotundum

Sphenopalatine foramen

Pterygopalatine fossa

Palatine bone

Lateral pterygoid plate

Maxillary sinus

Pyramidal process

Lacrimal bone

Inferior concha

A

7.91 Maxillary sinus

A. Lateral view. The inferior concha (*orange*) and palatine bone (*pink*) form part of the medial wall of the maxillary sinus. Note the ethmoid (*yellow*) and lacrimal (*blue*) bones of the medial wall of the orbital cavity and the sphenopalatine foramen opening into the nasal cavity from the pterygopalatine fossa. **B.** Partially opened sinus, medial view. **C.** Opened sinus, medial view.

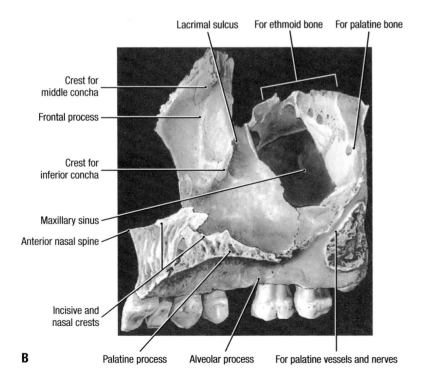

Lacrimal sulcus   For ethmoid bone   For palatine bone

Crest for middle concha

Frontal process

Crest for inferior concha

Maxillary sinus

Anterior nasal spine

Incisive and nasal crests

Palatine process   Alveolar process   For palatine vessels and nerves

B

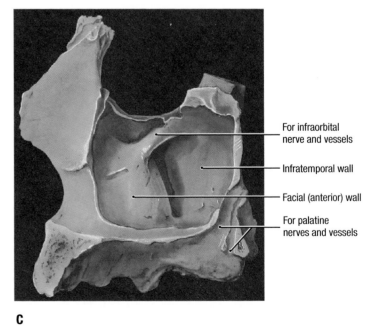

For infraorbital nerve and vessels

Infratemporal wall

Facial (anterior) wall

For palatine nerves and vessels

C

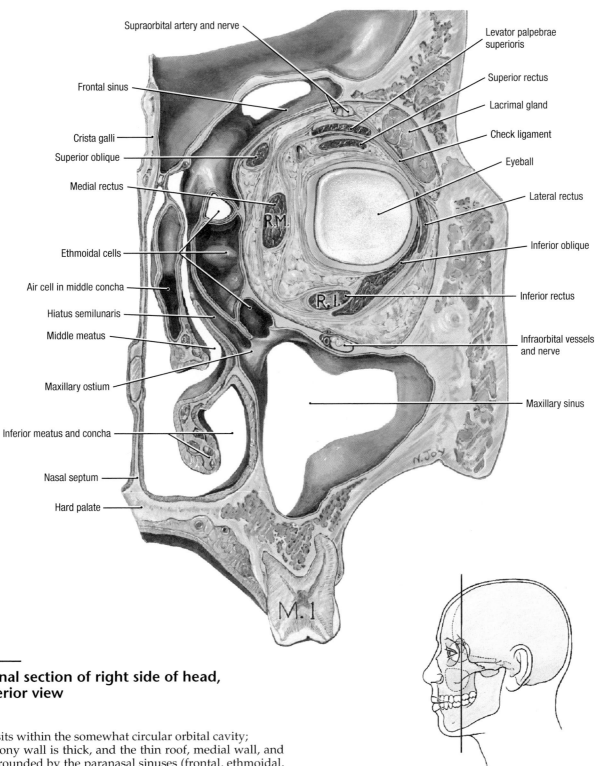

Supraorbital artery and nerve

Levator palpebrae superioris

Frontal sinus

Superior rectus

Lacrimal gland

Crista galli

Superior oblique

Check ligament

Medial rectus

Eyeball

R.M.

Lateral rectus

Ethmoidal cells

Inferior oblique

Air cell in middle concha

R.I.

Inferior rectus

Hiatus semilunaris

Middle meatus

Infraorbital vessels and nerve

Maxillary ostium

Maxillary sinus

Inferior meatus and concha

Nasal septum

Hard palate

N. Joy

M.1

7.92   Coronal section of right side of head, posterior view

OBSERVE:

1. The eyeball sits within the somewhat circular orbital cavity;
2. The lateral bony wall is thick, and the thin roof, medial wall, and floor are surrounded by the paranasal sinuses (frontal, ethmoidal, and maxillary);
3. The four recti and two oblique muscles are arranged around the bulb, and the inferior oblique is inserted by a tendon;
4. The levator palpebrae superioris is superior to the superior rectus muscle, and the check ligament passes from it;
5. The lacrimal gland lies between the check ligament and frontal bone;

6. The fascia unite the four recti, forming a circle around the bulb;
7. The entrance to the maxillary sinus is through the hiatus semilunaris, which is level with the roof of the sinus; the most inferior point of the sinus is inferior to the level of the floor of the nasal cavity.

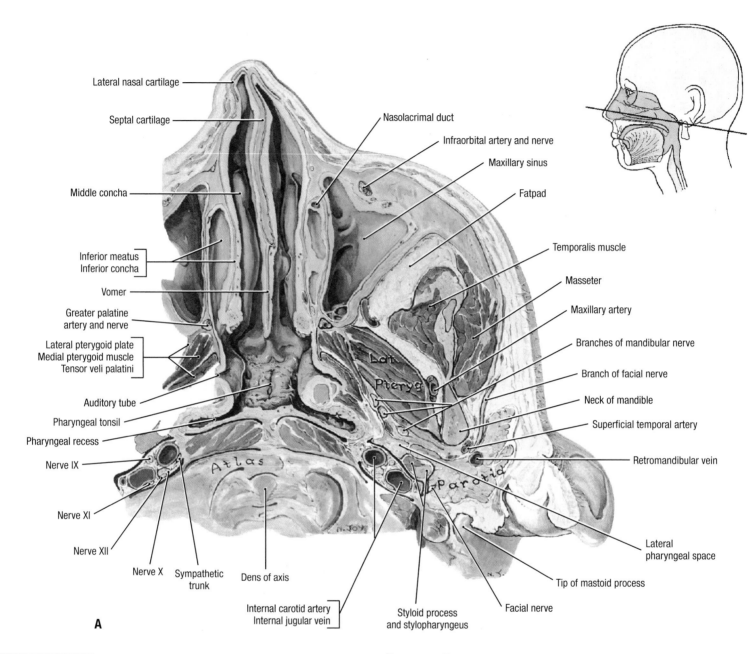

Lateral nasal cartilage

Septal cartilage

Middle concha

Inferior meatus
Inferior concha

Vomer

Greater palatine
artery and nerve

Lateral pterygoid plate
Medial pterygoid muscle
Tensor veli palatini

Auditory tube

Pharyngeal tonsil

Pharyngeal recess

Nerve IX

Nerve XI

Nerve XII

Nerve X   Sympathetic
trunk

Dens of axis

Internal carotid artery
Internal jugular vein

Styloid process
and stylopharyngeus

Facial nerve

Nasolacrimal duct

Infraorbital artery and nerve

Maxillary sinus

Fatpad

Temporalis muscle

Masseter

Maxillary artery

Branches of mandibular nerve

Branch of facial nerve

Neck of mandible

Superficial temporal artery

Retromandibular vein

Lateral
pharyngeal space

Tip of mastoid process

Lat.

Pteryg

Atlas

Parotid

A

7.93 **Sections passing through nose and paranasal sinuses**

A. Transverse section. **B.** Coronal section.

OBSERVE IN **A:**
1. The septal cartilage is continuous with the lateral nasal cartilages;
2. The nasolacrimal duct lies within the mucous membrane of the inferior meatus;
3. The infraorbital nerve and artery are anterior to the maxillary sinus, and the greater palatine nerve and artery are posterior to it;
4. The pharyngeal tonsil (adenoids);
5. The pharyngeal recess spreads laterally posterior to the opening of the auditory tube.

OBSERVE IN **B:**
6. The ethmoid bone is centrally positioned; its horizontal component forms the central part of the anterior cranial fossa superiorly and the roof of the nasal cavity inferiorly. The suspended ethmoidal cells give attachment to the superior and middle concha, and form part of the medial wall of the orbit. The perpendicular plate of the ethmoid forms part of the nasal septum;
7. The thin, orbital plate of the frontal bone forms a "roof" over the orbit and a "floor" for the anterior cranial fossa;
8. The palate forms the floor of the nasal cavity and the roof of the oral cavity;
9. The maxillary sinus forms the inferior part of the lateral wall of the nose; the middle concha shelters the hiatus semilunaris into which the maxillary sinus opens (*arrow*);
10. The mylohyoid muscle, slung between the right and left halves of the mandible, supports the structures of the oral cavity.

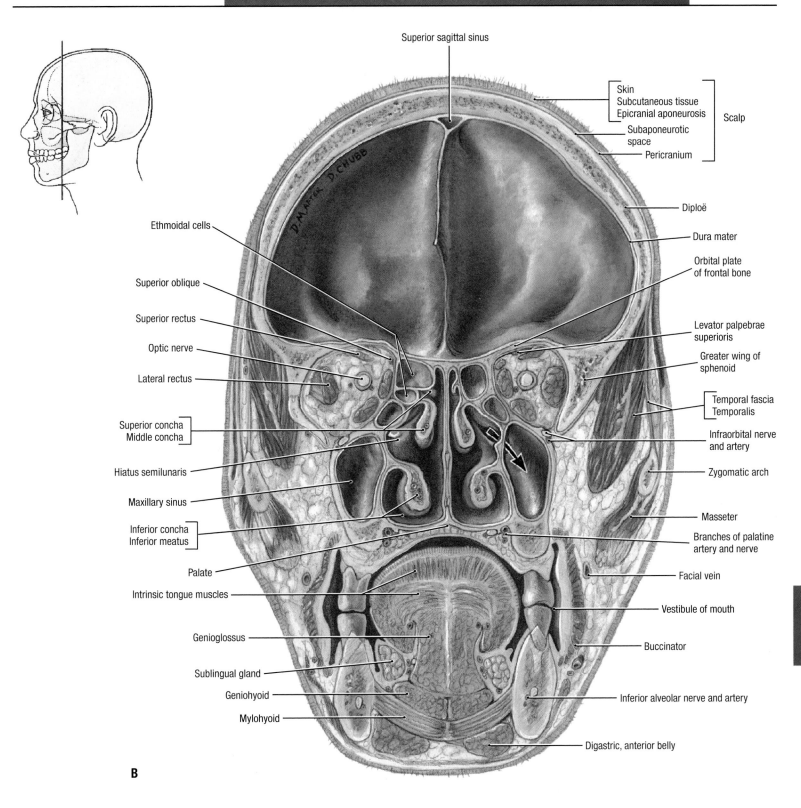

Superior sagittal sinus

Skin
Subcutaneous tissue
Epicranial aponeurosis   Scalp
Subaponeurotic space
Pericranium

Ethmoidal cells

Diploë

Dura mater

Orbital plate of frontal bone

Superior oblique

Superior rectus

Optic nerve

Levator palpebrae superioris

Greater wing of sphenoid

Lateral rectus

Temporal fascia
Temporalis

Superior concha
Middle concha

Infraorbital nerve and artery

Hiatus semilunaris

Zygomatic arch

Maxillary sinus

Masseter

Inferior concha
Inferior meatus

Branches of palatine artery and nerve

Palate

Facial vein

Intrinsic tongue muscles

Vestibule of mouth

Genioglossus

Buccinator

Sublingual gland

Geniohyoid

Inferior alveolar nerve and artery

Mylohyoid

Digastric, anterior belly

B

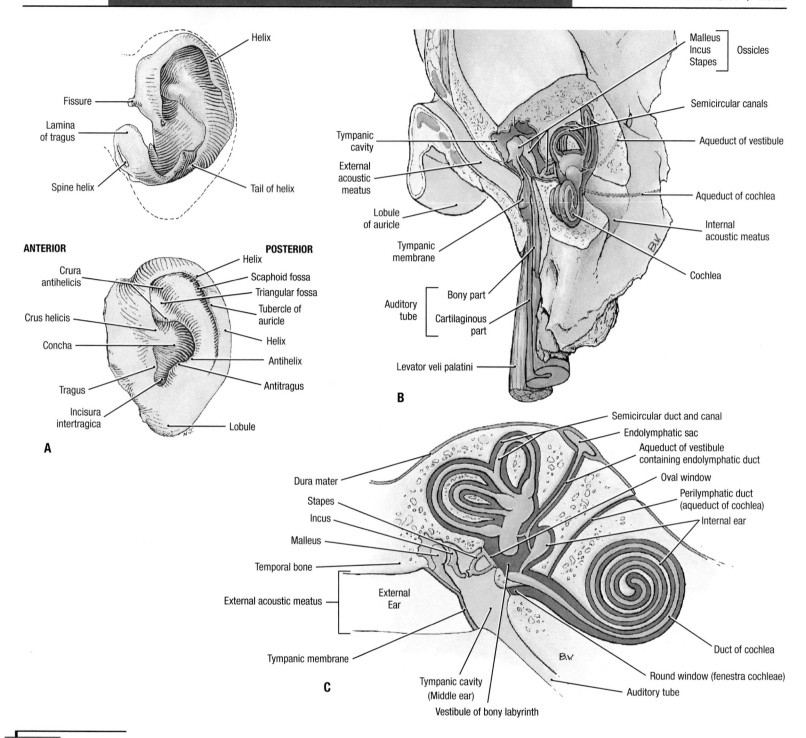

ANTERIOR   **POSTERIOR**

A

B

C

7.94   Ear and auricle

A. Left auricle cartilage (top) and surface anatomy (bottom), lateral views. **B.** Overview of ear, superior view. **C.** Middle and internal ear, schematic oblique section.

OBSERVE:

1. The ear is divisible into three parts: external, middle, and internal;
2. The external ear is comprised of the auricle and external acoustic (auditory) meatus;
3. The middle ear (tympanum) lies between the tympanic membrane and internal ear. Three ossicles (malleus, incus, and stapes) extend from the lateral to medial walls of the tympanum. Of these, the malleus is attached to the tympanic membrane. The stapes is attached by the anular ligament to the fenestra vestibuli (oval win-

dow), and the incus connects to the malleus and stapes. The auditory tube opens into the anterior wall of the tympanic cavity;
4. The internal ear is comprised of a closed system of membranous tubes and bulbs (the membranous labyrinth) that is filled with fluid (endolymph) and bathed in surrounding fluid, called perilymph (purple in **C**);
5. When the tympanic membrane vibrates, the malleus vibrates with it and transmits the vibrations through the incus to the stapes. The stapes, being attached to the margins of the fenestra vestibuli, transmits the vibrations to the perilymph within the vestibule. A secondary tympanic membrane, which closes the fenestra cochleae (round window), receives the vibrations transmitted to the incompressible perilymph and vibrates in turn.

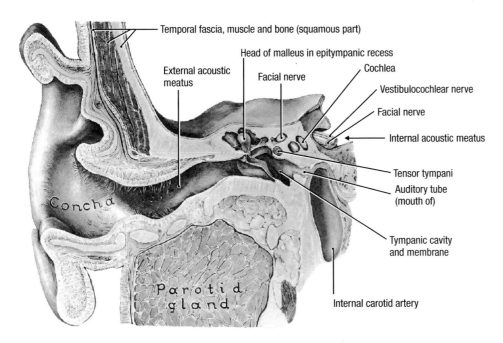

A

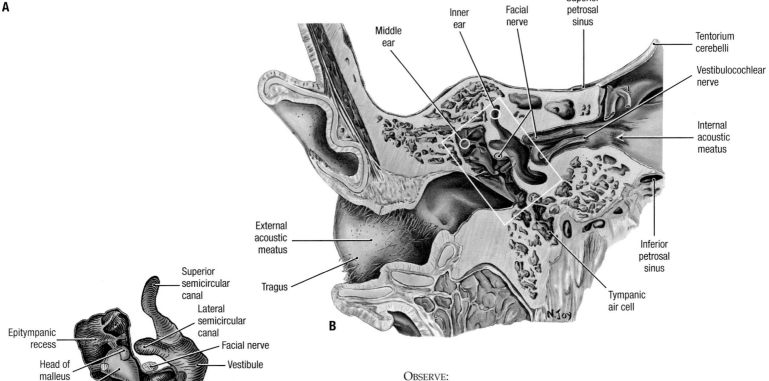

B

7.95 **Structure of ear**

A. Coronal section, anterior view. **B.** Coronal section, posterior view. The inner ear is blue, and the middle ear is pink; the inset drawing (outlined by the box) is an enlargement of the structures of the middle and inner ear.

OBSERVE:
1. The external acoustic meatus measures about 3 cm; half of its length is cartilaginous, and half is bony. It is narrowest near the tympanic membrane;
2. The external acoustic meatus is innervated by the auriculotemporal branch of the mandibular nerve (CN V3) and the auricular branches of the vagus nerve (CN X). *If the wall of the external acoustic meatus is irritated, reflex coughing or vomiting can occur; similarly, a toothache (CN V3 distribution) can refer pain to the ear;*
3. The cartilaginous part of the external acoustic meatus is lined with thick skin and has hairs and many gland openings; the bony part is lined with a thin epithelium that adheres to the periosteum and forms the outermost layer of the tympanic membrane;
4. The tympanic membrane is oblique. The middle ear, or tympanic cavity, is wide superiorly and narrow inferiorly.

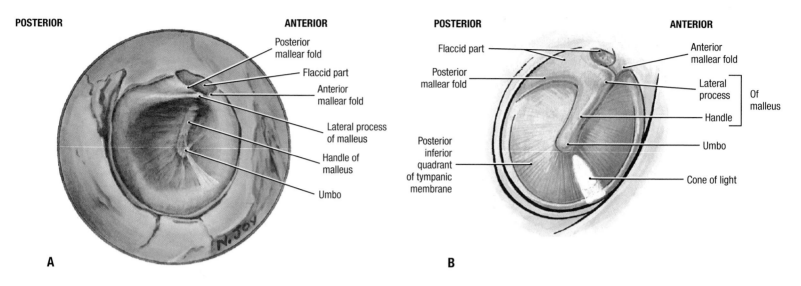

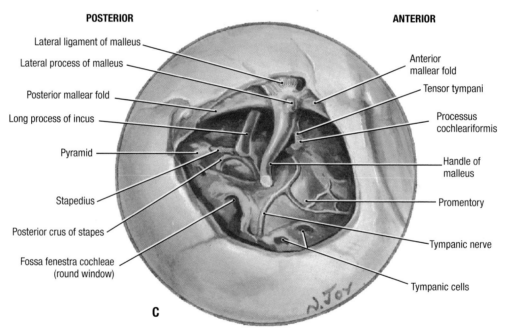

7.96   Tympanic membrane

A. Lateral view. **B.** Auriscopic view. **C.** Tympanic membrane removed, inferolateral view.

OBSERVE IN **A** AND **B**:

1. The oval tympanic membrane has a depressed part, the umbo, at the tip of the handle of the malleus; the handle of the malleus extends anteroinferior to the center of the membrane;
2. Superior to the lateral process of the malleus, the membrane is thin (the "flaccid part," or pars flaccida); the flaccid part lacks the radial and circular fibers present in the remainder of the membrane ("tense part," or pars tensa). The junction between the two parts is marked by anterior and posterior mallear folds;
3. The lateral surface of the tympanic membrane is innervated by the auricular branch of the auriculotemporal nerve (CN V3) and the auricular branch of the vagus nerve (CN X); medially, it is innervated by tympanic branches of the CN IX;

4. *In otitis media, to drain the middle ear, the tympanic membrane is incised in the posteroinferior quadrant to avoid the chorda tympani and auditory ossicles. The superior half of the tympanic membrane is also more vascular than the inferior half.*

OBSERVE IN **C**:

5. The handle of the malleus and long process of the incus, which lies posterior to it;
6. The posterior and anterior mallear folds of mucous membrane between the malleus and incus; the chorda tympani passes in these folds;
7. The promontory has grooves for the tympanic nerve (a branch of the glossopharyngeal nerve);

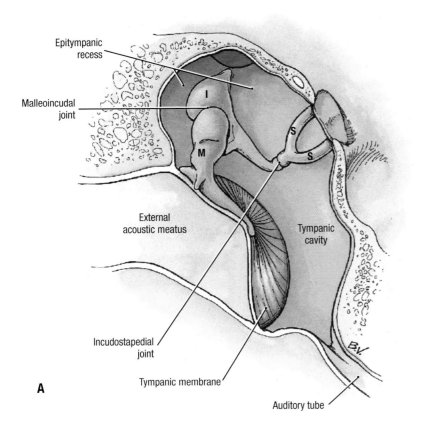

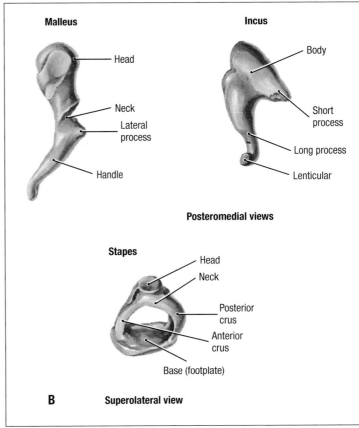

A. Ossicles in situ, coronal section. *M,* malleus; *I,* incus; *S,* stapes. **B.** Separated ossicles.

Labels (A): Epitympanic recess; Malleoincudal joint; External acoustic meatus; Incudostapedial joint; Tympanic membrane; Auditory tube; Tympanic cavity; BV

Labels (B): Malleus — Head, Neck, Lateral process, Handle; Incus — Body, Short process, Long process, Lenticular; **Posteromedial views**; Stapes — Head, Neck, Posterior crus, Anterior crus, Base (footplate); **Superolateral view**

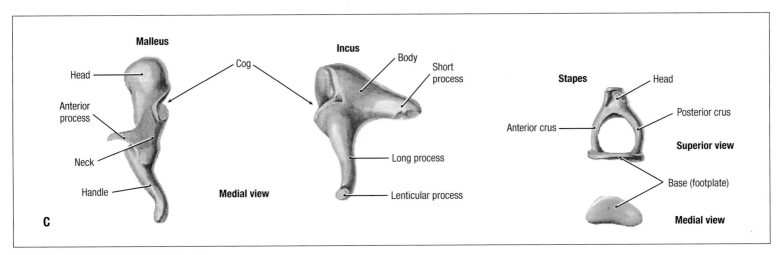

Labels (C): Malleus — Head, Cog, Anterior process, Neck, Handle, **Medial view**; Incus — Body, Short process, Long process, Lenticular process; Stapes — Head, Posterior crus, Anterior crus, Base (footplate), **Superior view**, **Medial view**

7.97 Ossicles of middle ear

A. Ossicles in situ, coronal section. *M,* malleus; *I,* incus; *S,* stapes. **B.** Separated ossicles. **C.** Ossicles of ear in their relative positions.

OBSERVE:

1. The head of the malleus and body and short process of the incus lie in the epitympanic recess;
2. The saddle-shaped articular surface of the head of the malleus and the reciprocally saddle-shaped articular surface of the body of the incus form the malleoincudal synovial joint;
3. The anterior process of the malleus and the short process of the incus are in line and anchored anteriorly and posteriorly by ligaments;

4. The handle of the malleus, from lateral process to tip, is embedded in the tympanic membrane;
5. The end of the long process of the incus has a convex articular facet at the incudostapedial synovial joint for articulation with the head of the stapes;
6. In the embryo, the hole in the stapes transmits an artery, the stapedial artery; the hole is later closed by a membrane. The superior border of the base (footplate) is convex and deeper anteriorly than posteriorly. The two crura are grooved; the anterior crus is more slender and straight, and it is fixed to a small area on the plate, whereas the posterior crus is attached to the whole depth of the plate.

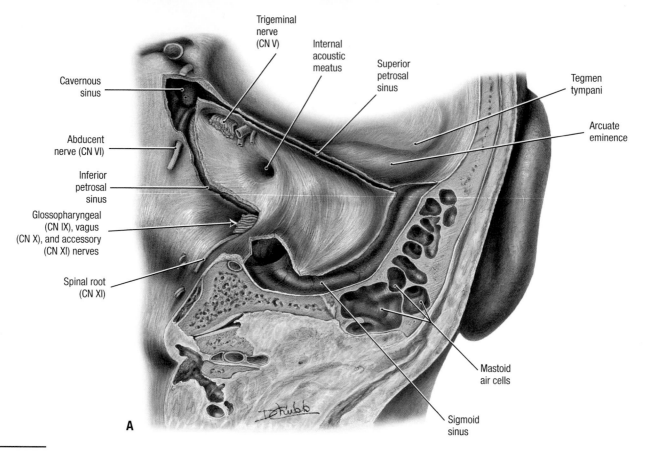

A

7.98 Petrous temporal bone, arcuate eminence, and tegmen tympani

A. Venous sinuses around the petrous temporal bone, posterior view.
B. Temporal bone, superior view.

OBSERVE IN **A:**

1. The mastoid air cells are lined with mucous membrane and occupy the diploë of the mastoid part of the petrous temporal bone;
2. The posterior surface of the petrous bone is encircled by three venous sinuses: sigmoid, superior petrosal, and inferior petrosal;
3. The superior and inferior petrosal sinuses drain the cavernous sinus;
4. The superior petrosal sinus bridges the trigemial nerve (CN V), occupying the attached margin of the tentorium cerebelli and ending in the sigmoid sinus;
5. The sigmoid sinus leaves the skull through the jugular foramen with cranial nerves IX, X, and XI, and the inferior petrosal sinus;
6. The abducent nerve (CN VI), within its dural sheath, passes through the inferior petrosal sinus and bends to enter the cavernous sinus;
7. The arcuate eminence is produced by the anterior semicircular canal of the internal ear;
8. The tegmen tympani is a thin plate of bone forming the roof of the middle ear.

OBSERVE IN **B:**

9. The parts of the temporal bone: squamous, petrous, and mastoid;
10. The grooves for the superior petrosal, inferior petrosal, and sigmoid sinuses;
11. The arcuate eminence of the inner ear and the tegmen typani of the middle ear;
12. The internal acoustic meatus for the facial nerve (CN VII), nervus intermedius (CN VII), vestibulocochlear nerve (CN VIII), and labyrinthine artery.

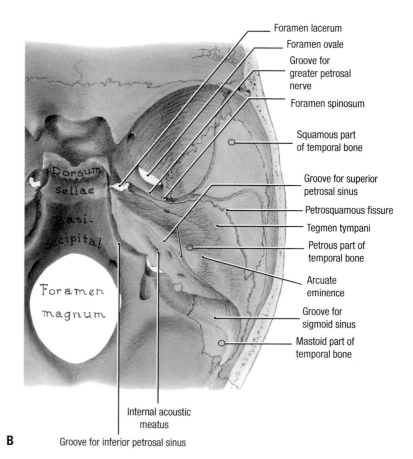

B

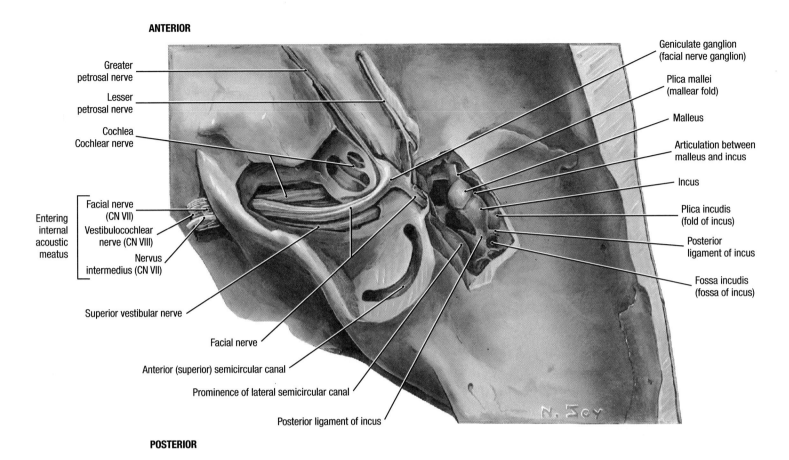

ANTERIOR

Greater petrosal nerve

Lesser petrosal nerve

Cochlea
Cochlear nerve

Entering internal acoustic meatus

Facial nerve (CN VII)
Vestibulocochlear nerve (CN VIII)
Nervus intermedius (CN VII)

Superior vestibular nerve

Facial nerve

Anterior (superior) semicircular canal

Prominence of lateral semicircular canal

Posterior ligament of incus

POSTERIOR

Geniculate ganglion (facial nerve ganglion)

Plica mallei (mallear fold)

Malleus

Articulation between malleus and incus

Incus

Plica incudis (fold of incus)

Posterior ligament of incus

Fossa incudis (fossa of incus)

7.99 Middle and inner ear in situ, superior view

The tegmen tympani has been removed to expose the middle ear; the arcuate eminence has been removed to expose the anterior semicircular canal; and the facial and vestibulocochlear nerves have been traced from the internal acoustic meatus through the internal ear.

OBSERVE:
1. The malleus, incus, and extensive folds of mucous membrane in the middle ear;
2. The facial nerve, the nervus intermedius, and the vestibulocochlear nerve enter and traverse the internal acoustic meatus;
3. The facial nerve, joined by the nervus intermedius, runs posterior to the cochlea to the geniculate ganglion;

4. At the ganglion, the facial nerve makes a right-angle bend, called the genu, and then curves posteroinferiorly within the bony facial canal; the papery lateral wall of the facial canal separates the facial nerve from the tympanic cavity of the middle ear;
5. The geniculate ganglion is the cell station of fibers of general sensation and taste;
6. Through the geniculate ganglion run fibers of the greater (superficial) petrosal nerve on their way to the pterygopalatine ganglion;
7. From the facial nerve, beyond the ganglion, a communicating branch goes to the lesser (superficial) petrosal nerve on its way to the otic ganglion.

7.100 Dissections of walls of tympanic cavity

These dissections were accomplished using a drill from the medial aspect of the tympanic cavity. **A.** Medial view. **B.** Lateral wall, medial view

OBSERVE IN **A**:

1. The tegmen tympani forms the roof of the tympanic cavity and mastoid antrum;
2. The internal carotid artery is the main feature of the anterior wall, the internal jugular vein is the main feature of the floor, and the facial nerve is the main feature of the posterior wall;
3. The superolateral part of the anterior wall leads to the auditory tube and tensor tympani; the superolateral part of the posterior wall leads to the mastoid antrum;
4. The tympanic membrane forms much of the lateral wall of the tympanic cavity; superior to it is the epitympanic recess in which are housed the larger parts of the malleus and incus.

OBSERVE IN **B**:

5. The oval tympanic membrane has a greater vertical than horizontal diameter; the margin of the membrane is fibrocartilaginous;
6. The handle of the malleus is incorporated in the membrane, with its end at the umbo;
7. The anterior process of the malleus is anchored anteriorly by the anterior ligament;
8. The facial nerve lies within its tough periosteal tube; the chorda tympani leaves the facial nerve and lies within two crescentic folds of mucous membrane, crossing the neck of the malleus superior to the tendon of tensor tympani and following the anterior process and anterior ligament of the malleus;
9. The tympanic membrane has three recesses: anterior, posterior, and superior (*arrowheads*).

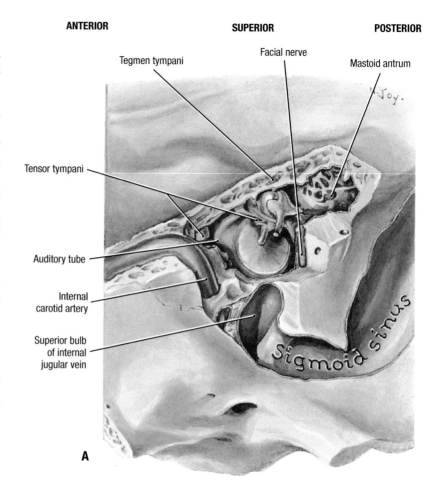

ANTERIOR   SUPERIOR   POSTERIOR

Tegmen tympani
Facial nerve
Mastoid antrum
Tensor tympani
Auditory tube
Internal carotid artery
Superior bulb of internal jugular vein
sigmoid sinus

A

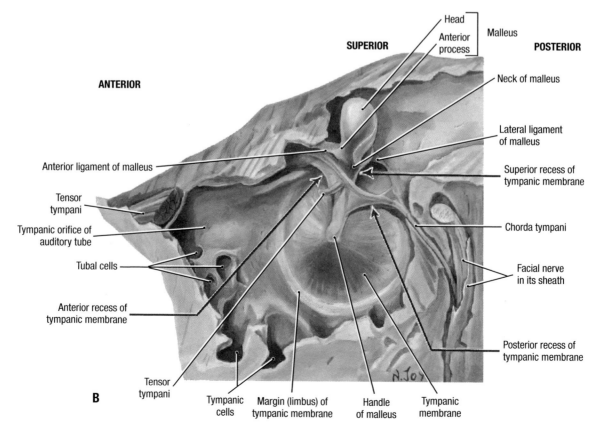

Head
Anterior process
Malleus
SUPERIOR
POSTERIOR

ANTERIOR

Neck of malleus
Lateral ligament of malleus
Superior recess of tympanic membrane
Chorda tympani
Facial nerve in its sheath
Posterior recess of tympanic membrane

Anterior ligament of malleus
Tensor tympani
Tympanic orifice of auditory tube
Tubal cells
Anterior recess of tympanic membrane

Tensor tympani
Tympanic cells
Margin (limbus) of tympanic membrane
Handle of malleus
Tympanic membrane

B

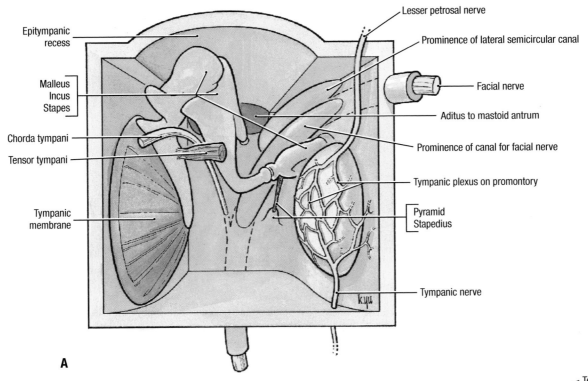

Epitympanic recess

Malleus
Incus
Stapes

Chorda tympani

Tensor tympani

Tympanic membrane

Lesser petrosal nerve

Prominence of lateral semicircular canal

Facial nerve

Aditus to mastoid antrum

Prominence of canal for facial nerve

Tympanic plexus on promontory

Pyramid
Stapedius

Tympanic nerve

A

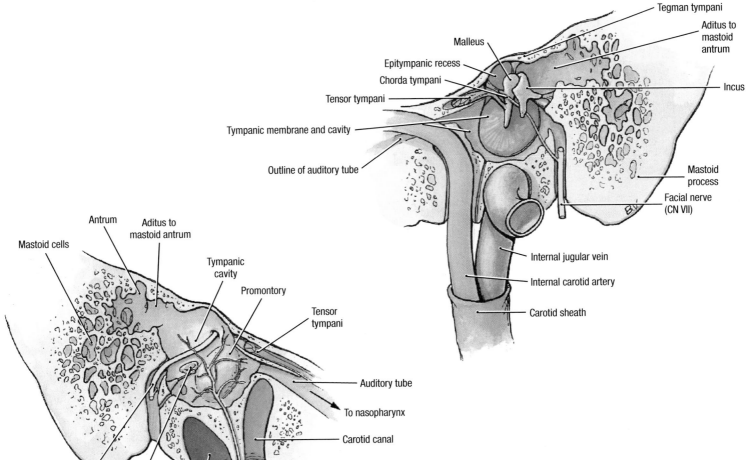

Tegman tympani

Aditus to mastoid antrum

Malleus

Epitympanic recess

Chorda tympani

Tensor tympani

Tympanic membrane and cavity

Outline of auditory tube

Incus

Mastoid process

Facial nerve (CN VII)

Internal jugular vein

Internal carotid artery

Carotid sheath

Antrum

Aditus to mastoid antrum

Mastoid cells

Tympanic cavity

Promontory

Tensor tympani

Auditory tube

To nasopharynx

Carotid canal

Tympanic nerve of CN IX

C

CN VII

Stapes, pyramid

Jugular foramen

7.101　Schematics of walls of tympanic cavity

A. Anterior wall removed, anterior view. **B.** Lateral wall, medial view. **C.** Medial wall, lateral view.

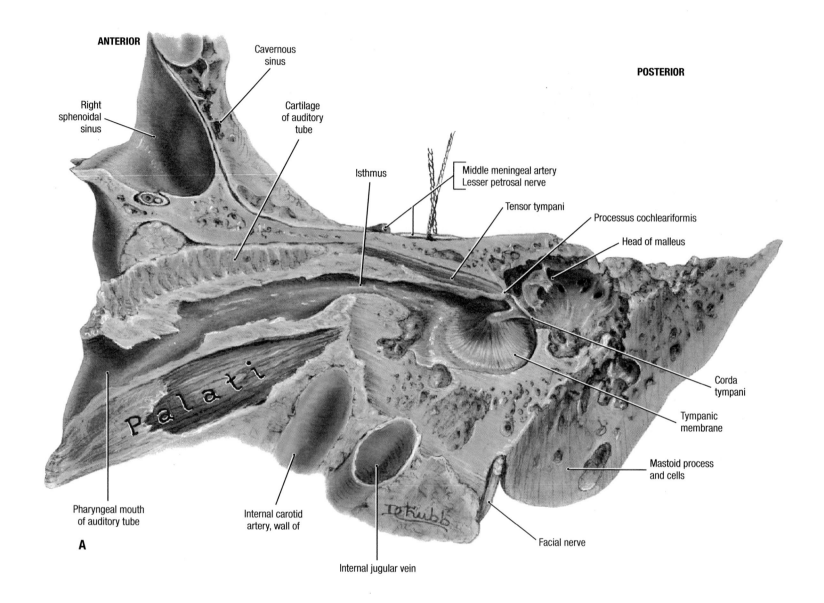

ANTERIOR

Cavernous sinus

Right sphenoidal sinus

Cartilage of auditory tube

POSTERIOR

Isthmus

Middle meningeal artery
Lesser petrosal nerve

Tensor tympani

Processus cochleariformis

Head of malleus

Corda tympani

Tympanic membrane

Mastoid process and cells

Pharyngeal mouth of auditory tube

Internal carotid artery, wall of

Facial nerve

Internal jugular vein

A

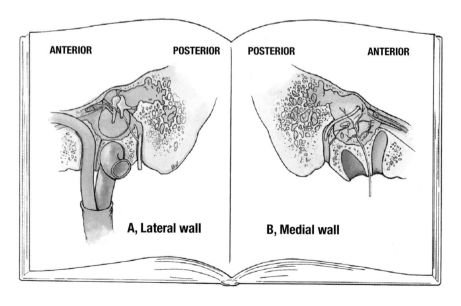

ANTERIOR   POSTERIOR   POSTERIOR   ANTERIOR

A, Lateral wall   **B, Medial wall**

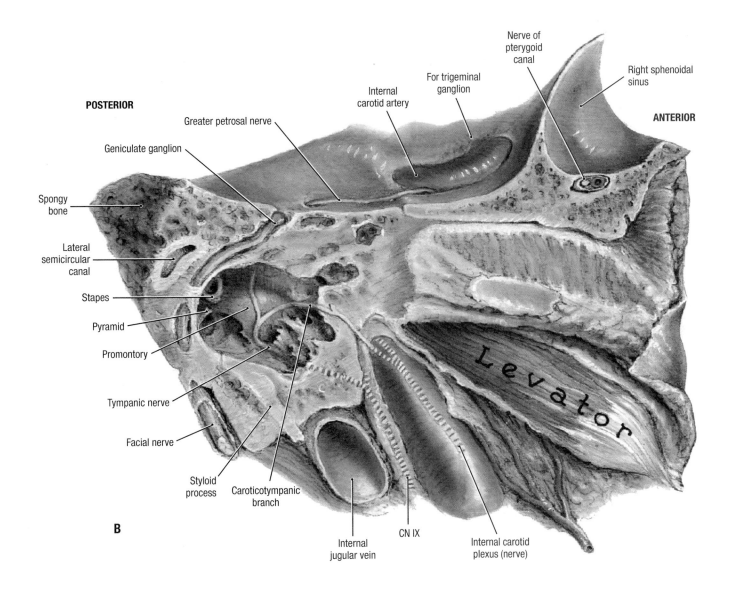

POSTERIOR

ANTERIOR

Nerve of
pterygoid
canal

For trigeminal
ganglion

Internal
carotid artery

Right sphenoidal
sinus

Greater petrosal nerve

Geniculate ganglion

Spongy
bone

Lateral
semicircular
canal

Stapes

Pyramid

Promontory

Tympanic nerve

Facial nerve

Styloid
process

Caroticotympanic
branch

Levator

Internal
jugular
vein

CN IX

Internal carotid
plexus (nerve)

B

| **7.102** | **Right auditory tube and tympanic cavity, split longitudinally** |

The cut surfaces of this longitudinally split specimen are displayed as pages in a book. **A.** Lateral part. **B.** Medial part.

OBSERVE:

1. The lateral wall of the cavity is dominated by the tympanic membrane, handle of the malleus, and chorda tympani nerve;
2. The medial wall has a broad bulge, the promontory, which overlies the first turn of the cochlea; on it, the tympanic nerve and caroticotympanic branches of the internal carotid plexus form the tympanic plexus, which supplies the region and gives off the lesser petrosal nerve;
3. The following structures are divided and seen on both medial and lateral parts: levator veli palatini, supporting the auditory tube; auditory tube, cartilaginous superiorly and medially, and membranous inferiorly and laterally; right sphenoidal sinus, with the pterygoid canal inferior to it; internal carotid artery; internal jugular vein; facial nerve; and a petrosal nerve, either greater or lesser.

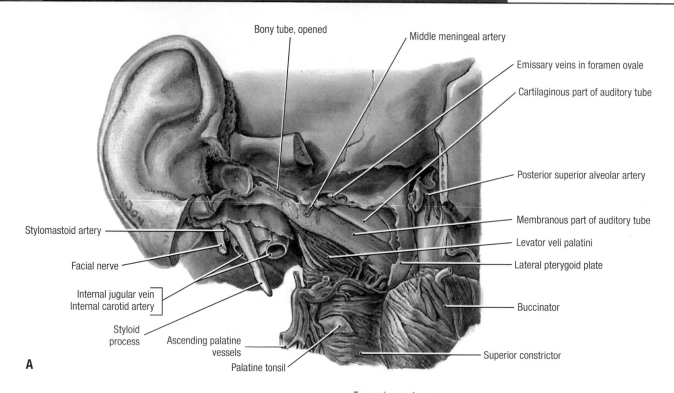

Bony tube, opened
Middle meningeal artery
Emissary veins in foramen ovale
Cartilaginous part of auditory tube
Posterior superior alveolar artery
Membranous part of auditory tube
Levator veli palatini
Lateral pterygoid plate
Buccinator
Superior constrictor
Stylomastoid artery
Facial nerve
Internal jugular vein
Internal carotid artery
Styloid process
Ascending palatine vessels
Palatine tonsil

A

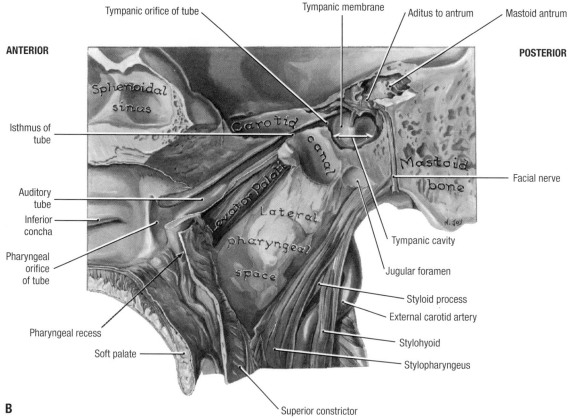

Tympanic orifice of tube
Tympanic membrane
Aditus to antrum
Mastoid antrum

ANTERIOR　　　　　　　　　　　　　　　**POSTERIOR**

Sphenoidal sinus
Carotid canal
Mastoid bone
Isthmus of tube
Levator Palati
Lateral pharyngeal space
Facial nerve
Auditory tube
Inferior concha
Pharyngeal orifice of tube
Tympanic cavity
Jugular foramen
Styloid process
External carotid artery
Stylohyoid
Stylopharyngeus
Pharyngeal recess
Soft palate
Superior constrictor

B

7.103 Auditory tube

A. Lateral aspect. **B.** Pharyngeal (medial) aspect.

OBSERVE:

1. The general direction of the tube is superior, posterior, and lateral from the nasopharynx to tympanic cavity;
2. The funnel-shaped pharyngeal orifice of the tube is situated just posterior to the inferior concha of the nose;

3. The cartilaginous part of the tube, rests throughout its length on the levator veli palatini muscle;
4. The bony part of the tube passes lateral to the carotid canal; it is narrow at the isthmus, where it joins the cartilaginous part, and wider at its tympanic orifice.

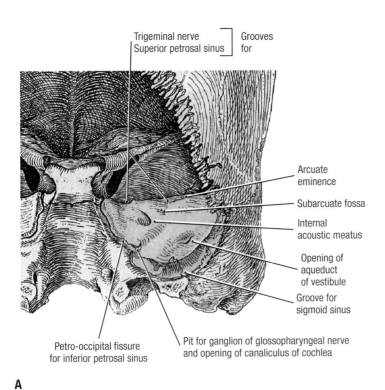

Grooves for
Trigeminal nerve
Superior petrosal sinus

Arcuate eminence

Subarcuate fossa

Internal acoustic meatus

Opening of aqueduct of vestibule

Groove for sigmoid sinus

Petro-occipital fissure for inferior petrosal sinus

Pit for ganglion of glossopharyngeal nerve and opening of canaliculus of cochlea

A

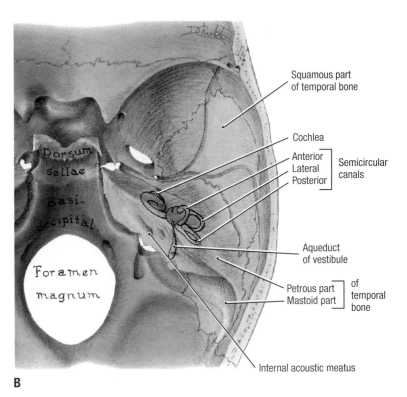

Squamous part of temporal bone

Cochlea

Anterior
Lateral
Posterior　Semicircular canals

Aqueduct of vestibule

Petrous part
Mastoid part　of temporal bone

Internal acoustic meatus

B

Arcuate eminence

Mastoid antrum

Anterior (superior) semicircular canal

Internal acoustic meatus

Posterior semicircular canal

Groove for sigmoid sinus

Aqueduct of vestibule

Mastoid cells

Canaliculus of cochlea

C

7.104　Location of cochlea and semicircular canals

A. Petrous and mastoid parts of temporal bone, posterior view. **B.** Osseous labyrinth in situ, superior view. **C.** Semicircular canals and aqueducts in situ, posterior view.

OBSERVE:

1. The aqueduct of the vestibule transmits the endolymphatic duct, which expands into a blind pouch, the endolymphatic sac (see Figures 7.94C); the sac is located deep to the dura mater on the posterior surface of the petrous part of the temporal bone and serves as a storage reservoir for excess endolymph formed by blood capillaries within the membranous labyrinth;

2. The perilymphatic duct (within the canaliculus of the cochlea) opens at the base of the pyramidal pit for the glossopharyngeal

ganglion; the duct runs from the scala vestibuli in the basal turn of the cochlea to an extension of the subarachnoid space around the glossopharyngeal, vagus, and accessory nerves (see Fig. 7.94C). This duct may allow the perilymph of the internal ear to mix with cerebrospinal fluid in the posterior cranial fossa, although there is evidence that it ends as a closed sac;

3. The anterior semicircular canal is set vertically below the arcuate eminence; it forms a right angle with the posterior surface of the petrous bone;

4. The posterior semicircular canal is nearly parallel to the posterior surface of the bone and close to the groove for the sigmoid sinus.

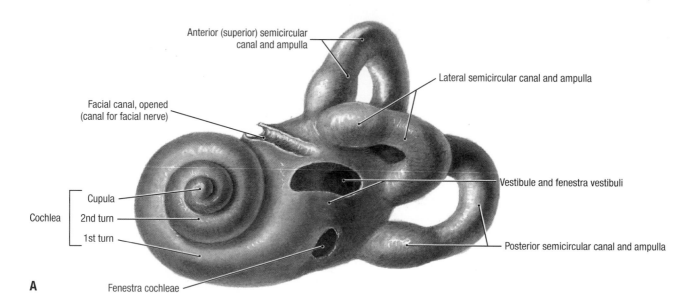

Anterior (superior) semicircular canal and ampulla

Lateral semicircular canal and ampulla

Facial canal, opened (canal for facial nerve)

Vestibule and fenestra vestibuli

Cochlea
- Cupula
- 2nd turn
- 1st turn

Posterior semicircular canal and ampulla

Fenestra cochleae

A

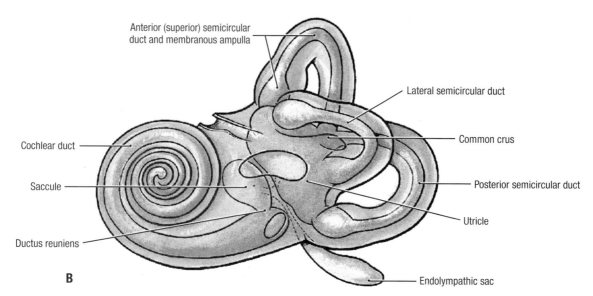

Anterior (superior) semicircular duct and membranous ampulla

Lateral semicircular duct

Cochlear duct

Common crus

Saccule

Posterior semicircular duct

Ductus reuniens

Utricle

Endolympathic sac

B

7.105   Labyrinth

A. Left bony labyrinth, lateral view. **B.** Left membranous labyrinth, superimposed on bony labyrinth, lateral view.

OBSERVE IN **A**:

1. The three parts of the bony internal ear, or bony labyrinth, are the cochlea, anteriorly; vestibule medially; and semicircular canals, posteriorly;
2. The cochlea takes 2.5 turns, or coils. The first, or basal, coil lies deep to the medial wall of the tympanic cavity and communicates with the tympanic cavity through the fenestra cochleae (round window); this fenestra is closed by the secondary tympanic membrane;
3. The vestibule is crossed superiorly by the facial canal and communicates with the tympanic cavity through the fenestra vestibuli (oval window); this window is closed by the base, or foot piece, of the stapes;
4. The three semicircular canals are: anterior, posterior, and lateral. The anterior and posterior canals set vertically at a right angle to each other; the lateral canal sets horizontally and at a right angle to the other two. Each canal forms approximately two thirds of a cir-

cle and has an ampulla at one end. The lateral canal is the shortest, and the posterior canal is the longest.

OBSERVE IN **B**:

5. The membranous labyrinth, or membranous internal ear, is contained within the bony labyrinth; it is a closed system of ducts and chambers that is filled with endolymph and surrounded with, or bathed in, perilymph;
6. The membranous labyrinth has three parts: the duct of the cochlea, within the cochlea; the saccule and utricle, within the vestibule; and the three semicircular ducts, within the three semicircular canals;
7. One end of the duct of the cochlea is closed; the other end communicates with the saccule through the ductus reuniens;
8. The saccule communicates with the utricle through the utriculosaccular duct (not shown); from this duct springs the endolymphatic duct, which occupies the aqueduct of the vestibule and ends in the endolymphatic sac. The three semicircular ducts have five openings into the utricle.

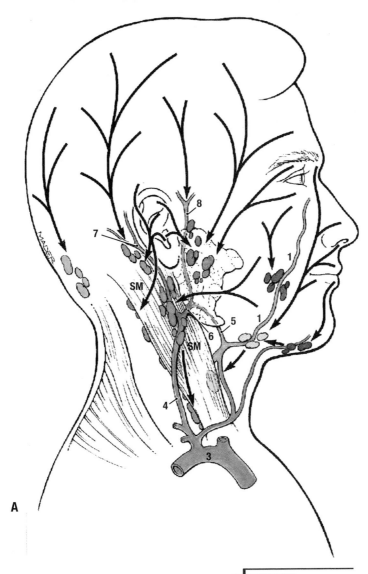

A

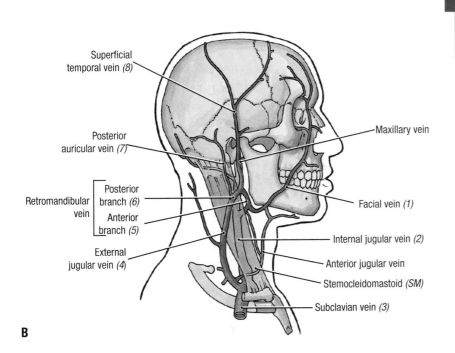

B

7.106 Drainage of head and neck

A. Superficial lymphatic drainage, lateral view. **B.** Venous drainage of head and neck, lateral view. **C.** Deep lymphatic drainage, lateral view. **D.** Lymphatic drainage of tongue, superior view.

OBSERVE:

1. All lymphatics from the head and neck drain into the deep cervical nodes, which lie in the connective tissue of the carotid sheath and are closely related to the internal jugular vein;

2. The deep cervical nodes drain into the jugular trunks, which drain into the thoracic duct (left side) and right lymphatic duct (right side);

3. The superficial nodes are clustered around the external and anterior jugular and facial veins and their tributaries; the superficial nodes drain into the deep cervical nodes;

4. The lymphatic drainage of the posterior third and central part of the anterior two thirds of the tongue is bilateral (see lines with *arrows* in **D**); *malignant tumors in these areas of the tongue have a poor prognosis;*

5. Lymphatics from the upper lip and lateral parts of the lower lip drain into the submandibular nodes, whereas the central part of the lower lip and chin drain into the submental lymph nodes.

Labels in figure B:
- Superficial temporal vein (8)
- Posterior auricular vein (7)
- Retromandibular vein — Posterior branch (6), Anterior branch (5)
- External jugular vein (4)
- Maxillary vein
- Facial vein (1)
- Internal jugular vein (2)
- Anterior jugular vein
- Sternocleidomastoid (SM)
- Subclavian vein (3)

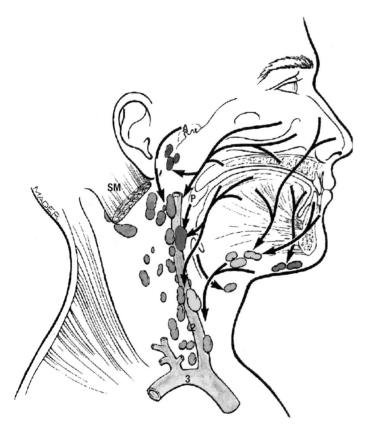

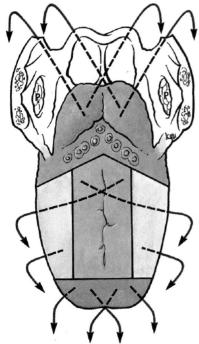

D

For A, C and D	
Nodes:	
☐ Occipital	☐ Retropharyngeal
☐ Retroauricular (mastoid)	☐ Deep cervical
☐ Parotid	☐ Jugulo-omohyoid
☐ Buccal	☐ Jugulodigastric
☐ Submental	☐ Submental
☐ Submandibular	☐ Submandibular
☐ Jugulo-omohyoid	☐ Infrahyoid
☐ Superficial cervical	**A** Pharyngeal tonsil
☐ Deep cervical	**P** Palatine tonsil

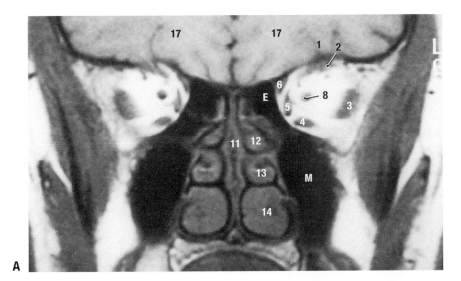

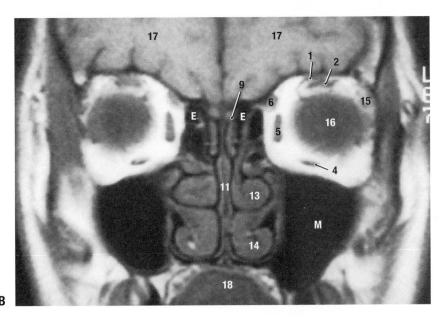

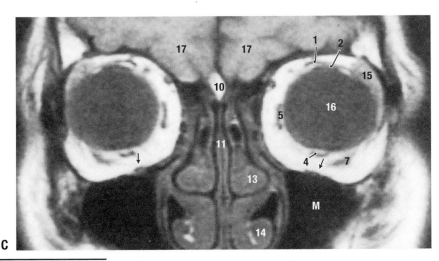

1	Levator palpabrae superioris
2	Superior rectus
3	Lateral rectus
4	Inferior rectus
5	Medial rectus
6	Superior oblique
7	Inferior oblique
8	Optic nerve
9	Olfactory bulb
10	Crista galli
11	Nasal septum
12	Superior concha
13	Middle concha
14	Inferior concha
15	Lacrimal gland
16	Eyeball
17	Frontal lobe
18	Tongue
19	Infraorbital vessels and nerve
M	Maxillary sinus
E	Ethmoidal sinus

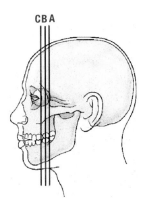

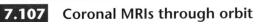

7.107   **Coronal MRIs through orbit**

See orientation drawing for site of scans **A–C.**

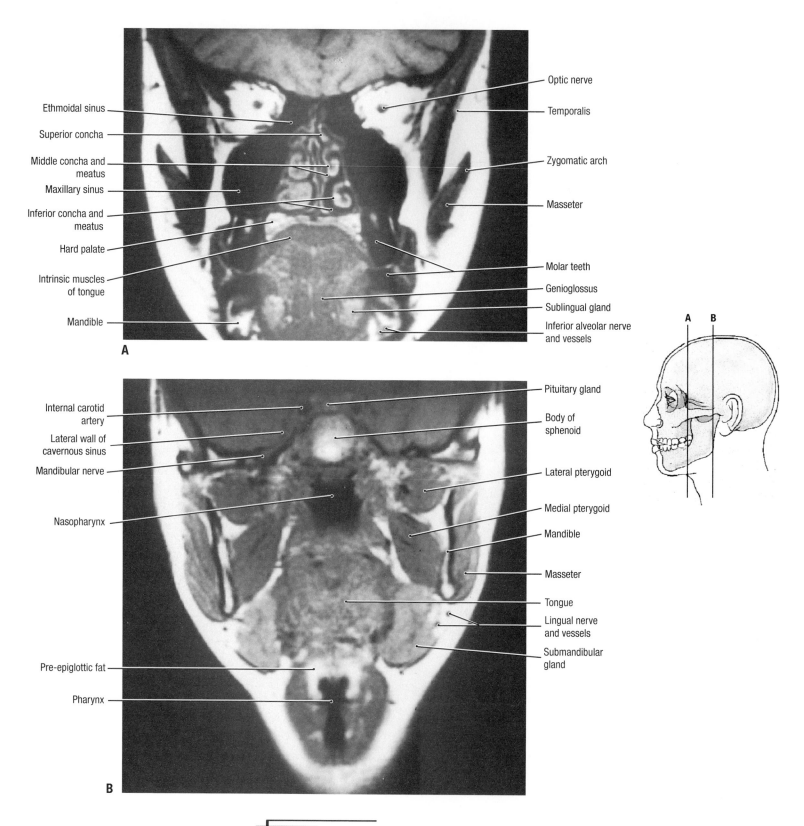

Ethmoidal sinus

Superior concha

Middle concha and meatus

Maxillary sinus

Inferior concha and meatus

Hard palate

Intrinsic muscles of tongue

Mandible

A

Optic nerve

Temporalis

Zygomatic arch

Masseter

Molar teeth

Genioglossus

Sublingual gland

Inferior alveolar nerve and vessels

Internal carotid artery

Lateral wall of cavernous sinus

Mandibular nerve

Nasopharynx

Pre-epiglottic fat

Pharynx

B

Pituitary gland

Body of sphenoid

Lateral pterygoid

Medial pterygoid

Mandible

Masseter

Tongue

Lingual nerve and vessels

Submandibular gland

7.108   **Coronal MRIs of head**

See orientation drawing for site of scans **A** and **B**.

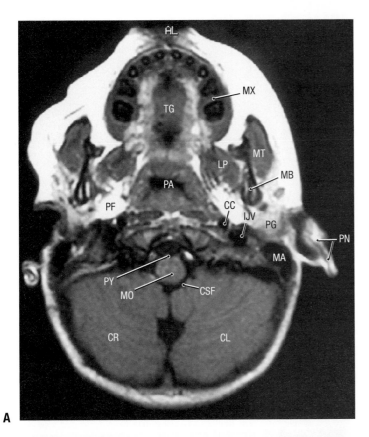

A

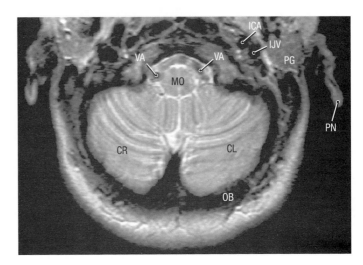

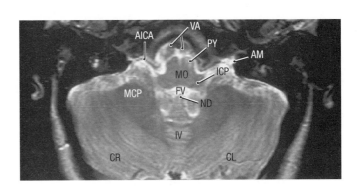

B

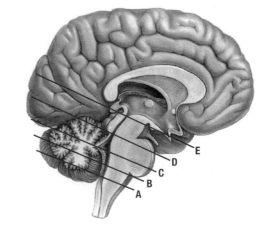

7.109 **Axial (transverse) MRIs through brainstem**

See orientation drawing for site of scans **A–C**. Images on left side of page aat T1 weighted, and images on the right side are T2 weighted.

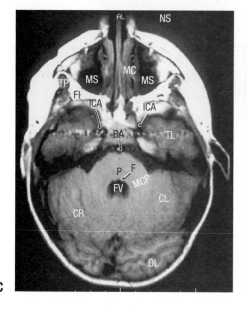

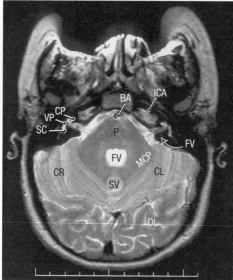

C

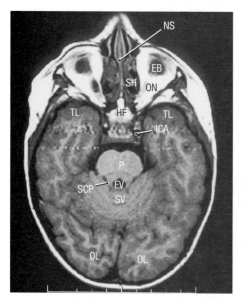

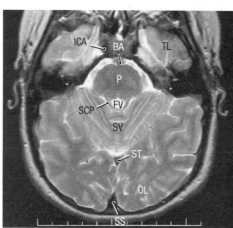

D

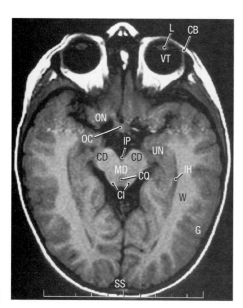

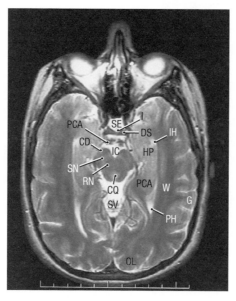

E

AICA	Anterior inferior cerebellar artery
AM	Internal auditory meatus
BA	Basilar artery
CA	Cerebral aqueduct
CB	Ciliary body
CC	Common carotid artery
CI	Colliculi
CL	Left cerebellar hemisphere
CP	Cochlear perilymph
CR	Right cerebellar hemisphere
CSF	Cerebrospinal fluid in subarachnoid space
DS	Dorsum sellae
EB	Eyeball
F	Facial (CN VII) and vestibulocochlear (CN VIII) nerves
FC	Facial colliculus
FI	Fat in infratemporal fossa
FL	Flocculus
FV	Fourth ventricle
G	Gray matter
HF	Hypophyseal fossa
HP	Hippocampus
I	Infundibulum
IC	Interpeduncular cistern
ICA	Internal carotid artery
ICP	Inferior cerebellar peduncle
IF	Inferior concha
IH	Inferior horn of lateral ventricle
IJV	Internal jugular vein
IP	Interpeduncular fossa
IV	Inferior vermis
L	Lens
LP	Lateral pterygoid
MA	Mastoid air cells
MB	Mandible
MC	Middle concha
MCP	Middle cerebellar peduncle
MD	Midbrain
MO	Medulla oblongata
MS	Maxillary sinus
MT	Masseter
MX	Maxilla
ND	Nodule of cerebellum
NS	Nasal septum
OB	Occipital bone
OC	Optic chiasma
OL	Occipital lobe
ON	Optic nerve (CNII)
P	Pons
PA	Pharynx
PCA	Posterior cerebral artery
PD	Cerebral peduncle
PF	Parapharyngeal fat
PG	Parotid gland
PH	Posterior horn of lateral ventricle
PN	Pinna
PY	Pyramid
RN	Red nucleus
SC	Semicircular canals
SCP	Superior cerebellar peduncle
SE	Suprasellar cistern
SH	Superior concha
SN	Substantia nigra
ST	Straight sinus
SV	Superior vermis
TG	Tongue
TL	Temporal lobe
To	Cerebellar tonsil
TP	Temporalis
UN	Uncus
VA	Vertebral artery
VP	Vestibular perilymph
VT	Vitreous body
W	White matter

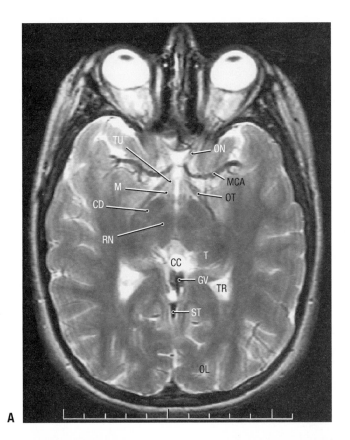

A

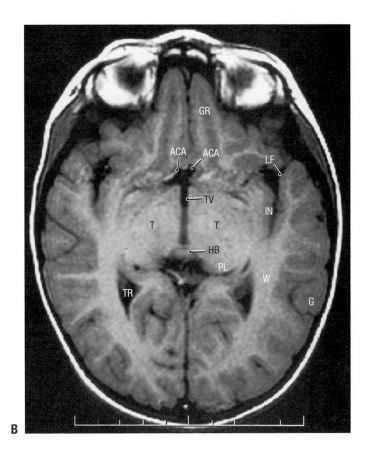

B

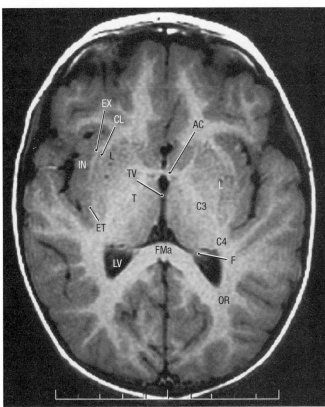

C

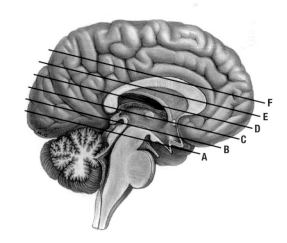

7.110 Axial (tranverse) MRIs through cerebral hemispheres

See orientation drawing for sites of scans **A–F. A** is T2 weighted, and **B–F** are T1 weighted.

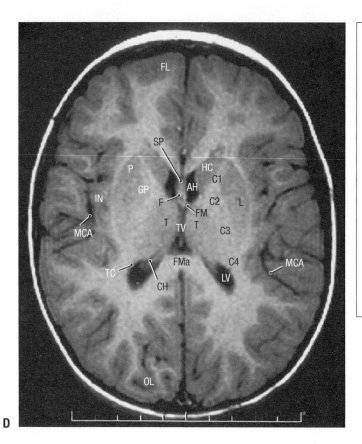

AC	Anterior commissure	EX	Extreme capsule	MCA	Middle cerebral artery
ACA	Anterior cerebral artery	F	Fornix		
		FC	Falx cerebri	OL	Occipital lobe
AH	Anterior horn of lateral ventricle	FL	Frontal lobe	ON	Optic nerve
		FM	Interventricular foramen	OR	Optic radiations
C1	Anterior limb of internal capsule			OT	Optic tract
		FMa	Forceps major	P	Putamen
C2	Genu of internal capsule	FMi	Forceps minor	PL	Pulvinar
		G	Gray matter	RN	Red nucleus
C3	Posterior limb of internal capsule	GL	Globus pallidus	SP	Septum pellucidum
		GR	Gyrus rectus	ST	Straight sinus
C4	Retrolenticular limb of internal capsule	HB	Habenular commissure	T	Thalamus
				TC	Tail of caudate nucleus
CC	Collicular cistern	HC	Head of caudate nucleus		
CD	Cerebral peduncle			TU	Tuber cinereum
CH	Choroid plexus	IN	Insular cortex	TR	Trigone of lateral ventricle
CL	Claustrum	L	Lentiform nucleus		
CN	Caudate nucleus	LF	Lateral fissure	TV	Third ventricle
CV	Great cerebral vein	LV	Lateral ventricle	W	White matter
ET	External capsule	M	Mamillary body		

D

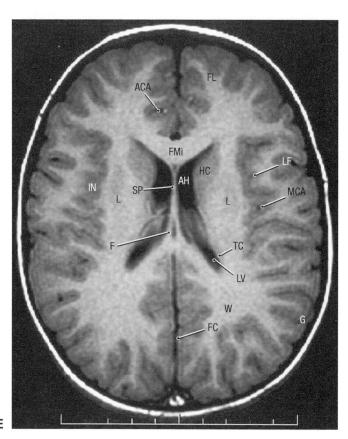

E

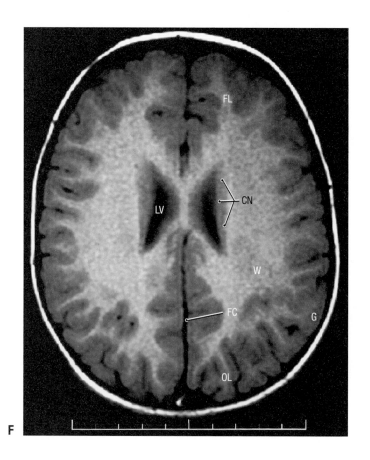

F

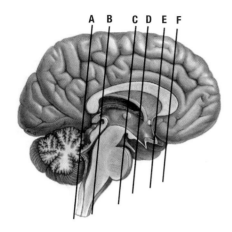

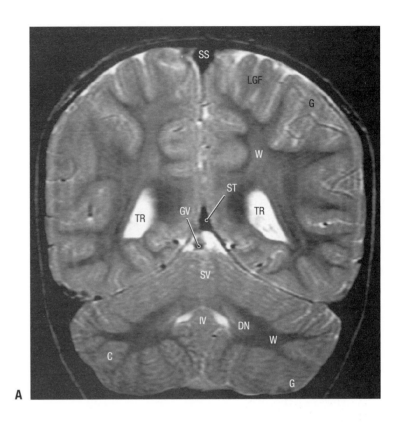

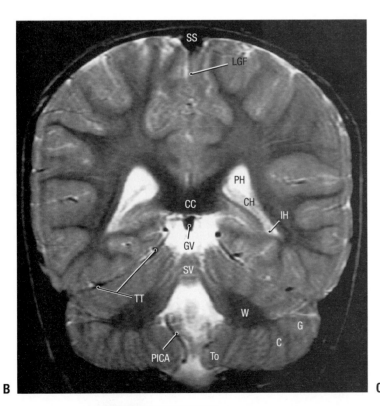

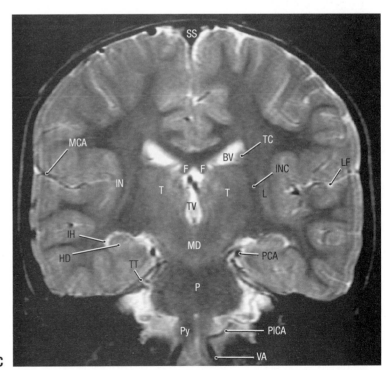

7.111   **Coronal MRIs of brain (T2 weighted)**

See orientation drawing for sites of scans A–F.

AA	Anterior communicating artery	LF	Lateral fissure
AC	Anterior commissure	LGF	Longitudinal fissure
ACA	Anterior cerebral artery	MCA	Middle cerebral artery
AH	Anterior horn of lateral ventricle	MD	Midbrain
BC	Body of caudate nucleus	MO	Medulla oblongata
BV	Body of lateral ventricle	OT	Optic tract
C	Cerebellum	P	Pons
CC	Corpus callosum	PCA	Posterior cerebral artery
CH	Choroid plexus	PH	Posterior horn of lateral ventricle
CS	Cavernous sinus		
CT	Corticospinal tract	PICA	Posterior inferior cerebellar artery
CV	Great cerebral vein		
DN	Dentate nucleus	PY	Pyramid
DS	Diaphragma sellae	SC	Supracerebellar cistern
F	Fornix	SCA	Superior cerebellar artery
FV	Fourth ventricle	SN	Substantia nigra
G	Gray matter	SP	Septum pellucidum
HC	Head of caudate nucleus	SS	Superior sagittal sinus
HP	Hippocampus	ST	Straight sinus
IC	Interpeduncular cistern	SV	Superior vermis
ICA	Internal carotid artery	T	Thalamus
IH	Inferior horn of lateral ventricle	TC	Tail of caudate nucleus
IN	Insular cortex	TL	Temporal lobe
INC	Internal capsule	To	Cerebellar tonsil
IV	Inferior vermis	TR	Trigone of lateral ventricle
IR	Intercerebral vein	TS	Transverse sinus
L	Lentiform nucleus	TT	Tentorium cerebelli
L1	Putamen	TV	Third ventricle
L2	External (lateral) segment of globus pallidus	VA	Vertebral artery
		W	White matter
L3	Internal (medial) segment of globus pallidus	Y	Hypophysis

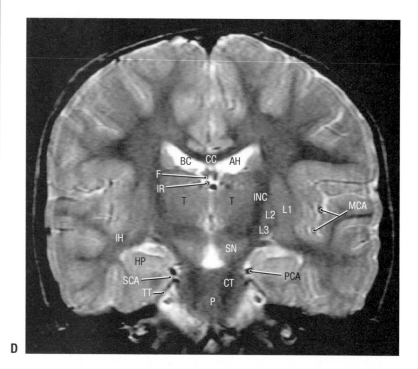

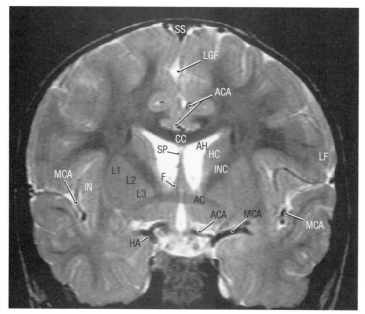

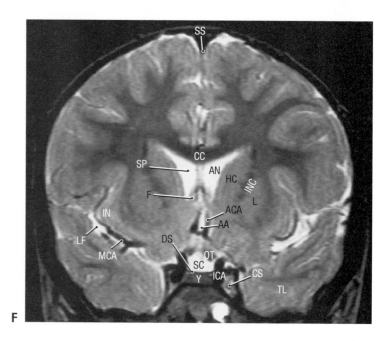

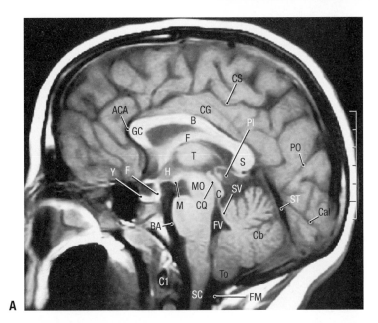

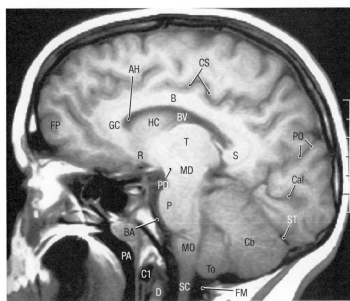

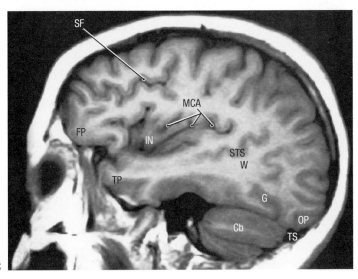

ACA	Anterior cerebral artery
AH	Anterior horn of lateral ventricle
B	Body of corpus callosum
BA	Basilar artery
BV	Body of lateral ventricle
C	Colliculus
Cb	Cerebellum
C1	Anterior tubercle of atlas
Cal	Calcarine sulcus
CG	Cingulate gyrus
CQ`	Cerebral aqueduct
CS	Cingulate sulcus
D	Dens (odontoid process)
F	Fornix
FM	Foramen magnum
FP	Frontal pole
FV	Fourth ventricle
G	Cerebral cortex (gray matter)
GC	Genu of corpus callosum
H	Hypothalamus
HC	Head of caudate nucleus
I	Infundibulum
IN	Insular cortex
M	Mamillary body
MCA	Middle cerebral artery
MD	Midbrain
MO	Medulla oblongata
OP	Occipital pole
P	Pons
PA	Pharynx
PI	Pineal
PD	Cerebral peduncle
PO	Parieto-occipital fissure
R	Rostrum of corpus callosum
S	Splenium of corpus callosum
SC	Spinal cord
SF	Superior frontal sulcus
ST	Straight sinus
STS	Superior temporal sulcus
SV	Superior medullary vellum
T	Thalamus
To	Cerebellar tonsil
TP	Temporal pole
TS	Transverse sinus
W	White matter
Y	Hypophysis

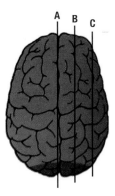

7.112　**Sagittal MRIs of brain (T1 weighted)**

See orientation drawing for site of scans **A–C.**

C H A P T E R 8

Neck

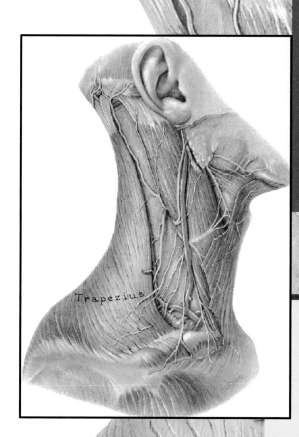

Trapezius

Trapezius

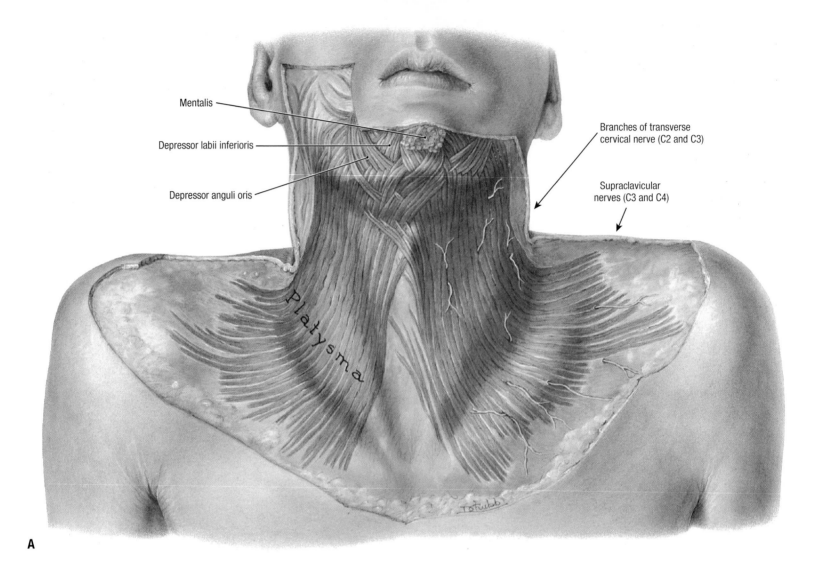

Mentalis

Depressor labii inferioris

Depressor anguli oris

Branches of transverse cervical nerve (C2 and C3)

Supraclavicular nerves (C3 and C4)

Platysma

A

8.1 Platysma muscle, anterior views

A. Dissection. **B.** Surface anatomy.

OBSERVE:

1. The platysma muscle spreads subcutaneously like a "sheet" that is pierced by cutaneous nerves;
2. The platysma muscle attaches superiorly to the inferior border of the mandible and to the skin and subcutaneous tissues of the lower face, and blends inferiorly with the fascia covering the superior parts of the pectoralis major and deltoid muscles to the level of the 1st or 2nd rib and to the acromion;
3. The anterior borders of the muscle decussate posterior to the chin in the submental region and diverge inferiorly, leaving the median part of the neck uncovered;
4. The posterior borders cover the anteroinferior part of the posterior triangle and continue superiorly across the inferior border of the mandible to the angles of the mouth;
5. The mentalis, depressor labii inferioris, and depressor anguli oris muscles blend with the platysma.

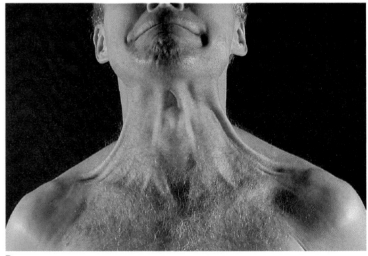

B

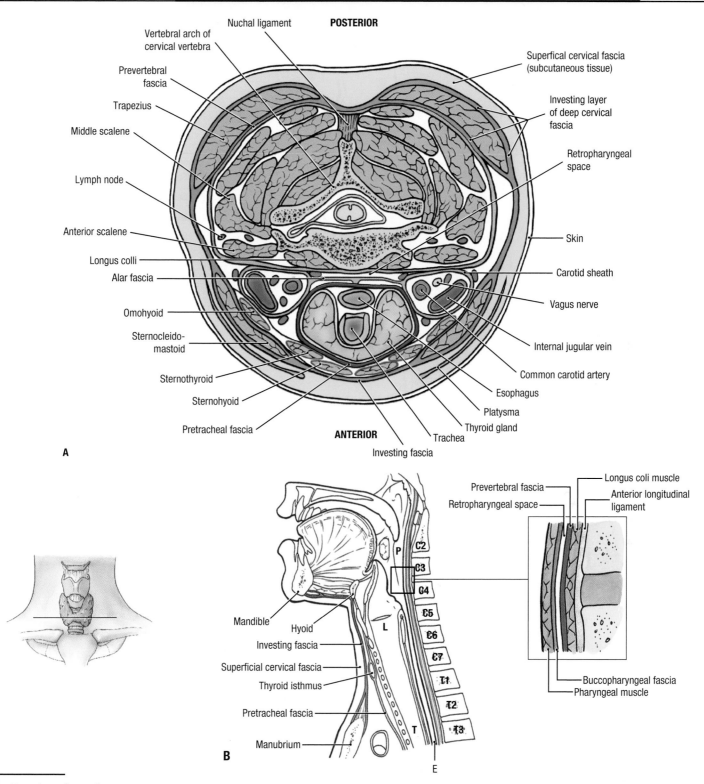

A. Transverse section through thyroid gland. **B.** Pretracheal fascia and carotid sheath, anterior view.

A

B

8.2   Fascia of neck

A. Transverse section through thyroid gland. **B.** Pretracheal fascia and carotid sheath, anterior view.

OBSERVE:

1. The deep cervical fascia consists of the investing, pretracheal, and prevertebral fasciae;
2. The investing fascia surrounds the neck and envelopes the trapezius and sternocleidomastoid muscles;
3. The prevertebral fascia is tubular, surrounding the vertebral col-

umn and associated musculature; at vertebral level T3, the prevertebral fascia fuses with the anterior longitudinal ligament and extends laterally as the axillary sheath;

4. The pretracheal fascia is limited to the anterior part of the neck and extends inferiorly to blend with the fibrous pericardium; it surrounds the thyroid, trachea, pharynx, and esophagus;
5. The tubular carotid sheath contains the common (internal) carotid arteries, internal jugular vein, and vagus (CN X) nerve.

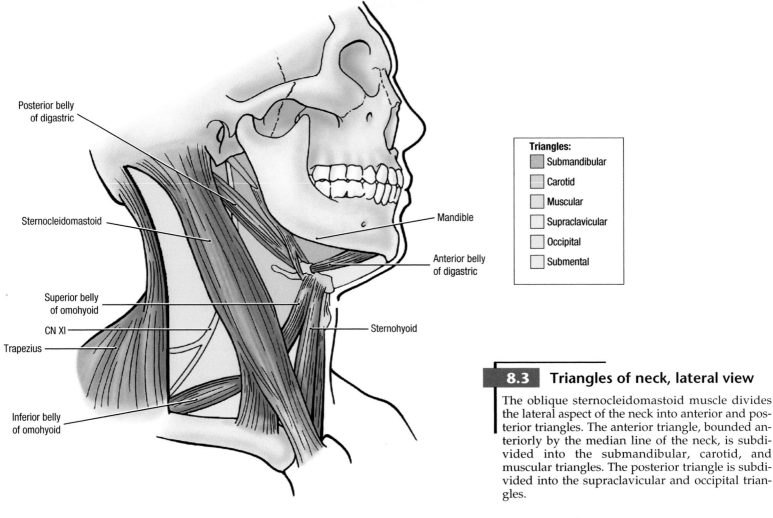

Posterior belly
of digastric

Sternocleidomastoid

Superior belly
of omohyoid

CN XI

Trapezius

Inferior belly
of omohyoid

Mandible

Anterior belly
of digastric

Sternohyoid

Triangles:
- Submandibular
- Carotid
- Muscular
- Supraclavicular
- Occipital
- Submental

8.3   Triangles of neck, lateral view

The oblique sternocleidomastoid muscle divides the lateral aspect of the neck into anterior and posterior triangles. The anterior triangle, bounded anteriorly by the median line of the neck, is subdivided into the submandibular, carotid, and muscular triangles. The posterior triangle is subdivided into the supraclavicular and occipital triangles.

8.4   Bony landmarks of neck, lateral view

OBSERVE:

1. The external occipital protuberance and mastoid process for the attachment of the trapezius and sternocleidomastoid muscles;

2. *The transverse process of the atlas, the most prominent of the cervical transverse processes, can be palpated with the fingertip by pressing superiorly between the angle of the mandible and the mastoid process;*

3. The body of the hyoid bone lies at the angle between the floor of the mouth and the anterior aspect of the neck at the level of C3/C4; *the greater horn of one side of the hyoid bone is palpable only when the greater horn of the opposite side is steadied;*

4. The arch of the cricoid cartilage projects further anteriorly than the rings of the trachea; it is the guide to the level of C6.

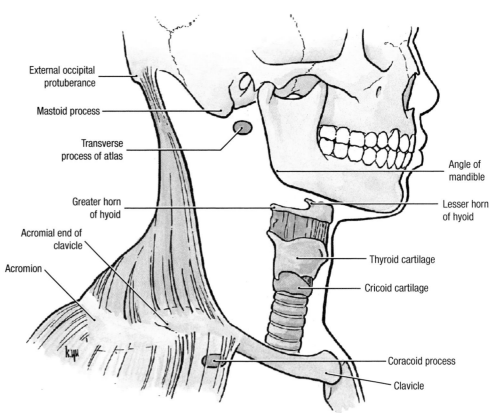

External occipital
protuberance

Mastoid process

Transverse
process of atlas

Greater horn
of hyoid

Acromial end of
clavicle

Acromion

Angle of
mandible

Lesser horn
of hyoid

Thyroid cartilage

Cricoid cartilage

Coracoid process

Clavicle

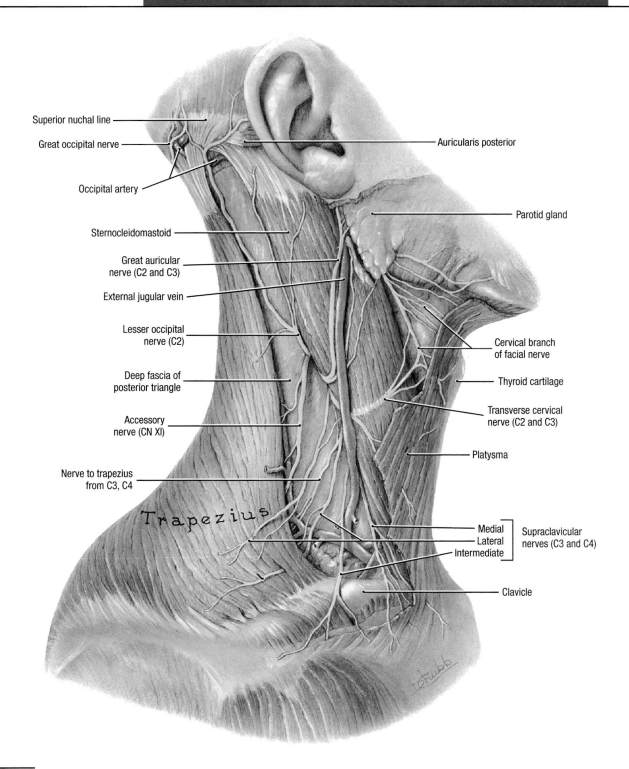

Superior nuchal line

Great occipital nerve

Occipital artery

Sternocleidomastoid

Great auricular
nerve (C2 and C3)

External jugular vein

Lesser occipital
nerve (C2)

Deep fascia of
posterior triangle

Accessory
nerve (CN XI)

Nerve to trapezius
from C3, C4

Trapezius

Auricularis posterior

Parotid gland

Cervical branch
of facial nerve

Thyroid cartilage

Transverse cervical
nerve (C2 and C3)

Platysma

Medial
Lateral   Supraclavicular
Intermediate   nerves (C3 and C4)

Clavicle

8.5   Posterior triangle of neck—I, lateral view

OBSERVE:

1. The three sides of the posterior triangle are the trapezius muscle, sternocleidomastoid muscle, and middle one third of the clavicle; the apex is where the aponeuroses of the two muscles blend just inferior to the superior nuchal line;
2. The platysma muscle (partly cut away) covers the inferior part of the triangle;
3. The external jugular vein descends vertically from posterior to the angle of the mandible, across the sternocleidomastoid muscle, to its posterior border where it pierces the deep fascia approximately one inch superior to the clavicle;
4. The "fascial carpet" covers the muscular floor;
5. The accessory nerve (CN XI), the only motor nerve superficial to the "fascial carpet," descends within the deep fascia and disappears approximately 2 fingersbreadth superior to the clavicle;
6. The cutaneous nerves (C2, C3, C4) radiate from the posterior border of the sternocleidomastoid muscle, inferior to the accessory nerve.

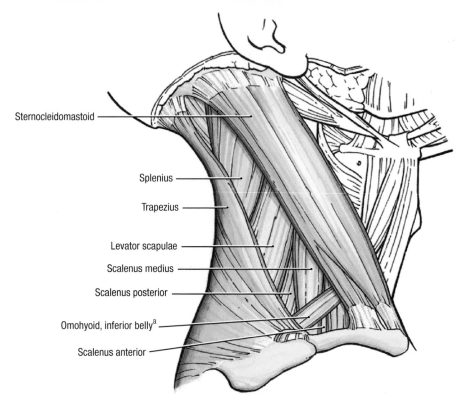

Sternocleidomastoid

Splenius

Trapezius

Levator scapulae

Scalenus medius

Scalenus posterior

Omohyoid, inferior belly[a]

Scalenus anterior

Table 8.1 Muscles of Posterior Triangle

Muscle	Origin	Insertion	Innervation	Actions
Trapezius	Medial third of superior nuchal line, external occipital protuberance, ligamentum nuchae, spinous processes of C7–T12 vertebrae, and lumbar and sacral spinous processes	Lateral third of clavicle, acromion and spine of scapula	Spinal root of accessory nerve (CN XI) and C3 and C4 nerves	Elevates, retracts, and rotates scapula
Sternocleidomastoid	Lateral surface of mastoid processes of temporal bone and lateral half of superior nuchal line	*Sternal head:* anterior surface of manubrium of sternum *Clavicular head:* superior surface of medial third of clavicle	Spinal root of accessory nerve (CN XI) and C2 and C3 nerves	Tilts head to one side (i.e., laterally); flexes neck and rotates it so face is turned superiorly toward opposite side; acting together, the two muscles flex the neck
Splenius capitis	Inferior half of ligamentum nuchae and spinous processes of superior six thoracic vertebrae	Lateral aspect of mastoid process and lateral third of superior nuchal line	Dorsal rami of middle cervical spinal nerves	Laterally flexes and rotates head and neck to same side; acting bilaterally, they extend head and neck
Levator scapulae	Posterior tubercles of transverse processes of C1–C4 vertebrae	Superior part of medial border of scapula	Dorsal scapular nerve (C5) and cervical spinal nerves (C3 and C4)	Elevates scapula and tilts its glenoid cavity inferiorly by rotating scapula
Scalenus posterior	Posterior tubercles of transverse processes of C4–C6 vertebrae	External border of 2nd rib	Ventral rami of cervical nerves (C7 and C8)	Flexes neck laterally; elevates 2nd rib during forced inspiration
Scalenus medius	Posterior tubercles of transverse processes of C2–C7 vertebrae	Superior surface of 1st rib, posterior to groove for subclavian artery	Ventral rami of cervical spinal nerves (C3 and C8)	Flexes neck laterally; elevates 1st rib during forced inspiration
Scalenus anterior	Anterior tubercles of transverse processes of C3–C6 vertebrae	Scalene tubercle of 1st rib	Ventral rami of cervical spinal nerves (C5 to C7)	

[a]Omohyoid, see Table 8.2.

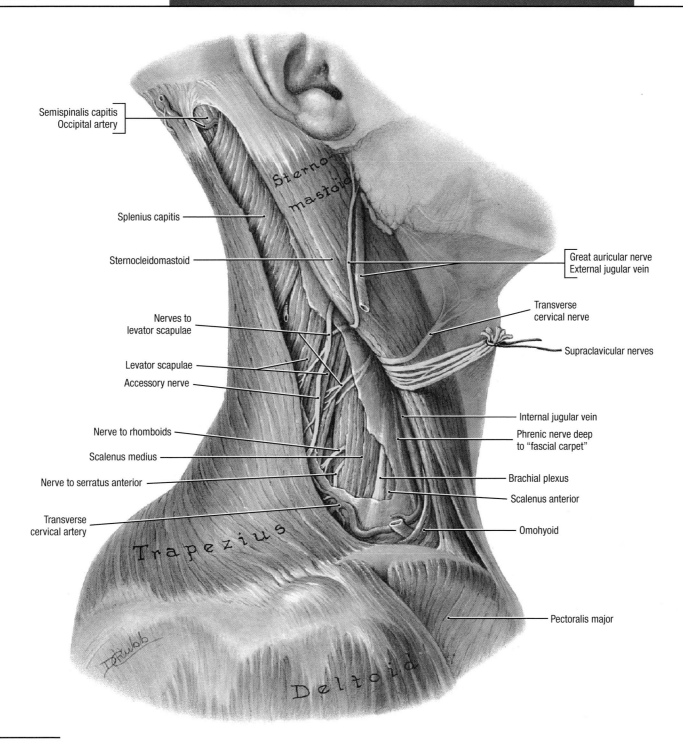

Semispinalis capitis
Occipital artery

Splenius capitis

Sterno-mastoid

Sternocleidomastoid

Great auricular nerve
External jugular vein

Transverse
cervical nerve

Nerves to
levator scapulae

Supraclavicular nerves

Levator scapulae
Accessory nerve

Internal jugular vein
Phrenic nerve deep
to "fascial carpet"

Nerve to rhomboids
Scalenus medius

Nerve to serratus anterior

Brachial plexus
Scalenus anterior

Transverse
cervical artery

Omohyoid

Trapezius

Pectoralis major

Deltoid

8.6   Posterior triangle of neck—II, lateral view

The motor nerves and superior part of the floor of the triangle have been dissected.

OBSERVE:

1. The muscles that form the floor superiorly are the semispinalis capitis, splenius capitis, and levator scapulae;
2. The accessory nerve supplies the sternocleidomastoid and trapezius muscles; it lies along the levator scapulae muscle but is separated from it by the "fascial carpet" (partially removed);
3. Motor nerves to the levator scapulae (C3, C4), the rhomboids (C5), and the serratus anterior (C5, C6); the branch from C7 lies protected posterior to the plexus;

4. *Two structures of clinical importance, situated just beyond the geometric confines of the triangle are: a) the phrenic nerve to the diaphragm (C3, C4, C5), located between the fascial carpet and the floor; and b) the internal jugular vein, superficial to the carpet. Severance of a phrenic nerve results in paralysis of the corresponding half of the diaphragm. To produce a short period of paralysis of the diaphragm (e.g., for a long surgery), a phrenic nerve block is performed. The anesthetic is injected where the nerve lies on the anterior surface of the middle one third of the scalenus anterior. Pulsations of the internal jugular vein caused by contraction of the right ventricle of the heart can be palpable superior to the medial end of the clavicle in the root of the neck. The internal jugular pulse increases with conditions such as mitral valve disease.*

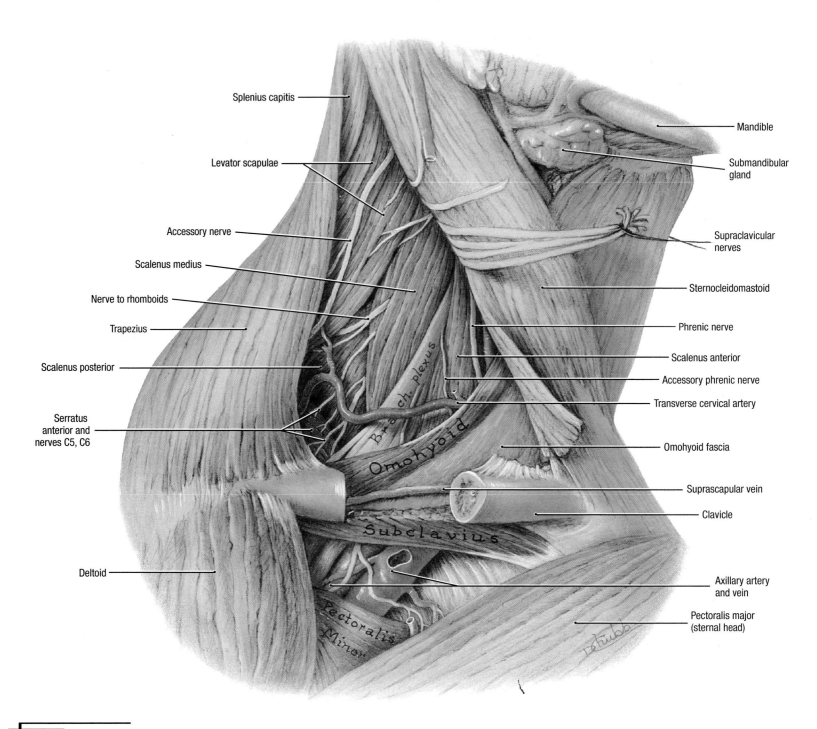

Splenius capitis

Levator scapulae

Accessory nerve

Scalenus medius

Nerve to rhomboids

Trapezius

Scalenus posterior

Serratus anterior and nerves C5, C6

Deltoid

Mandible

Submandibular gland

Supraclavicular nerves

Sternocleidomastoid

Phrenic nerve

Scalenus anterior

Accessory phrenic nerve

Transverse cervical artery

Omohyoid fascia

Suprascapular vein

Clavicle

Axillary artery and vein

Pectoralis major (sternal head)

Brach plexus

Omohyoid

Subclavius

Pectoralis Minor

8.7 Posterior triangle of neck—III, lateral view

In this dissection of the omohyoid and its fascia, the clavicular head of the pectoralis major muscle and part of the clavicle have been excised.

OBSERVE:

1. The omohyoid fascia lies between the omohyoid and subclavius muscles;
2. The brachial plexus appears between the scalenus anterior and

scalenus medius muscles and gives off an accessory phrenic nerve from C5;

3. The posterior border of the scalenus anterior muscle is nearly parallel to the posterior border of the sternocleidomastoid muscle and slightly posterior to it.

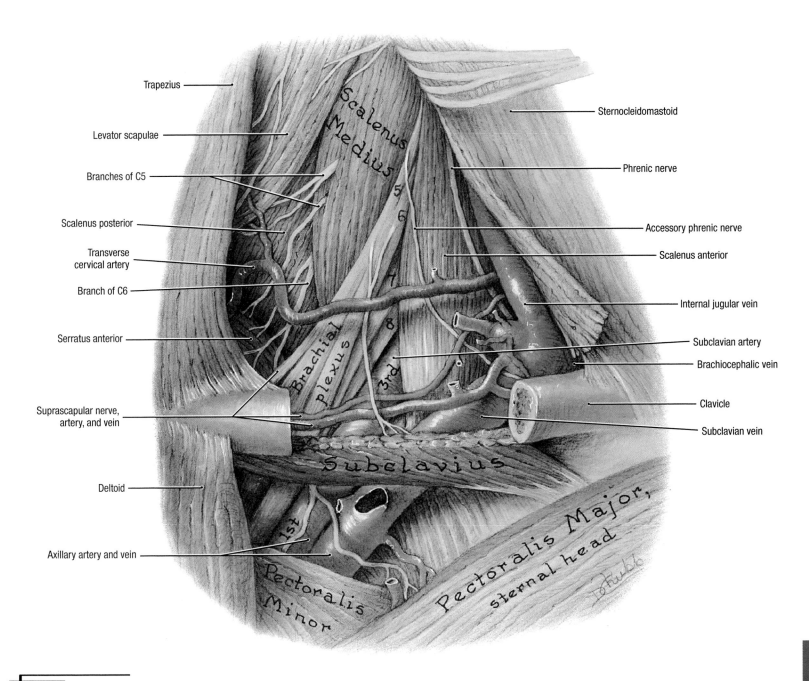

8.8 Posterior triangle of neck—IV, lateral view

The brachial plexus and subclavian vessels have been dissected.

OBSERVE:

1. The third part of the subclavian artery and first part of the axillary artery are labeled;
2. The scalene (posterior, medius, and anterior) and serratus anterior muscles form the floor of the inferior part of the triangle;
3. The ventral primary rami of C5–C8 (T1 not visible) form the brachial plexus; the brachial plexus and subclavian artery emerge between the scalenus medius and scalenus anterior muscles; the most inferior root of the plexus (T1) is concealed by the third part of the subclavian artery;

4. The subclavian vein is separated from the second part of the subclavian artery by the scalenus anterior muscle;
5. *The subclavius is unimportant as a muscle, but valuable as a buffer between a fractured clavicle and the subclavian vessels;*
6. *The subclavian vein is often used for insertion of a central venous catheter for recording venous pressure, giving hyperalimentation fluids, placing cardiac pacemaker leads (electrodes), and inserting right cardiac catheters. Therefore, the relationships of the subclavian vein to the sternocleidomastoid muscle, clavicle, 1st rib, and cupula of pleura (see Fig. 8.32) are of clinical importance.*

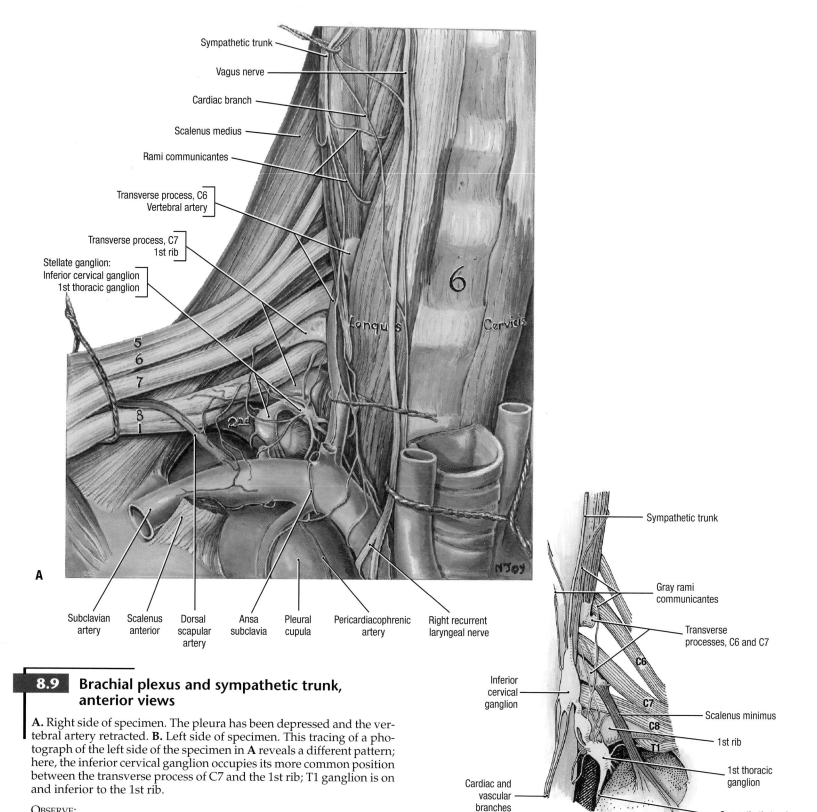

A. Right side of specimen. The pleura has been depressed and the vertebral artery retracted. **B.** Left side of specimen. This tracing of a photograph of the left side of the specimen in **A** reveals a different pattern; here, the inferior cervical ganglion occupies its more common position between the transverse process of C7 and the 1st rib; T1 ganglion is on and inferior to the 1st rib.

OBSERVE:

1. The inferior trunk of the branchial plexus (C8 and T1) is raised from the groove it occupies on the 1st rib posterior to the subclavian artery; the dorsal scapular artery passes through the plexus;

2. The sympathetic trunk (retracted laterally) sends a communicating branch to the vagus, gray rami communicantes to the cervical nerves, and cardiac branches;

8.9   Brachial plexus and sympathetic trunk, anterior views

3. The vertebral artery is retracted medially to uncover the stellate ganglion (the combined inferior cervical and 1st thoracic ganglia);

4. Fine branches pass from the stellate ganglion to nerves C7, C8, and T1, and to adjacent arteries.

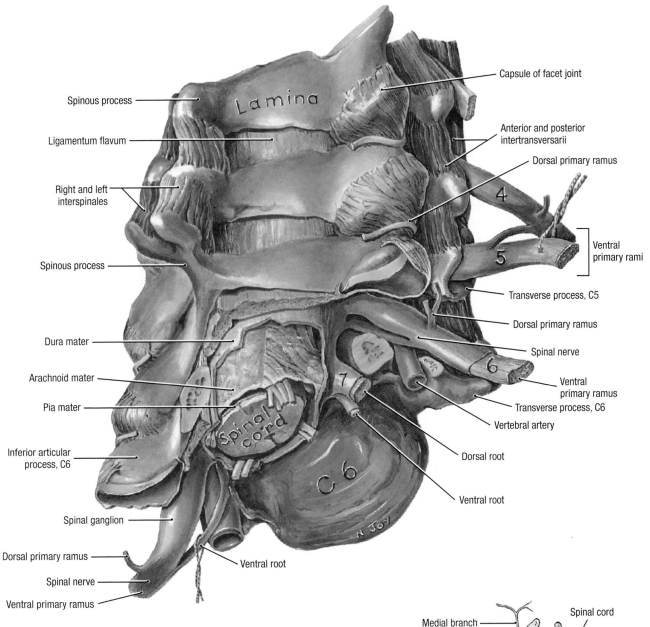

Spinous process

Ligamentum flavum

Right and left interspinales

Spinous process

Dura mater

Arachnoid mater

Pia mater

Inferior articular process, C6

Spinal ganglion

Dorsal primary ramus

Spinal nerve

A Ventral primary ramus

Ventral root

Capsule of facet joint

Anterior and posterior intertransversarii

Dorsal primary ramus

Ventral primary rami

Transverse process, C5

Dorsal primary ramus

Spinal nerve

Ventral primary ramus

Transverse process, C6

Vertebral artery

Dorsal root

Ventral root

8.10 Cervical nerves

 A. Cervical spinal nerves in situ, posteroinferior view. B. Relationships of spinal cord and spinal nerve to a cervical vertebra, superior view. *This diagram illustrates the vulnerability of the vertebral artery, spinal cord, and nerve roots to arthritic expansion from articular processes and the vertebral body, particularly the lateral edge of the superior surface of the body, the uncovertebral joint (joint of Luschka).*

OBSERVE:

1. The dura mater is adjacent to the ligamentum flavum; the arachnoid mater is applied to the dura mater and separated from the pia mater by the subarachnoid space, which contains cerebrospinal fluid;
2. The swelling of a dorsal root is the spinal (dorsal root) ganglion. The ventral and dorsal roots, each in a separate dural sheath, unite beyond the ganglion to form a spinal nerve; the spinal nerve, approximately 1 cm long, divides into a small dorsal and large ventral primary ramus;

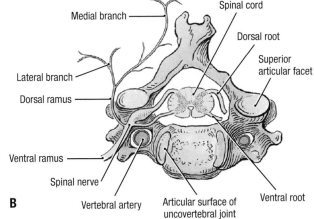

Medial branch

Lateral branch

Dorsal ramus

Ventral ramus

Spinal nerve

B   Vertebral artery

Spinal cord

Dorsal root

Superior articular facet

Articular surface of uncovertebral joint

Ventral root

3. The roots and spinal nerve cross posterior to the vertebral artery. The dorsal primary ramus curves dorsally around the superior articular process; the ventral primary ramus rests on the transverse process, which is grooved to support it.

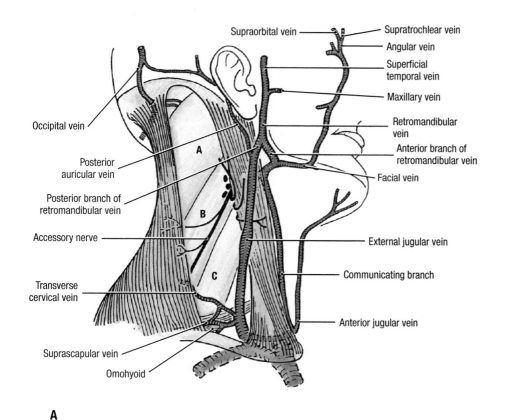

A

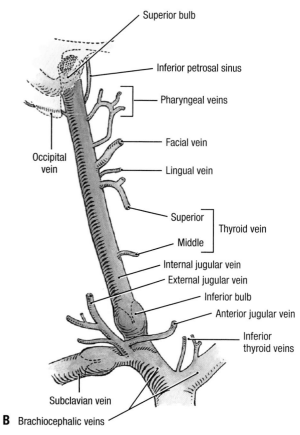

B Brachiocephalic veins

8.11 Superficial and deep veins, lateral views

A. Superficial veins. Outside the skull, superficial temporal and maxillary veins form the retromandibular vein, whose posterior division unites with the posterior auricular vein to form the external jugular vein. The facial vein receives the anterior division of the retromandibular vein before emptying into the internal jugular vein. (*A,* Splenius muscle; *B,* Levator scapulae muscle; *C,* Scalenus medius and scalenus posterior muscles.) **B.** Internal jugular vein and its tributaries. Note the dilation, or bulb, at each end of the internal jugular vein. The superior bulb is separated from the floor of the middle ear by a delicate bony plate. The inferior bulb, like the corresponding bulb at the end of the subclavian vein, contains a bicuspid valve that permits the flow of blood toward the heart. There are no valves in the brachiocephalic veins or superior vena cava. **C.** Variable relationships of accessory nerves, phrenic nerves, and ansa cervicalis to the great veins. Studies in the laboratory showed the accessory nerve crossing anterior to the internal jugular vein in 70% of 188 specimens, and crossing posterior to it in 30%. The phrenic nerve (C3, C4, and C5) passes posterior to the site of union of the subclavian, internal jugular, and brachiocephalic veins, but occasionally the branch from C5 or, less commonly, the entire phrenic nerve, passes anterior to the subclavian vein.

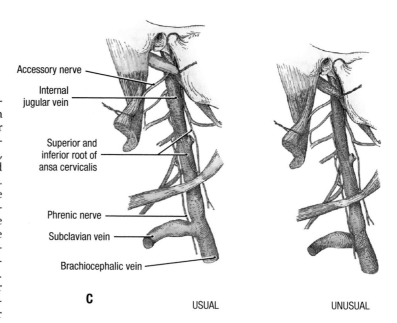

C

USUAL   UNUSUAL

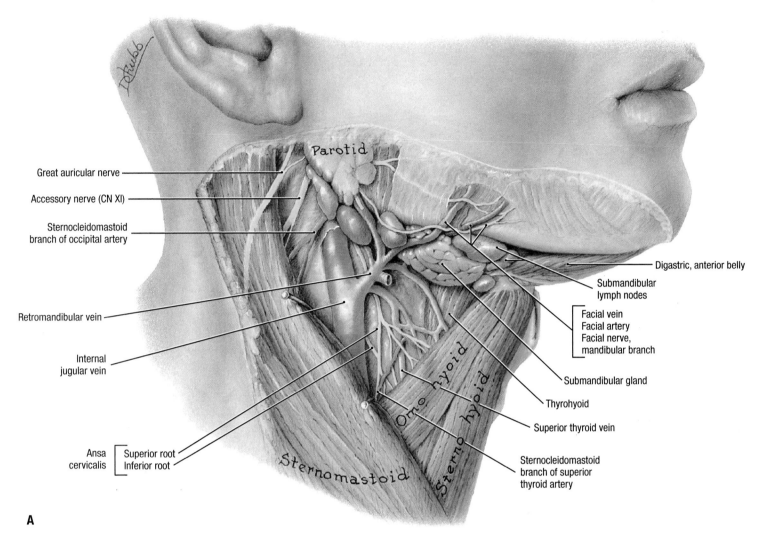

A

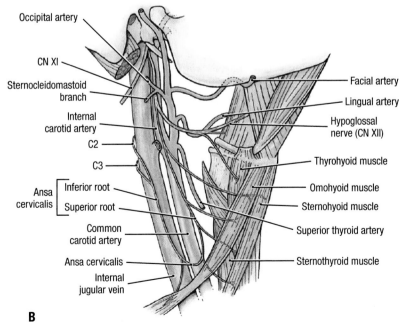

B

8.12 Anterior triangle of neck—I, lateral views

A. Superficial dissection. **B.** Ansa cervicalis. The ansa cervicalis is a nerve loop in the neck that innervates the infrahyoid muscles. Branches of the C1 and C2 nerves join the hypoglossal nerve at the base of the skull, travel with it for a short distance, and then form the superior root of the ansa cervicalis. The superior root travels anterior to the internal and common carotid arteries. The inferior root, from the C2 and C3 nerves, travels posterior to the carotid sheath to join the superior root lateral or medial to the internal jugular vein. Branches of the ansa innervate the infrahyoid (strap) muscles.

OBSERVE:

1. The accessory nerve enters the deep surface of the sternocleidomastoid muscle and is joined along its inferior border by the sternocleidomastoid branch of the occipital artery;
2. The internal jugular vein is joined anteriorly by several veins, notably the facial vein near the level of the hyoid bone;
3. The sternocleidomastoid branch of the superior thyroid artery descends near the superior border of the omohyoid muscle;

4. The retromandibular and facial veins run superficial to the submandibular gland;
5. The submandibular lymph nodes.

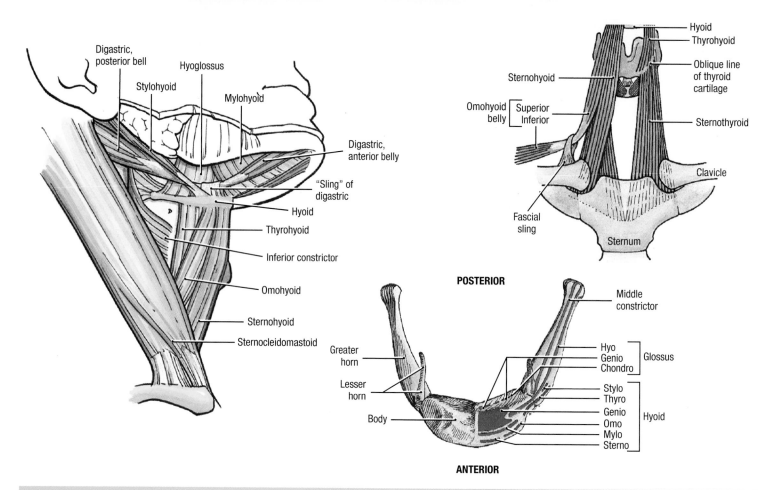

Table 8.2 Suprahyoid and Infrahyoid Muscles

Muscle	Origin	Insertion	Innervation	Actions
Mylohyoid	Mylohyoid line of mandible	Raphe and body of hyoid bone	Mylohyoid nerve, a branch of inferior alveolar nerve (CN V3)	Elevates hyoid bone, floor of mouth, and tongue during swallowing and speaking
Geniohyoid	Inferior mental spine of mandible	Body of hyoid bone	C1 through the hypoglossal nerve (CN XII)	Pulls hyoid bone anterosuperiorly, shortens floor of mouth, and widens pharynx
Stylohyoid	Styloid process of temporal bone	Body of hyoid bone	Cervical branch of facial nerve (CN VII)	Elevates and retracts hyoid bone, thereby elongating floor of mouth
Digastric	*Anterior belly:* digastric fossa of mandible *Posterior belly:* mastoid notch of temporal bone	Intermediate tendon to body and superior (greater) horn of hyoid bone	*Anterior belly:* mylohyoid nerve, a branch of inferior alveolar nerve (CN V3) *Posterior belly:* facial nerve (CN VII)	Depresses mandible; raises hyoid bone and steadies it during swallowing and speaking
Sternohyoid	Manubrium of sternum and medial end of clavicle	Body of hyoid bone	C1–C3 from ansa cervicalis	Depresses hyoid bone after it has been elevated during swallowing
Sternothyroid	Posterior surface of manubrium of sternum	Oblique line of thyroid cartilage	C2 and C3 by a branch of ansa cervicalis	Depresses hyoid bone and larynx
Thyrohyoid	Oblique line of thyroid cartilage	Inferior border of body and superior (greater) horn of hyoid bone	C1 through hypoglossal nerve (CN XII)	Depresses hyoid bone and elevates larynx
Omohyoid	Superior border of scapula near suprascapular notch	Inferior border of hyoid bone	C1–C3 by a branch of ansa cervicalis	Depresses, retracts, and steadies hyoid bone

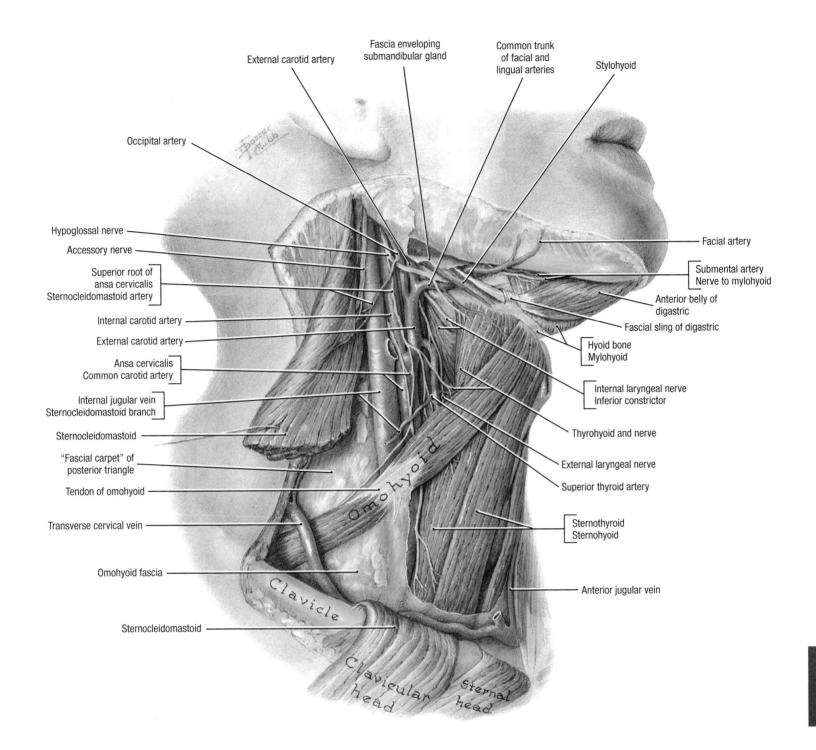

Occipital artery

External carotid artery

Fascia enveloping submandibular gland

Common trunk of facial and lingual arteries

Stylohyoid

Facial artery

Hypoglossal nerve

Accessory nerve

Superior root of ansa cervicalis

Sternocleidomastoid artery

Internal carotid artery

External carotid artery

Ansa cervicalis

Common carotid artery

Internal jugular vein

Sternocleidomastoid branch

Sternocleidomastoid

"Fascial carpet" of posterior triangle

Tendon of omohyoid

Transverse cervical vein

Omohyoid fascia

Sternocleidomastoid

Submental artery

Nerve to mylohyoid

Anterior belly of digastric

Fascial sling of digastric

Hyoid bone

Mylohyoid

Internal laryngeal nerve

Inferior constrictor

Thyrohyoid and nerve

External laryngeal nerve

Superior thyroid artery

Sternothyroid

Sternohyoid

Anterior jugular vein

Omohyoid

Clavicle

Clavicular head

Sternal head

8.13 **Anterior triangle of neck—II, lateral view**

OBSERVE:

1. The tendon of the digastric muscle is held down to the hyoid bone by a fascial sling; the tendon of the omohyoid muscle is similarly held down to the clavicle;

2. The facial and lingual arteries arise from a common trunk and pass deep to the stylohyoid and digastric muscles;

3. The thyrohyoid and inferior constrictor muscles form the floor, or medial wall, of the carotid triangle (see Fig. 8.3);

4. The hypoglossal nerve passes deep to the digastric muscle twice, crossing the internal and external carotid arteries and giving off two branches: the superior root of the ansa cervicalis and the nerve to the thyrohyoid muscle;

5. The internal and external laryngeal nerves are deep to the external carotid artery;

6. *The common carotid artery lies in a groove between the trachea and the strap muscles. The carotid pulse is routinely checked during cardiopulmonary resuscitation (CPR); the absence of a carotid pulse indicates cardiac arrest.*

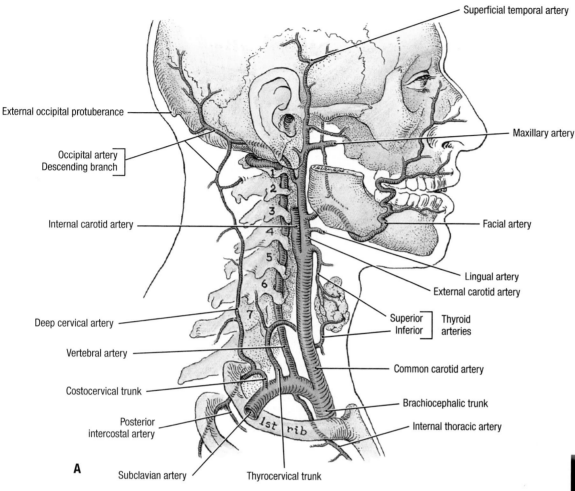

Superficial temporal artery

External occipital protuberance

Maxillary artery

Occipital artery
Descending branch

Internal carotid artery

Facial artery

Lingual artery
External carotid artery

Superior
Inferior
Thyroid
arteries

Deep cervical artery

Vertebral artery

Common carotid artery

Costocervical trunk

Brachiocephalic trunk

Posterior
intercostal artery

Internal thoracic artery

A

Subclavian artery   Thyrocervical trunk

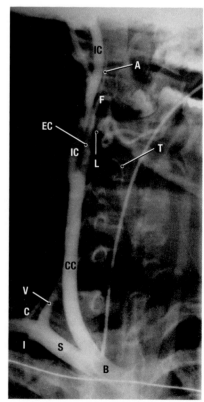

B

8.14   Arteries of neck

A. Overview, lateral view. **B.** Carotid arteriogram, oblique. (*B*, Brachiocephalic artery; *S*, Subclavian artery; *V*, Vertebral artery; *I*, Internal thoracic artery; *C*, Thyrocervical trunk; *CC*, Common carotid artery; *IC*, Internal carotid artery; *EC*, External carotid artery; *T*, Superior thyroid artery; *F*, Facial artery; *L*, Lingual artery; *A*, Ascending pharyngeal artery.)

OBSERVE:
1. The common carotid and subclavian arteries supply blood to the head;
2. The vertebral artery, a branch of the subclavian artery, enters the foramen magnum and contributes to the cerebral arterial circle (of Willis);
3. The common carotid artery terminates as the internal and external carotid arteries. In general, the internal carotid supplies structures inside the head, and the external carotid supplies the exterior. However, the ophthalmic artery (from the internal carotid) sends supraorbital and supratrochlear arteries to the forehead;
4. The deep cervical artery (from the costocervical trunk) anastomoses with the descending branch of the occipital artery and branches of the vertebral artery.

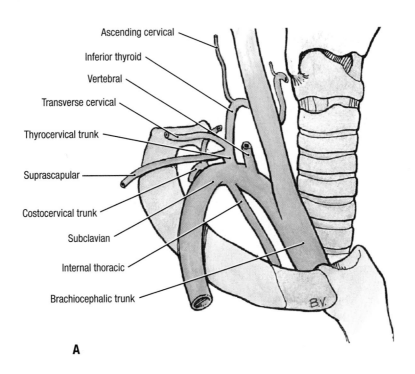

A

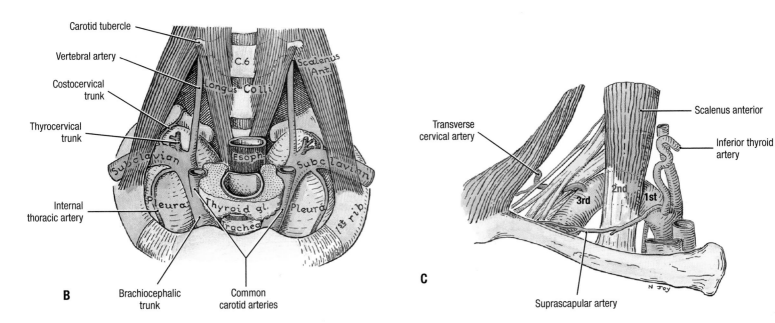

B

C

8.15 Subclavian artery

A. Subclavian artery and its branches, lateral view. **B.** Origin of vertebral artery, anterior view. The vertebral artery arises from the dorsal superior aspect of the subclavian artery and in this specimen enters the foramen transversarium of C6 vertebra; in other cases it may enter a more superior foramen. **C.** Branches of third part of subclavian artery, anterolateral view. The scalenus anterior divides the subclavian artery into three parts. Some branches from the second or third part (most commonly, the dorsal scapular and, less frequently, the transverse cervical and suprascapular arteries) pass laterally through the brachial plexus (see Figs. 8.8 and 8.32A).

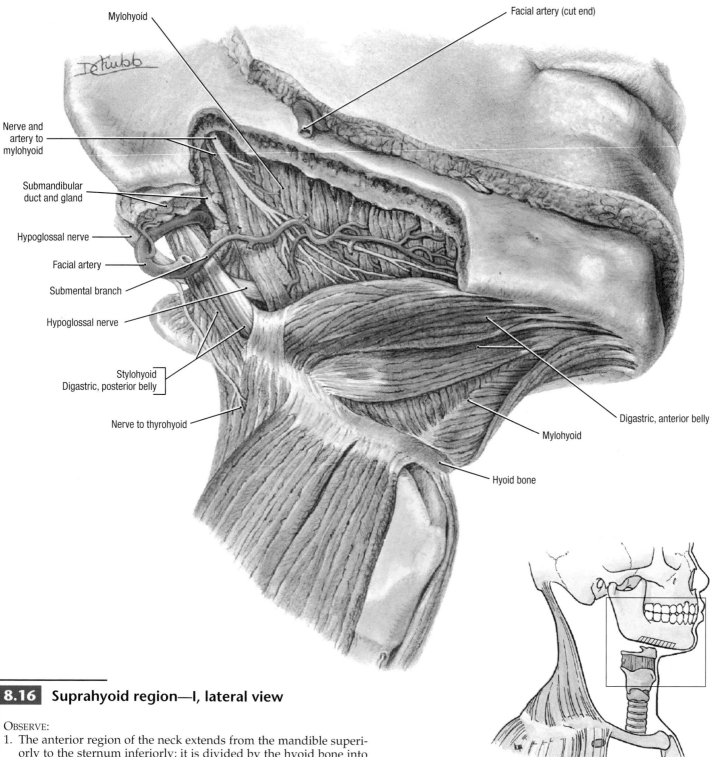

Mylohyoid

Facial artery (cut end)

Nerve and artery to mylohyoid

Submandibular duct and gland

Hypoglossal nerve

Facial artery

Submental branch

Hypoglossal nerve

Stylohyoid
Digastric, posterior belly

Nerve to thyrohyoid

Digastric, anterior belly

Mylohyoid

Hyoid bone

8.16   Suprahyoid region—I, lateral view

OBSERVE:
1. The anterior region of the neck extends from the mandible superiorly to the sternum inferiorly; it is divided by the hyoid bone into suprahyoid and infrahyoid parts;
2. The stylohyoid and posterior belly of the digastric muscle form the posterior border of the submandibular triangle; the facial artery arches superficial to these muscles;
3. The anterior belly of the digastric muscle forms the anterior border of the submandibular triangle. In this specimen, the anterior belly has an extra origin from the hyoid bone;
4. The mylohyoid muscle forms the medial wall of the triangle and has a free, thick posterior border;

5. The nerve to the mylohyoid, which supplies the mylohyoid muscle and anterior belly of the digastric muscle, is accompanied by the mylohyoid branch of the inferior alveolar artery posteriorly and the submental branch of the facial artery anteriorly;
6. The hypoglossal nerve and the submandibular gland and duct pass anteriorly deep to the posterior border of the mylohyoid muscle.

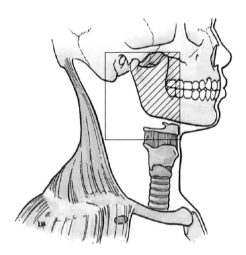

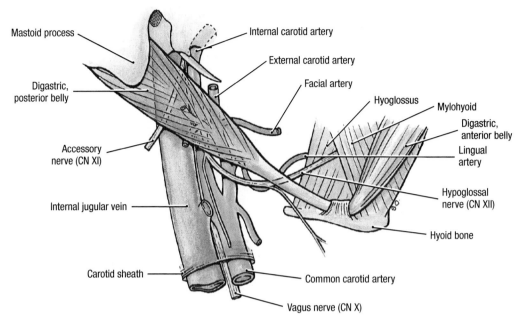

Mastoid process

Internal carotid artery

Digastric, posterior belly

External carotid artery

Facial artery

Hyoglossus

Mylohyoid

Digastric, anterior belly

Accessory nerve (CN XI)

Lingual artery

Hypoglossal nerve (CN XII)

Internal jugular vein

Hyoid bone

Carotid sheath

Common carotid artery

Vagus nerve (CN X)

A

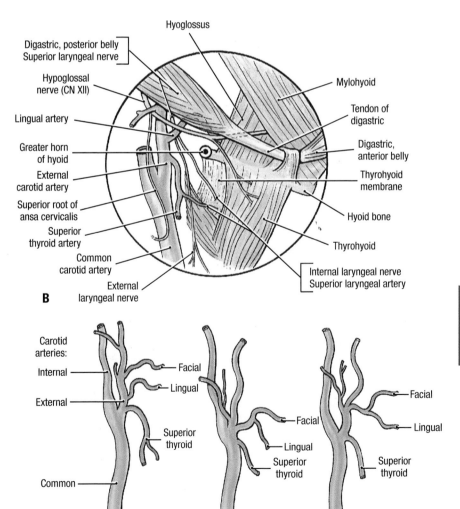

Hyoglossus

Digastric, posterior belly
Superior laryngeal nerve

Mylohyoid

Hypoglossal nerve (CN XII)

Tendon of digastric

Lingual artery

Digastric, anterior belly

Greater horn of hyoid

Thyrohyoid membrane

External carotid artery

Superior root of ansa cervicalis

Hyoid bone

Superior thyroid artery

Thyrohyoid

Common carotid artery

Internal laryngeal nerve
Superior laryngeal artery

External laryngeal nerve

B

8.17 Relationships of muscles, nerves, and vessels to hyoid bone, lateral views

A. Structures related to posterior belly of digastric muscle. **B.** Hypoglossal, internal and external laryngeal nerves. The tip of the greater horn of the hyoid bone is the reference point for many structures. **C.** Origin of lingual artery. Variation in origin was studied in 211 specimens. In 80%, the superior thyroid, lingual, and facial arteries arose separately (left); in 20%, the lingual and facial arteries arose from a common stem inferiorly (middle) or high on the external carotid artery (right). In one specimen, the superior thyroid and lingual arteries arose from a common stem.

OBSERVE:
1. The superficial position of the posterior belly of the digastric muscle, which runs from the mastoid process to the hyoid bone;
2. All vessels and nerves cross deep to this belly, except the cervical branches of the facial nerve, the facial branches of the great auricular nerve, and the external jugular vein and its connections.

Carotid arteries:

Internal

Facial

Lingual

External

Facial

Facial

Lingual

Superior thyroid

Lingual

Superior thyroid

Common

Superior thyroid

C

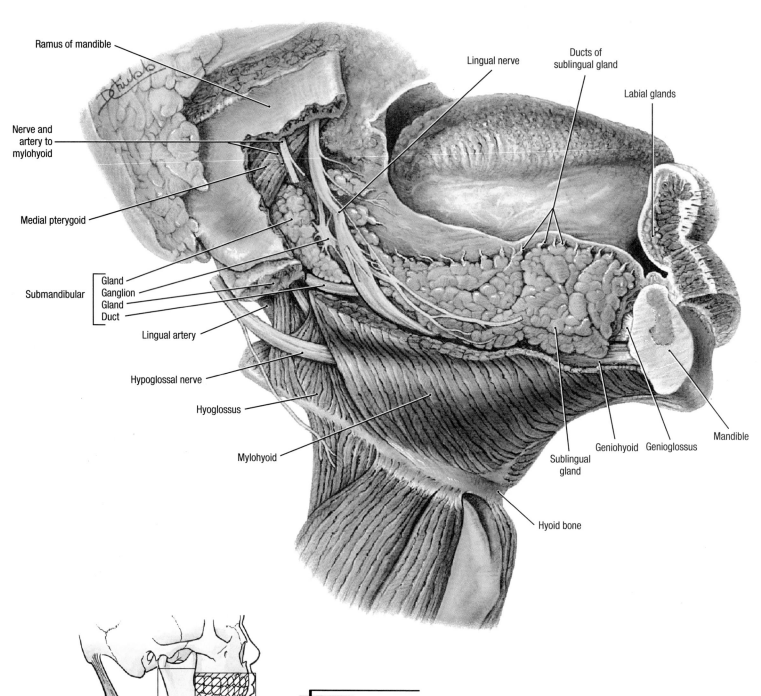

Ramus of mandible

Nerve and artery to mylohyoid

Medial pterygoid

Submandibular
- Gland
- Ganglion
- Gland
- Duct

Lingual artery

Hypoglossal nerve

Hyoglossus

Mylohyoid

Lingual nerve

Ducts of sublingual gland

Labial glands

Sublingual gland

Geniohyoid   Genioglossus

Mandible

Hyoid bone

8.18   **Suprahyoid region—II, lateral view**

OBSERVE:
1. The cut surface of the mylohyoid muscle becomes progressively thinner anteriorly;
2. The sublingual salivary gland lies posterior to the mandible and is in contact with the deep part of the submandibular gland posteriorly;
3. Twelve or more fine ducts pass from the superior border of the sublingual gland to open on the sublingual fold;
4. Several individual or detached lobules of the sublingual gland, each with a fine duct, lie posterior to the main mass of the gland; there are labial glands in the lip;
5. The nerve and artery (cut short) to the mylohyoid and the lingual nerve lie between the medial pterygoid muscle and ramus of the mandible;
6. The lingual nerve lies between the sublingual gland and the deep part of the submandibular gland; the submandibular ganglion is suspended from this nerve.

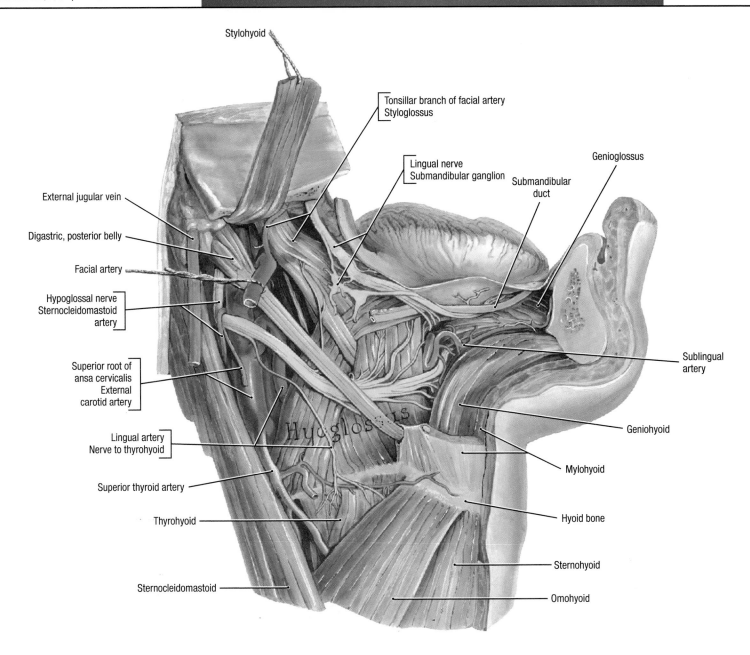

Stylohyoid

Tonsillar branch of facial artery
Styloglossus

Lingual nerve
Submandibular ganglion

Submandibular duct

Genioglossus

External jugular vein

Digastric, posterior belly

Facial artery

Hypoglossal nerve
Sternocleidomastoid artery

Superior root of ansa cervicalis
External carotid artery

Lingual artery
Nerve to thyrohyoid

Superior thyroid artery

Thyrohyoid

Sternocleidomastoid

Hyoglossus

Sublingual artery

Geniohyoid

Mylohyoid

Hyoid bone

Sternohyoid

Omohyoid

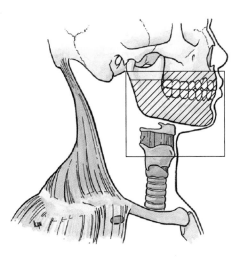

8.19   Suprahyoid region—III, lateral view

The stylohyoid muscle is reflected superiorly, and the posterior belly of the digastric muscle is left in situ as a landmark.

OBSERVE:
1. The hyoglossus muscle ascends from the greater horn and body of the hyoid bone to the side of the tongue. The styloglossus muscle is crossed by the tonsillar branch of the facial artery posterosuperiorly and interdigitates with bundles of the hyoglossus muscle. The genioglossus muscle fans out into the tongue anteriorly. The hyoglossus, styloglossus, and genioglossus are extrinsic muscles of the tongue;
2. The hypoglossal nerve supplies all of the muscles of the tongue, both extrinsic and intrinsic, except the palatoglossus muscle; the branches of the hypoglossal nerve leave its inferior border, thus it is best to dissect along the superior border;
3. The submandibular duct runs anteriorly across the hyoglossus and genioglossus muscles to its orifice;
4. The lingual nerve is in contact with the mandible posteriorly, making a partial spiral around the submandibular duct and ending in the tongue. The submandibular ganglion is suspended from the lingual nerve, and twigs leave the nerve to supply the mucous membrane.

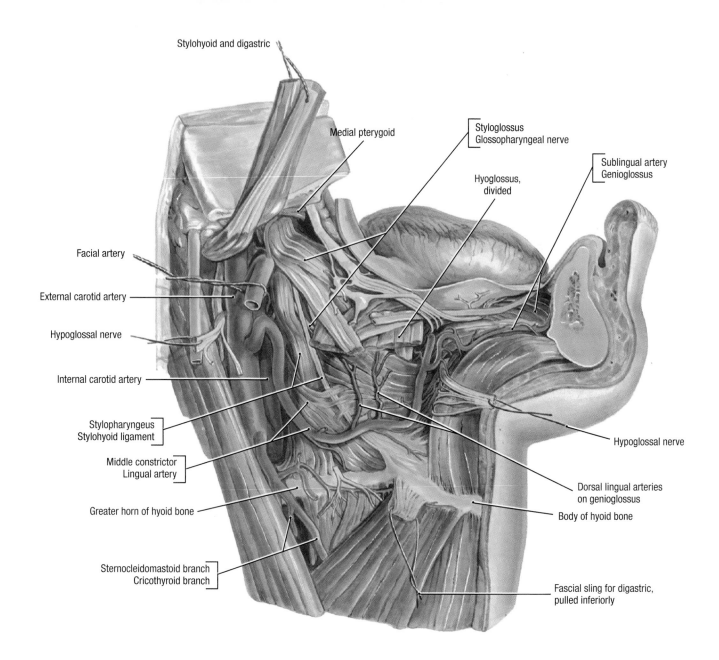

Stylohyoid and digastric

Medial pterygoid

Styloglossus
Glossopharyngeal nerve

Sublingual artery
Genioglossus

Hyoglossus,
divided

Facial artery

External carotid artery

Hypoglossal nerve

Internal carotid artery

Stylopharyngeus
Stylohyoid ligament

Middle constrictor
Lingual artery

Greater horn of hyoid bone

Hypoglossal nerve

Dorsal lingual arteries
on genioglossus

Body of hyoid bone

Sternocleidomastoid branch
Cricothyroid branch

Fascial sling for digastric,
pulled inferiorly

8.20   Suprahyoid region—IV, lateral view

The stylohyoid and posterior belly of the digastric muscle are reflected superiorly, the hypoglossal nerve is divided, and the hyoglossus muscle is mostly removed.

OBSERVE:

1. The lingual artery, crossed twice by the hypoglossal nerve, passes deep to the hyoglossus muscle, parallel to the greater horn of the hyoid, and lies on the middle constrictor muscle, stylohyoid ligament, and genioglossus muscle. It finally ascends at the anterior

border of the hyoglossus muscle, which partly overlaps it, and turns into the tongue as the deep lingual arteries (see Fig. 8.18 B);

2. The branches of the lingual artery: a) muscular; b) dorsal lingual, which reach the tonsil bed; and c) sublingual, which supplies the sublingual gland and anterior part of the floor of the mouth;

3. The stylopharyngeus muscle appears deep to the styloglossus muscle and disappears deep to the middle constrictor muscle;

4. The glossopharyngeal nerve does not make the usual spiral descent lateral to the stylopharyngeus muscle, but descends medial to it.

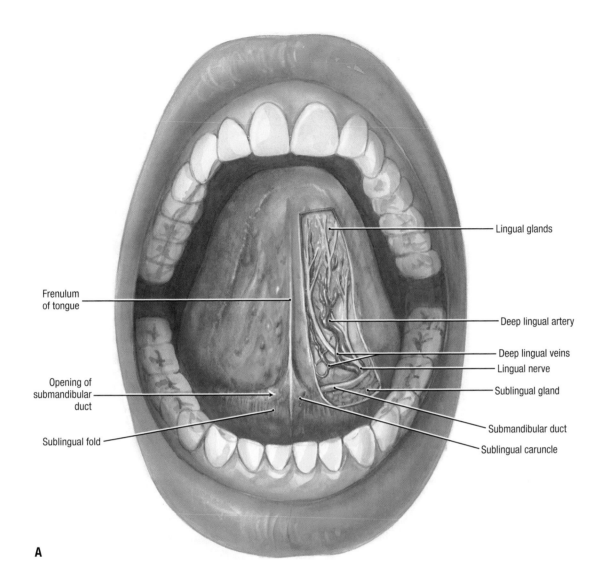

A

8.21 Sublingual gland and lingual artery

A. Floor of mouth and inferior surface of tongue. **B.** Course of lingual artery, lateral view.

OBSERVE IN A:
1. The inferior (sublingual) surface of the tongue is covered by a mucous membrane through which the underlying deep lingual veins can be seen;
2. The sublingual caruncle, a papilla on each side of the frenulum, marks the location of the opening of the submandibular duct.

OBSERVE IN **B**:
3. The deep lingual artery supplies the body of the tongue, the dorsal lingual artery supplies the root of the tongue and palatine tonsil, and the sublingual branch supplies the floor of the mouth.

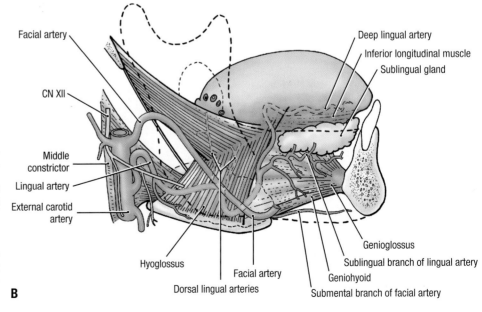

B

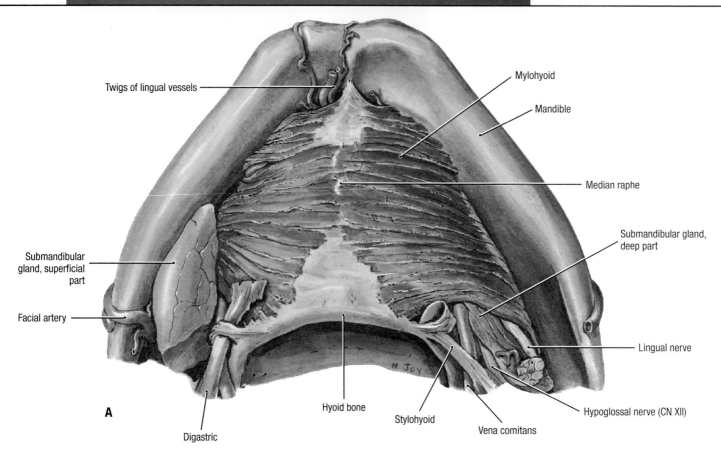

Twigs of lingual vessels

Mylohyoid

Mandible

Median raphe

Submandibular gland, deep part

Submandibular gland, superficial part

Facial artery

Lingual nerve

Digastric

Hyoid bone

Stylohyoid

Vena comitans

Hypoglossal nerve (CN XII)

A

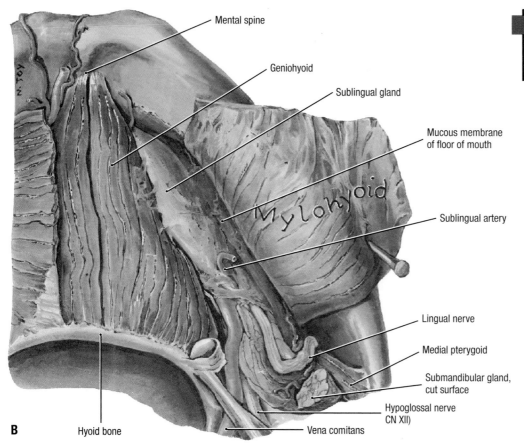

Mental spine

Geniohyoid

Sublingual gland

Mucous membrane of floor of mouth

Sublingual artery

Lingual nerve

Medial pterygoid

Submandibular gland, cut surface

Hypoglossal nerve CN XII)

Lingual nerve

Vena comitans

Hyoid bone

B

8.22 Floor of mouth, inferior views

A. Mylohyoid muscles. The anterior bellies of the digastric muscle have been removed. **B.** Geniohyoid muscles. The left mylohyoid muscle and part of the right are reflected.

OBSERVE IN **A**:
1. The right and left mylohyoid muscles, which together form the "oral diaphragm," attach to the mylohyoid line of the mandible, a median raphe, and the hyoid bone;
2. The submandibular gland arches around the posterior border of the mylohyoid muscle;
3. The hypoglossal nerve and its companion vein (vena comitans) pass deep to the posterior border of the mylohyoid; the lingual nerve is adjacent to the mandible.

OBSERVE IN **B**:
4. The geniohyoid muscle extends from the mental spine of the mandible to the body of the hyoid bone;
5. The hypoglossal nerve, deep part of the submandibular gland, and lingual nerve;
6. The areolar covering of the sublingual gland and, lateral to it, the mucous membrane of the mouth with twigs of the sublingual artery.

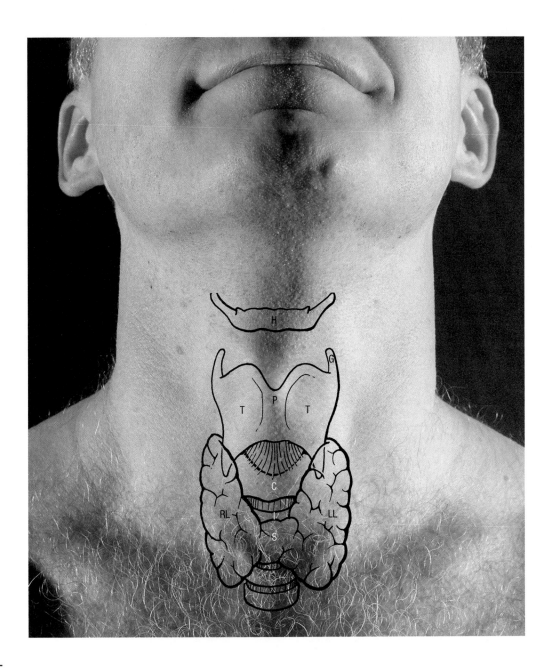

8.23   **Anterior neck—I, surface anatomy, anterior view**

OBSERVE:

1. The hyoid bone (*H*) lies at the angle between the floor of the mouth and anterior aspect of the neck;
2. The laminae of the thyroid cartilage (*T*) project anteriorly from their point of union to form the laryngeal prominence (*P*); the superior horn (*G*) is palpable;
3. The arch of the cricoid cartilage (*C*) projects further anteriorly than the rings of the trachea and lies at the level of C6;
4. The first tracheal ring (*I*);

5. The thyroid gland consists of right (*RL*) and left (*LL*) lobes and a connecting isthmus (*S*);
6. *A vertical, or transverse, incision through the neck and anterior wall of the trachea (tracheostomy) can be performed to establish an airway in patients with upper airway obstruction or respiratory failure. The infrahyoid muscles are retracted laterally, and the isthmus of the thyroid gland is divided or retracted superiorly. An opening is made in the trachea between the first and second tracheal rings or through the second to fourth rings. The tracheostomy tube is then inserted into the trachea.*

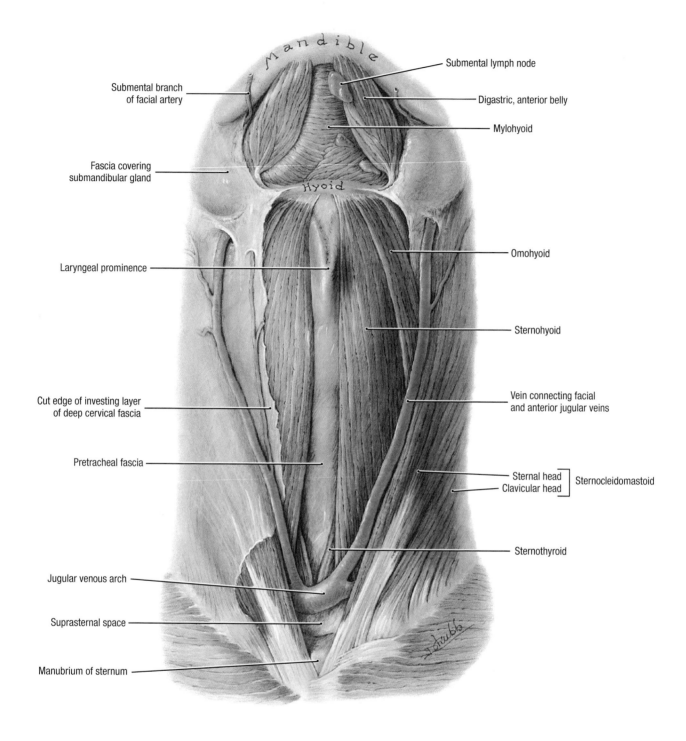

8.24 **Anterior neck—II, superficial dissection, anterior view**

OBSERVE:
1. The anterior bellies of the digastric muscles form the sides of the suprahyoid part, or submental triangle (floor of the mouth); the hyoid bone is its base, the mylohyoid muscles are its floor, and some submental lymph nodes are the contents;
2. The infrahyoid part, shaped like an elongated diamond, is bounded by the sternohyoid muscle superiorly and sternothyroid muscle inferiorly;
3. The suprasternal (fascial) space contains a cross-connecting vein, the jugular venous arch. In this specimen, the anterior jugular veins are absent in the median part of the neck, but present superior to the clavicles.

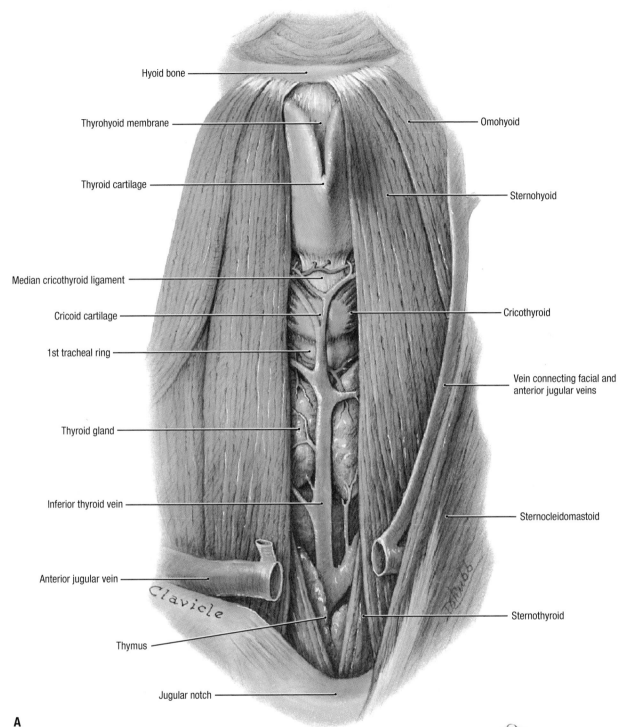

Hyoid bone

Thyrohyoid membrane

Thyroid cartilage

Median cricothyroid ligament

Cricoid cartilage

1st tracheal ring

Thyroid gland

Inferior thyroid vein

Anterior jugular vein

Clavicle

Thymus

Jugular notch

Omohyoid

Sternohyoid

Cricothyroid

Vein connecting facial and anterior jugular veins

Sternocleidomastoid

Sternothyroid

A

8.25   Anterior neck—III, intermediate dissection, anterior views

A. Superficial infrahyoid (strap) muscles. **B.** Connecting vein. The connecting vein that lies along the anterior border of the sternocleidomastoid muscle and connects the facial vein to the anterior jugular vein can vary in size; it can be as large as the internal jugular vein and is sometimes mistaken for it.

OBSERVE:
1. The enlarged thymus projects superiorly from the thorax;
2. The two superficial depressors of the larynx ("strap muscles") are the omohyoid (superior belly) and sternohyoid.

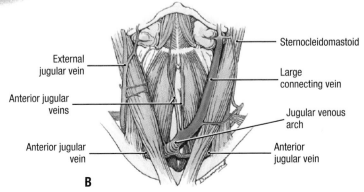

External jugular vein

Anterior jugular veins

Anterior jugular vein

Sternocleidomastoid

Large connecting vein

Jugular venous arch

Anterior jugular vein

B

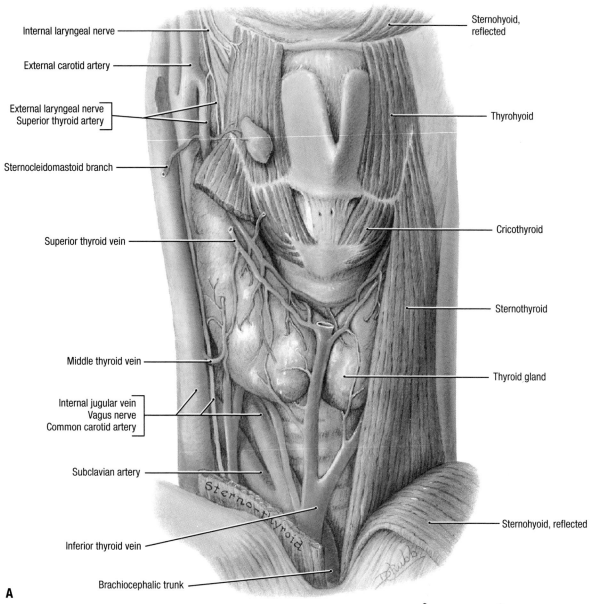

A

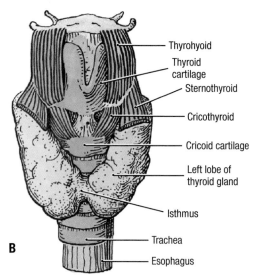

B

8.26   Anterior neck—IV, deep dissection, anterior views

A. Thyroid gland. On the left side of the specimen, the sternohyoid and omohyoid muscles are reflected, exposing the deep sternothyroid and the thyrohyoid muscles; on the right side of the specimen, the sternothyroid muscle is largely excised. **B.** Relations of thyroid gland and deep strap muscles.

OBSERVE:
1. The two lobes of the thyroid gland are united across the median plane by an isthmus;
2. The surface network of veins on the gland is drained by the superior, middle, and inferior thyroid veins;
3. The right lobe of the gland lies over the common carotid artery;
4. The superior thyroid artery and external laryngeal nerve;
5. An accessory thyroid gland, or detached lobule, is occasionally present.

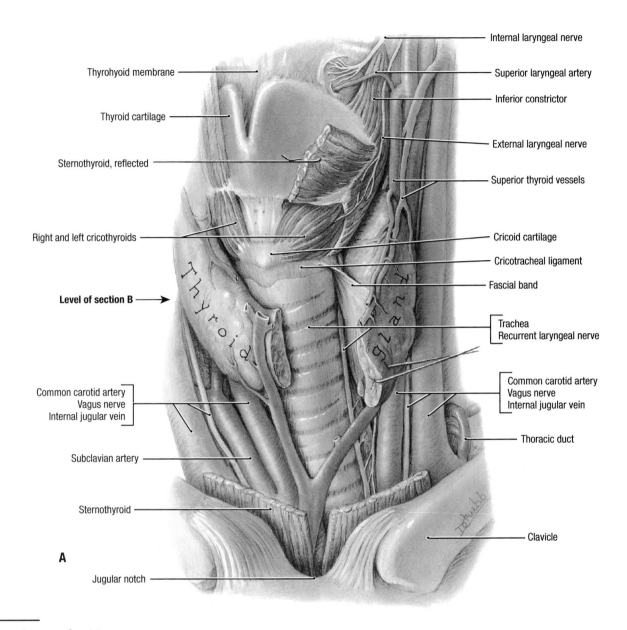

Internal laryngeal nerve

Thyrohyoid membrane

Superior laryngeal artery

Thyroid cartilage

Inferior constrictor

External laryngeal nerve

Sternothyroid, reflected

Superior thyroid vessels

Right and left cricothyroids

Cricoid cartilage

Cricotracheal ligament

Fascial band

Level of section B →

Trachea
Recurrent laryngeal nerve

Common carotid artery
Vagus nerve
Internal jugular vein

Common carotid artery
Vagus nerve
Internal jugular vein

Subclavian artery

Thoracic duct

Sternothyroid

Clavicle

A

Jugular notch

8.27   Anterior neck—V

A. Thyroid gland retracted, anterolateral view. The isthmus of the thyroid gland is divided, and the left lobe is retracted. **B.** Relations of thyroid gland, transverse section.

OBSERVE:
1. The retaining fascial band attaches the capsule of the thyroid gland to the cricotracheal ligament and cricoid cartilage;
2. The left recurrent laryngeal nerve ascends on the lateral aspect of the trachea, just anterior to the angle between the trachea and esophagus, and posterior to the fascial band;
3. The internal laryngeal nerve runs along the superior border of the inferior constrictor muscle and pierces the thyrohyoid membrane with several branches;
4. The external laryngeal nerve lies adjacent to the inferior constrictor muscle, runs along the anterior border of the superior thyroid

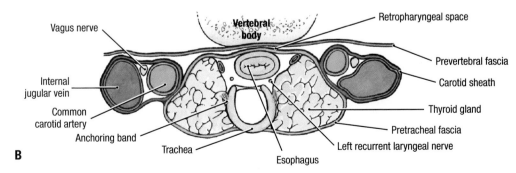

Vagus nerve

Retropharyngeal space

Vertebral body

Prevertebral fascia

Internal jugular vein

Carotid sheath

Common carotid artery

Thyroid gland

Anchoring band

Pretracheal fascia

Left recurrent laryngeal nerve

Trachea

Esophagus

B

artery, passes deep to the insertion of the sternothyroid muscle, and gives twigs to the inferior constrictor muscle, piercing it before ending in the cricothyroid muscle.

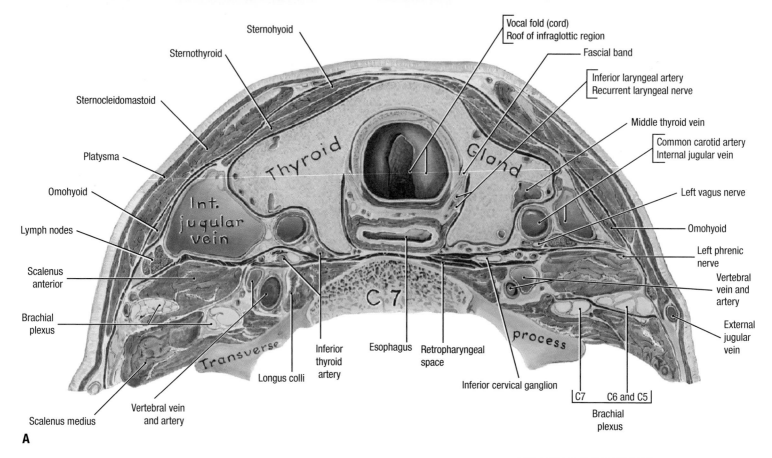

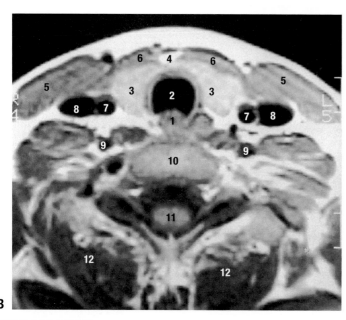

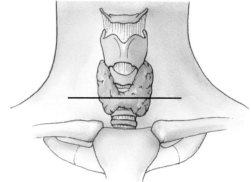

8.28 Transverse section of neck through thyroid gland

A. Illustration. **B.** MRI

OBSERVE:

1. The thyroid gland is asymmetrically enlarged within its sheath; it lies anterior to the carotid sheath and its contents; the internal jugular veins and vertebral arteries are asymmetric;

2. The vertebral artery and vein lie between the longus colli and scalenus anterior muscles;

3. The brachial plexus passes inferolaterally between the scalenus anterior and scalenus medius muscles;

4. The fascial band retains the thyroid gland and, posterior to it, the recurrent laryngeal nerve and inferior laryngeal artery; *1,* Esophagus; *2,* Trachea; *3,* Lobes of thyroid gland; *4,* Thyroid isthmus; *5,* Sternocleidomastoid; *6,* Strap muscles; *7,* Common carotid artery; *8,* Internal jugular vein; *9,* Vertebral artery; *10,* Vertebral body; *11,* Spinal cord in cerebrospinal fluid; *12,* Deep muscles of back; *13,* Retropharyngeal space.

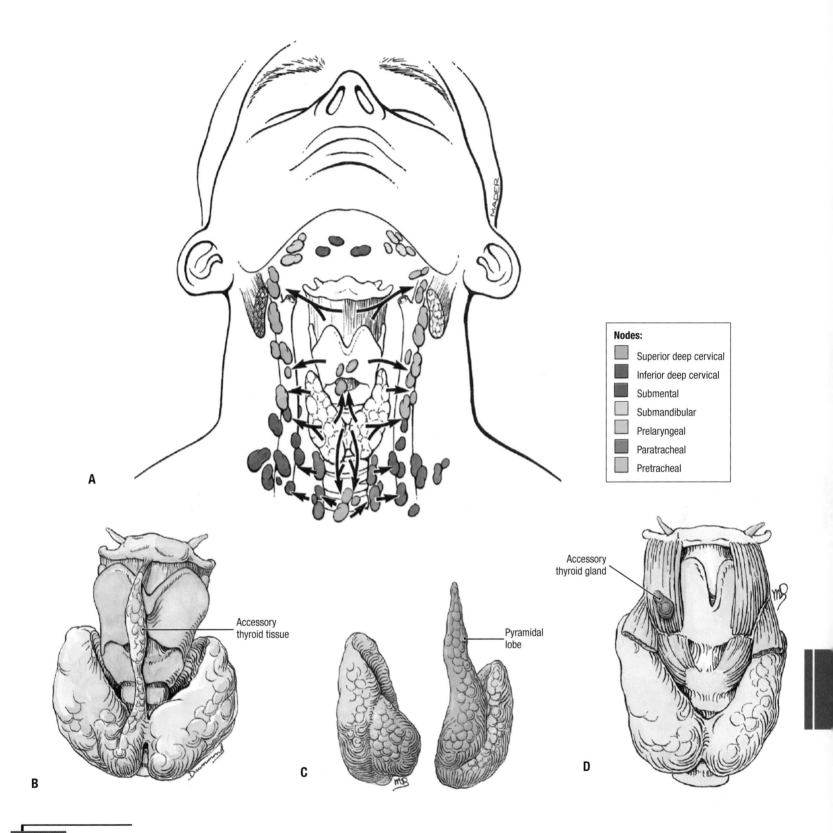

Nodes:
- Superior deep cervical
- Inferior deep cervical
- Submental
- Submandibular
- Prelaryngeal
- Paratracheal
- Pretracheal

Accessory thyroid tissue

Pyramidal lobe

Accessory thyroid gland

| 8.29 | **Thyroid gland and variations** |

A. Lymphatic drainage of the thyroid gland, larynx, and trachea. **B.** Accessory thyroid tissue. This can occur along the course of the thyroglossal duct. **C.** Pyramidal lobe, or absence of isthmus. Approximately 50% of glands have a pyramidal lobe that extends from near the isthmus to or toward the hyoid bone; the isthmus is occasionally absent, in which case the gland is in two parts. **D.** Accessory thyroid gland. This can occur between the suprahyoid region and arch of the aorta.

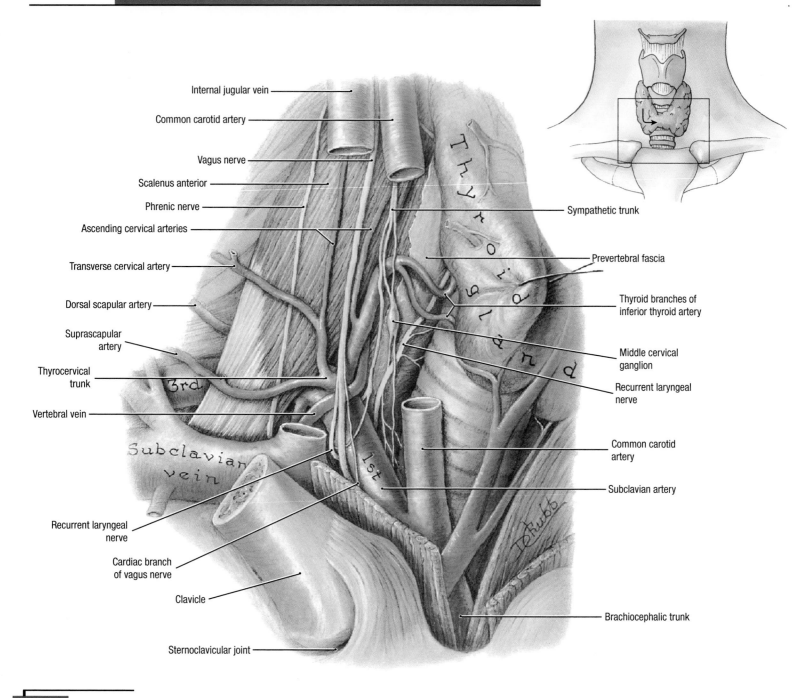

Internal jugular vein

Common carotid artery

Vagus nerve

Scalenus anterior

Phrenic nerve

Ascending cervical arteries

Transverse cervical artery

Dorsal scapular artery

Suprascapular artery

Thyrocervical trunk

Vertebral vein

Recurrent laryngeal nerve

Cardiac branch of vagus nerve

Clavicle

Sternoclavicular joint

Sympathetic trunk

Prevertebral fascia

Thyroid branches of inferior thyroid artery

Middle cervical ganglion

Recurrent laryngeal nerve

Common carotid artery

Subclavian artery

Brachiocephalic trunk

8.30　**Root of neck, right side of specimen, anterolateral view**

The clavicle is removed, sections are taken from the common carotid artery and internal jugular vein, and the right lobe of the thyroid gland is retracted.

OBSERVE:

1. The brachiocephalic trunk divides posterior to the sternoclavicular joint into the right common carotid and right subclavian arteries;
2. The scalenus anterior muscle divides the subclavian artery into three parts and separates the second part from the subclavian vein; this vein lies anteroinferior to the artery and joins the internal jugular vein at the medial border of the scalenus anterior muscle to form the brachiocephalic vein;
3. Running vertically on the oblique scalenus anterior muscle are: a) the common carotid artery, internal jugular vein, and vagus nerve (inside the carotid sheath); b) sympathetic trunk posterior to the common carotid artery (outside the sheath); c) ascending cervical artery (here represented by two vessels); and d) most lateral, the phrenic nerve;
4. The right vagus nerve crosses the first part of the subclavian artery and gives off an inferior cardiac branch and the right recurrent laryngeal nerve; the latter recurs inferior to the subclavian artery, passing posterior to the common carotid artery on its way to the lateral aspect of the trachea, giving twigs to the trachea and esophagus, and receiving twigs from the sympathetic trunk;
5. The middle cervical (sympathetic) ganglion;
6. The thyrocervical trunk divides into the inferior thyroid, transverse cervical, and suprascapular arteries;
7. The dorsal scapular branch of the transverse cervical artery branches from the second or third part of the subclavian artery; the vertebral vein crosses the first part of the artery.

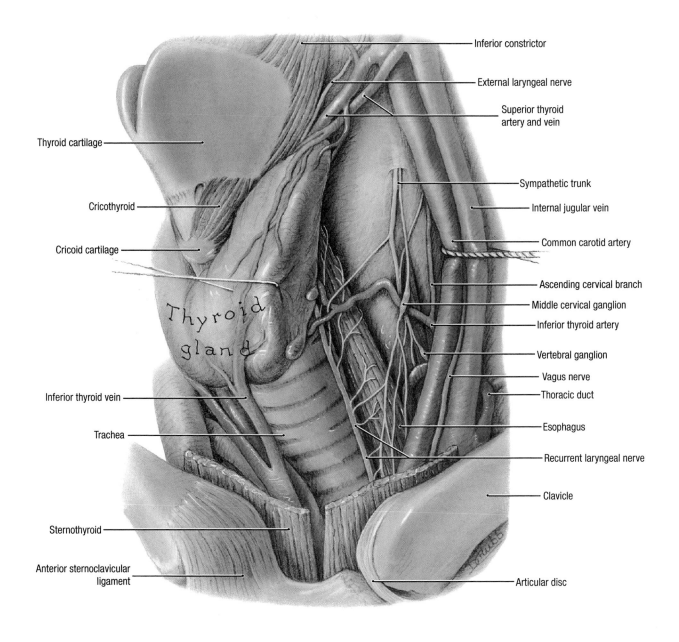

Inferior constrictor

External laryngeal nerve

Superior thyroid artery and vein

Thyroid cartilage

Sympathetic trunk

Cricothyroid

Internal jugular vein

Cricoid cartilage

Common carotid artery

Thyroid gland

Ascending cervical branch

Middle cervical ganglion

Inferior thyroid artery

Vertebral ganglion

Vagus nerve

Inferior thyroid vein

Thoracic duct

Trachea

Esophagus

Recurrent laryngeal nerve

Clavicle

Sternothyroid

Anterior sternoclavicular ligament

Articular disc

8.31   **Root of neck, left side of specimen, anterolateral view**

OBSERVE:

1. The three structures contained in the carotid sheath (internal jugular vein, common carotid artery, and vagus nerve) are retracted;
2. The esophagus bulges to the left of the trachea;
3. The left recurrent laryngeal nerve ascends on the lateral aspect of the trachea, just anterior to the angle between the trachea and esophagus, giving twigs to the esophagus and trachea, and receiving twigs from the sympathetic trunk. *The recurrent laryngeal nerves are vulnerable to injury during thyroidectomy and other surgeries in the anterior triangles of the neck. Because the inferior laryngeal nerve innervates the muscles moving the vocal folds, paralysis of the vocal folds results when this nerve is injured;*
4. The thoracic duct passes from the lateral aspect of the esophagus to its termination by arching immediately posterior to the three structures contained in the carotid sheath;

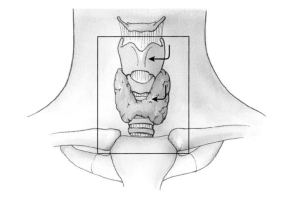

5. The middle cervical (sympathetic) ganglion in this specimen is in two parts: one is anterior to the inferior thyroid artery, and the other, the vertebral ganglion, is just superior to the thoracic duct.

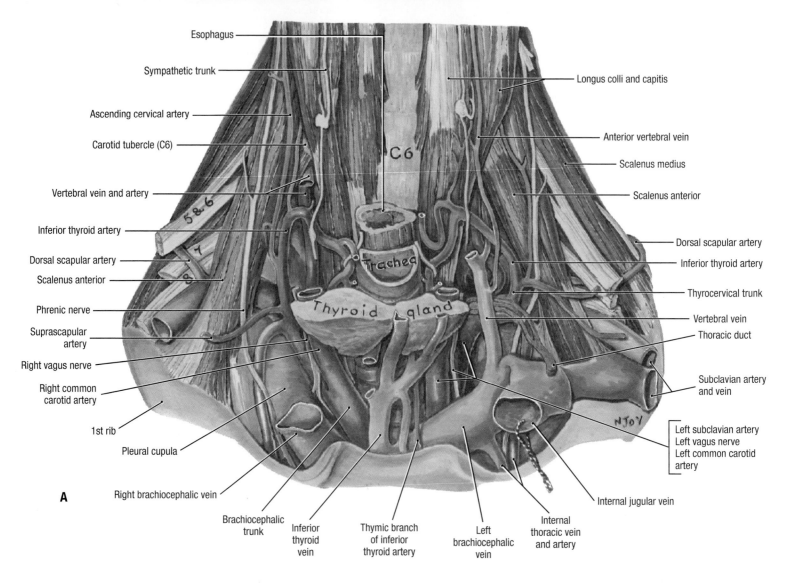

Esophagus
Sympathetic trunk
Ascending cervical artery
Carotid tubercle (C6)
Vertebral vein and artery
Inferior thyroid artery
Dorsal scapular artery
Scalenus anterior
Phrenic nerve
Suprascapular artery
Right vagus nerve
Right common carotid artery
1st rib
Pleural cupula
Right brachiocephalic vein

Longus colli and capitis
Anterior vertebral vein
Scalenus medius
Scalenus anterior
Dorsal scapular artery
Inferior thyroid artery
Thyrocervical trunk
Vertebral vein
Thoracic duct
Subclavian artery and vein
Left subclavian artery
Left vagus nerve
Left common carotid artery
Internal jugular vein

C6
Trachea
Thyroid gland
NJoY

A

Brachiocephalic trunk
Inferior thyroid vein
Thymic branch of inferior thyroid artery
Left brachiocephalic vein
Internal thoracic vein and artery

8.32   Root of neck, anterior views

A. Dissection. **B.** Termination of thoracic duct. The thoracic duct arches laterally in the neck to pass posterior to the carotid sheath and anterior to the vertebral and subclavian arteries, entering the left brachiocephalic vein at the junction of the subclavian and internal jugular veins.

OBSERVE:
1. Laterally, the pleural cupola rises superior to the sternal end of the 1st rib. The subclavian artery arches over the pleura; the third part of the artery and the brachial plexus appear between the scalenus anterior and scalenus medius muscles;
2. The phrenic nerve descends almost vertically to cross the scalenus anterior muscle, lies on the pleura, and crosses anterior to the internal thoracic artery;
3. In the median plane, the esophagus is anterior to the vertebral column, the trachea is anterior to the esophagus, and the thyroid gland is anterior to the trachea;
4. Lateral to these median structures, the carotid sheath surrounds the artery, vein, and nerve. The vagus nerves descend on the lateral side of the common carotid artery. The inferior thyroid artery arches medially to reach the thyroid gland as two branches, a su-

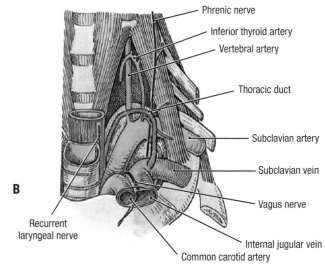

Phrenic nerve
Inferior thyroid artery
Vertebral artery
Thoracic duct
Subclavian artery
Subclavian vein
Vagus nerve
Internal jugular vein
Common carotid artery
Recurrent laryngeal nerve

B

perior and inferior; the recurrent laryngeal nerve bears a varying relationship to these arteries;
5. The thoracic duct is pulled inferiorly by the reflected internal jugular vein.

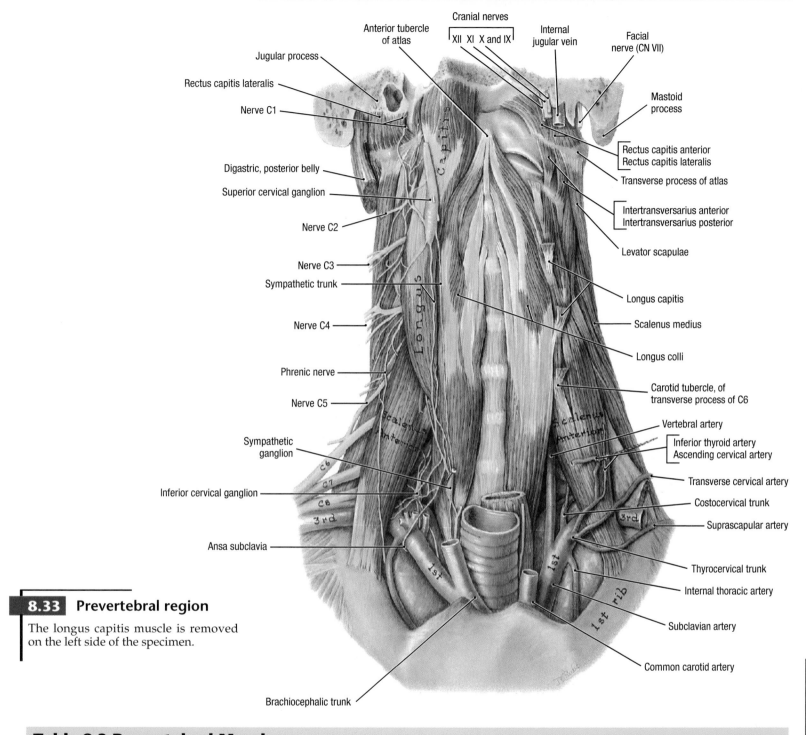

8.33 Prevertebral region

The longus capitis muscle is removed on the left side of the specimen.

Table 8.3 Prevertebral Muscles

Muscle	Superior Attachment	Inferior Attachment	Innervation	Main Actions
Longus colli	Anterior tubercle of C1 vertebra (axis)	Body of T3 vertebra with attachments to bodies of C1–C3 and transverse processes of C3–C6 vertebrae	Ventral rami of C2–C6 spinal nerves	Flexes neck
Longus capitis	Basilar part of occipital bone	Anterior tubercles of C3–C6 transverse processes	Ventral rami of C2 and C3 spinal nerves	Flexes head
Rectus capitis anterior	Base of skull, just anterior to occipital condyle	Anterior surface of lateral mass of C1 vertebra (atlas)	Branches from loop between C1 and C2 spinal nerves	Flexes head
Rectus capitis lateralis	Jugular process of occipital bone	Transverse process of C1 vertebra (atlas)		Flexes head and helps to stabilize the head

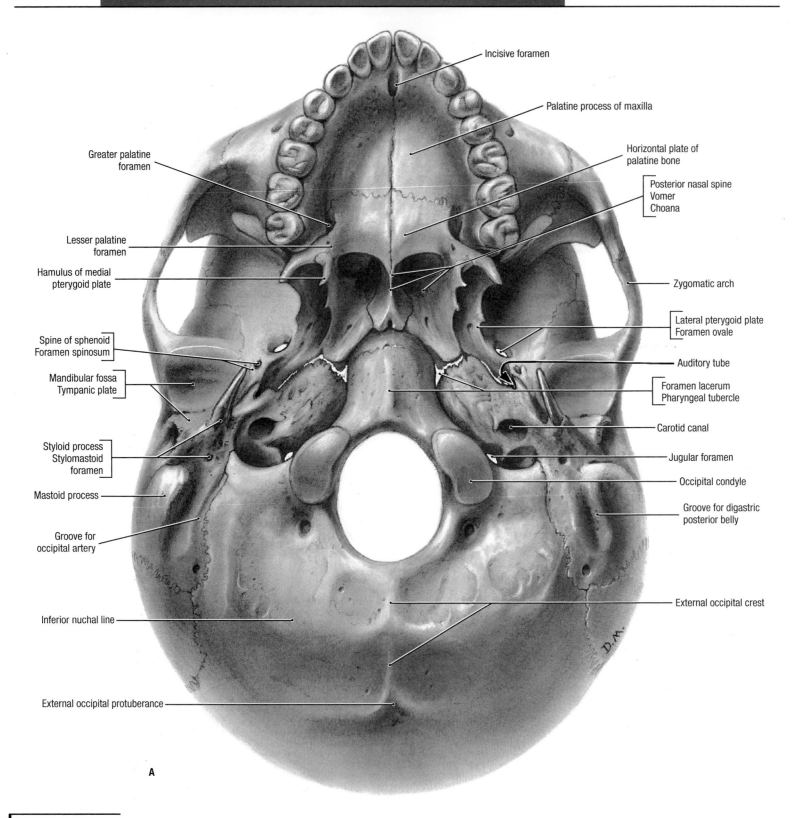

Incisive foramen

Palatine process of maxilla

Greater palatine foramen

Horizontal plate of palatine bone

Posterior nasal spine
Vomer
Choana

Lesser palatine foramen

Hamulus of medial pterygoid plate

Zygomatic arch

Lateral pterygoid plate
Foramen ovale

Spine of sphenoid
Foramen spinosum

Auditory tube

Mandibular fossa
Tympanic plate

Foramen lacerum
Pharyngeal tubercle

Carotid canal

Styloid process
Stylomastoid foramen

Jugular foramen

Occipital condyle

Mastoid process

Groove for digastric posterior belly

Groove for occipital artery

External occipital crest

Inferior nuchal line

External occipital protuberance

A

8.34 Base of skull, inferior views

A. Features. **B.** Bones.

OBSERVE:
1. The foramen ovale is at the root of the lateral pterygoid plate;
2. The foramen lacerum is at the root of the medial pterygoid plate;
3. A small foramen, not clearly seen between the carotid canal and

jugular foramen, transmits the tympanic branch of the glossopharyngeal nerve (CN IX);
4. The spine of the sphenoid is for attachment of the sphenomandibular ligament, the hamulus of the medial pterygoid plate is for the pterygomandibular ligament, and the styloid process is for the stylomandibular and stylohyoid ligaments.

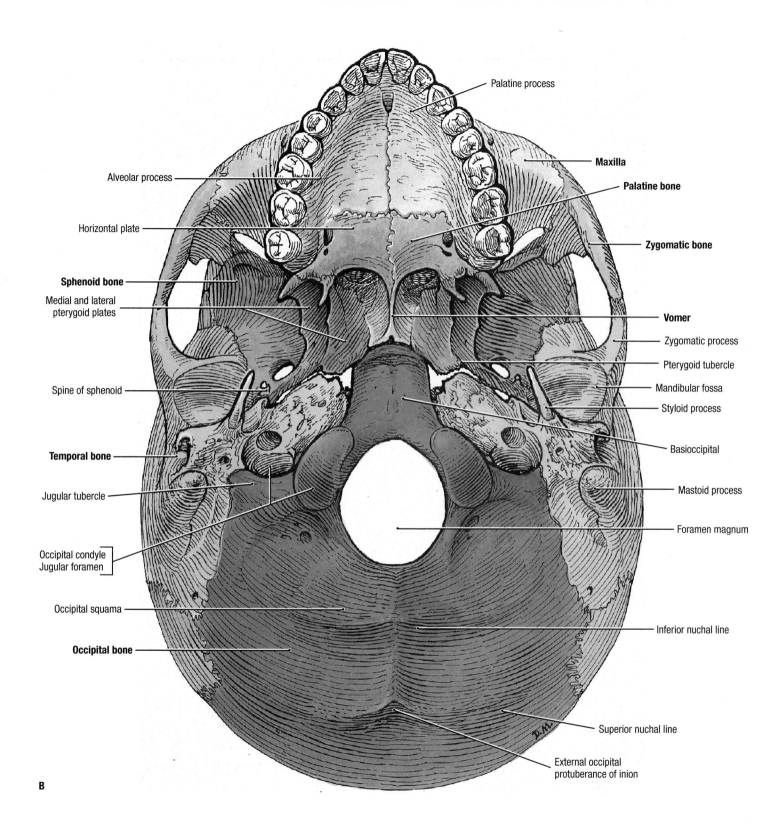

Palatine process

Maxilla

Alveolar process

Palatine bone

Horizontal plate

Zygomatic bone

Sphenoid bone

Medial and lateral
pterygoid plates

Vomer

Zygomatic process

Pterygoid tubercle

Spine of sphenoid

Mandibular fossa

Styloid process

Basioccipital

Temporal bone

Mastoid process

Jugular tubercle

Foramen magnum

Occipital condyle
Jugular foramen

Occipital squama

Inferior nuchal line

Occipital bone

Superior nuchal line

External occipital
protuberance of inion

B

5. *A blow delivered to the side of the mandible does not drive the mandible under the cranium because the head of the mandible would have to descend the steep, medial wall of the mandibular fossa and the spine of the sphenoid.*

6. The spine of the sphenoid "guards" four strategic points: a) anteri-orly, the foramen spinosum for the middle meningeal artery; b) posteriorly, the entrance to the carotid canal; c) medially, the entrance to the bony auditory tube; and d) laterally, the mandibular fossa for the head of the mandible.

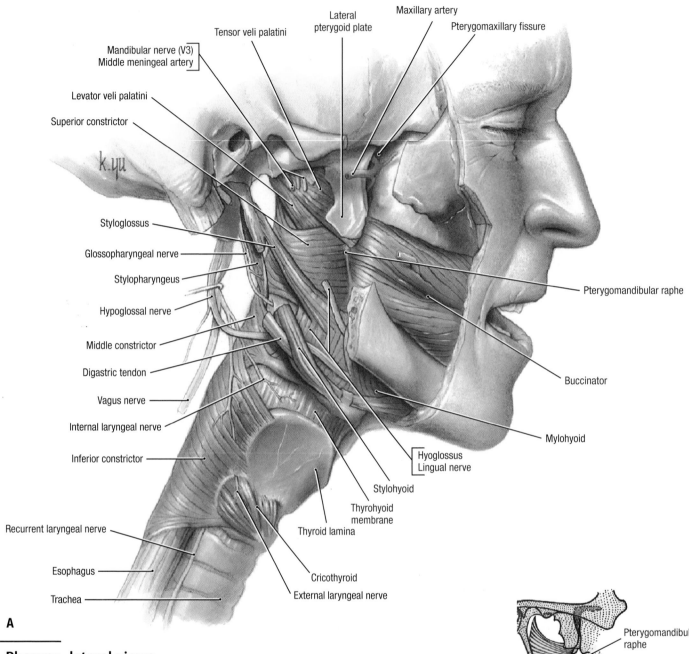

Lateral pterygoid plate

Maxillary artery

Pterygomaxillary fissure

Tensor veli palatini

Mandibular nerve (V3)
Middle meningeal artery

Levator veli palatini

Superior constrictor

k.yu

Styloglossus

Glossopharyngeal nerve

Stylopharyngeus

Hypoglossal nerve

Middle constrictor

Digastric tendon

Vagus nerve

Internal laryngeal nerve

Inferior constrictor

Recurrent laryngeal nerve

Esophagus

Trachea

Pterygomandibular raphe

Buccinator

Mylohyoid

Hyoglossus
Lingual nerve

Stylohyoid

Thyrohyoid membrane

Thyroid lamina

Cricothyroid

External laryngeal nerve

A

8.35 Pharynx, lateral views

A. Dissection. **B.** Constrictor muscles. **C.** Schematic illustration.

OBSERVE:

1. The wall of the pharynx is composed of two layers of muscles: an external, circular layer formed by the three constrictor muscles, and a deeper, longitudinal layer formed by the palatopharyngeus, stylopharyngeus, and salpingopharyngeus muscles;
2. The inferior constrictor muscle overlaps the middle constrictor, and the middle constrictor overlaps the superior constrictor;
3. There are four gaps in the pharyngeal musculature that allow for the entry of structures: a) superior to the superior constrictor muscle for the levator veli palatini muscle and auditory tube; b) between the superior and middle constrictors for the stylopharyngeus muscle, CN IX, and the stylohyoid ligament; c) between the middle and inferior constrictors for the internal laryngeal nerve and superior laryngeal artery and nerve; and d) inferior to the inferior constrictor muscle for the recurrent laryngeal nerve.

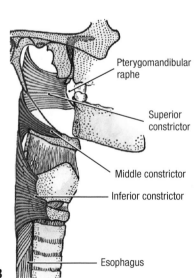

Pterygomandibular raphe

Superior constrictor

Middle constrictor

Inferior constrictor

Esophagus

B

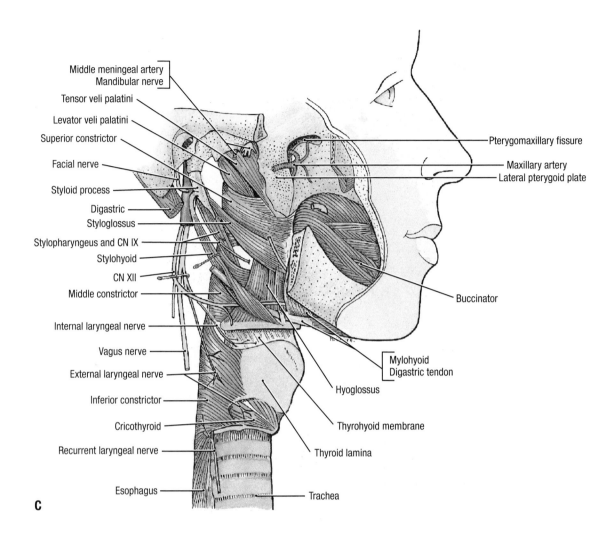

Middle meningeal artery
Mandibular nerve
Tensor veli palatini
Levator veli palatini
Superior constrictor
Facial nerve
Styloid process
Digastric
Styloglossus
Stylopharyngeus and CN IX
Stylohyoid
CN XII
Middle constrictor
Internal laryngeal nerve
Vagus nerve
External laryngeal nerve
Inferior constrictor
Cricothyroid
Recurrent laryngeal nerve
Esophagus

Pterygomaxillary fissure
Maxillary artery
Lateral pterygoid plate
Buccinator
Mylohyoid
Digastric tendon
Hyoglossus
Thyrohyoid membrane
Thyroid lamina
Trachea

C

Table 8.4 Muscles of Pharynx

Muscle	Origin	Insertion	Innervation	Main Action(s)
Superior constrictor	Pterygoid hamulus, pterygomandibular raphe, posterior end of mylohyoid line of mandible, and side of tongue	Median raphe of pharynx and pharyngeal tubercle	Pharyngeal and superior laryngeal branches of vagus (CN X) through pharyngeal plexus	Constrict wall of pharynx during swallowing
Middle constrictor	Stylohyoid ligament and superior (greater) and inferior (lesser) horns of hyoid bone	Median raphe of pharynx		
Inferior constrictor	Oblique line of thyroid cartilage and side of cricoid cartilage			
Palatopharyngeus	Hard plate and palatine aponeurosis	Posterior border of lamina of thyroid cartilage and side of pharynx and esophagus	Glossopharyngeal nerve (CN IX)	Elevate pharynx and larynx during swallowing and speaking
Salpingopharyngeus	Cartilaginous part of auditory tube	Blends with palatopharyngeus		
Stylopharyngeus	Styloid process of temporal bone	Posterior and superior borders of thyroid cartilage with palatopharyngeus		

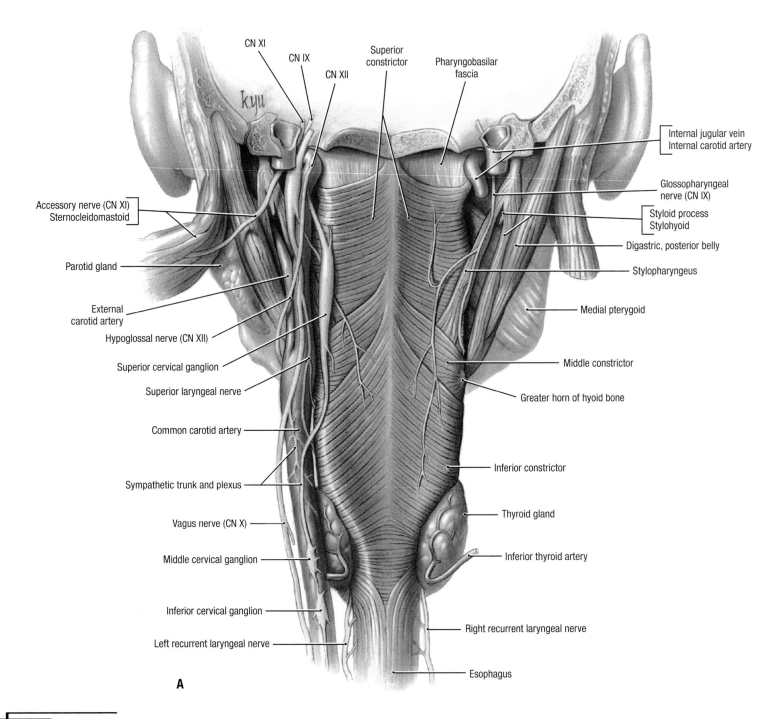

A

8.36   Pharynx, exterior, posterior views

A. Dissection. **B.** Schematic illustration.

OBSERVE IN **A:**

1. The three pharyngeal constrictor muscles overlap one another; the posterior aspect is flat, and even slightly concave;
2. On the right side of the specimen, the stylopharyngeus muscle passes from the medial side of the styloid process anteromedially to the interval between the superior and middle constrictor muscles. The stylohyoid muscle passes from the lateral side anterolaterally

and is split on its way to the hyoid bone by the digastric. The glossopharyngeal nerve spirals around the stylopharyngeus muscle, and both enter the pharyngeal wall;

3. On the left side of the specimen, note cranial nerves IX, X, XI, and XII; the sympathetic trunk and the superior, middle, and inferior sympathetic ganglia; and the common carotid artery, which branches into the internal and external carotid arteries.

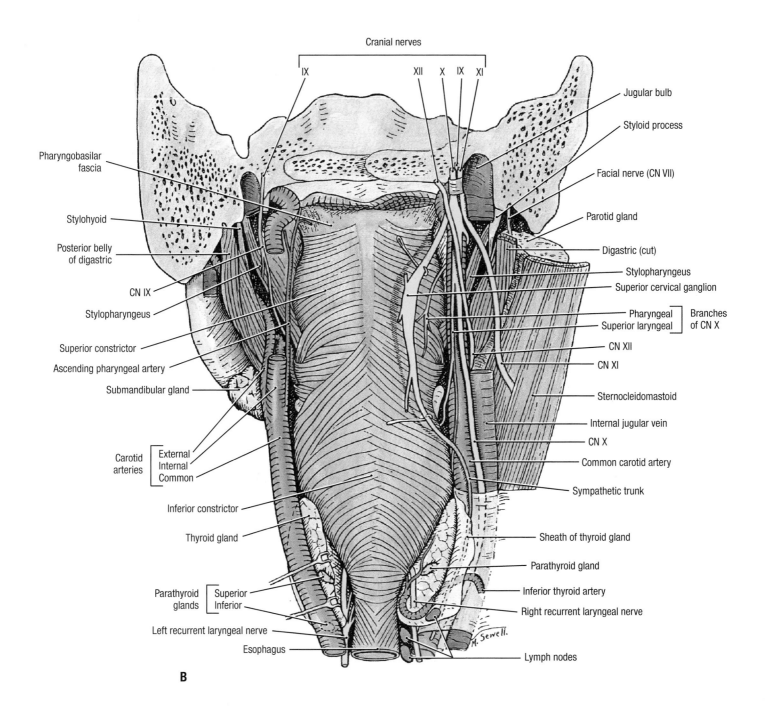

Cranial nerves

IX   XII   X IX XI

Pharyngobasilar fascia

Stylohyoid

Posterior belly of digastric

CN IX

Stylopharyngeus

Superior constrictor

Ascending pharyngeal artery

Submandibular gland

Carotid arteries — External / Internal / Common

Inferior constrictor

Thyroid gland

Parathyroid glands — Superior / Inferior

Left recurrent laryngeal nerve

Esophagus

B

Jugular bulb

Styloid process

Facial nerve (CN VII)

Parotid gland

Digastric (cut)

Stylopharyngeus

Superior cervical ganglion

Pharyngeal / Superior laryngeal — Branches of CN X

CN XII

CN XI

Sternocleidomastoid

Internal jugular vein

CN X

Common carotid artery

Sympathetic trunk

Sheath of thyroid gland

Parathyroid gland

Inferior thyroid artery

Right recurrent laryngeal nerve

Lymph nodes

M. Sewell.

OBSERVE IN **B**:

4. The narrowest and least distensible part of the digestive tract is where the pharynx becomes the esophagus;

5. Between the superior constrictor muscle and the base of the skull, the pharyngobasilar fascia attaches the pharynx to the occipital bone;

6. The nerves and vein that emerge from the foramina are: the facial nerve (stylomastoid foramen), internal jugular vein, and last four cranial nerves (jugular foramen and hypoglossal canal); of the four nerves, IX lies anterior to X and XI, and XII is the most medial;

7. Lying posterior to the internal carotid artery are the sympathetic trunk and the elongated superior cervical ganglion, whose fibers (the internal carotid nerve,) accompany the internal carotid artery into the skull.

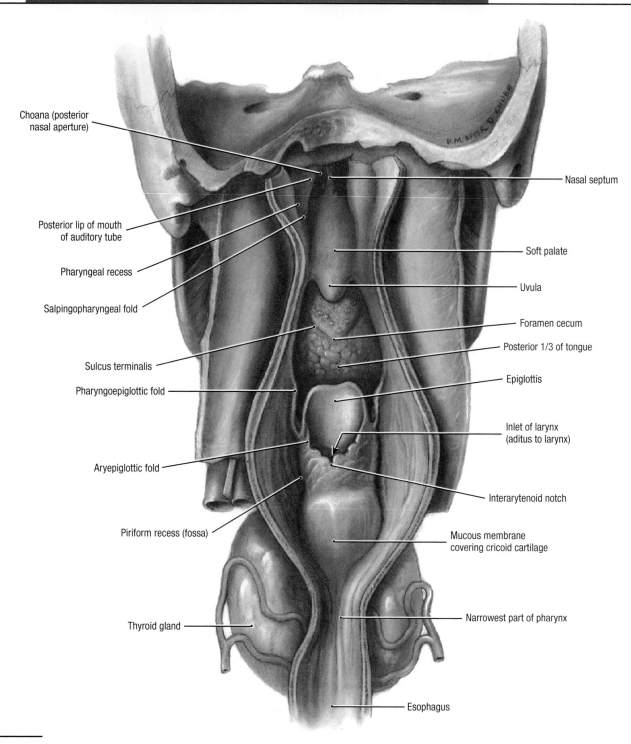

Choana (posterior nasal aperture)

Posterior lip of mouth of auditory tube

Pharyngeal recess

Salpingopharyngeal fold

Sulcus terminalis

Pharyngoepiglottic fold

Aryepiglottic fold

Piriform recess (fossa)

Thyroid gland

Nasal septum

Soft palate

Uvula

Foramen cecum

Posterior 1/3 of tongue

Epiglottis

Inlet of larynx (aditus to larynx)

Interarytenoid notch

Mucous membrane covering cricoid cartilage

Narrowest part of pharynx

Esophagus

8.37   Interior of pharynx—I, posterior view

OBSERVE:

1. The pharynx extends from the base of the skull to the inferior border of the cricoid cartilage, where it narrows to become the esophagus;
2. The soft palate ends posteroinferiorly in the uvula;
3. The larynx extends superiorly to the tip of the epiglottis;
4. The three parts of the pharynx: nasal, oral, and laryngeal;
5. The nasal part (nasopharynx) lies superior to the level of the soft palate and is continuous anteriorly, through the choanae, with the nasal cavities;
6. The oral part (oropharynx) lies between the levels of the soft palate

and larynx, communicates anteriorly with the oral cavity, and has the posterior one third of the tongue as its anterior wall;

7. The posterior one third of the tongue is studded with lymph follicles (collectively called the lingual tonsil) and demarcated from the anterior two thirds by the foramen cecum and V-shaped sulcus terminalis;
8. The laryngeal part (laryngopharynx) lies posterior to the larynx and communicates with the cavity of the larynx through the aditus; on each side of the inlet, separated from it by the aryepiglottic fold, is a piriform recess.

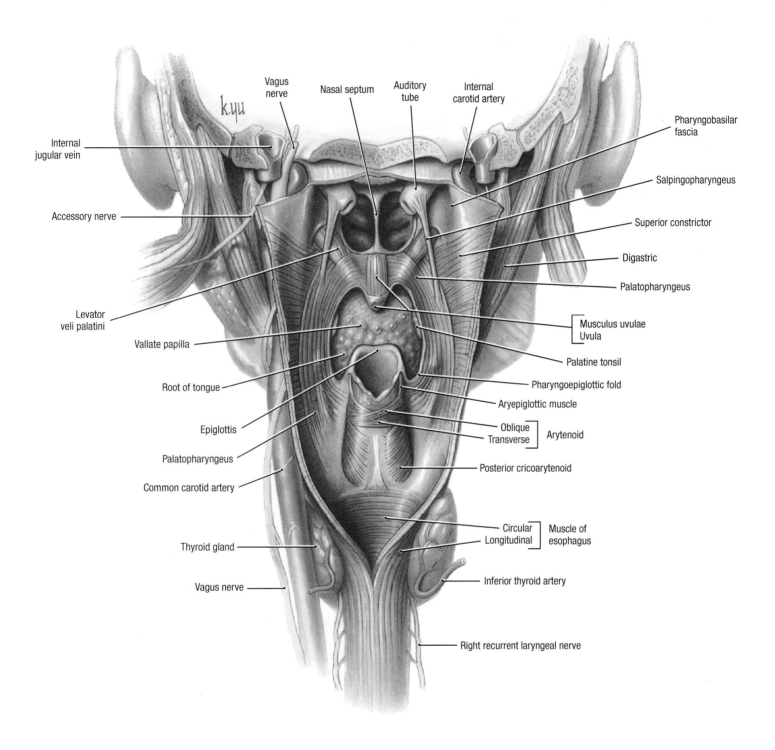

8.38 **Interior of pharynx—II, posterior view**

The posterior wall of the pharynx has been cut in the midline and reflected laterally to reveal the interior of the pharynx and the nasal, oral, and laryngeal orifices. The mucous membrane was removed to expose the underlying musculature.

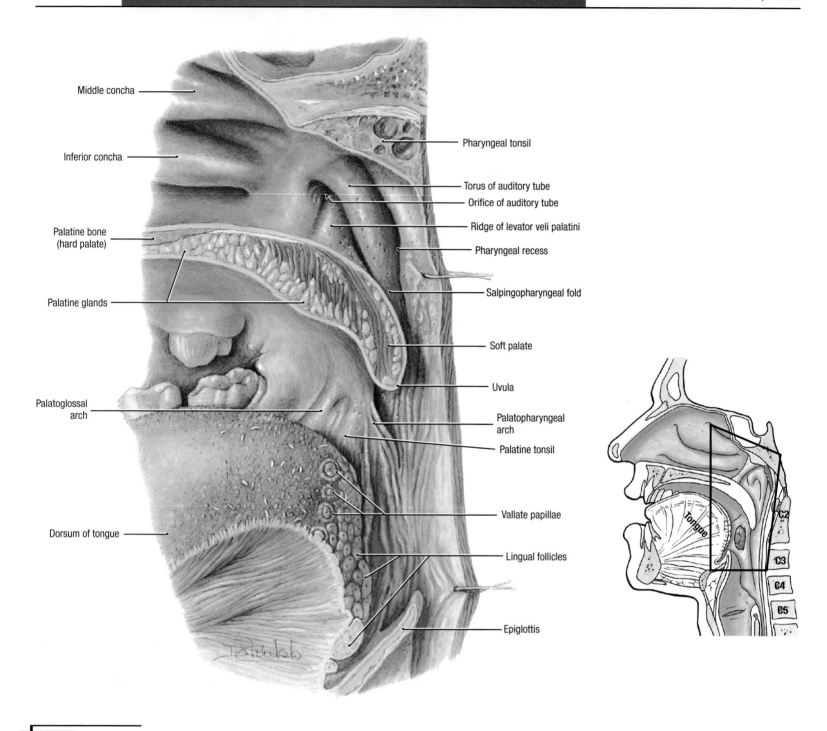

Middle concha

Inferior concha

Palatine bone
(hard palate)

Palatine glands

Palatoglossal
arch

Dorsum of tongue

Pharyngeal tonsil

Torus of auditory tube

Orifice of auditory tube

Ridge of levator veli palatini

Pharyngeal recess

Salpingopharyngeal fold

Soft palate

Uvula

Palatopharyngeal
arch

Palatine tonsil

Vallate papillae

Lingual follicles

Epiglottis

8.39   Interior of pharynx—I, median section

OBSERVE:
1. The prominent torus of the auditory tube and the salpingopha-ryngeal fold, which descends from the torus;
2. The orifice of the auditory tube is located approximately 1 cm pos-terior to the inferior concha;
3. The ridge produced by the levator veli palatini muscle;
4. The deep pharyngeal recess posterior to the torus of the auditory tube;
5. The numerous pinpoint orifices of the ducts of the mucous glands about the torus;
6. The pharyngeal tonsil in the mucous membrane of the roof and posterior wall of the nasopharynx;

7. The considerable proportion of glandular tissue, the palatine glands, in the soft palate;
8. The palatoglossal and palatopharyngeal arches, which, in this specimen, are not the sharp folds commonly seen; the palatine ton-sil lies between them;
9. Each lingual follicle has the duct of a mucous gland opening on to its surface; collectively, the follicles are known as the lingual tonsil;
10. The sensory supply of the pharynx (not shown): the pharyngeal branch of the maxillary nerve to the roof, lesser palatine nerves to the anterior parts of the soft palate, and internal laryngeal nerve to the inferior part of the pharynx and to the surroundings of the la-ryngeal orifice.

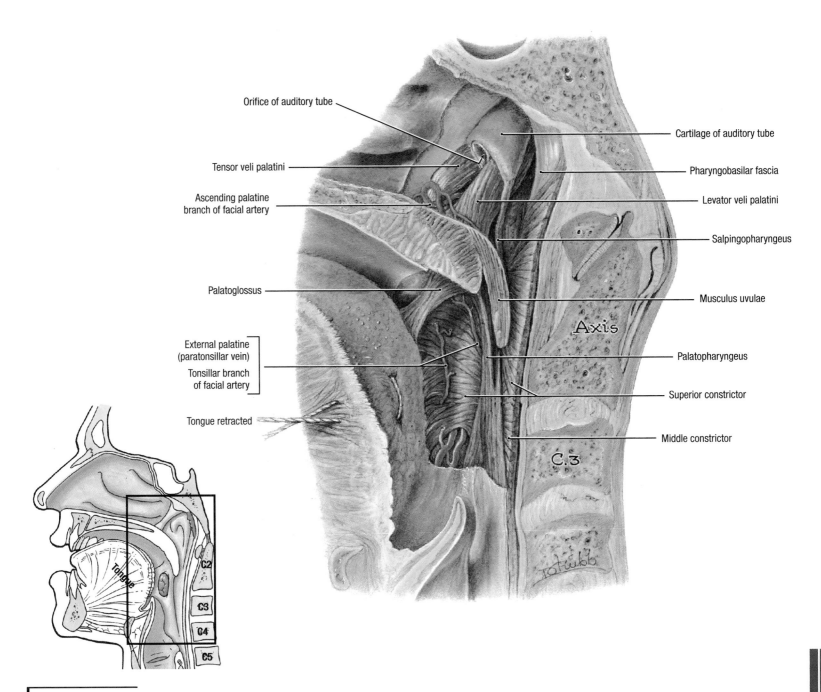

Orifice of auditory tube

Tensor veli palatini

Ascending palatine branch of facial artery

Palatoglossus

External palatine (paratonsillar vein)

Tonsillar branch of facial artery

Tongue retracted

Cartilage of auditory tube

Pharyngobasilar fascia

Levator veli palatini

Salpingopharyngeus

Musculus uvulae

Axis

Palatopharyngeus

Superior constrictor

C.3

Middle constrictor

Tongue

C2

C3

C4

C5

8.40   Interior of pharynx—II, median section

The palatine and pharyngeal tonsils and mucous membrane have been removed. The submucous pharyngobasilar fascia, which attaches the pharynx to the basilar part of the occipital bone, is thick superiorly and thin posteriorly. It was also removed, except at the superior, arched border of the superior constrictor.

OBSERVE:

1. The curved cartilage of the auditory tube, and the pharyngeal orifice of the tube;
2. The salpingopharyngeus muscle descends from the posterior lip to join the palatopharyngeus muscle;
3. The ascending palatine branch of the facial artery descends with the levator veli palatini muscle to the soft palate;
4. The five paired muscles of the palate: tensor veli palatini; levator

veli palatini, which provides most of the muscle fibers in the sectioned soft palate; uvular muscle (musculus uvulae), a finger-like bundle that arises mostly from the palatine aponeurosis at the posterior nasal spine; palatoglossus, in this specimen a substantial band, but commonly a thin muscle with free anterior and posterior borders; and palatopharyngeus;

5. A thin sheet of pharyngobasilar fascia has been removed from the tonsil bed, exposing the palatopharyngeus and superior constrictor muscles. The bed of the palatine tonsil extends far into the soft palate;
6. The tonsillar branch of the facial artery is long and large. The paratonsillar vein, descending from the soft palate to join the pharyngeal plexus of veins, is a close lateral relation of the tonsil.

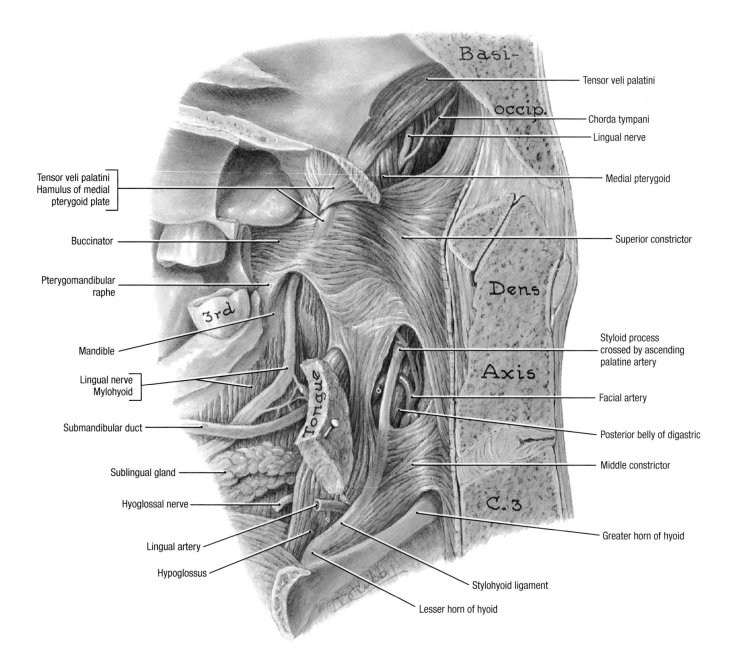

Basi-
occip.
Dens
Axis
C.3
3rd
Tongue

Tensor veli palatini
Chorda tympani
Lingual nerve
Medial pterygoid
Superior constrictor
Styloid process crossed by ascending palatine artery
Facial artery
Posterior belly of digastric
Middle constrictor
Greater horn of hyoid
Stylohyoid ligament
Lesser horn of hyoid

Tensor veli palatini
Hamulus of medial pterygoid plate
Buccinator
Pterygomandibular raphe
Mandible
Lingual nerve
Mylohyoid
Submandibular duct
Sublingual gland
Hyoglossal nerve
Lingual artery
Hypoglossus

8.41   Interior of pharynx—III, median section

OBSERVE:

1. The superior constrictor muscle arises from: a) the pterygo-mandibular raphe, which unites it to the buccinator muscle; b) the bones at each end of the raphe (the hamulus of the medial ptery-goid plate superiorly and the mandible inferiorly); and c) the root (posterior part) of the tongue;
2. The arched superior and inferior borders of the superior constrictor muscle extend to the median plane, where the muscle meets the superior constrictor of the opposite side;
3. The middle constrictor muscle arises from the angle formed by the

greater and lesser horns of the hyoid bone and from the stylohyoid ligament; in this specimen, the styloid process is long and, there-fore, a lateral relation of the tonsil;
4. The facial artery arches superior to the posterior belly of the digas-tric muscle, and the lingual artery arches just inferior to it;
5. The tendon of the tensor veli palatini muscle hooks around the hamulus;
6. The lingual nerve is joined by the chorda tympani, disappears at the posterior border of the medial pterygoid muscle, reappears at the anterior border, and then follows the mandible.

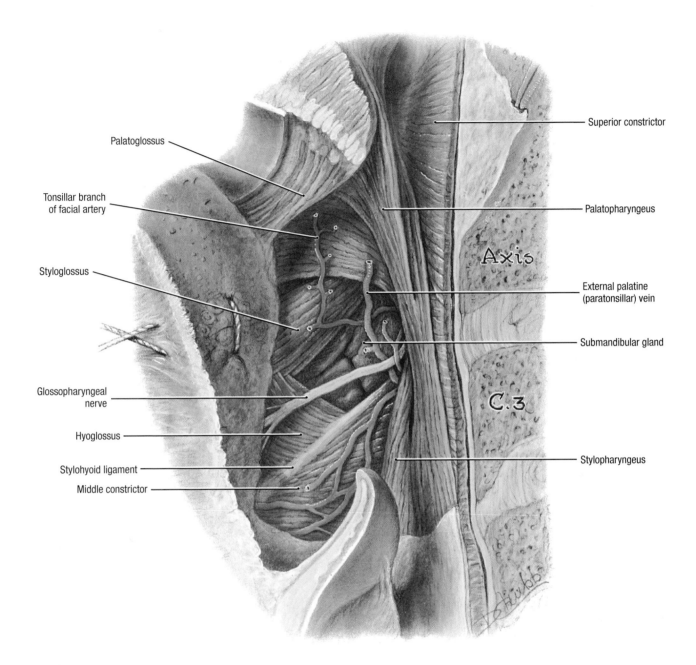

Palatoglossus

Tonsillar branch
of facial artery

Stylaglossus

Glossopharyngeal
nerve

Hyoglossus

Stylohyoid ligament

Middle constrictor

Superior constrictor

Palatopharyngeus

Axis

External palatine
(paratonsillar) vein

Submandibular gland

C.3

Stylopharyngeus

8.42   Interior of the pharynx—IV, median section

In this deep dissection of the tonsil bed, the tongue was pulled anteriorly, and the inferior part of the origin of the superior constrictor muscle was cut away.

OBSERVE:

1. The styloglossus muscle passes to the anterior two thirds of the tongue, where it interdigitates with the hyoglossus muscle. The glossopharyngeal nerve passes to the posterior one third of the tongue and lies anterior to the stylopharyngeus muscle. The sty-lopharyngeus muscle descends along the anterior border of the palatopharyngeus muscle;

2. The tonsillar branch of the facial artery sends a branch (cut short) to accompany the glossopharyngeal nerve to the tongue; the submandibular gland is seen lateral to the artery and paratonsillar vein;

3. The palatopharyngeus and stylopharyngeus muscles form the longitudinal muscle "coat" of the pharynx; the constrictor muscles form the circular coat.

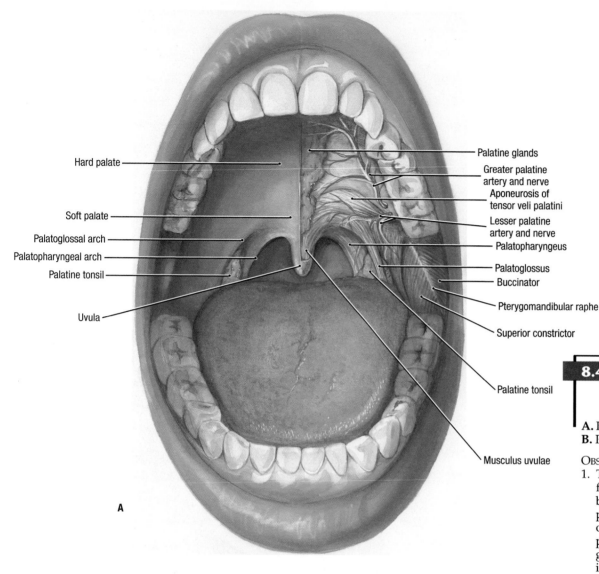

Hard palate

Soft palate

Palatoglossal arch

Palatopharyngeal arch

Palatine tonsil

Uvula

Palatine glands

Greater palatine artery and nerve

Aponeurosis of tensor veli palatini

Lesser palatine artery and nerve

Palatopharyngeus

Palatoglossus

Buccinator

Pterygomandibular raphe

Superior constrictor

Palatine tonsil

Musculus uvulae

A

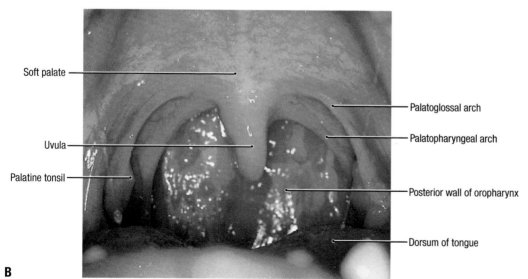

Soft palate

Uvula

Palatine tonsil

Palatoglossal arch

Palatopharyngeal arch

Posterior wall of oropharynx

Dorsum of tongue

B

8.43 Oral cavity and palatine tonsils, anterior views

A. Roof of mouth and palatine tonsils.
B. Palatine tonsils, in situ

OBSERVE:

1. The fauces (throat), the passage from the mouth to the pharynx, bounded superiorly by the soft palate, inferiorly by the root (base) of the tongue, and laterally by the palatoglossal and palatopharyngeal arches; the soft palate extending posteroinferiorly as a curved margin from which hangs the uvula;

2. The palatine tonsils located between the palatoglossal and palatopharyngeal arches; the tonsillar bed formed by the superior constrictor and palatopharyngeus muscles;

3. Deep to the mucosa of the hard palate the mucus-secreting palatine glands;

4. The soft palate consisting of an aponeurotic part (palatine aponeurosis), formed by the expanded tendon of the tensor veli palatini, and a muscular part, consisting of the tensor and levator (not shown) veli palatini, palatoglossus, palatopharyngeus, and musculus uvulae;

5. The greater and lesser palatine nerves and vessels emerging from the greater and lesser palatine foramina, respectively, to supply the hard and soft palates.

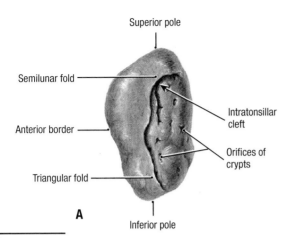

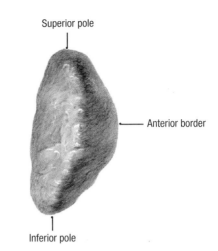

8.44   Palatine tonsil

A. Medial view. **B.** Lateral view.

OBSERVE:

1. The long axis runs vertically;
2. The fibrous capsule forms the lateral, or attached, surface of the tonsil; in removing the tonsil, the loose areolar tissue lying between the capsule and the thin pharyngobasilar fascia that forms the immediate bed of the tonsil, was easily traversed;

3. The capsule extends around the anterior border and slightly over the medial surface as a thin, free fold, covered with mucous membrane on both surfaces; the superior part of this fold is the semilunar fold; the inferior part is the triangular fold;
4. On the medial, or free, surface, the dozen orifices of the crypts extend right through the organ to the capsule; the intratonsillar cleft extends toward the superior pole.

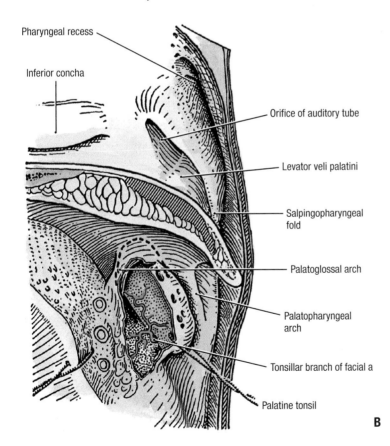

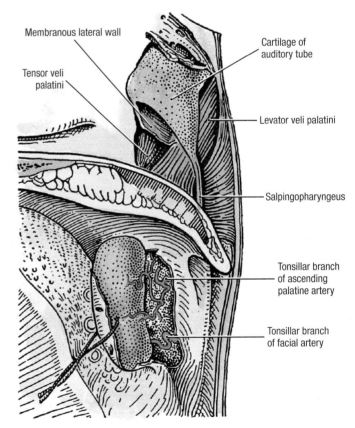

8.45   Removal of tonsil, median section of pharynx

A. First stage. The mucous membrane was incised along the palatoglossal arch, and the areolar space lateral to the fibrous capsule of the tonsil was entered. **B.** Second stage. The anterior border of the tonsil was freed, and the superior part, which extends far into the soft palate, was shelled out. The mucous membrane along the palatopharyngeal arch was cut through.

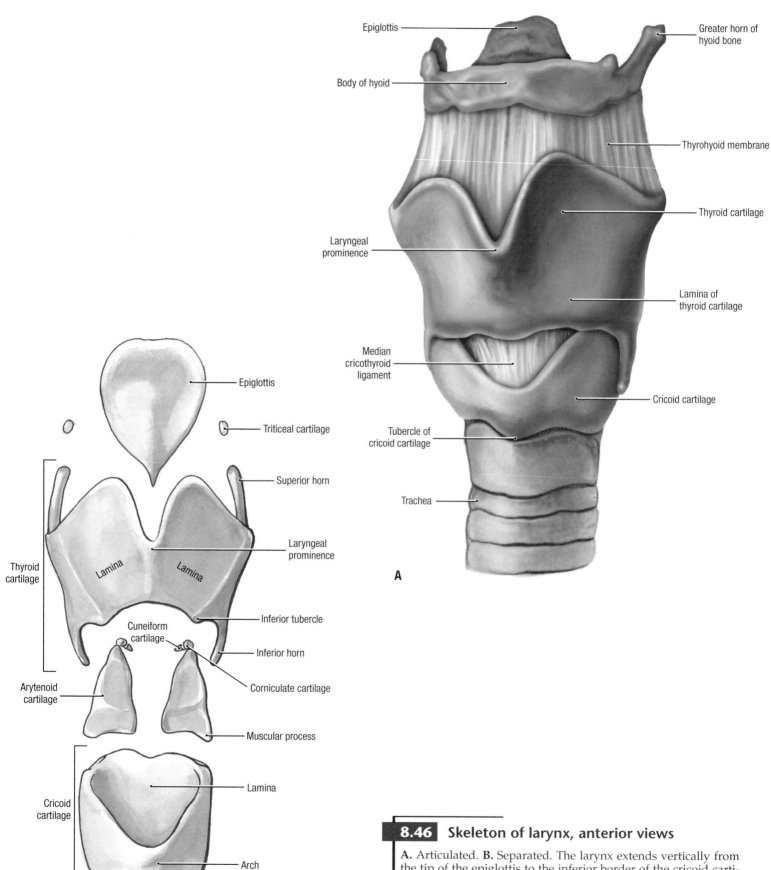

A

B

8.46 **Skeleton of larynx, anterior views**

A. Articulated. **B.** Separated. The larynx extends vertically from the tip of the epiglottis to the inferior border of the cricoid cartilage. The hyoid bone is not regarded as part of the larynx.

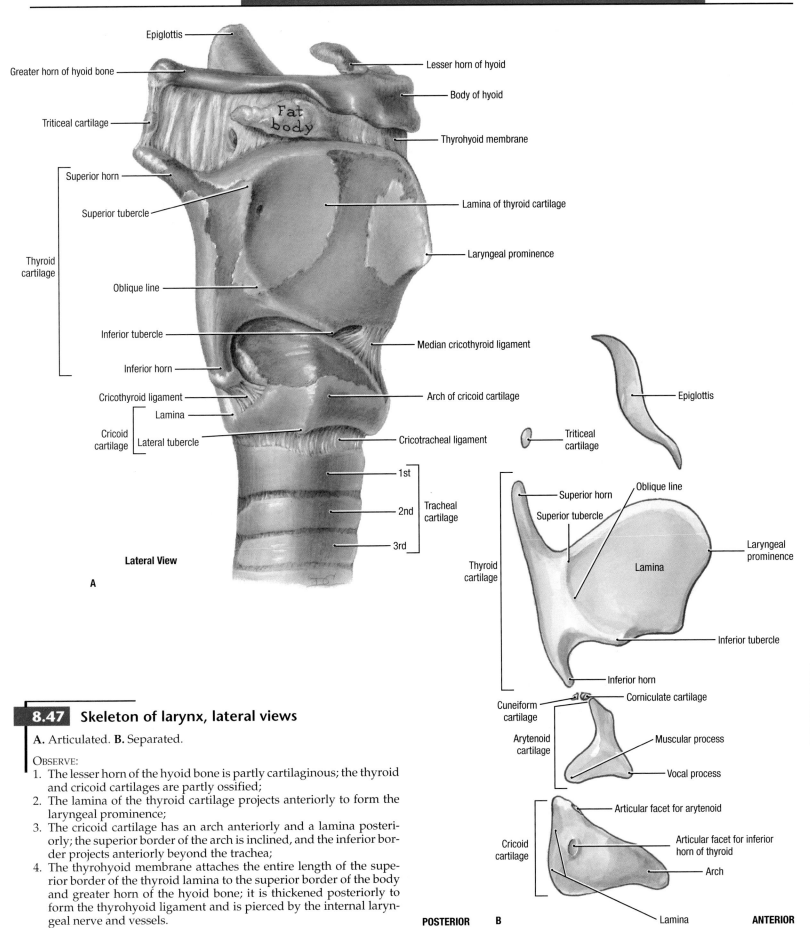

Lateral View

A

POSTERIOR   **B**   **ANTERIOR**

8.47 Skeleton of larynx, lateral views

A. Articulated. **B.** Separated.

OBSERVE:

1. The lesser horn of the hyoid bone is partly cartilaginous; the thyroid and cricoid cartilages are partly ossified;
2. The lamina of the thyroid cartilage projects anteriorly to form the laryngeal prominence;
3. The cricoid cartilage has an arch anteriorly and a lamina posteriorly; the superior border of the arch is inclined, and the inferior border projects anteriorly beyond the trachea;
4. The thyrohyoid membrane attaches the entire length of the superior border of the thyroid lamina to the superior border of the body and greater horn of the hyoid bone; it is thickened posteriorly to form the thyrohyoid ligament and is pierced by the internal laryngeal nerve and vessels.

8.48   Skeleton of larynx, posterior view

OBSERVE:

1. The thyroid cartilage shields the smaller cartilages of the larynx (epiglottic, arytenoid, corniculate, and cuneiform);
2. The rounded posterior border of the thyroid cartilage and its superior and inferior horns; the inferior horn articulates with the cricoid cartilage at the cricothyroid joint;
3. The quadrangular membrane connects the border of the epiglottic cartilage to the arytenoid and corniculate cartilages.

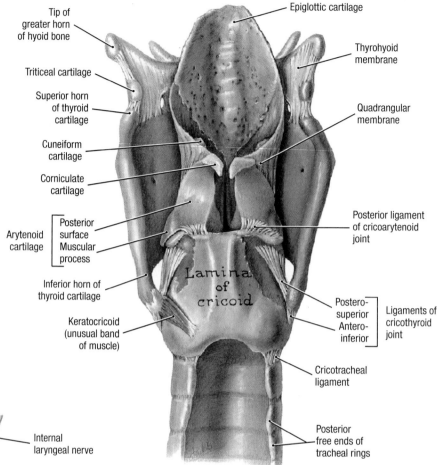

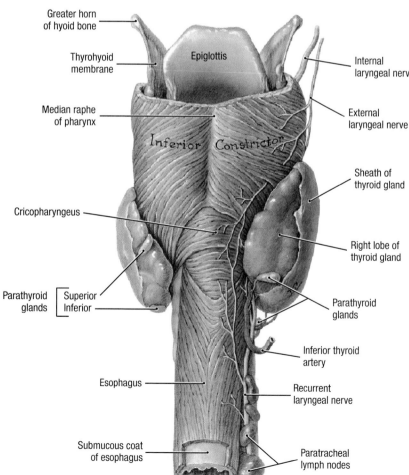

8.49   Thyroid gland and laryngeal nerves, posterior view

OBSERVE:

1. The superior parathyroid gland lies in a crevice on the posterior border of the lobes of the thyroid gland. On the right side of the specimen, both parathyroid glands are low;
2. The internal laryngeal nerve innervates the mucous membrane superior to the vocal folds, and the external laryngeal nerve supplies the inferior constrictor and cricothyroid muscles. The recurrent laryngeal nerve supplies the esophagus, trachea, and inferior constrictor muscle, and then continues into the larynx. At the larynx, it supplies sensory innervation to the area inferior to the vocal folds (cords) and motor innervation to all of the intrinsic muscles of the larynx, except the cricothyroid.

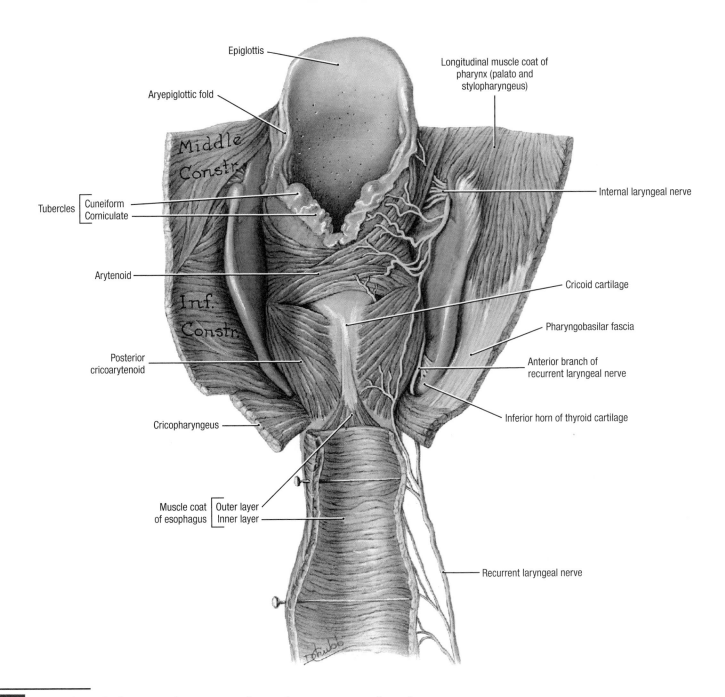

8.50   Muscles of pharynx, larynx, and esophagus, posterior view

The mucous membrane of the pharynx and esophagus, as well as the left palatopharyngeus muscle, were removed. The constrictor muscles are thereby uncovered.

OBSERVE:

1. The pinpoint orifices of the glands that occupy the epiglottic cartilage;
2. The palatopharyngeus and stylopharyngeus muscles together constitute the inner, or longitudinal, muscle coat of the pharynx and insert into the pharyngobasilar fascia and thyroid cartilage;
3. The esophagus has inner, circularly arranged muscle fibers and outer, longitudinally arranged fibers; the latter suspend the esophagus from the cricoid cartilage;
4. The inferior constrictor muscle is attached to the oblique line and

tubercles of the thyroid cartilage; its lowest fibers, the cricopharyngeus, are attached to the cricoid cartilage and act as a sphincter;
5. The posterior cricoarytenoid muscle is fan-shaped; its superior fibers rotate the arytenoid cartilage laterally, and its lower fibers pull the cartilage inferiorly;
6. The arytenoid (interarytenoid) muscle has transverse and oblique fibers that are continued into the aryepiglottic fold as aryepiglottic muscle;
7. The recurrent laryngeal nerve enters the larynx as two branches; the anterior branch runs immediately posterior to the cricothyroid joint;
8. The internal laryngeal nerve pierces the thyrohyoid membrane as several diverging branches.

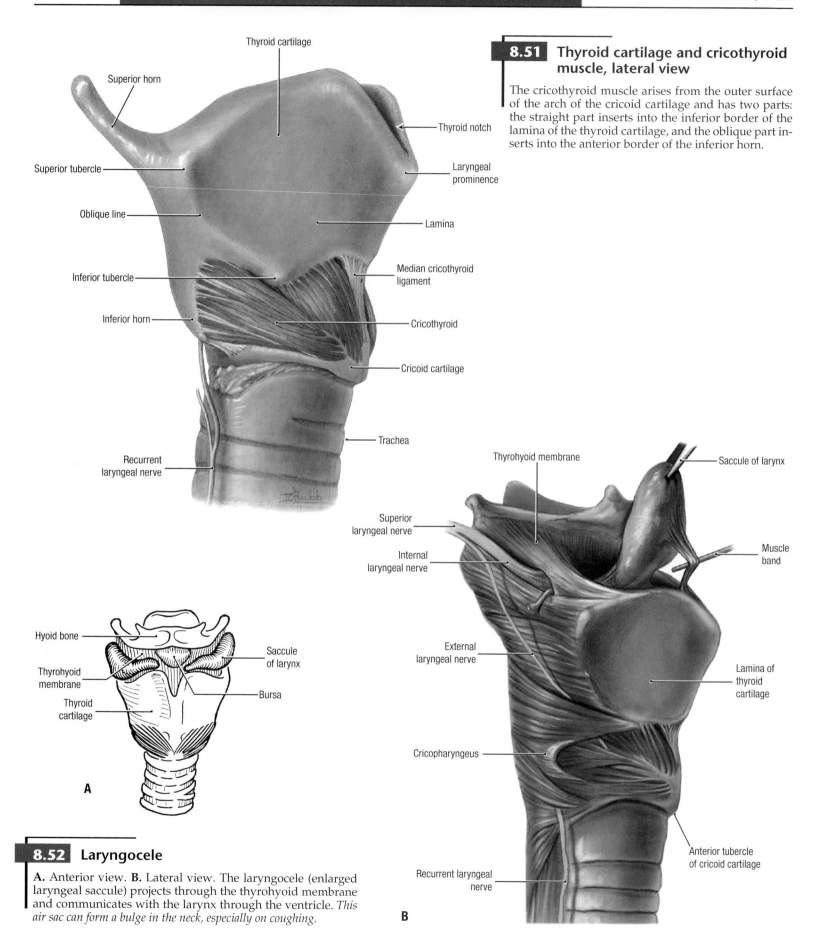

Thyroid cartilage

Superior horn

Superior tubercle

Oblique line

Inferior tubercle

Inferior horn

Recurrent
laryngeal nerve

Thyroid notch

Laryngeal
prominence

Lamina

Median cricothyroid
ligament

Cricothyroid

Cricoid cartilage

Trachea

8.51   Thyroid cartilage and cricothyroid muscle, lateral view

The cricothyroid muscle arises from the outer surface of the arch of the cricoid cartilage and has two parts: the straight part inserts into the inferior border of the lamina of the thyroid cartilage, and the oblique part inserts into the anterior border of the inferior horn.

Hyoid bone

Thyrohyoid
membrane

Thyroid
cartilage

Saccule
of larynx

Bursa

A

8.52   Laryngocele

A. Anterior view. **B.** Lateral view. The laryngocele (enlarged laryngeal saccule) projects through the thyrohyoid membrane and communicates with the larynx through the ventricle. *This air sac can form a bulge in the neck, especially on coughing.*

Thyrohyoid membrane

Superior
laryngeal nerve

Internal
laryngeal nerve

External
laryngeal nerve

Cricopharyngeus

Recurrent laryngeal
nerve

Saccule of larynx

Muscle
band

Lamina of
thyroid
cartilage

Anterior tubercle
of cricoid cartilage

B

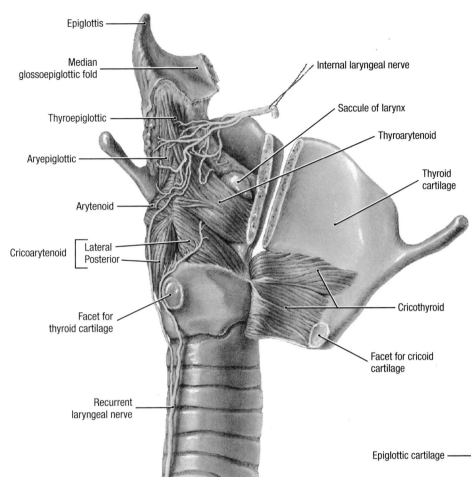

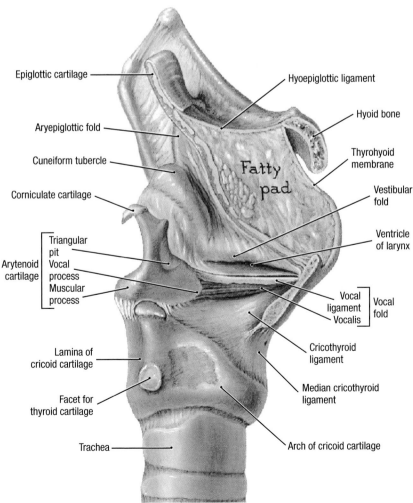

8.53 Muscles and nerves of larynx, and cricothyroid joint, lateral view

The thyroid cartilage was sawed through in the median plane, the cricothyroid joint was opened, and the right lamina of the thyroid cartilage was turned anteriorly, stripping the cricothyroid muscle off the arch of the cricoid cartilage.

OBSERVE:
1. The lateral cricoarytenoid muscle;
2. The thyroarytenoid muscle inserts with the arytenoid muscle into the lateral border of the arytenoid cartilage; its superior fibers continue to the epiglottis as the thyroepiglottic muscle;
3. The internal and recurrent laryngeal nerves.

8.54 Larynx, lateral view

Superior to the vocal folds, the larynx was sectioned near the median plane to reveal the interior of its left side. Inferior to this level, the right side of the larynx was dissected.

OBSERVE:
1. A fat pad and glands fill the triangular space between the hyoepiglottic ligament, thyrohyoid membrane, and epiglottic cartilage;
2. The raised, circular facet on the lateral aspect of the cricoid cartilage for the inferior horn of the thyroid cartilage; superior to this is the sloping facet for the arytenoid cartilage.
3. The vocal fold (true vocal cord) consists of the vocal ligament and vocalis (vocal muscle), which is part of the thyroarytenoid muscle.

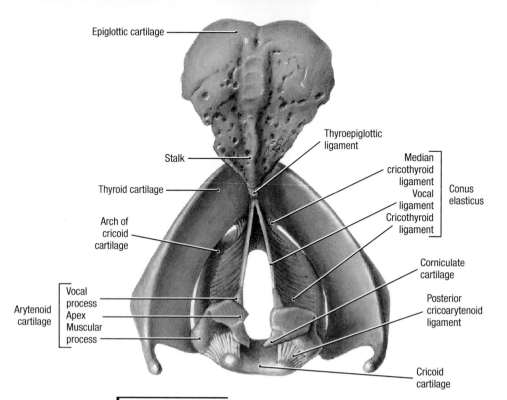

8.55   Skeleton of larynx, superior view

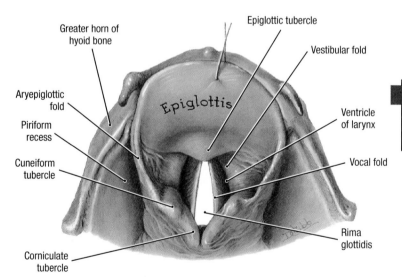

8.56   Larynx, superior view

OBSERVE:
1. The inlet, or aditus, to the larynx is bounded anteriorly by the epiglottis; posteriorly by the arytenoid cartilages, the corniculate cartilages that cap them, and the interarytenoid fold that unites them; and on each side by the aryepiglottic fold, which contains the superior end of the cuneiform cartilage;
2. The vocal folds are closer together than the vestibular folds;
3. The rima glottidis is the aperature between the vocal folds. *During normal respiration, it is narrow and wedge shaped; during forced respiration, it is wide. Variation in the tension and length of the vocal folds, in the width of the rima glottidis, and in the intensity of the expiratory effort produce changes in the pitch of the voice.*

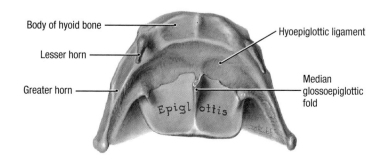

8.57   Epiglottis and hyoepiglottic ligament, superior view

OBSERVE:
1. The hyoepiglottic ligament unites the epiglottic cartilage to the hyoid bone;
2. The body, lesser, and greater horns of the hyoid bone.

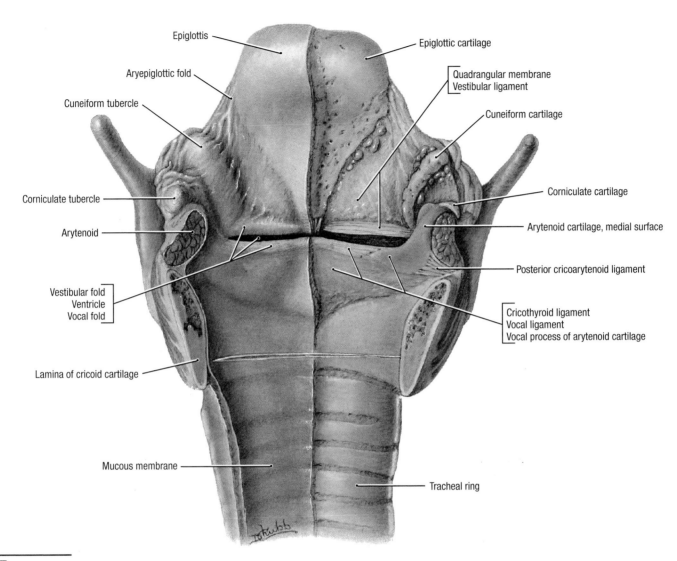

Epiglottis

Aryepiglottic fold

Cuneiform tubercle

Corniculate tubercle

Arytenoid

Vestibular fold
Ventricle
Vocal fold

Lamina of cricoid cartilage

Mucous membrane

Epiglottic cartilage

Quadrangular membrane
Vestibular ligament

Cuneiform cartilage

Corniculate cartilage

Arytenoid cartilage, medial surface

Posterior cricoarytenoid ligament

Cricothyroid ligament
Vocal ligament
Vocal process of arytenoid cartilage

Tracheal ring

8.58 Interior of larynx, posterior view

The posterior wall of the larynx was split in the median plane, and the two sides were held apart. On the left side of the specimen, the mucous membrane, which is the innermost coat of the larynx, is intact; on the right side of the specimen, the mucous and submucous coats were peeled off, and the next coat, consisting of cartilages, ligaments, and fibroelastic membrane, was uncovered.

OBSERVE:

1. The arytenoid muscle and lamina of the cricoid cartilage are divided posteriorly;
2. The entrance to the larynx is oblique; the inferior limit, at the inferior border of the cricoid cartilage where the trachea begins, is horizontal;
3. The three compartments of the larynx: a) the superior compartment of the vestibule, superior to the level of the vestibular folds (false cords); b) the middle, between the levels of the vestibular and vocal folds; and c) the inferior, or infraglottic, cavity, inferior to the level of the vocal folds;
4. The mucous membrane is smooth and adherent over the epiglottic cartilage and vocal ligaments, and loose and wrinkled about the arytenoid cartilages;

5. The two parts of the fibroelastic membrane: a) superior quadrangular and b) inferior triangular. The superior part, the quadrangular membrane, is thickened inferiorly to form the vestibular ligament; the inferior part, the cricothyroid ligament (conus elasticus), begins inferiorly as the strong median cricothyroid ligament and ends superiorly as the vocal ligament. Between the vocal and vestibular ligaments, the membrane, lined with mucous membrane, is evaginated to form the wall of the ventricle;
6. The cuneiform cartilage, composed of elastic cartilage and glands, is attached to the arytenoid cartilage near the posterior end of the vestibular ligament;
7. The posterior ligament of the cricoarytenoid joint anchors the arytenoid cartilage; the submucous surface of the arytenoid cartilage is flat and medial.
8. *When foreign objects such as food contact the epithelium of the vestibular epithelium, violent coughing occurs in an attempt to expel them. If this fails, the foreign material can lodge in the rima glottidis, causing laryngeal obstruction (choking). Compression of the abdomen (Heimlich maneuver) causes the diaphragm to elevate and the lungs to compress, expelling air from the trachea into the larynx. This maneuver can dislodge the trapped material.*

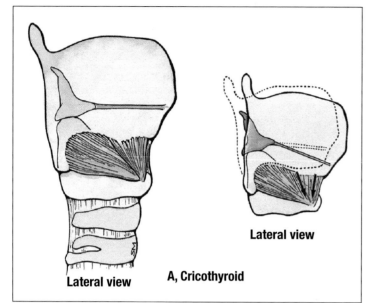

Lateral view

Lateral view

A, Cricothyroid

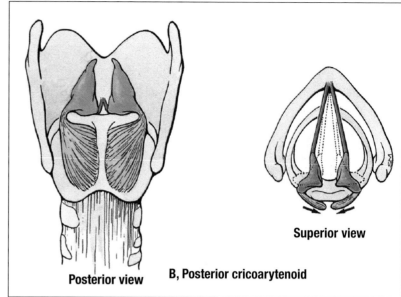

Superior view

Posterior view

B, Posterior cricoarytenoid

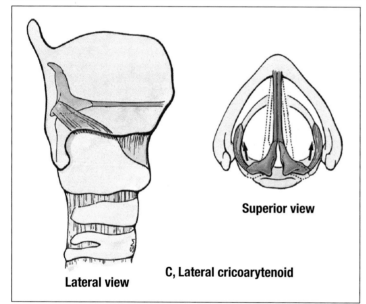

Superior view

Lateral view

C, Lateral cricoarytenoid

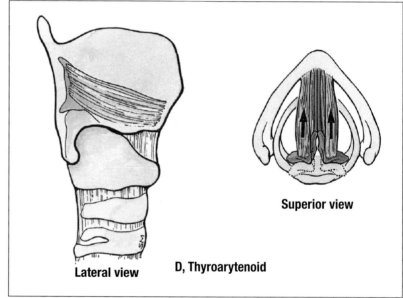

Superior view

Lateral view

D, Thyroarytenoid

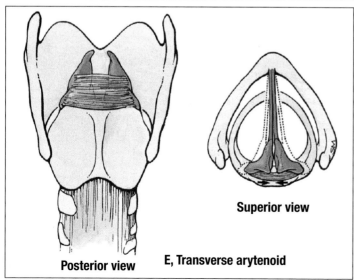

Superior view

Posterior view

E, Transverse arytenoid

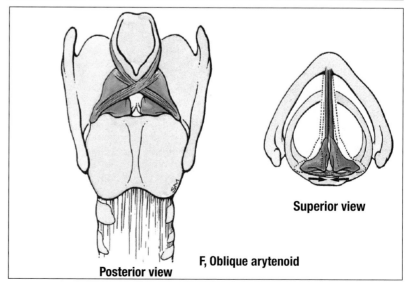

Superior view

Posterior view

F, Oblique arytenoid

Table 8.5 Muscles of Larynx[a]

Muscle	Origin	Insertion	Innervation	Main Action(s)
Cricothyroid **(A)**	Anterolateral part of cricoid cartilage	Inferior margin and inferior horn of thyroid cartilage	External laryngeal nerve	Stretches and tenses vocal fold
Posterior cricoarytenoid **(B)**	Posterior surface of laminae of cricoid cartilage	Muscular process of arytenoid cartilage		Abducts vocal fold
Lateral cricoarytenoid **(C)**	Arch of cricoid cartilage			Adducts vocal fold
Tyroarytenoid[b] **(D)**	Posterior surface of thyroid cartilage	Muscular process of arytenoid process	Recurrent laryngeal nerve	Relaxes vocal fold
Transverse **(E)** and oblique **(F)** arytenoids[c]	One arytenoid cartilage	Opposite arytenoid cartilage		Close inlet of larynx by approximating arytenoid cartilages
Vocalis[d]	Angle between laminae of thyroid cartilage	Vocal process of arytenoid cartilage		Alters vocal fold during phonation

[a]Letters in muscle column correspond to figures on opposite page.
[b]Superior fibers of the thyroarytenoid muscle pass into the aryepiglottic fold, and some of them reach the epiglottic cartilage. These fibers constitute the thyroepiglottic muscle, which widens inlet of larynx.
[c]Some fibers of oblique arytenoid muscle continue as aryepiglottic muscle.
[d]This slender muscular slip is derived from inferior deeper fibers of the thyroarytenoid muscle.

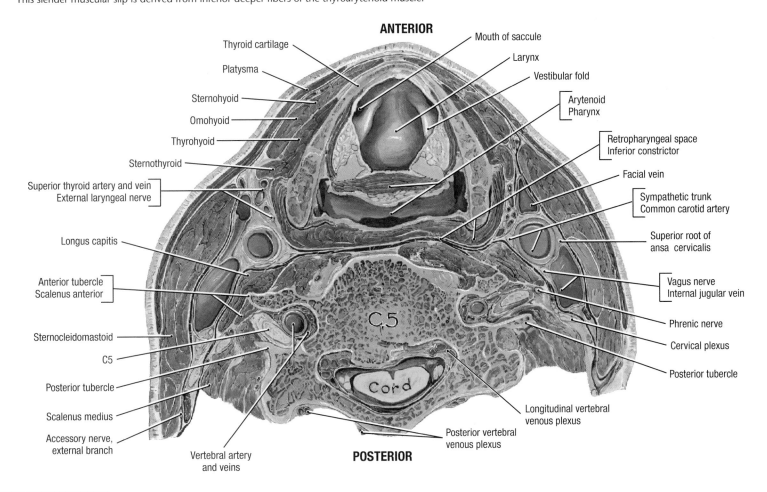

8.59   Transverse section of neck through middle of larynx, inferior view

OBSERVE:
1. The thyroid cartilage shields the larynx and pharynx;
2. The arytenoid muscle was cut obliquely, and therefore appears wide;
3. The three contents of the carotid sheath: common carotid artery, internal jugular vein, and, posteriorly between them, vagus nerve;
4. The sympathetic trunk is posteromedial to the carotid artery and medial to the vagus nerve;
5. The retropharyngeal space is between the pretracheal fascia, which covers the inferior constrictor muscle, and the prevertebral fascia, which covers the longi colli and capitis muscles;
6. The vertebral artery is surrounded with a venous plexus that inferiorly becomes the vertebral vein.

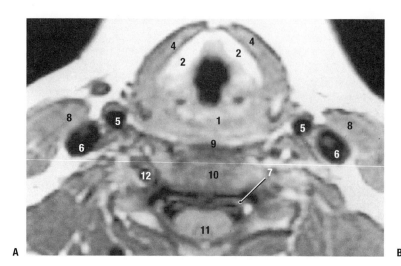

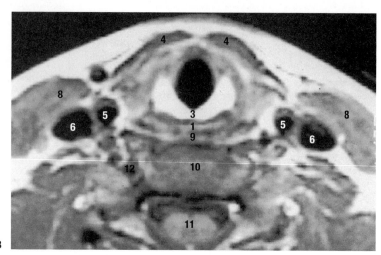

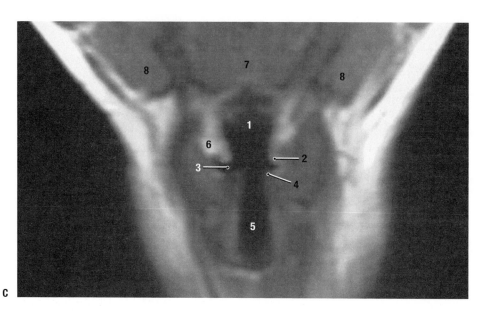

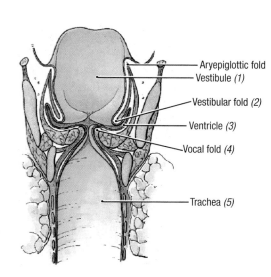

Aryepiglottic fold
Vestibule *(1)*

Vestibular fold *(2)*

Ventricle *(3)*

Vocal fold *(4)*

Trachea *(5)*

8.60   Imaging of larynx

A. Transverse (axial) MRI through thyroid cartilage. **B.** Transverse (axial) MRI through cricoid cartilage. For **A** and **B:** *1,* Esophagus; *2,* Thyroid cartilage; *3,* Lamina of cricoid cartilage; *4,* Strap muscles; *5,* Common carotid artery; *6,* Internal jugular vein; *7,* Ventral root; *8,* Sternocleidomastoid; *9,* Inferior constrictor; *10,* Vertebral body; *11,* Spinal cord in cerebrospinal fluid; *12,* Vertebral artery. **C.** Coronal MRI (left) and diagram (right) through larynx and trachea. For **C:** Numbers in parentheses on diagram refer to numbered structures on MRI; *6,* Preepiglottic fat; *7,* Tongue; *8,* Submandibular gland.

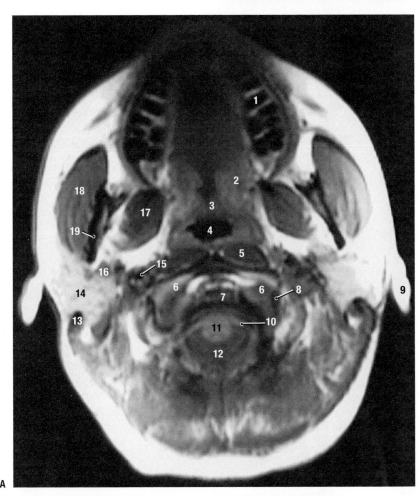

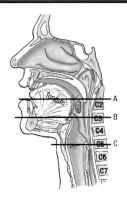

1	Tooth	23	Genioglossus
2	Sublingual gland	24	Buccal fat
3	Uvula	25	Submandibular gland
4	Oropharynx	26	Intrinsic muscles of tongue
5	Longus capitis and colli	27	Vertebral body
6	Lateral mass of atlas	28	Lamina
7	Dens (odontoid process)	29	Semispinalis cervicis
8	Vertebral artery	30	Semispinalis capitis
9	Pinna	31	Splenius capitis
10	Ventral rootlet	32	Trapezius
11	Spinal cord	33	Sternocleidomastoid
12	Cerebrospinal fluid in subarachnoid space	34	Internal jugular vein
13	Mastoid process	35	Bifurcation of common carotid artery
14	Parotid gland	36	Levator scapulae
15	Internal carotid artery	37	External jugular vein
16	Retromandibular vein	38	Common carotid artery
17	Medial pterygoid	39	Rima glottidis
18	Masseter	40	Vocal fold
19	Ramus of mandible	41	Thyrohyoid
20	Body of mandible	42	Thyroid cartilage
21	Mylohyoid		
22	Hyoglossus		

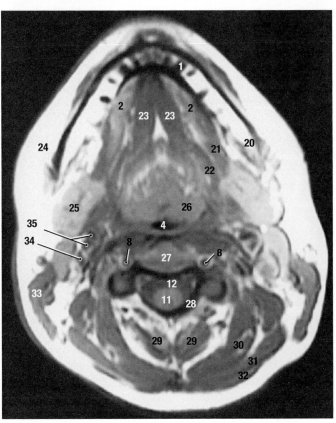

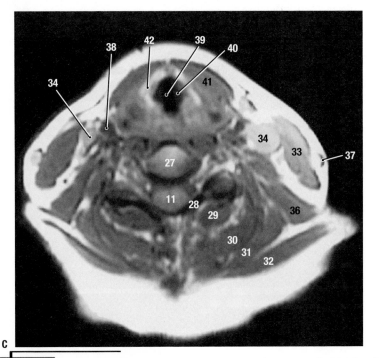

8.61   **Median magnetic resonance images (MRIs) of the neck**

8.62 Head and neck, median section

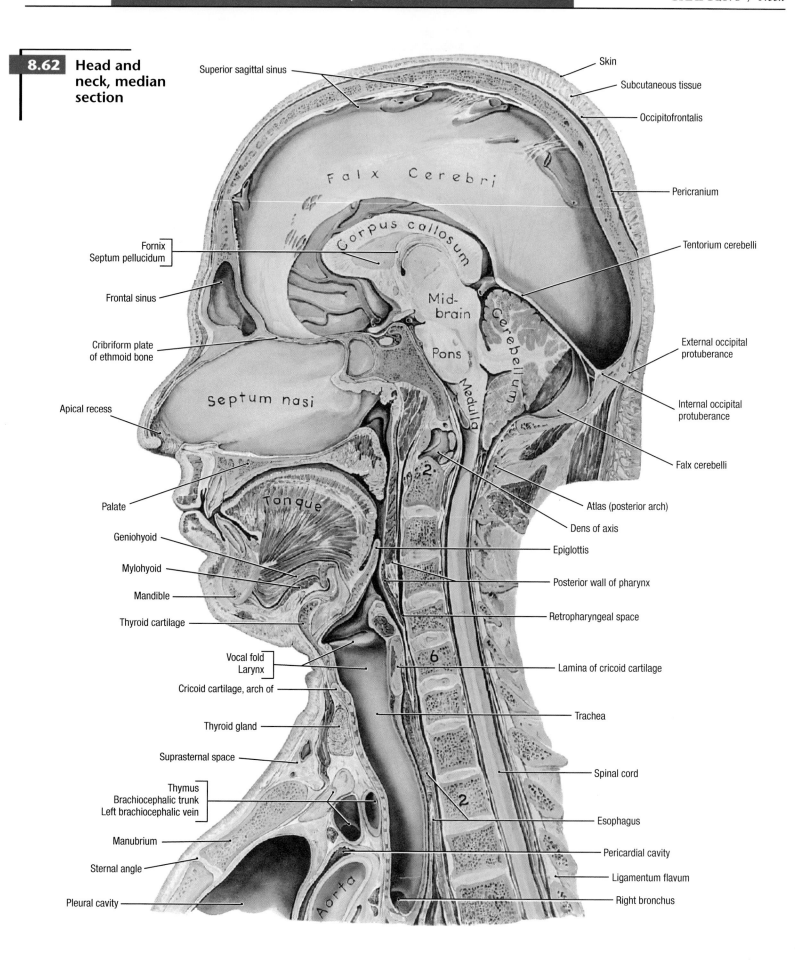

Superior sagittal sinus

Skin

Subcutaneous tissue

Occipitofrontalis

Falx Cerebri

Pericranium

Fornix
Septum pellucidum

Corpus callosum

Tentorium cerebelli

Frontal sinus

Mid-brain

Cerebellum

Pons

Medulla

External occipital protuberance

Cribriform plate of ethmoid bone

Septum nasi

Internal occipital protuberance

Apical recess

Falx cerebelli

Tongue

Atlas (posterior arch)

Palate

Dens of axis

Geniohyoid

Epiglottis

Mylohyoid

Posterior wall of pharynx

Mandible

Retropharyngeal space

Thyroid cartilage

Vocal fold
Larynx

Lamina of cricoid cartilage

Cricoid cartilage, arch of

Thyroid gland

Trachea

Suprasternal space

Thymus
Brachiocephalic trunk
Left brachiocephalic vein

Spinal cord

Manubrium

Esophagus

Sternal angle

Pericardial cavity

Aorta

Ligamentum flavum

Pleural cavity

Right bronchus

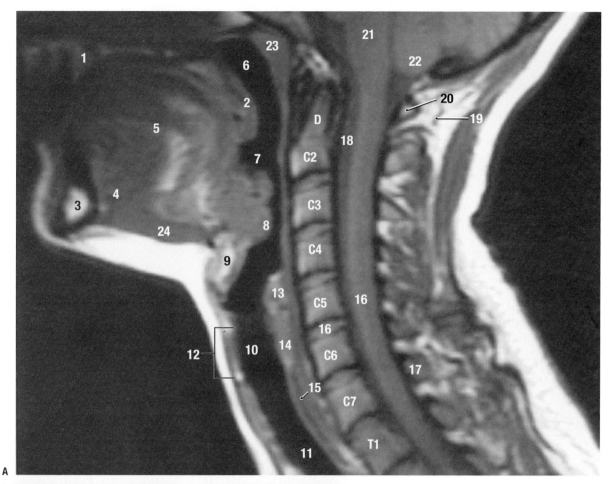

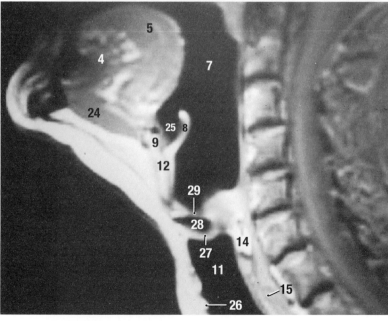

1	Hard palate	16	Intervertebral disc
2	Soft palate	17	Spinous process
3	Mandible	18	Cerebrospinal fluid in
4	Genioglossus		subarachnoid space
5	Tongue	19	Ligamentum nuchae
6	Nasopharynx	20	Posterior arch of atlas
7	Oropharynx	21	Medulla oblongata
8	Epiglottis	22	Tonsil of cerebellum
9	Hyoid bone	23	Pharyngeal tonsil (adenoid)
10	Laryngopharynx	24	Geniohyoid
11	Trachea	25	Vallecula
12	Thyroid cartilage	26	Tracheal ring
13	Arytenoid cartilage	27	Vocal fold
14	Cricoid cartilage	28	Ventricle
15	Esophagus	29	Vestibular fold

8.63   Coronal MRIs of the neck

The line diagram indicates the location of the section of the MRIs.
A. Compartments of larynx, coronal section. These are: a vestibule, a middle compartment having a right and a left ventricle, and an infraglottic cavity. **B.** Coronal MRI through oropharynx, larynx, and trachea

CHAPTER 9

Cranial Nerves

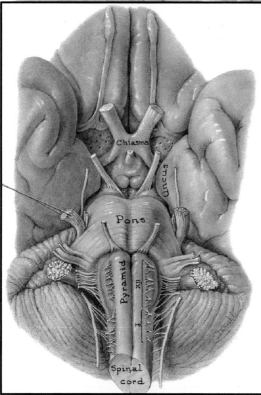

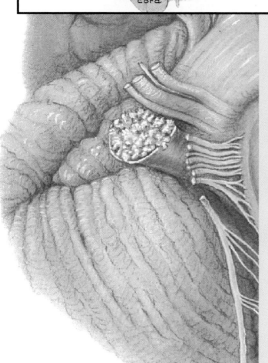

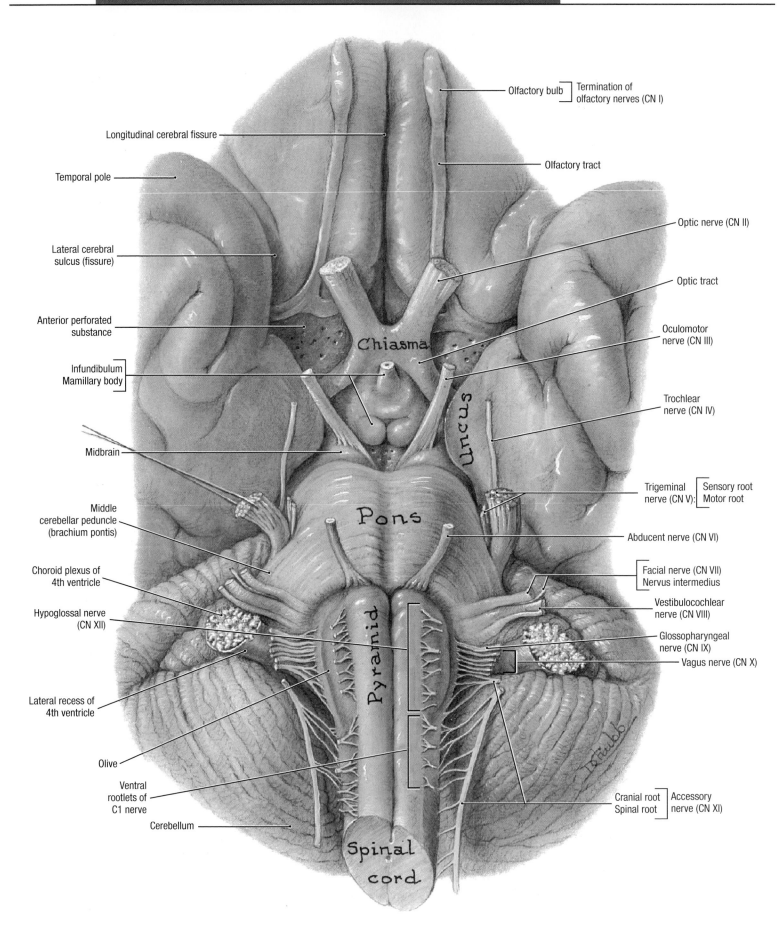

Olfactory bulb ⎤ Termination of
⎦ olfactory nerves (CN I)

Longitudinal cerebral fissure

Olfactory tract

Temporal pole

Optic nerve (CN II)

Lateral cerebral
sulcus (fissure)

Optic tract

Anterior perforated
substance

Oculomotor
nerve (CN III)

Chiasma

Infundibulum
Mamillary body

Uncus

Trochlear
nerve (CN IV)

Midbrain

Trigeminal ⎤ Sensory root
nerve (CN V): ⎦ Motor root

Middle
cerebellar peduncle
(brachium pontis)

Pons

Abducent nerve (CN VI)

⎤ Facial nerve (CN VII)
⎦ Nervus intermedius

Choroid plexus of
4th ventricle

Vestibulocochlear
nerve (CN VIII)

Hypoglossal nerve
(CN XII)

Pyramid

Glossopharyngeal
nerve (CN IX)

Vagus nerve (CN X)

Lateral recess of
4th ventricle

Olive

Ventral
rootlets of
C1 nerve

Cranial root ⎤ Accessory
Spinal root ⎦ nerve (CN XI)

Cerebellum

Spinal
cord

Table 9.1. Functional Components of the Cranial Nerves

No.	Name	SSA	GSA	GVA	SVA	GSE	SVE	GVE
I	Olfactory				•			
II	Optic	•						
III	Oculomotor					•		•
IV	Trochlear					•		
V	Trigeminal		•				•	
VI	Abducent					•		
VII	Facial		•	•	•		•	•
VIII	Vestibulocochlear	•						
IX	Glossopharyngeal		•	•	•		•	•
X	Vagus		•	•	•		•	•
XI	Accessory						•	
XII	Hypoglossal					•		

9.1   Base of brain: superficial origins of cranial nerves, inferior view

OBSERVE:

1. There are 12 pairs of cranial nerves that are named and numbered in rostrocaudal sequence to their attachment to the brain;
2. The olfactory nerves (not shown) end in the olfactory bulb;
3. The rootlets of the hypoglossal nerve arise between the pyramid and olive.

Cranial nerves carry one or more of the following functional components:

- Special somatic afferent (*SSA*) include the special senses of vision, hearing, and balance
- General somatic afferent (*GSA*) carry general sensation from skin and mucous membranes
- General visceral afferent (*GVA*) carry visceral sensation from parotid gland, carotid body and sinus, middle ear, pharynx, larynx, trachea, bronchi, lungs, heart, esophagus, and intestines as far as the left colic flexure
- Special visceral afferent (*SVA*) include taste and smell; olfactory stimuli arouse emotions and induce visceral responses
- General somatic efferent (*GSE*) supply muscles derived from the myotome regions of the embryonic somites (e.g., muscles of the orbit and tongue)
- Special visceral efferent (*SVE*) supply muscles derived from embryonic branchial arches (e.g., muscles of the larynx and pharynx)
- General visceral efferent (*GVE*) consist of the cranial parasympathetic system

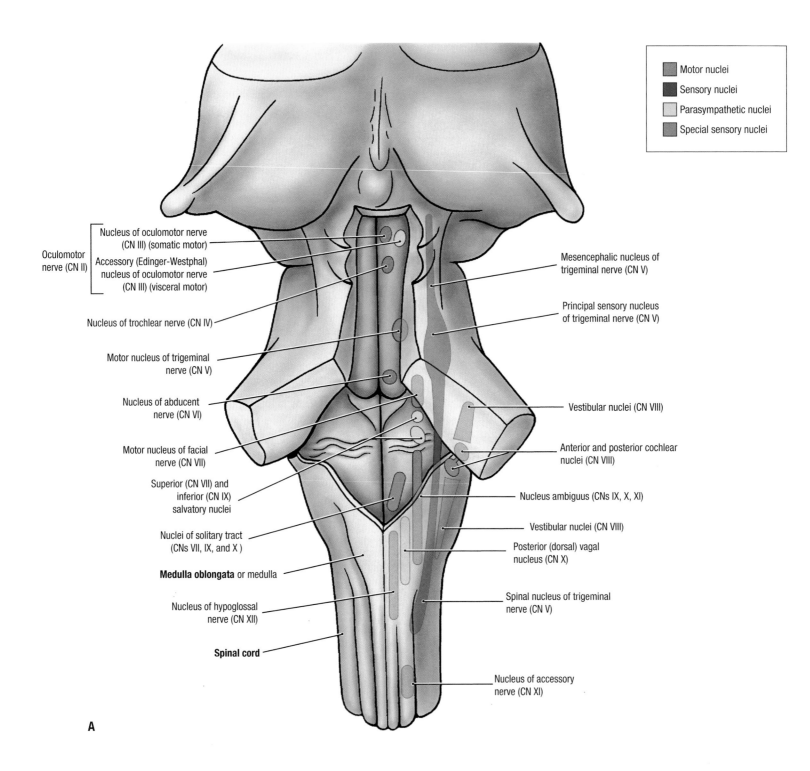

Motor nuclei

Sensory nuclei

Parasympathetic nuclei

Special sensory nuclei

Oculomotor nerve (CN II)

Nucleus of oculomotor nerve (CN III) (somatic motor)

Accessory (Edinger-Westphal) nucleus of oculomotor nerve (CN III) (visceral motor)

Nucleus of trochlear nerve (CN IV)

Motor nucleus of trigeminal nerve (CN V)

Nucleus of abducent nerve (CN VI)

Motor nucleus of facial nerve (CN VII)

Superior (CN VII) and inferior (CN IX) salvatory nuclei

Nuclei of solitary tract (CNs VII, IX, and X)

Medulla oblongata or medulla

Nucleus of hypoglossal nerve (CN XII)

Spinal cord

Mesencephalic nucleus of trigeminal nerve (CN V)

Principal sensory nucleus of trigeminal nerve (CN V)

Vestibular nuclei (CN VIII)

Anterior and posterior cochlear nuclei (CN VIII)

Nucleus ambiguus (CNs IX, X, XI)

Vestibular nuclei (CN VIII)

Posterior (dorsal) vagal nucleus (CN X)

Spinal nucleus of trigeminal nerve (CN V)

Nucleus of accessory nerve (CN XI)

A

9.2   Cranial nerve nuclei

A. Dorsal view. The fibers of the cranial nerves are connected to nuclei (groups of nerve cell bodies in the central nervous system [CNS]), in which afferent (sensory) fibers terminate and from which efferent (motor) fibers originate. The cochlear nerve and nuclei, and fibers of the abducens and hypoglossal nuclei that exit ventrally are not shown. **B.** Midsagittal view. The brainstem is represented as a hollow shell except for the cranial nerves and nuclei.

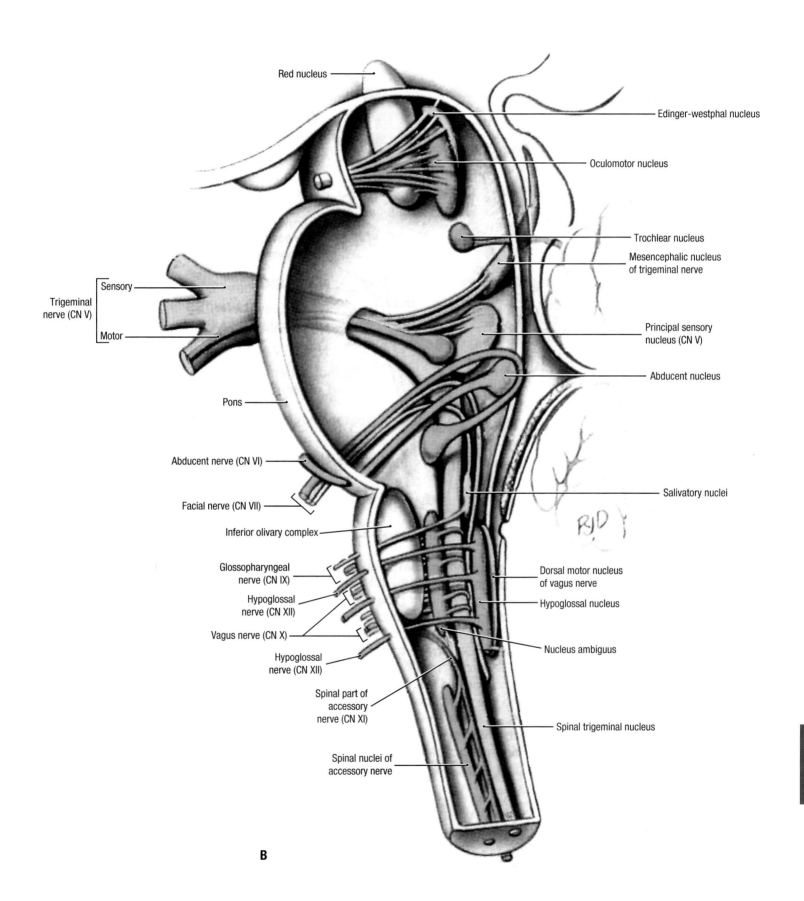

Red nucleus

Edinger-westphal nucleus

Oculomotor nucleus

Trochlear nucleus

Mesencephalic nucleus of trigeminal nerve

Sensory

Trigeminal nerve (CN V)

Motor

Principal sensory nucleus (CN V)

Abducent nucleus

Pons

Abducent nerve (CN VI)

Facial nerve (CN VII)

Salivatory nuclei

Inferior olivary complex

Glossopharyngeal nerve (CN IX)

Dorsal motor nucleus of vagus nerve

Hypoglossal nerve (CN XII)

Hypoglossal nucleus

Vagus nerve (CN X)

Hypoglossal nerve (CN XII)

Nucleus ambiguus

Spinal part of accessory nerve (CN XI)

Spinal trigeminal nucleus

Spinal nuclei of accessory nerve

B

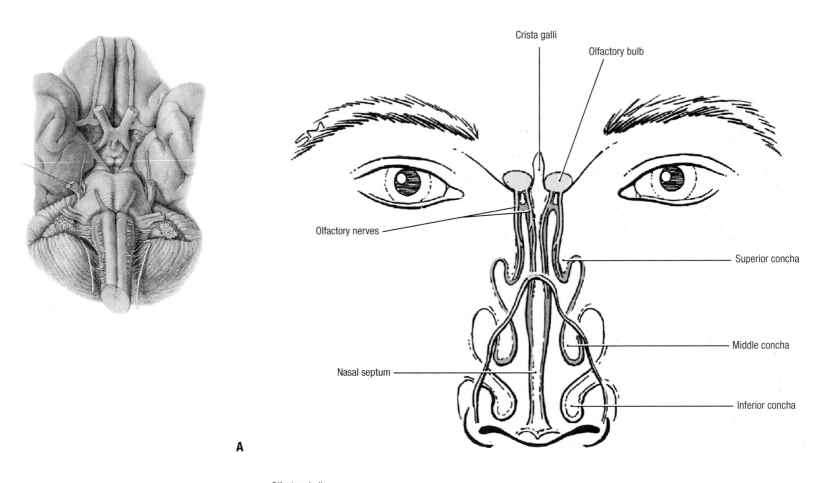

Crista galli

Olfactory bulb

Olfactory nerves

Superior concha

Middle concha

Nasal septum

Inferior concha

A

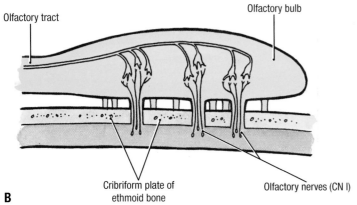

Olfactory tract

Olfactory bulb

Cribriform plate of
ethmoid bone

Olfactory nerves (CN I)

B

9.3   Distribution of olfactory nerve (CN I)

A. Anterior view. **B.** Enlargement of olfactory area, lateral view. Bundles of olfactory nerve fibers arise from the olfactory epithelium, pass through the cribriform plate and synapse with neurons in the olfactory bulb. **C.** Lateral wall of nose and septum, sagittal section. The sagittal section through the nasal cavity enables the lateral wall of the nose and the nasal septum to be displayed as pages in a book. *S*, superior concha; *M*, middle concha; *I*, inferior concha.

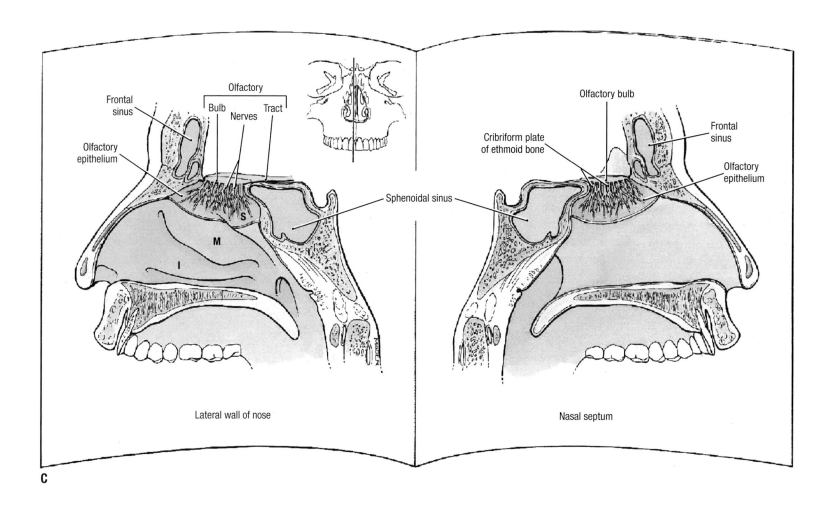

Lateral wall of nose

Nasal septum

C

Table 9.2. Olfactory Nerve (CN I)

Nerve	Functional Components	Cells of Origin/Termination	Cranial Exit	Distribution and Functions
Olfactory	SVA	Olfactory epithelium (olfactory cells/ olfactory bulb)	Foramina in cribriform plate of ethmoid bone	Smell from nasal mucosa of roof of each nasal cavity and superior sides of nasal septum and superior concha

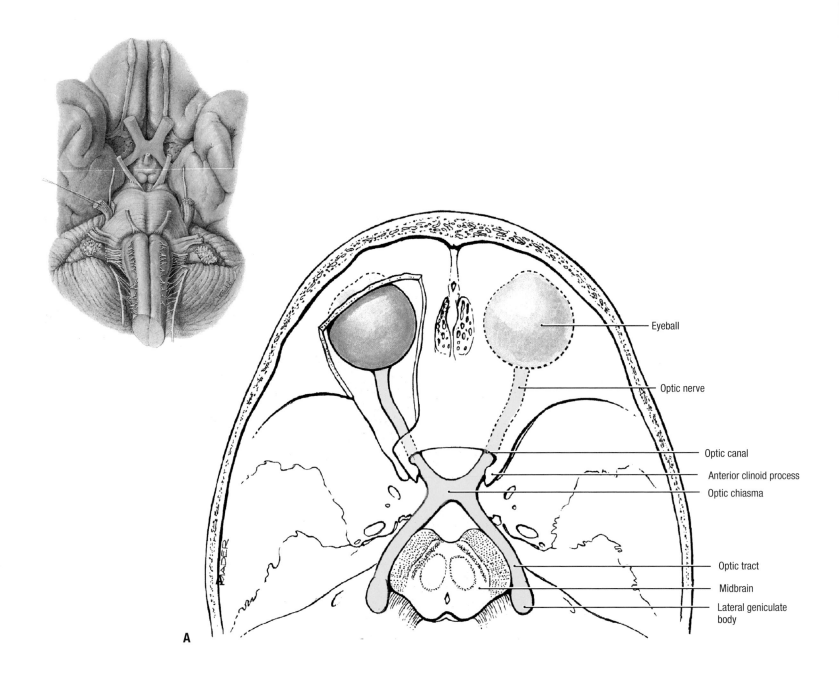

A

Table 9.3. Optic Nerve (CN II)

Nerve	Functional Components	Cells of Origin/Termination	Cranial Exit	Distribution and Functions
Optic	SSA	Retina (ganglion cells)/lateral geniculate body (nucleus)	Optic canal	Vision from retina

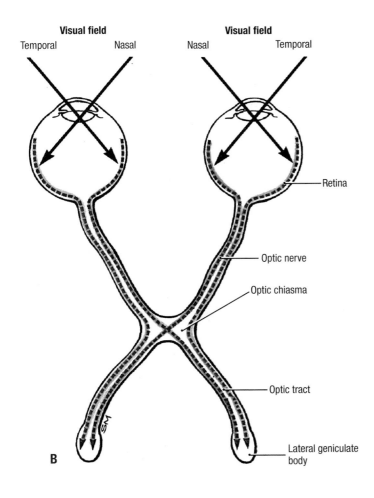

Visual field
Temporal   Nasal

Visual field
Nasal   Temporal

Retina

Optic nerve

Optic chiasma

Optic tract

Lateral geniculate body

B

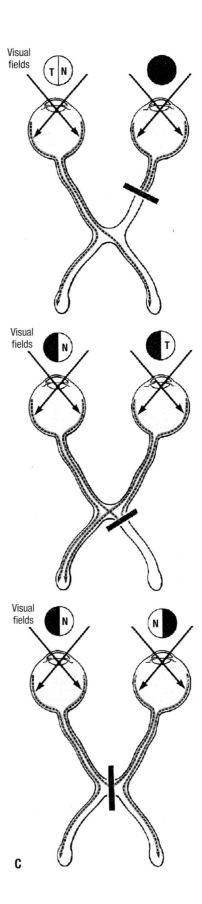

Visual fields

Visual fields

Visual fields

C

9.4   Distribution of optic nerve (CN II)

A. Optic nerve in situ, superior view. **B.** Schematic of visual system, horizontal section. Neurons from the retina of the eyeball travel through the optic nerve to the optic chiasma, where the fibers from the nasal half of the retina cross the midline and join the optic tract of the opposite side. The *large arrows* represent rays of light from the nasal (*N*) and temporal (*T*) halves of the field of vision. The rays of light from the right half of the field of vision stimulate receptors in the left half of the retina of both eyes and reach the brain through the left optic tract. **C.** Schematic of lesions of visual system, horizontal sections. *A lesion of the right optic nerve (top) would result in blindness of the right eye (monocular blindness); a lesion of the right optic tract (middle) would eliminate vision from the left visual fields of both eyes (homonymous hemianopia); and a lesion of the optic chiasma (bottom) would reduce peripheral vision (bitemporal hemianopia or tunnel vision). The pituitary gland lies just posterior to the optic chiasma; expansion of this gland by a tumor would put pressure on these crossing-over fibers.*

9.5   Distribution of oculomotor (CN III), trochlear (CN IV), and abducent nerves (CN VI), lateral views

A. Somatic motor (GSE) and parasympathetic (GVE) innervation of orbit. **B.** Overview of innervation of orbit and eyeball (CN III, IV, V1, VI, and sympathetic nerves). **C.** Parasympathetic (GVE) innervation of eyeball (CN III). **D.** Sympathetic innervation of eyeball. **E.** Sensory (GSA) innervation of eyeball (CN V1 nasociliary branch).

A

Table 9.4. Oculomotor (CNIII), Trochlear (CN IV), and Abducent (CN VI) Nerves[a]

Nerve	Functional Components	Cells of Origin/Termination	Cranial Exit	Distribution and Functions
Oculomotor	GSE	Oculomotor nucleus	Superior orbital fissure	Motor to superior, inferior, and medial rectus, inferior oblique, and levator palpebrae superioris muscles; raises upper eyelid; turns eyeball superiorly, inferiorly, and medially
	GVE	Preganglionic: midbrain (Edinger-Westphal nucleus); postganglionic: ciliary ganglion		Parasympathetic innervation to sphincter pupillae and ciliary muscle; constricts pupil and accommodates lens of eye
Trochlear	GSE	Trochlear nucleus		Motor to superior oblique that assists in turning eye inferolaterally
Abducent	GSE	Abducent nucleus		Motor to lateral rectus that turns eye laterally

[a]See also Table 9.15.

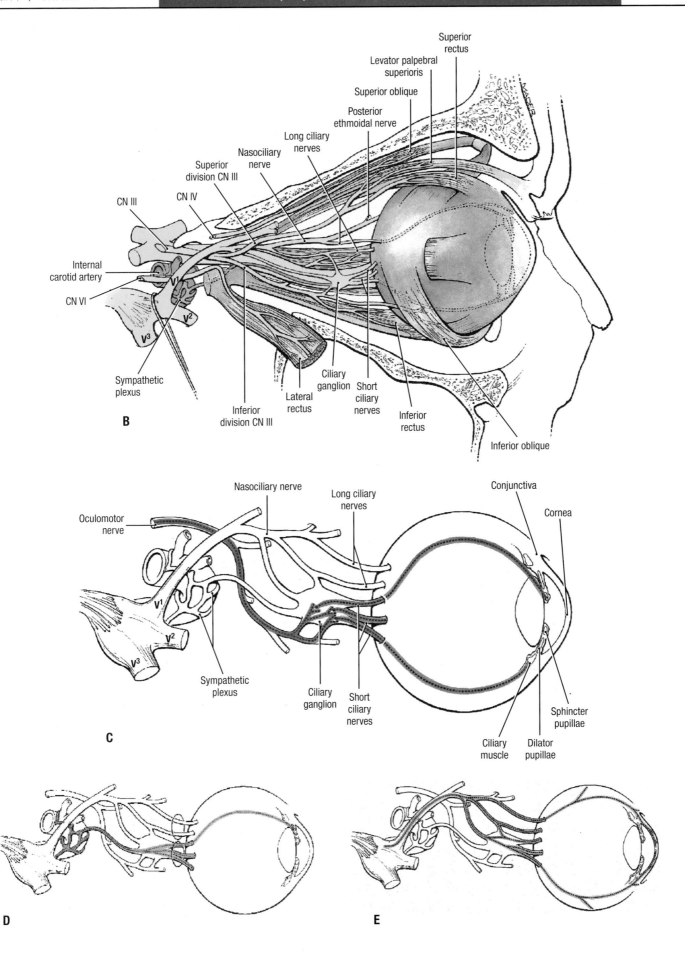

B

Superior rectus

Levator palpebral superioris

Superior oblique

Posterior ethmoidal nerve

Long ciliary nerves

Nasociliary nerve

Superior division CN III

CN III

CN IV

Internal carotid artery

CN VI

V¹

V²

V³

Sympathetic plexus

Inferior division CN III

Lateral rectus

Ciliary ganglion

Short ciliary nerves

Inferior rectus

Inferior oblique

C

Oculomotor nerve

Nasociliary nerve

Long ciliary nerves

Conjunctiva

Cornea

V¹

V²

V³

Sympathetic plexus

Ciliary ganglion

Short ciliary nerves

Ciliary muscle

Dilator pupillae

Sphincter pupillae

D

E

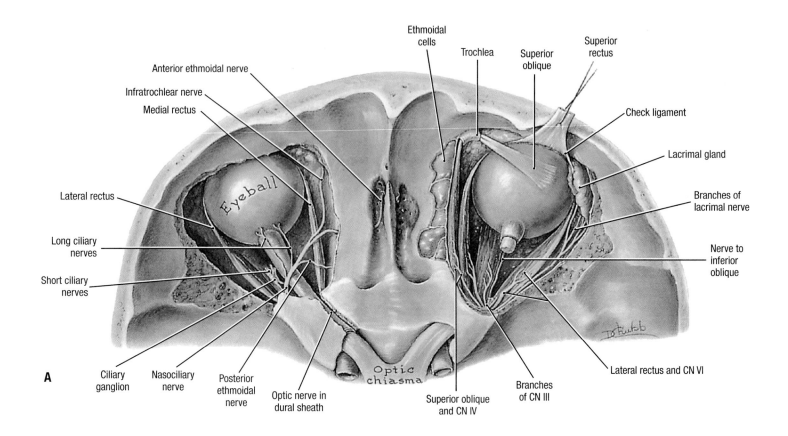

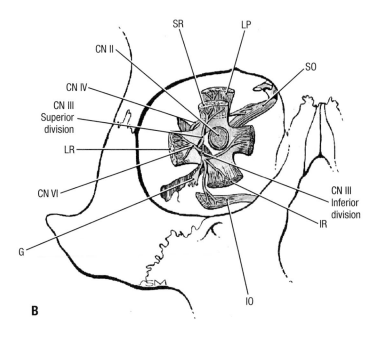

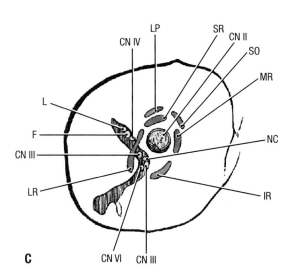

9.6   Overview of muscles and nerves of orbit

A. Orbital cavity, dissected superiorly. **B.** Structures of apex and orbit, anterior view. **C.** Relationship of muscle attachments and nerves at apex of orbit, anterior view. *L*, lacrimal nerve (CN V1); *F*, frontal nerve (CN V1); *NC*, nasociliary nerve (CN V1); *LR*, lateral rectus; *LP*, levator palpebrae superioris; *SO*, superior oblique; *SR*, superior rectus; *MR*, medial rectus; *IR*, inferior rectus; *IO*, inferior oblique; *G*, ciliary ganglion.

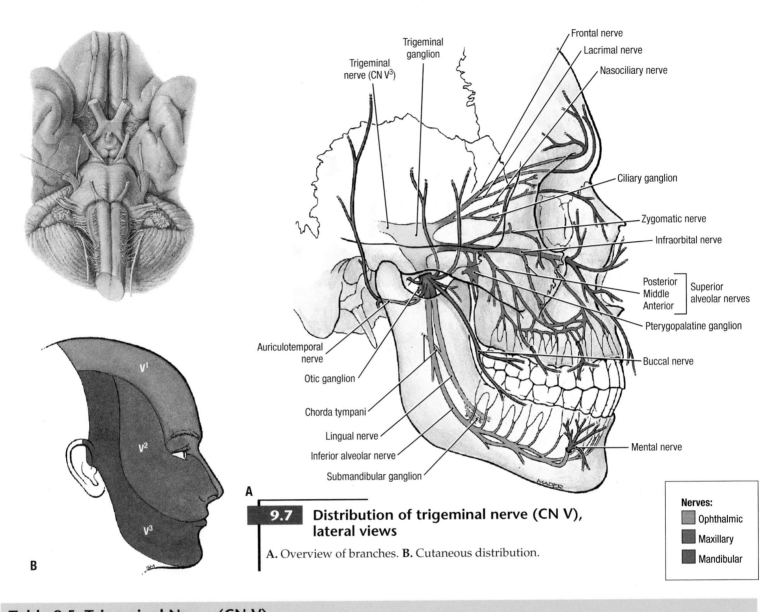

9.7 **Distribution of trigeminal nerve (CN V), lateral views**

A. Overview of branches. **B.** Cutaneous distribution.

Nerves:
- Ophthalmic
- Maxillary
- Mandibular

Table 9.5. Trigeminal Nerve (CN V)

Nerve Division	Functional Components	Cells of Origin/ Termination	Cranial Exit	Distribution and Functions
Ophthalmic division (CN V¹)	GSA	Trigeminal ganglion/spinal, principal and mesencephalic nucleus of CN V	Superior orbital fissure	Sensation from cornea, skin of forehead, scalp, eyelids, nose, and mucosa of nasal cavity and paranasal sinuses
Maxillary division (CN V²)	GSA		Foramen rotundum	Sensation from skin of face over maxilla including upper lip, maxillary teeth, mucosa of nose, maxillary sinuses, and palate
Mandibular division (CN V³)	GSA		Foramen ovale	Sensation from the skin over mandible, including lower lip and side of head, mandibular teeth, temporomandibular joint, and mucosa of mouth and anterior two thirds of tongue
	SVE	Trigeminal motor nucleus	Foramen ovale	Motor to muscles of mastication, mylohyoid, anterior belly of digastric, tensor veli palatini, and tensor tympani

9.8   Ophthalmic nerve (CN V¹)

A. Superior view. **B.** Lateral view.

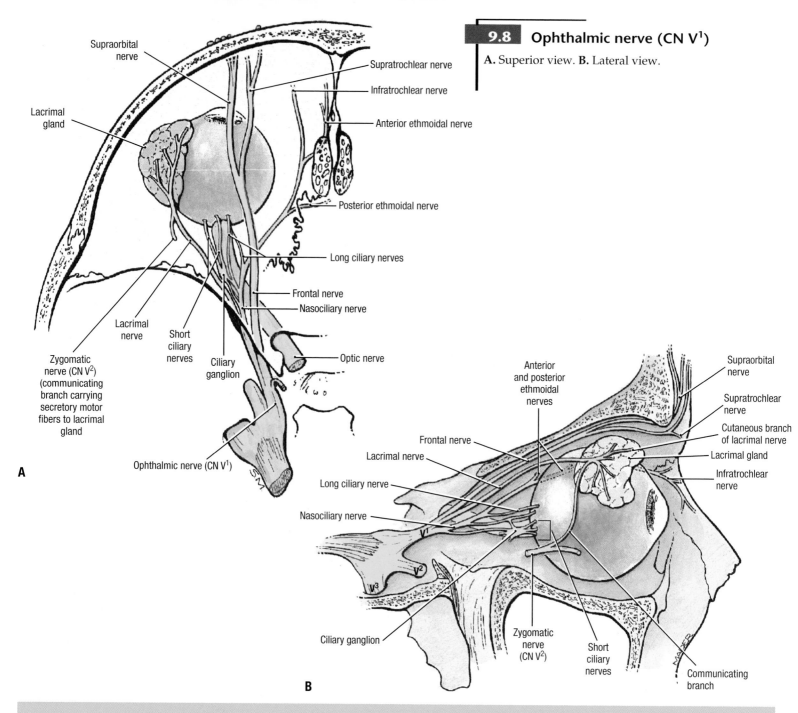

A

Supraorbital nerve
Supratrochlear nerve
Infratrochlear nerve
Anterior ethmoidal nerve
Lacrimal gland
Posterior ethmoidal nerve
Long ciliary nerves
Frontal nerve
Nasociliary nerve
Lacrimal nerve
Short ciliary nerves
Ciliary ganglion
Optic nerve
Zygomatic nerve (CN V²) (communicating branch carrying secretory motor fibers to lacrimal gland)
Ophthalmic nerve (CN V¹)

B

Anterior and posterior ethmoidal nerves
Supraorbital nerve
Supratrochlear nerve
Cutaneous branch of lacrimal nerve
Lacrimal gland
Infratrochlear nerve
Frontal nerve
Lacrimal nerve
Long ciliary nerve
Nasociliary nerve
Ciliary ganglion
Zygomatic nerve (CN V²)
Short ciliary nerves
Communicating branch

Table 9.6. Branches of Ophthalmic Nerve (CN V¹)

Function	Branches

The ophthalmic nerve is a sensory nerve passing through the superior orbital fissure that supplies the eyeball and conjunctiva, lacrimal gland and sac, nasal mucosa, frontal sinus, external nose, upper eyelid, forehead, and scalp	Lacrimal nerve
	Frontal nerve
	  Supraorbital nerve
	  Supratrochlear nerve
	Nasociliary nerve
	  Short ciliary nerves
	  Long ciliary nerves
	  Infratrochlear nerve
	  Anterior and posterior ethmoidal nerves

9.9　**Maxillary nerve (CN V^2)**

A. Lateral view.

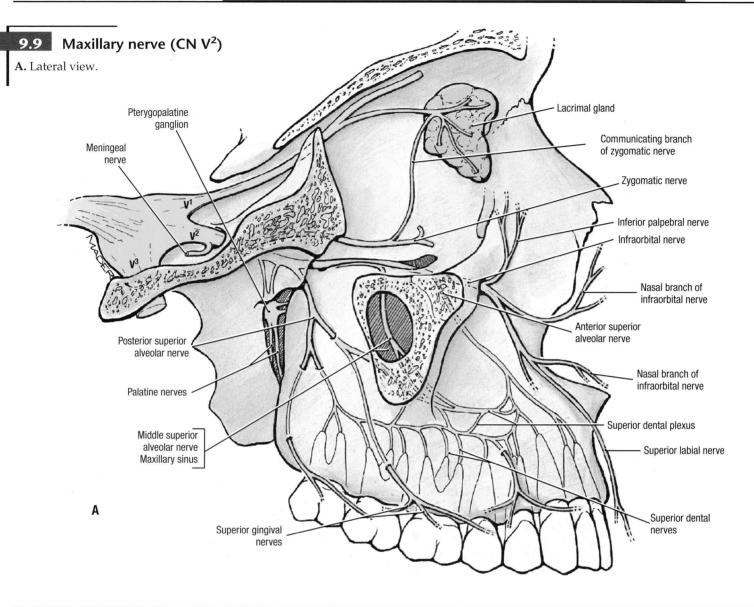

Pterygopalatine ganglion

Meningeal nerve

Lacrimal gland

Communicating branch of zygomatic nerve

Zygomatic nerve

Inferior palpebral nerve

Infraorbital nerve

Nasal branch of infraorbital nerve

Anterior superior alveolar nerve

Nasal branch of infraorbital nerve

Posterior superior alveolar nerve

Palatine nerves

Middle superior alveolar nerve Maxillary sinus

Superior dental plexus

Superior labial nerve

Superior dental nerves

Superior gingival nerves

A

Table 9.7. Branches of Maxillary Nerve (CN V^2)

Function	*Branches*
The maxillary nerve is a sensory nerve passing through the foramen rotundum that supplies sensation to the face, upper teeth and gums, mucous membrane of the nasal cavity, palate and roof of the pharynx, maxillary ethmoidal and sphenoidal sinuses, and secretory fibers from the pterygopalatine ganglion, which pass with the zygomatic and lacrimal nerves to the lacrimal gland.	Meningeal nerve Zygomatic nerve 　Zygomaticofacial nerve 　Zygomaticotemporal nerve Posterior superior alveolar nerves Infraorbital nerve 　Anterior and middle superior alveolar nerves 　Superior labial nerves 　Inferior palpebral nerves 　External and internal nasal nerves Greater palatine nerve 　Posterior inferior lateral nasal nerves Lesser palatine nerve Posterior superior lateral nasal nerves Nasopalatine nerve Pharyngeal nerve

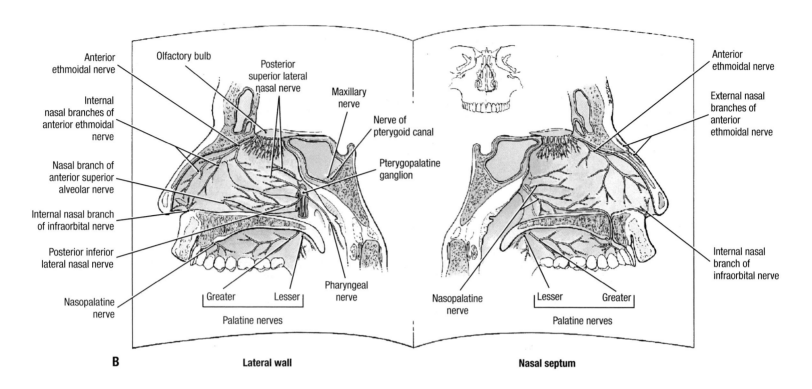

B   **Lateral wall**   **Nasal septum**

B. Lateral wall of nose and nasal septum, sagittal section through nasal cavity. The lateral wall of the nose and nasal septum are displayed as pages in a book, following sagittal sectioning of the nose through the nasal cavity.

Table 9.8. Branches of Mandibular Nerve (CN V³)

Function	Branches

The mandibular nerve is a sensory and motor nerve passing through the foramen ovale. General sensory branches (GSA) supply the lower teeth, gums, lip, auricle, external acoustic meatus, outer surface of tympanic membrane, cheek, anterior two thirds of tongue, and floor of mouth. CN V3 also conveys secretory fibers from the otic ganglion to the parotid gland. Taste to the anterior two thirds of the tongue and secretory motor fibers to the submandibular ganglion are conveyed by the chorda tympani. Postsynaptic fibers from the submandibular ganglion terminate in the submandibular and sublingual glands.	Meningeal nerve
	Buccal nerve
	Auriculotemporal nerve
	Inferior alveolar nerve
	   Inferior dental nerves
	   Mental nerve
	   Incisive nerve
	Lingual nerve

Motor branches (SVE) supply the muscles of mastication and other muscles derived from the embryonic brachial arches.	Masseter Temporalis Medial and lateral pterygoids Tensor veli palatini Mylohyoid Anterior belly of digastric Tensor tympani

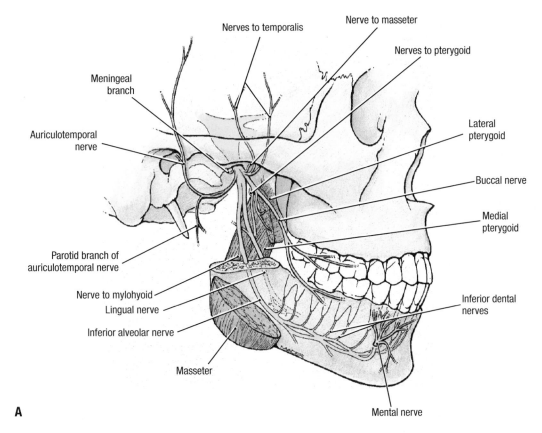

Nerves to temporalis

Nerve to masseter

Nerves to pterygoid

Meningeal branch

Auriculotemporal nerve

Lateral pterygoid

Buccal nerve

Medial pterygoid

Parotid branch of auriculotemporal nerve

Nerve to mylohyoid

Lingual nerve

Inferior alveolar nerve

Inferior dental nerves

Masseter

Mental nerve

A

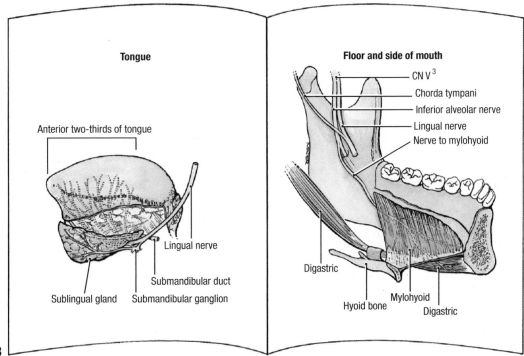

Tongue

Anterior two-thirds of tongue

Lingual nerve

Submandibular duct

Sublingual gland　　Submandibular ganglion

Floor and side of mouth

CN V ^{3}

Chorda tympani

Inferior alveolar nerve

Lingual nerve

Nerve to mylohyoid

Digastric

Hyoid bone　　Mylohyoid

Digastric

B

9.10　**Mandibular nerve (CN V³)**

A. Overview of branches, lateral view. **B.** Branches to tongue, lateral view, and floor and side of mouth, medial view. The tongue has been separated from the floor and side of the mouth. The lateral surface of the tongue and medial view of the side and floor of the mouth are displayed as pages in a book.

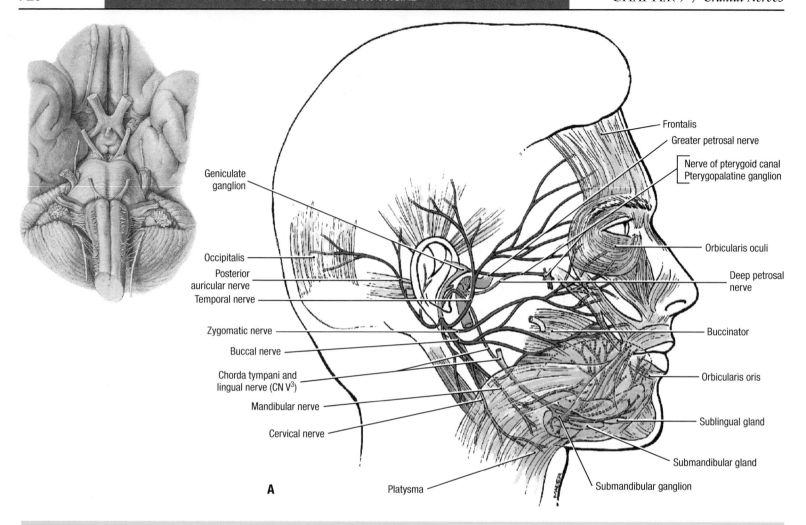

A

Table 9.9. Facial Nerve (CN VII), Including Motor Root and Nervus Intermedius[a]

Nerve Branch	Functional Components	Cells of Origin/ Termination	Cranial Exit	Distribution and Functions
Temporal, zygomatic, buccal, mandibular, cervical, posterior auricular nerves, nerve to posterior belly of digastric, nerve to stylohyoid, nerve to stapedius	SVE	Facial motor nucleus	Stylomastoid foramen; nerve to stapedius facial canal (9)	Motor to muscles of facial expression and scalp; also supplies stapedius of middle ear, stylohyoid, and posterior belly of digastric
Nervus intermedius through chorda tympani	SVA	Geniculate ganglion/ solitary nucleus	Facial canal/ petrotympanic fissure	Taste from anterior two thirds of tongue, floor of mouth, and palate
Nervus intermedius	GSA	Geniculate ganglion/ spinal trigeminal nucleus	N/A	Sensation from skin of external acoustic meatus
Nervus intermedius through greater petrosal nerve	GVA	Solitary nucleus	Facial canal/ foramen for greater petrosal nerve	Mucous membranes of nasopharynx and palate
Greater petrosal nerve (1) Chorda tympani (2)	GVE	*Preganglionic*: superior salivatory nucleus *Postganglionic*: pterygopalatine ganglion (1) and submandibular ganglion (2)	Facial canal/ foramen for greater petrosal nerve (1), petrotympanic fissure (2)	Parasympathetic innervation to lacrimal gland and glands of the nose and palate (1); submandibular and sublingual salivary glands (2)

[a]See also Table 9.15.

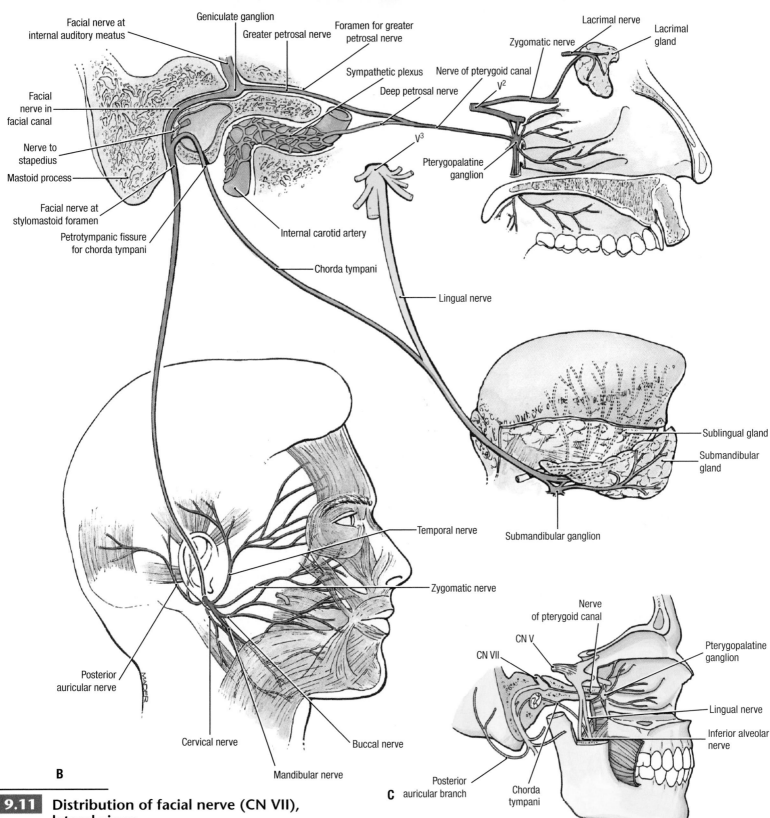

9.11 Distribution of facial nerve (CN VII), lateral views

A. Face, lateral view. The facial nerve emerges as two roots, the larger motor root and the smaller nervus intermedius that carries taste and parasympathetic and sensory fibers. The facial nerve traverses the internal acoustic meatus, facial canal, and parotid gland. Within the facial canal, CN VII gives rise to the greater petrosal nerve, nerve to stapedius, and the chorda tympani, and then the nerve emerges from the stylomastoid foramen and divides into the temporal, zygomatic, buccal, mandibular, cervical, and posterior auricular nerves. **B.** Overview of innervation. Top left: ear. Top right: lacrimal gland, nose, and palate. Lower left: face. Lower right: tongue. **C.** Chorda tympani and nerve of pterygoid canal, lateral view.

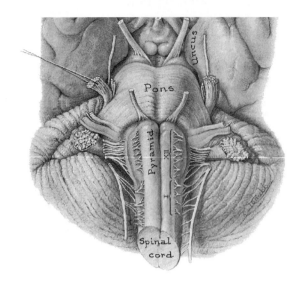

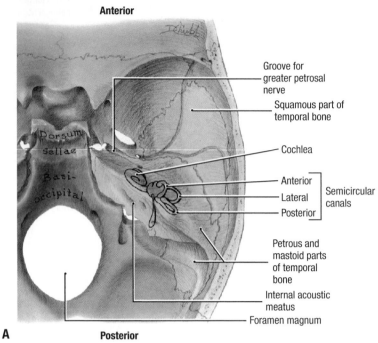

Anterior

Groove for greater petrosal nerve

Squamous part of temporal bone

Cochlea

Anterior
Lateral — Semicircular canals
Posterior

Petrous and mastoid parts of temporal bone

Internal acoustic meatus

Foramen magnum

A   **Posterior**

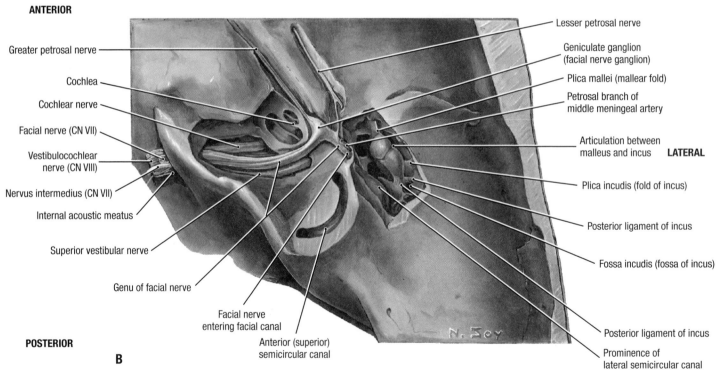

ANTERIOR

Greater petrosal nerve

Cochlea

Cochlear nerve

Facial nerve (CN VII)

Vestibulocochlear nerve (CN VIII)

Nervus intermedius (CN VII)

Internal acoustic meatus

Superior vestibular nerve

Genu of facial nerve

Facial nerve entering facial canal

Anterior (superior) semicircular canal

POSTERIOR

B

Lesser petrosal nerve

Geniculate ganglion (facial nerve ganglion)

Plica mallei (mallear fold)

Petrosal branch of middle meningeal artery

Articulation between malleus and incus   **LATERAL**

Plica incudis (fold of incus)

Posterior ligament of incus

Fossa incudis (fossa of incus)

Posterior ligament of incus

Prominence of lateral semicircular canal

Table 9.10. Vestibulocochlear Nerve (CN VIII)

Part of Vestibulocochlear Nerve	Functional Components	Cells of Origin/ Termination	Cranial Exit	Distribution and Functions
Vestibular nerve	SSA	Vestibular ganglion/ vestibular nuclei	Internal auditory meatus	Vestibular sensation from semicircular ducts, utricle, and saccule related to position and movement of head
Cochlear nerve	SSA	Spiral ganglion/ cochlear nuclei	Internal auditory meatus	Hearing from spiral organ

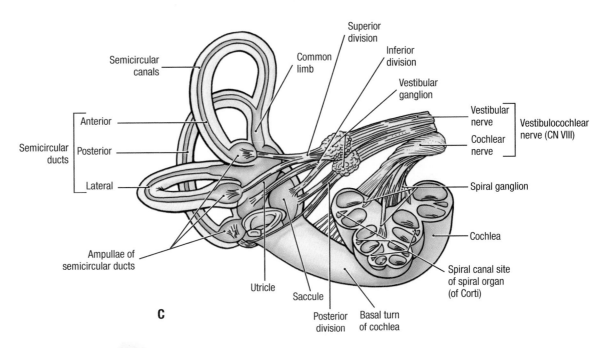

C

9.12 Distribution of vestibulocochlear nerve (CN VIII)

A. Cochlea and semicircular canals in situ, superior view. **B.** Dissection of vestibulocochlear and facial nerve, superior view. **C.** Labyrinthine and cochlear apparatus: nerves and ganglia, lateral view. The cochlea has been rotated inferolaterally to expose the vestibular ganglia. **D.** Schematic of axial section through cochlea. The inset drawing is an axial section of the cochlea; the large drawing shows details of the marked area.

OBSERVE IN **B**:
1. The facial nerve, nervus intermedius, and vestibulocochlear nerve enter the internal acoustic meatus;
2. The facial nerve runs posterior to the cochlea and across the roof of the vestibule to the geniculate ganglion; at the ganglion, it makes a right-angle bend, called a genu, and then curves posteroinferiorly within the bony facial canal;
3. The vestibulocochlear nerve in the internal acoustic meatus divides into the cochlear nerve anteriorly and the vestibular nerve posteriorly.

OBSERVE IN **C**:
4. The cochlear nerve's fibers transmit impulses from the spinal organ of Corti in the cochlear duct; their cell bodies form the spiral ganglion;
5. The three divisions of the vestibular nerve: the superior division from the utricle and ampullae of the anterior and lateral semicircular ducts, the inferior division from the saccule, and the posterior division from the ampulla of the posterior semicircular duct;

OBSERVE IN **D**:
6. The cochlear duct is a spiral tube fixed to the internal and external walls of the cochlear canal by the spiral ligament;

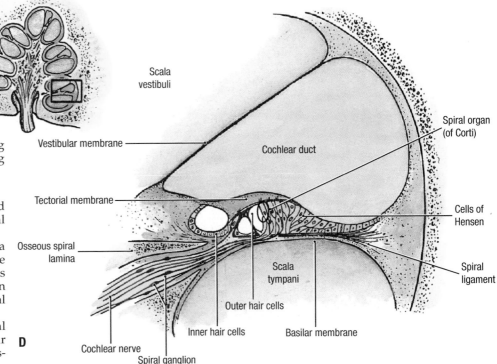

D

7. The triangular cochlear duct lies between the osseous spiral lamina and the external wall of the cochlear canal;
8. The roof of the cochlear duct is formed by the vestibular membrane, and the floor by the basilar membrane and osseous spiral lamina;
9. The receptor of auditory stimuli is the spiral organ (of Corti), situated on the basilar membrane; it is overlaid by the gelatinous tectorial membrane;
10. The spiral organ contains hair cells that respond to vibrations induced in the endolymph by sound waves;
11. The fibers of the cochlear nerve are axons of neurons in the spiral ganglion; the peripheral processes enter the spiral organ (of Corti).

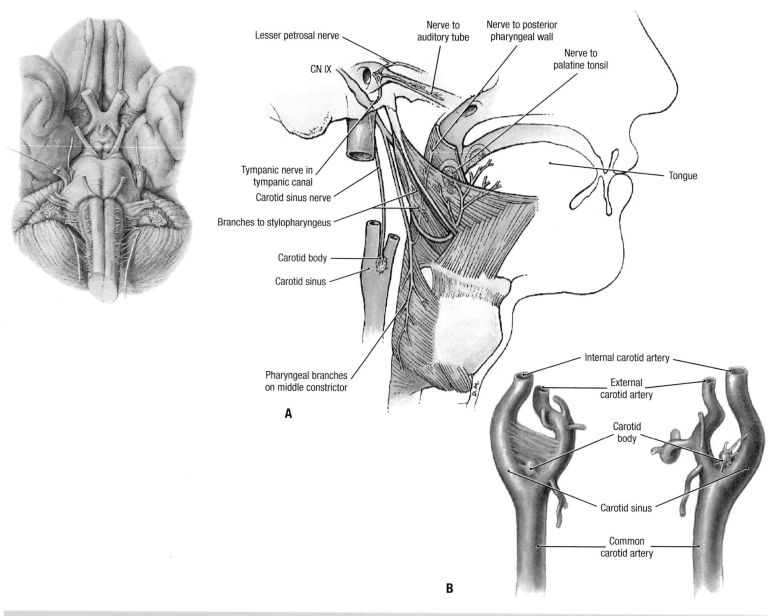

A

B

Table 9.11. Glossopharyngeal nerve (CN IX)[a]

Nerve	Functional Components	Cells of Origin/Termination	Cranial Exit	Distribution and Functions
Glossopharyngeal	SVE	Nucleus ambiguus	Jugular foramen	Motor to stylopharyngeus that assists with swallowing
	GVE	Preganglionic: inferior salivatory nucleus Postganglionic: otic ganglion		Parasympathetic innervation to parotid gland
	GVA	Solitary nucleus, spinal trigeminal nucleus/superior ganglion		Visceral sensation from parotid gland, carotid body and carotid sinus, pharynx, and middle ear
	SVA	Solitary nucleus/inferior ganglion		Taste from posterior third of tongue
	GSA	Spinal trigeminal nucleus/inferior ganglion		Cutaneous sensation from external ear

[a]See also Table 9.15.

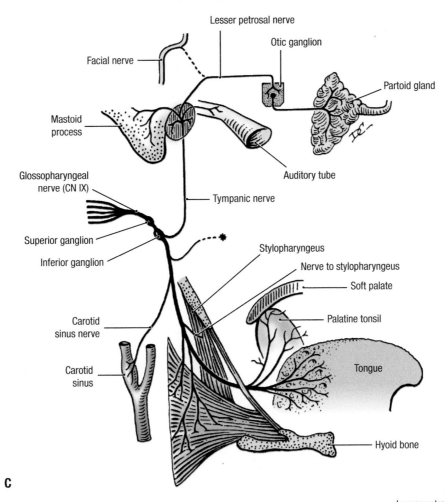

Lesser petrosal nerve

Otic ganglion

Facial nerve

Partoid gland

Mastoid process

Auditory tube

Glossopharyngeal nerve (CN IX)

Tympanic nerve

Superior ganglion

Inferior ganglion

Stylopharyngeus

Nerve to stylopharyngeus

Soft palate

Palatine tonsil

Carotid sinus nerve

Carotid sinus

Tongue

Hyoid bone

C

9.13   Distribution of glossopharyngeal nerve (CN IX)

A. Larynx and pharynx, lateral view. **B.** Carotid body and carotid sinus, posterior views. The carotid sinus is a dilation of the proximal part of the internal carotid artery and is a blood pressure regulating area. The wall of the carotid sinus contains modified end organs that respond to blood pressure changes. The carotid body is a small, ovid mass of tissue located at the bifurcation of the common carotid artery. It is a chemoreceptor that responds to decreasing levels of PO2 and increasing levels of PCO_2 in the blood. Innervation is mainly by the carotid sinus nerve, a branch of CN IX, but also by the vagus nerve and sympathetic fibers. **C.** Schematic overview of structures innervated by the glossopharyngeal nerve, lateral view. **D.** Connections of otic ganglion, lateral view. The tympanic nerve arises from CN IX before it emerges from the jugular foramen and then enters the middle ear to join the tympanic plexus. From the tympanic plexus, the tympanic nerve continues as the lesser petrosal nerve, which emerges from the superior part of the petrous temporal bone to enter the middle cranial fossa. The lesser petrosal nerve exits through the foramen ovale, and the parasympathetic fibers synapse in the otic ganglion. Postsynaptic fibers from the otic ganglion innervate the parotid gland via the auriculotemporal nerve (CN V³).

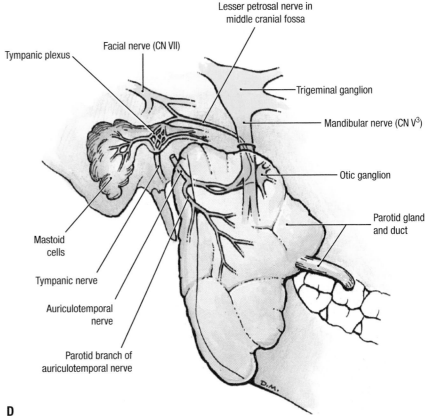

Lesser petrosal nerve in middle cranial fossa

Facial nerve (CN VII)

Tympanic plexus

Trigeminal ganglion

Mandibular nerve (CN V³)

Otic ganglion

Parotid gland and duct

Mastoid cells

Tympanic nerve

Auriculotemporal nerve

Parotid branch of auriculotemporal nerve

D

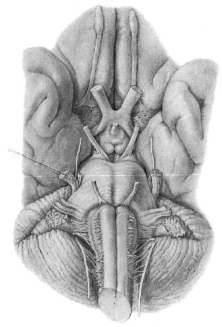

Right vagus nerve

Superior laryngeal nerve

Sinus nerve

Laryngeal nerve [Internal / External]

Superior cardiac branch

Right recurrent laryngeal nerve

Inferior cardiac branches

Pulmonary plexus

Esophageal plexus

Posterior gastric nerve

Celiac ganglion and plexus

Superior mesenteric ganglion

Pyloric branch

Renal plexus

Hepatic flexure

Pharyngeal branch of vagus nerve

Left vagus nerve

Left recurrent laryngeal nerve

Cardiac plexus

Branches of cardiac plexus

Anterior gastric nerve

Gastric nerves

Splenic nerves

Pancreatic nerves

Splenic flexure

Branches to the small and large intestine as far as the splenic flexure

9.14   Distribution of vagus nerve (CN X)

A. Schematic overview of course and structures innervated by the vagus nerve, anterior view. The branches of the vagus nerve before it exits through the jugular foramen are: meningeal nerve and auricular nerve; in neck: pharyngeal nerve, superior laryngeal nerve, right recurrent laryngeal nerve, and cardiac nerves; in thorax: left recurrent laryngeal nerve, cardiac nerves, pulmonary nerves to bronchi and lungs, and esophageal nerves; in abdomen: esophageal nerves, gastric nerves, nerves to gallbladder; nerves to intestine as far as left colic flexure. **B.** Innervation of pharynx, larynx, and palate, lateral view. **C.** Relationships of internal jugular vein and internal carotid artery to CN IX, X, and XI at jugular foramen, anterior view.

A

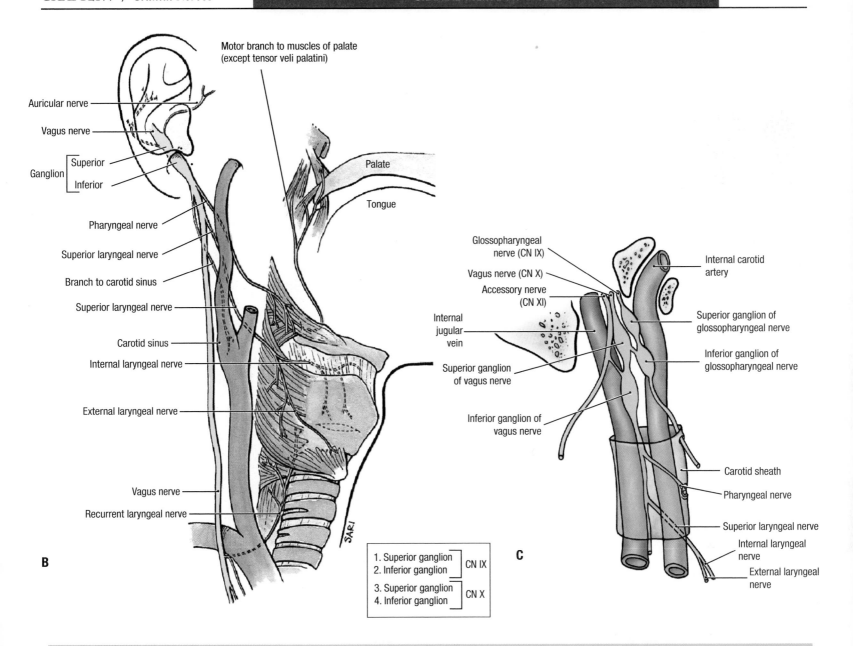

Motor branch to muscles of palate (except tensor veli palatini)

Auricular nerve

Vagus nerve

Ganglion { Superior / Inferior }

Palate

Tongue

Pharyngeal nerve

Superior laryngeal nerve

Branch to carotid sinus

Superior laryngeal nerve

Carotid sinus

Internal laryngeal nerve

External laryngeal nerve

Vagus nerve

Recurrent laryngeal nerve

B

Glossopharyngeal nerve (CN IX)

Vagus nerve (CN X)

Accessory nerve (CN XI)

Internal jugular vein

Superior ganglion of vagus nerve

Inferior ganglion of vagus nerve

Internal carotid artery

Superior ganglion of glossopharyngeal nerve

Inferior ganglion of glossopharyngeal nerve

Carotid sheath

Pharyngeal nerve

Superior laryngeal nerve

Internal laryngeal nerve

External laryngeal nerve

C

1. Superior ganglion } CN IX
2. Inferior ganglion

3. Superior ganglion } CN X
4. Inferior ganglion

Table 9.12. Vagus Nerve (CN X)

Nerve	Functional Components	Cells of Origin/Termination	Cranial Exit	Distribution and Functions
Vagus	SVE	Nucleus ambiguus		Motor to constrictor muscles of pharynx, intrinsic muscles of larynx, and muscles of palate, except tensor veli palatini, and striated muscle in superior two thirds of esophagus
	GVE	*Preganglionic*: dorsal vagal nucleus *Postganglionic*: neurons in, on, or near viscera		Parasympathetic innervation to smooth muscle of trachea, bronchi, digestive tract, and cardiac muscle
	GVA	Solitary nucleus, spinal trigeminal nucleus/superior ganglion	Jugular foramen	Visceral sensation from base of tongue, pharynx, larynx, trachea, bronchi, heart, esophagus, stomach, and intestine
	SVA	Solitary nucleus/inferior ganglion		Taste from epiglottis and palate
	GSA	Spinal trigeminal nucleus/superior ganglion		Sensation from auricle, external acoustic meatus, and dura mater of posterior cranial fossa

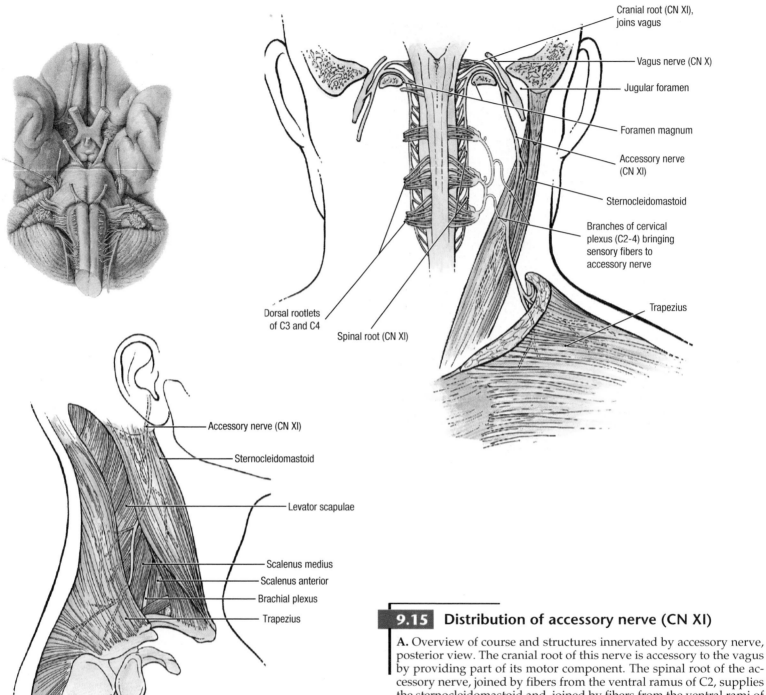

Cranial root (CN XI),
joins vagus

Vagus nerve (CN X)

Jugular foramen

Foramen magnum

Accessory nerve
(CN XI)

Sternocleidomastoid

Branches of cervical
plexus (C2-4) bringing
sensory fibers to
accessory nerve

Trapezius

Dorsal rootlets
of C3 and C4

Spinal root (CN XI)

Accessory nerve (CN XI)

Sternocleidomastoid

Levator scapulae

Scalenus medius

Scalenus anterior

Brachial plexus

Trapezius

B

9.15 **Distribution of accessory nerve (CN XI)**

A. Overview of course and structures innervated by accessory nerve,
posterior view. The cranial root of this nerve is accessory to the vagus
by providing part of its motor component. The spinal root of the accessory nerve, joined by fibers from the ventral ramus of C2, supplies
the sternocleidomastoid and, joined by fibers from the ventral rami of
C3 and C4, supplies the trapezius muscle. **B.** Accessory nerve in posterior triangle, lateral view.

Table 9.13. Accessory nerve (CN XI)

Part of Accessory Nerve	Functional Components	Cells of Origin/Termination	Cranial Exit	Distribution and Functions
Cranial root	SVE	Nucleus ambiguus	Jugular foramen	Motor to striated muscles of soft palate, pharynx, and larynx through fibers that join CN X
Spinal root	GSE	Accessory nucleus of spinal cord		Motor to sternocleidomastoid and trapezius

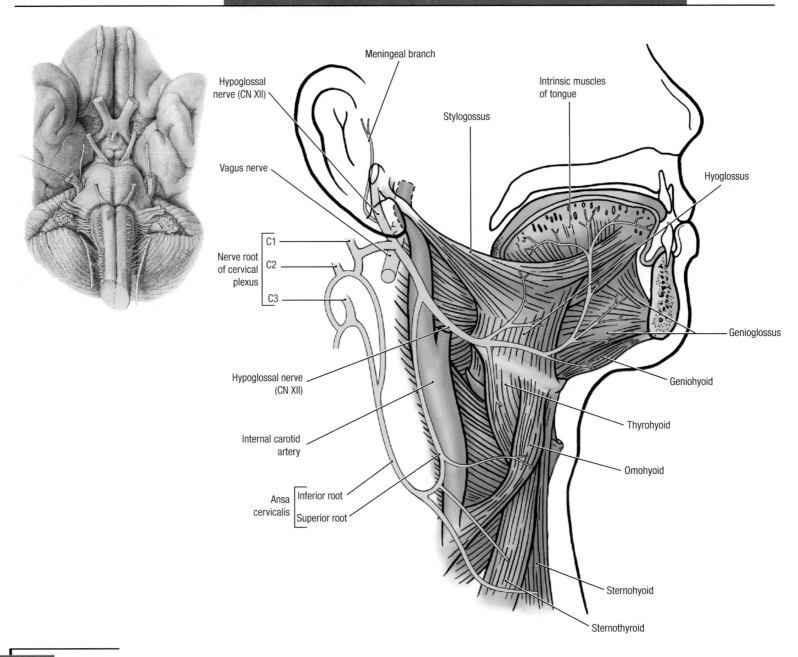

9.16 Distribution of hypoglossal nerve (CN XII), lateral views

Innervation of tongue by hypoglossal nerve and overview of course and structures innervated by hypoglossal nerve and ansa cervicales.

OBSERVE:
1. The hypoglossal nerve receives a mixed (motor and sensory) branch from the loop between the ventral rami of C1 and C2;
2. The sensory fibers of C1 and C2 take a recurrent course and end in the dura mater of the posterior cranial fossa;

3. The C1 and C2 fibers travel with the hypoglossal nerve for a short distance and then leave it as a descending branch (superior root of the ansa cervicalis) that unites with a descending branch of C2 and C3 (inferior root of the ansa cervicalis) to form a loop, the ansa cervicalis. The superior and inferior roots of the ansa cervicalis innervate the geniohyoid, thyrohyoid, omohyoid, sternohyoid, and sternothyroid muscles.

Table 9.14. Hypoglossal nerve CN XII

Nerve	Functional Components	Cells of Origin/Termination	Cranial Exit	Distribution and Functions
Hypoglossal	GSE	Hypoglossal nucleus	Hypoglossal canal	Motor to muscles of tongue (except palatoglossus)

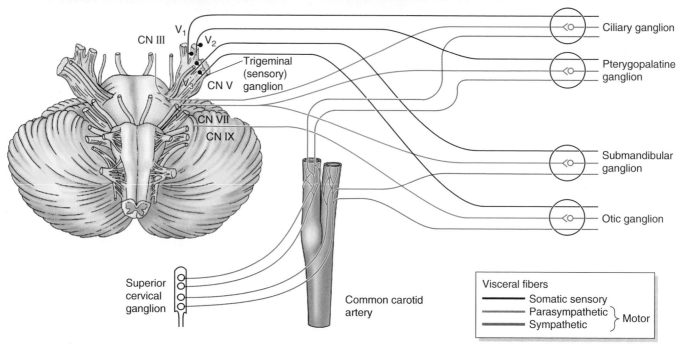

Table 9.15. Autonomic Ganglia of the Head

Ganglion	Location	Parasympathetic Root (Nucleus of Origin)[a]	Sympathetic Root	Main Distribution
Ciliary	Located between optic nerve and lateral rectus, close to apex of orbit	Inferior branch of oculomotor nerve (Edinger-Westphal nucleus)	Branch from internal carotid plexus in cavernous sinus	Parasympathetic postganglionic fibers from ciliary ganglion pass to ciliary muscle and sphincter pupillae of iris; sympathetic postganglionic fibers from superior cervical ganglion pass to dilator pupillae and blood vessels of eye
Pterygopalatine	Located in pterygopalatine fossa, where it is attached by pterygopalatine branches of maxillary nerve; located just anterior to opening of pterygoid canal and inferior to CN V^2	Greater petrosal nerve from facial nerve (superior salivatory nucleus)	Deep petrosal nerve, a branch of internal carotid plexus that is continuation of postsynaptic fibers of cervical sympathetic trunk; fibers from superior cervical ganglion pass through pterygopalatine ganglion and enter branches of CN V^2	Parasympathetic postganglionic fibers from pterygopalatine ganglion innervate lacrimal gland through zygomatic branch of CN V^2; sympathetic postganglionic fibers from superior cervical ganglion accompany those branches of pterygopalatine nerve that are distributed to the nasal cavity, palate, and superior part of the pharynx
Otic	Located between tensor veli palatini and mandibular nerve; lies inferior to foramen ovale sphenoid bone	Tympanic nerve from glossopharyngeal nerve; from tympanic plexus, tympanic nerve continues as lesser petrosal nerve (inferior salivatory nucleus)	Fibers from superior cervical ganglion come from plexus on middle meningeal artery	Parasympathetic postganglionic fibers from otic ganglion are distributed to parotid gland through auriculotemporal nerve (branch of CN V^3); sympathetic postganglionic fibers from superior cervical ganglion pass to parotid gland and supply its blood vessels
Submandibular	Suspended from lingual nerve by two short roots; lies on surface of hyoglossus muscle inferior to submandibular duct	Parasympathetic fibers join facial nerve and leave it in its chorda tympani branch, which unites with lingual nerve (superior salivatory nucleus)	Sympathetic fibers from superior cervical ganglion come from the plexus on facial artery	Postganglionic parasympathetic fibers from submandibular ganglion are distributed to the sublingual and submandibular glands; sympathetic fibers supply sublingual and submandibular glands and appear to be secretomotor

[a]For location of nuclei, see Figure 9.2.

Table 9.16. Summary of Cranial Nerve Lesions

Nerve	Type and/or Site of Lesion	Abnormal Findings
CN 1	Fracture of cribiform plate	Anosmia (loss of smell); Cerebrospinal fluid (CSF) rhinorrhea (leakage of CSF through nose)
CN II	Direct trauma to orbit or eyeball; fracture involving optic canal	Loss of pupillary constriction
	Pressure on optic pathway; laceration or intracerebral clot in the temporal, parietal, or occipital lobes of brain	Visual field defects
	Increased CSF pressure	Swelling of optic disc (papilledema)
CN III	Pressure from herniating uncus on nerve; fracture involving cavernous sinus; aneurysms	Dilated pupil, ptosis, eye turns down and out; pupillary reflex on the side of the lesion will be lost
CN IV	Stretching of nerve during its course around brainstem; fracture of orbit	Inability to look down when the eye is adducted
CN V	Injury to terminal branches (particularly CN V^2) in roof of maxillary sinus; pathologic processes (tumors, aneurysms, infections) affecting trigeminal nerve	Loss of pain and touch sensations/ paraesthesia on face; loss of corneal reflex (blinking when cornea touched); paralysis of muscles of mastication; deviation of mandible to side of lesion when mouth is opened
CN VI	Base of brain or fracture involving cavernous sinus or orbit	Eye does not move laterally; diplopia on lateral gaze
CN VII	Laceration or contusion in parotid region	Paralysis of facial muscles; eye remains open; angle of mouth droops; forehead does not wrinkle
	Fracture of temporal bone	As above, plus associated involvement of cochlear nerve and chorda tympani; dry cornea and loss of taste on anterior two thirds of tongue
	Intracranial hematoma ("stroke")	Weakness (paralysis) of lower facial muscles contralateral to the lesion, upper facial muscles are not affected because they are bilaterally innervated
CN VIII	Tumor of nerve	Progressive, unilateral hearing loss; tinnitus (noises in ear); vertigo (loss of balance)
CN IX[a]	Brainstem lesion or deep laceration of neck	Loss of taste on posterior third of tongue; loss of sensation on affected side of soft palate; loss of gag reflex on affected side
CN X	Brainstem lesion or deep laceration of neck	Sagging of soft palate; deviation of uvula to unaffected side; hoarseness owing to paralysis of vocal fold; difficulty in swallowing and speaking
CN XI	Laceration of neck	Paralysis of sternocleidomastoid and superior fibers of trapezius; drooping of shoulder
CN XII	Neck laceration; basal skull fractures	Protruded tongue deviates toward affected side; moderate dysarthria (disturbance of articulation)

[a]Isolated lesions of CN IX are uncommon; usually, CN IX, X, and XI are involved together as they pass through the jugular foramen.

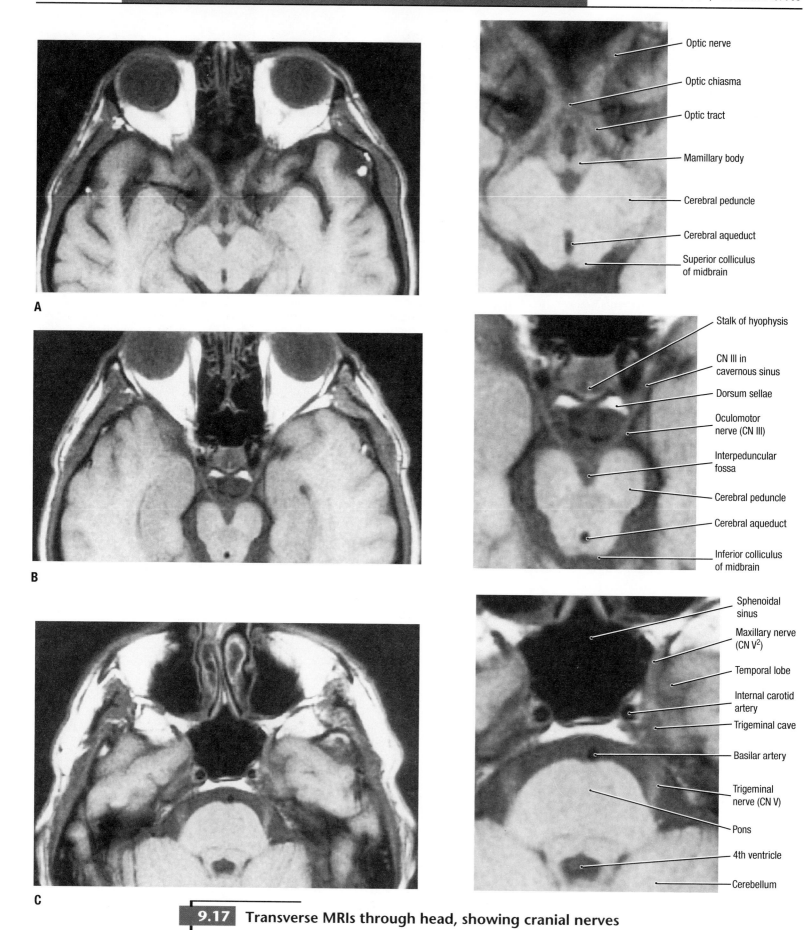

9.17 Transverse MRIs through head, showing cranial nerves

Optic nerve

Optic chiasma

Optic tract

Mamillary body

Cerebral peduncle

Cerebral aqueduct

Superior colliculus of midbrain

A

Stalk of hyophysis

CN III in cavernous sinus

Dorsum sellae

Oculomotor nerve (CN III)

Interpeduncular fossa

Cerebral peduncle

Cerebral aqueduct

Inferior colliculus of midbrain

B

Sphenoidal sinus

Maxillary nerve (CN V^2)

Temporal lobe

Internal carotid artery

Trigeminal cave

Basilar artery

Trigeminal nerve (CN V)

Pons

4th ventricle

Cerebellum

C

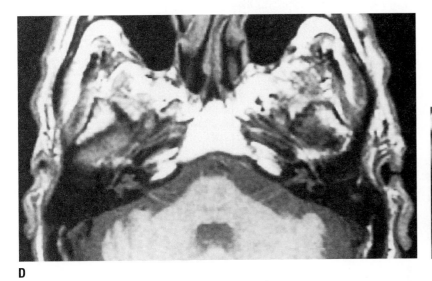

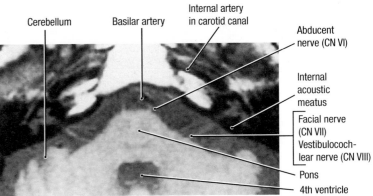

Cerebellum　Basilar artery　Internal artery in carotid canal

Abducent nerve (CN VI)

Internal acoustic meatus

Facial nerve (CN VII)

Vestibulocochlear nerve (CN VIII)

Pons

4th ventricle

D

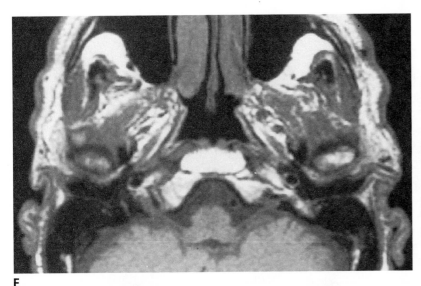

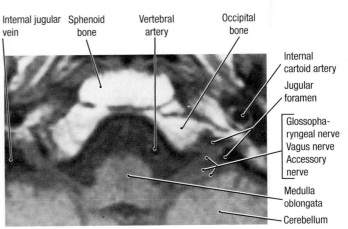

Internal jugular vein　Sphenoid bone　Vertebral artery　Occipital bone

Internal cartoid artery

Jugular foramen

Glossopharyngeal nerve
Vagus nerve
Accessory nerve

Medulla oblongata

Cerebellum

E

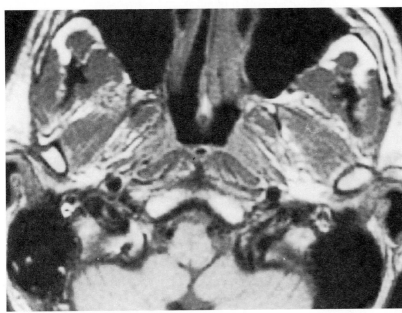

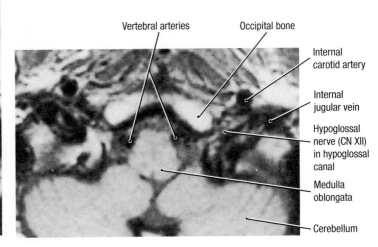

Vertebral arteries　Occipital bone

Internal carotid artery

Internal jugular vein

Hypoglossal nerve (CN XII) in hypoglossal canal

Medulla oblongata

Cerebellum

F

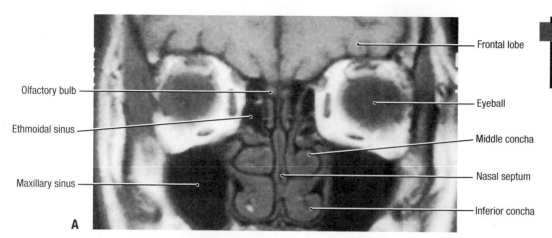

Frontal lobe

Olfactory bulb

Eyeball

Ethmoidal sinus

Middle concha

Maxillary sinus

Nasal septum

Inferior concha

A

9.18 Coronal MRIs through head, showing cranial nerves

There are four autonomic ganglia in the head: ciliary, pterygopalatine, otic, and submandibular. Each receives three types of fibers: sensory (GSA), from a branch of the trigeminal nerve; parasympathetic (GVE), from cranial nerves III, VII, or IX (these nerves synapse in the ganglion); and sympathetic, from the sympathetic trunk, "hitchhiking" on the wall of the closest artery.

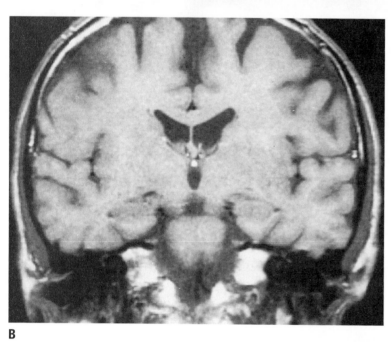

B

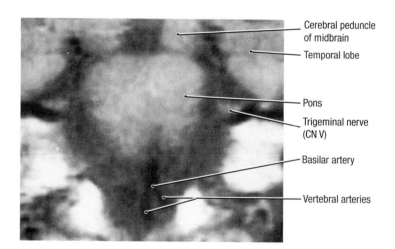

Cerebral peduncle of midbrain

Temporal lobe

Pons

Trigeminal nerve (CN V)

Basilar artery

Vertebral arteries

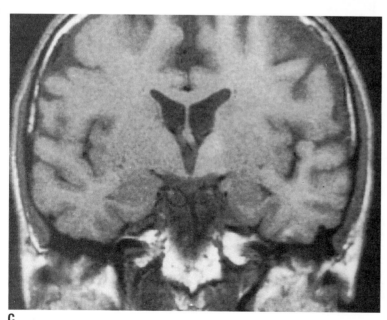

C

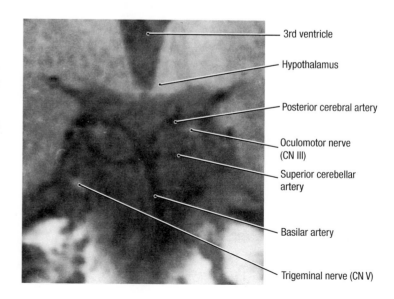

3rd ventricle

Hypothalamus

Posterior cerebral artery

Oculomotor nerve (CN III)

Superior cerebellar artery

Basilar artery

Trigeminal nerve (CN V)

INDEX